toxicology

The National Veterinary Medical Series for Independent Study

toxicology

Gary D. Osweiler, D.V.M., Ph.D., D.A.B.V.T.

Professor
College of Veterinary Medicine
Veterinary Diagnostic Laboratory
Iowa State University
Ames, Iowa

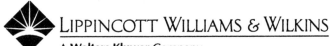

LIPPINCOTT WILLIAMS & WILKINS
A **Wolters Kluwer** Company
Philadelphia • Baltimore • New York • London
Buenos Aires • Hong Kong • Sydney • Tokyo

Senior Acquisitions Editor: Elizabeth A. Nieginski
Development Editor: Melanie Cann
Managing Editor: Amy G. Dinkel
Production Coordinator: Peter J. Carley
Series Editor, Basic Sciences: John P. Kluge, DVM, PhD

The publisher gratefully acknowledges the support of the Iowa State University College of Veterinary Medicine in the initiation of the National Veterinary Medical Series.

The publisher gratefully acknowledges the Professional Examination Service (PES) for providing information about the format and content of the National Board Examination (NBE) for Veterinary Medical Licensing.

Copyright © 1996
Lippincott Williams & Wilkins
Suite 5025
Rose Tree Corporate Center
Building Two
1400 N. Providence Road
Media, PA 19063 USA

RECYCLED

Printed in the United States of America

Library of Congress Cataloging-in-Publication Data
Osweiler, Gary D.
    Toxicology / Gary D. Osweiler.
        p.   cm. — (The national veterinary medical series for
    independent study)
    Includes index.
    ISBN 0-683-06664-1
    1. Veterinary toxicology—Outlines, syllabi, etc.   2. Veterinary
toxicology—Examinations, questions, etc.   I. Title.   II. Series.
SF757.5.O89   1995
636.089'59'0076—dc20   94-49123
                                                           CIP

Contents

Preface

In veterinary medicine, the discipline of toxicology concerns the protection of companion animals, wildlife, and food-producing animals. Animals are exposed to natural toxicants in their native environments, as well as to synthetic chemicals and drugs. The practicing veterinarian and the diagnostic or clinical veterinary toxicologist are often the first to respond to these problems, which may appear as a clinical syndrome of unknown cause. Because toxicoses may occur infrequently in any specific practice, but are often extensive and explosive, ready access to information in addition to a well-developed plan of action are important in the response to intoxications. To that end, this book is divided into three sections. The first section covers general principles of toxicology. The second section discusses how toxicants affect major body systems at the clinical level, which is how the veterinarian first encounters and must deal with a toxicologic problem, and the third section discusses specific agents.

A discussion of all potential toxicants is well beyond the scope of this book. Many toxicoses are regional and related to cultural practices or specific exposure scenarios. The topics chosen are representative of those considered important in contemporary veterinary toxicology, based on the author's experience as a diagnostic veterinary toxicologist and the opinions and advice of colleagues over many years. The intended audience is veterinary students or others who may desire a focused review of veterinary toxicology issues and agents. This book is intended as a review or update in toxicology and is most effective when used in conjunction with more extensive and targeted texts, reviews, or monographs.

Acknowledgments

I would like to thank Elizabeth Nieginski and Williams & Wilkins for providing me with the opportunity to participate in this new series, which promises to make a significant contribution to veterinary education. Early editorial direction from Jane Velker was much appreciated, as were Melanie Cann's patience and attention to the manuscript throughout the editorial process.

PART I

GENERAL TOXICOLOGY

Chapter 1
Introduction

I. TOXICOLOGY CONCEPTS AND TERMINOLOGY

A. **Definition of toxicology.** Toxicology is the study of poisons. It includes the identification of poisons, their chemical properties, and their biologic effects as well as the treatment of disease conditions that they cause.

1. Pharmacology and toxicology share many common principles, including biodynamics of uptake and elimination, mechanisms of action, principles of treatment, and dose–response relationships.

2. Therapeutic drugs and essential nutrients can become poisons under certain conditions.

3. The veterinary toxicologist deals with many different chemicals, feed additives, environmental contaminants, pesticides, and natural toxins of plant and animal origin, which may adversely affect the health of animals.
   a. The clinical veterinary toxicologist is a specialist in the cause, identification, and treatment of animal poisonings.
   b. The toxicologist may have training in human medicine, pharmacology, physiology, pathology, and chemistry, and the integration of these areas of knowledge is applied toward solving practical problems.

B. **Poison.** A poison is any solid, liquid, or gas that, through either oral or topical routes, can interfere with life processes of cells of the organism. This interference occurs by the inherent qualities of the poison without mechanical action and irrespective of temperature.

1. Another term for **poison is toxicant.**

2. The term **toxin** is used to describe poisons that originate from biologic processes; these are generally classified as **biotoxins.**

3. The term **toxic** is used to describe the **effects of a poison** on living systems.

4. **Toxicosis** describes the disease state that results from exposure to a poison. The term toxicosis is often used interchangeably with the terms poisoning and intoxication.

C. **Toxicity.** The amount of a poison that, under a specific set of conditions, causes toxic effects or results in detrimental biologic changes is referred to as toxicity.

1. A major concept in toxicity is the relationship of **dose and response.**
   a. A toxic or adverse reaction to a chemical has a **threshold dose,** above which detrimental effects can be measured.
   b. Most toxic responses increase in degree or severity (known as a **graded response**) as the amount or dosage of toxicant increases.

2. Toxicity is usually expressed as milligrams (mg) of toxicant per kilogram (kg) of body weight that will produce a defined biologic effect.
   a. The amount of toxicant per unit of animal weight is **dosage.**
   b. The total amount of toxicant received per animal is the **dose.**

3. In some species, such as wildlife or fish, toxicity may be expressed as the concentration of the substance in the feed or water, where dosage is directly correlated with concentration when the material is freely available.
   a. The **lethal concentration (LC)** is the lowest concentration of compound in feed (or in water in the case of fish) that causes death. It is expressed as milligrams of compound per kilogram of feed and water.
   b. The **acute lethal toxicity** is expressed as the LC_{50}, or concentration of compound in feed or water that will kill 50% of animals exposed.

4. Other terms are sometimes used to define toxicity.
   a. The **highest nontoxic dose (HNTD)** is the largest dose that does not result in clinical or pathologic drug-induced alterations.
   b. **Toxic dose–low (TDL)** is the lowest dose that will produce alterations; administration of twice this dose is not lethal.
   c. The **toxic dose–high (TDH)** is the dose that will produce drug-induced alterations and administration of twice this dose is lethal.
   d. The **lethal dose (LD)** is the lowest dose that causes death in any animal during the period of observation. Various percentages can be attached to the LD value to indicate doses required to kill 1% (LD_1), 50% (LD_{50}), or 100% (LD_{100}) of the test animals. LD_{50} is a commonly used measure of toxicity (see I F 1 a).
   e. **Median lethal dose (MLD)** is equivalent to the LD_{50} and can be used interchangeably with it.
   f. The **ED_{50} (Effective Dose 50)** is the dosage of a drug or therapeutic agent that produces the desired effect in half of a population.

D. **Expressions of safety for drugs** are given by comparisons of the LD_{50} to the ED_{50}.

1. The **therapeutic index (TI)** is defined by the ratio of the LD_{50} to the ED_{50}:

$$TI = \frac{LD_{50}}{ED_{50}}$$

2. The **standard safety margin (SSM)** is a more conservative estimate than the TI. The SSM is the ratio of the LD_1 to the ED_{99}:

$$SSM = \frac{LD_1}{ED_{99}}$$

E. General guidelines have been developed to classify the relative toxicities of compounds within defined ranges on a milligram or gram per kilogram basis (Table 1-1).

F. Exposure to toxicants and the expression of effects of toxicants are often defined according to the frequency and duration of exposure. These are generally defined as acute, subacute, subchronic, and chronic.

1. **Acute toxicity** is a term that describes the effects of a single dose or multiple doses during a 24-hour period.
   a. The acute LD_{50} is a patterned toxicity study designed to compare the most reproducible part of the dose–response curve for different chemicals under closely defined

TABLE 1-1. Guidelines for the Classification of Relative Toxicities

Classification	Toxicity
Extremely toxic	< 1 mg/kg
Highly toxic	1–50 mg/kg
Moderately toxic	50–500 mg/kg
Slightly toxic	0.5–5 g/kg
Practically nontoxic	5–15 g/kg
Relatively harmless	> 15 g/kg

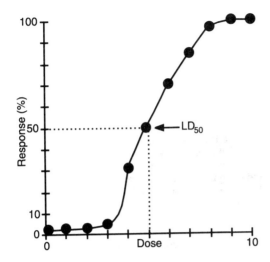

FIGURE 1-1. Cumulative response is the total response of all animals to each successive increasing dosage. Notice that there are low dosages with no response (below the threshold or LD_0), followed by dosages with a rapidly increasing response, and finally a maximal effect to which all possible animals have responded (LD_{100}). The result is a sigmoid dose–response curve; the most nearly linear and reproducible responses occur in the middle range of dosages.

conditions of exposure. Recently, toxicology organizations and government regulatory agencies have greatly reduced reliance on the LD_{50} in order to reduce the number of animals needed for testing.

b. The LD_{50} value is based on the effects of exposure to successively increasing dosage levels, which often are spaced at logarithmic or geometric intervals.

(1) The LD_{50} defines a dosage that is lethal to 50% of animals exposed to a specific toxicant under defined conditions, including species, route of exposure, and duration of exposure.

(2) The LD_{50} value does not pertain to the severity of clinical signs observed or the characteristic changes caused by the toxicant.

(3) The LD_{50} bears no relationship to chronic toxicity or to other adverse effects such as reproductive hazard or cancer risk.

(4) The LD_{50} is based on a "quantal" (all-or-none) response of a population of animals and is the cumulative response to increasing dosage. It is a sigmoid graph when plotted on linear coordinates as shown in Figure 1-1. Response is most nearly linear at the LD_{50} and is most rapidly and reliably affected by dosage in this area.

(5) The LD_{50} can be transformed to a straight line on semilogarithmic or probit paper. By using probits, each standard deviation above and below the mean can be expressed as a positive whole number (Figure 1-2).

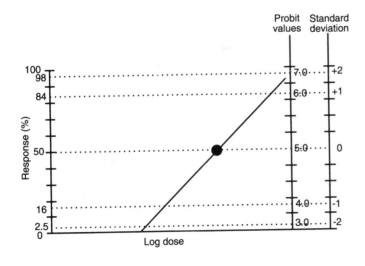

FIGURE 1-2. When dose versus response is plotted as the log of the dose given versus the percent cumulative response, the graph is a straight line. The probit scale is a weighted number assigned to the percent cumulative response in order to simplify calculations by using whole numbers that correspond to one or more standard deviations from the LD_{50}.

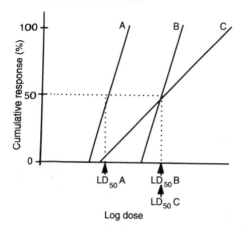

FIGURE 1-3. The slope of the dose–response curve defines the margin between minimal and maximal response. Compounds can have different slopes but the same LD_{50} (B and C); and, in other cases, the LD_{50} can be different, but the slopes are similar (A and B)

    (6) The slope of the dose–response curve defines the margin between minimal and maximal toxic response (Figure 1-3).

2. Subacute toxicity refers to repeated exposure and effects observed for 30 days or less.

3. Subchronic toxicity is the study of exposure and effects for 1 to 3 months. Studies of 3 months are considered adequate to express all forms of toxicosis except carcinogenic effects and multigenerational (reproductive) effects.

4. Chronic toxicity is produced by prolonged exposure for 3 months or longer.
    a. Compounds that are rapidly metabolized have about the same chronic LD_{50} as the single-dose LD_{50}, because the rapidly excreted compound has little opportunity to accumulate in the body.
    b. Prolonged exposure to a toxicant may allow animals to develop **tolerance** to the toxicant so that the size of the dose required to produce lethality upon repeated exposure increases. This is often due to an increase in the metabolic detoxification of the compound.
    c. The ratio of the acute to chronic LD_{50} doses is the **chronicity factor** (Table 1-2).
        (1) Compounds with cumulative effects have a high chronicity factor.
        (2) Table 1-2 compares chronicity factors for a cumulative toxin (warfarin) and a rapidly excreted toxin (caffeine).
        (3) A chronicity factor greater than 2.0 indicates a relatively cumulative toxicant.
    d. Hazard (or **risk**) is the probability that a chemical will cause harm under specific conditions of use.
        (1) Compounds of high inherent toxicity may pose little risk if access or exposure of animals is limited.
        (2) Materials of low toxicity may be dangerous if used extensively or carelessly.
        (3) The ratio between inherent toxicity and use or exposure level can be used to compare relative risk. Table 1-3 compares the risk of urea toxicosis with the risk of monensin toxicosis, two substances that are commonly added to cattle feeds.

TABLE 1-2. Chronicity Factors for Two Toxicants*

Compound	Acute LD_{50}	90-day LD_{50}	Chronicity Factor
Warfarin	1.6	0.077	21.0
Caffeine	192.0	150.0	1.3

*Chronicity factor = $\dfrac{\text{Acute } LD_{50}}{\text{90-day } LD_{50}}$

TABLE 1-3. Comparison of Risk (Hazard)*

Chemical	Toxicity	Use Level	Risk Ratio
Urea	300 mg/kg	100 mg/kg	3:1
Monensin	20 mg/kg	1 mg/kg	20:1

*Risk is defined by a comparison of toxicity and conditions of use. Monensin is much more toxic than urea; however, the rate of monensin use is much lower than that for urea. Comparison of the ratios of toxicity to use level for these two substances shows that the risk of urea toxicosis would be much higher than the risk of monensin toxicosis.

II. CALCULATIONS IN TOXICOLOGY

A. **Manipulation of numbers and estimation of dosage** are basic to the practice of medicine (Table 1-4).

1. Calculating concentrations and estimating dosages are essential to the interpretation of toxicology data resulting from laboratory analyses or estimates of probable exposure. The toxicologist calculates drug dosages based on estimates of body weight and food consumption (Table 1-5). The practitioner must determine if clinical poisoning is probable by relating a level of contamination in feed or forage to a known toxic dosage.

TABLE 1-4. Conversion Factors Useful in Veterinary Toxicology

Unit	Abbreviation or Symbol	Equivalent
LENGTH		
1 inch	in	2.54 centimeters
1 meter	m	39.37 inches
1 micron	μm	1×10^{-6} meters, 1×10^{-3} millimeters
1 angstrom	Å	1×10^{-5} microns
AREA		
1 acre	. . .	43,560 square feet
1 hectare	. . .	2.471 acres, 10,000 square meters
WEIGHT		
1 ounce	oz	28.35 grams
1 gram	g	15.43 grains
1 pound	lb	453.6 grams
1 kilogram	kg	2.205 pounds
1 short ton	. . .	907.2 kilograms
1 metric ton	. . .	2000 kilograms
LIQUID		
1 ounce	oz	29.6 milliliters
1 quart	qt	0.946 liter, 57.75 cubic inches
1 gallon	gal	3.785 liters
1 gallon (water)	gal	8.35 pounds
1 cubic foot	cu ft	7.48 gallons, 28.32 liters
1 bushel	bu	9.31 gallons
1 liter	L	1.057 quarts, 0.264 gallon
1 teaspoon	tsp	5 milliliters
1 tablespoon	T	15 milliliters
1 acre-foot	. . .	3.259×10^5 gallons
DRY MEASURE		
1 bushel	bu	8 gallons, 35.24 liters, 1.24 cubic feet
1 cubic meter	m^3	35.3 cubic feet

TABLE 1-5. Estimated Food Intake for Animals*

Animal	Daily Dry Food Intake (% Body Weight)
Cat	
Kitten	8.0
Adult	4.0
Dog	
Puppy (small)	8.0
Adolescent	6.0
Adult	3.0
Beef cattle	
Yearling (350 kg)	2.5
Finishing cattle (600 kg)	1.5
Dairy cow	
Gestating	1.8
Lactating	2.0–3.0
Sheep	
Ewe (lactating)	4.0
Ewe (nonlactating)	2.5
Lamb (30 kg)	4.0
Swine	
Sow (lactating)	3.0–4.0
Feeder pig (15 kg)	7.0
Finishing pig (70 kg)	4.5
Horse	
Mature	2.0
Colt	3.0

*Intakes are only estimates, and amounts will vary widely depending on nutrient density, animal age and weight, physical exercise, lactation, and environmental temperature. For more precise calculations, the Nutrient Requirement Data published by the National Academy of Sciences should be consulted. National Academy of Sciences, National Research Council, National Academy Press, 2101 Constitution Avenue, Washington, DC 20418.

2. Failure to consider dose versus response is a common problem in clinical toxicology.

3. Toxicology calculations require familiarity with the metric system. Useful metric units and abbreviations used in toxicology calculations are listed in Table 1-6.

B. Expressions of chemical concentrations in clinical toxicology

1. Chemical concentrations in clinical toxicology are often expressed in **parts per million (ppm), parts per billion (ppb)** or **parts per trillion (ppt).**
   a. These universal expressions of concentration are multiples of 1000 compared to one another.
   - **(1)** 1 ppm = 1000 ppb
   - **(2)** 1 ppb = 1000 ppt
   - **(3)** 1 ppm = 1,000,000 ppt

TABLE 1-6. Metric Units Used in Toxicology Calculations

Unit	Abbreviation	Equivalent
Megagram	M	1×10^{6} gram
Kilogram	kg	1×10^{3} gram
Milligram	mg	1×10^{-3} gram
Microgram	μg	1×10^{-6} gram
Nanogram	ng	1×10^{-9} gram
Picogram	pg	1×10^{-9} gram
Femtogram	fg	1×10^{-12} gram

b. For chemical analysis, these common relative expressions of concentration are replaced by absolute values.

(1) 1 ppm = 1 mg/kg = 1 µg/g
(2) 1 ppb = 1 µg/kg = 1 ng/g
(3) 1 ppt = 1 ng/kg = 1 pg/g

c. There is a direct relationship between percentage concentration and parts per million. It can be determined by the percentage equivalent of 1 ppm (1 mg/kg).

(1) 1 ppm = 1 mg/kg = 1 mg/1000 g = 1 mg/1,000,000 mg
(2) 1 mg is a fractional part of 1,000,000 given by:

$$\frac{1}{1,000,000} = 0.000001$$

   (a) This fraction is multiplied by 100 to convert to percent; therefore:

$$0.000001 \times 100 = 0.0001\%$$

   (b) Thus, 1 ppm is equivalent to 0.0001%.
   (c) It should be noted that moving the decimal point for ppm four places to the left converts ppm to percentage.

(i) 1,000,000 ppm	=	100%
(ii) 10,000 ppm	=	1.0%
(iii) 1,000 ppm	=	0.1%
(iv) 100 ppm	=	0.01%
(v) 1 ppm	=	0.0001%

   (d) To convert percentage to ppm, the decimal place is moved four places to the right (i.e., 1.0% = 10,000 ppm).

2. Concentrations of drugs and chemicals are often expressed for commercial uses in the **English system of ounces and pounds**. For example, concentrations of drugs and micronutrients in animal feeds are expressed as pounds or grams of drug per ton of feed; however, toxicology data and analytical results are usually given in the metric system as mg/kg or µg/g or ng/g. Interpretation of a toxic exposure is possible only when the equivalent units are compared.

a. For concentrations expressed as pounds per ton
   (1) A fractional relationship should be established for 1 pound of drug per 1 ton of feed (i.e., 1 lb in 2000 lbs).
   (2) The fractional relationship should be calculated and converted to a percentage so that:

$$1 \text{ lb}/2000 \text{ lb}$$
$$= 0.0005 \text{ (fractional portion)} \times 100$$
$$= 0.05\%$$

   (3) The percentage is then converted to ppm (i.e., the decimal point is moved four places to the right):

$$\text{mg/kg} = 0.05\% \times 10,000 = 500 \text{ ppm}$$

b. For concentrations expressed as grams per ton
   (1) Tons should be converted to kilograms:

$$2000 \text{ lb/ton} \div 2.2 \text{ lb/kg} = 907 \text{ kg/ton}$$

   (2) To express grams of chemical as a fractional part of 907 kg, convert 907 kg to the same units as the drug (i.e., grams). Thus:

$$454 \text{ g/ton} \div 907 \text{ kg/ton} = 454 \text{ g}/907,000 \text{ g}$$

   (3) The fractional relationship is then calculated and converted to a percentage:

$$454 \text{ g}/907,000 \text{ g} = 0.0005 \times 100 = 0.05\%$$

   (4) The percentage is converted to ppm or mg/kg (i.e., the decimal point is moved four places to the right), so that:

$$0.05\% \times 10,000$$
$$= 500 \text{ ppm}$$
$$= 500 \text{ mg/kg}$$

(5) It should be noted that:

$$
\begin{aligned}
1\,g/ton \;=\; & 1g/907{,}000\ g \\
=\; & 0.00011\% \\
=\; & 1.1\ ppm \\
=\; & 1.1\ mg/kg
\end{aligned}
$$

Therefore, a useful rule for quick calculation is that 1 gram of chemical per ton of feed is equal to 1.1 ppm.

C. **Estimating exposure to animals on a body weight basis when concentrations are given in feed or water**

1. When toxicity data for animals are given, they are often provided as a dosage per kilogram of body weight (bw) [i.e., mg drug per kg bw], but estimated exposure in feed or forage is presented as a concentration in the feedstuff. These are not equivalent values, and feed and water concentrations must be interpreted by how much they contribute to dosage.

   a. Essential information for calculations includes:
      (1) The concentration of chemical in the feed
      (2) The weight of the exposed animal (alternatively, the calculations can be done on the basis of one kilogram of body weight)
      (3) The portion of animal body weight that is consumed as feed, water, or bait, which must be determined by measurement or estimated by consulting appropriate references

   b. For example, if a feed containing 100 ppm of a toxic chemical is fed to animals that typically consume food at 3% of their body weight each day, and if each kilogram of animal weight requires 3% as food, then: 1 kg × 0.03 = 0.03 kg of food daily. If the food contains 100 ppm (mg/kg) of the chemical, and 0.03 kg of food is required, then 3 mg of chemical are supplied per kg of animal weight (i.e., the dosage is 3 mg drug per kg body weight).

      (1) This relationship can be expressed in the formula:

   $$
   \text{mg drug/kg bw} \;=\; \frac{(\text{feed level [ppm]}) \times \text{kg feed eaten}}{\text{bw in kg}}
   $$

      (2) Adjusting this formula allows determination of the feed level that will cause toxicosis.

   $$
   \text{feed level (ppm)} \;=\; \frac{\text{mg drug/kg bw} \times \text{bw(kg)}}{\text{kg feed eaten}}
   $$

      (3) If the percentage of body weight consumed as feed is known, then the formula can be simplified as:

   $$
   \text{feed level (ppm)} \;=\; \frac{\text{mg drug/kg bw}}{\text{percentage bw consumed as food}}
   $$

   $$
   \text{For example: ppm} \;=\; \frac{3\ \text{mg/kg bw} = 100\ \text{ppm}}{0.03}
   $$

   Note that the percentage term is expressed as a fraction (0.03), rather than as a whole number (3%).

2. As shown, accurate calculations require reasonable estimates of feed intake.
   a. Feed intake varies widely among various species and sizes and ages of animals and according to exercise, ambient temperature, and specific conditions such as lactation and pregnancy.
   b. Estimates of the average amount of feed consumed by common domestic animals during various stages of the life cycle are published by the National Academy of Sciences, National Research Council.
   c. Toxicity may vary if feed or water is consumed quickly at one time, rather than evenly throughout the day.
      (1) Slower intake allows metabolic detoxification and excretion and usually increases tolerance to acute poisoning.

(2) Conversely, toxicants may accumulate in the body from dosages provided daily in the feed.

d. Average water intake values (by weight) for various animals are approximately twice the amount of feed consumed.

(1) Water consumption varies widely, depending on weather, exercise, health status, palatability, and other variables.

(2) Any estimate of the role of water in toxic exposure must be done with these environmental and physiological factors in mind.

D. **Estimating dosages when exposure is based on consumption of green forage that has been sprayed**

1. Forage crops used for hay or pasture may be sprayed with a potential toxicant prior to use by animals for food and resulting residues may be suspected of causing toxicosis.

2. Sampling and analysis can provide an estimate of exposure, but sometimes an immediate, "on site" estimate can be useful in interpreting the probability of poisoning.

a. Information used to estimate chemical intake from sprayed forages includes:

(1) Amount of forage eaten by animals at risk

(2) Application rate of chemical per acre or hectare

(3) Yield of forage per unit of land sprayed

b. The contribution of 1 lb of chemical per acre to the diet of a forage-consuming animal can be calculated as follows:

(1) One acre of land = 43,560 square feet, and 1 lb = 454 g.

(2) 454 g
$$= 454{,}000 \text{ mg} \div 43{,}560 \text{ sq ft}$$
$$= 10.4 \text{ mg chemical per sq ft.}$$

(3) The forage yield should be estimated at 2 tons per acre (or actual values should be used if they are known).
$$2 \text{ tons} \times 907 \text{ kg/ton}$$
$$= 1814 \text{ kg} \times 43{,}560 \text{ sq ft} = 0.042 \text{ kg}$$
$$= 42 \text{ g forage/sq ft.}$$

(4) Thus:
$$(1000 \text{ g/kg} \div 42 \text{ sq ft}) \times 10.4 \text{ mg chemical per sq ft}$$
$$= 248 \text{ mg chemical per kg of forage.}$$

(5) Therefore, under the conditions specified, 1 lb of chemical on 1 acre of forage at 2 tons yield per acre provides 248 ppm of chemical in the forage.

(6) mg/kg body weight
$$= \text{forage level (ppm)} \times \% \text{ bw eaten as forage}$$
$$= 248 \text{ mg/kg} \times 0.03$$
$$= 7.4 \text{ mg/kg body weight.}$$

(7) Thus, under the conditions described, and assuming all sprayed chemical remains on the forage and is not lost to decomposition or metabolism, animals allowed to graze the sprayed forage would receive approximately 7 mg/kg body weight for each pound of applied chemical.

III. TOXICOKINETICS: THE ABSORPTION, DISTRIBUTION, AND EXCRETION OF TOXICANTS

A. **Definition.** Toxicokinetics is the movement and disposition of toxicants in the organism.

1. Response to chemicals is affected by toxicokinetic influence on:

a. Rate and amount of absorption

b. Distribution of chemical within the body

c. Biotransformation (see Chapter 3 III A)

d. Rate of excretion

2. Most transport of toxicants is initially by blood, and once absorbed, distribution depends on several factors:

    a. Blood flow to different organs or regions can vary significantly.

    b. Different biological membranes are traversed and the nature of those membranes can affect absorption.

    c. Accumulation of chemical in an area or organ may not always be associated with toxicosis. Some organs or tissues act as inert storage sites for specific toxicants, for example:

        (1) Chlorinated hydrocarbons are stored in body fat without toxic effects.

        (2) Lead may be stored in bone and cause no clinical effects.

        (3) Arsenic accumulation in hair causes no adverse effects.

B. **Chemical transport.** Passage across membranes may be by passive diffusion, active transport, facilitated diffusion, or endocytosis (phagocytosis), and each mechanism is defined by certain principles and characteristics.

    1. Passive transport or simple diffusion is the **most common means of toxicant transport**. Rate of passage is dependent on several factors.

    a. Chemicals move across membranes along a concentration gradient in proportion to the differences in concentration.

    b. Molecular size of molecules relative to size of pores or channels is a physical barrier. Pore diameter of some cells may be as small as 4 Å whereas other cells, such as glomerular capillaries, are 40–80 Å and allow passage of molecules as large as serum albumin (molecular weight, 69,000).

    c. Greater lipid solubility allows greater dissolution and passage through the largely lipid cell membrane. Molecules cross the lipid membrane best in the uncharged form. Ionization of compounds that are weak acids or bases retards absorption.

        (1) The tendency for a weak acid or weak base to ionize is defined by its tendency to be a proton donor or acceptor.

            (a) An acid is a substance that acts as a proton donor.

            (b) A base is a substance that accepts protons.

        (2) Protonated acids are un-ionized while protonated bases are ionized. The Henderson-Hasselbalch equation is used to quantify this relationship as follows:

$$\text{Acids } pK'_a - pH = \log \frac{\textbf{[un-ionized chemical]}}{\text{[ionized chemical]}}$$

$$\text{Bases } pK_a - pH = \log \frac{\textbf{[ionized chemical]}}{\text{[un-ionized chemical]}}$$

        where [ ] defines the concentration of either acid or base.

            (a) pK is the negative logarithm of K (–log K) and is equal to the pH at which half of the acid molecules are dissociated and half are undissociated.

            (b) K_a is the apparent dissociation constant.

        (3) For example, for an acid with pK_a of 3, in the stomach where the pH is 2, the ionized portion is $3 - 2 = \log_{10} 1 = 10$. Thus, in an acid medium, the ratio of un-ionized to ionized chemicals is 10:1, and the chemical could be readily absorbed.

        (4) Both pH of body fluids and pK'_a interact to affect ionization in the body. As shown above, chemicals with acidic pK_a are least ionized in an acidic medium, while those with basic pK_a are least ionized in a basic environment.

    2. Active transport is a specialized form of membrane passage. It is important for removal of toxicants after absorption. Specific transport systems exist for organic acids, organic bases, and neutral compounds.

    a. The chemicals move against a concentration gradient.

    b. Systems are selective and specific based on chemical structure and can become saturated or overwhelmed.

    c. Metabolic energy is required.

    d. Competitive inhibition can occur.

3. **Facilitated diffusion,** which is not a common transport system for xenobiotics (i.e., for-eign chemicals), has some characteristics of both passive diffusion and active transport.
   a. Compounds move along a concentration gradient.
   b. Energy is not required.
   c. The transport system can be saturated.

4. **Endocytosis (phagocytosis)** is a relatively uncommon specialized system at the cell sur-face, useful for some large molecules that may not pass membranes by other mechanisms.

C. **Distribution** of chemicals is dependent on many factors, including membrane passage, biotransformation, affinity for storage sites, and mode of excretion.

1. The apparent **volume of distribution (V_D)** defines the fluid volume in which a chemical seems to be dissolved.
   a. It is determined by the formula:
   $$V_D = \frac{\text{Weight of chemical distributed in the body}}{\text{Plasma concentration of chemical at equilibrium}}$$
   b. If V_D for a chemical is consistent with the known volume of a body compartment, the chemical is likely confined to that compartment.
   c. A V_D greater than the total body volume suggests that the chemical is accumulated in a tissue depot (Figure 1-4).

2. **Storage of toxicants in tissues** can alter both the toxicokinetics and the biologic effects of the toxicant.
   a. When chemicals are concentrated in specific tissues, storage can have two effects.
      (1) Storage can be at a site with susceptible receptors (e.g., accumulation of paraquat in the lung, where the chemical can act as an agonist).
      (2) Storage can be at an inert site without receptors or effectors that respond to the chemical (e.g., storage of arsenic in hair).
   b. Storage may affect excretion by slowing the availability of drug for renal filtration.
   c. Binding to plasma proteins represents a form of dynamic storage.
      (1) A bound toxicant is not free to pass the glomerulus.
      (2) Bound material may be available for active transport or for secretion.
      (3) Bound chemical may be displaced by another chemical, making it free to react with receptors or to be filtered by the glomerulus.

D. **Excretion.** Xenobiotic excretion occurs mainly from the kidneys (urine) and liver (bile); however, it can occur as well via lungs, intestines, sweat, saliva, and milk.

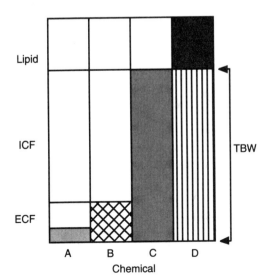

FIGURE 1-4. Volume of distribution (V_D) may define the presence of chemicals (*A, B, C,* and *D*) in differ-ent body compartments, such as plasma (*PL*), extra-cellular fluids (*ECF*), intracellular fluids (*ICF*), or total body water (*TBW*). If storage occurs, as shown for fat, the volume of distribution may be overesti-mated.

1. **Routes of elimination.** Renal excretion may be by either glomerular filtration or active tubular secretion.
   a. The glomeruli filter compounds up to the size of plasma albumin (molecular weight, 69,000). Only free compounds (not bound by plasma proteins) are filtered by the glomeruli.
   b. Tubular reabsorption affects the amount of filtered xenobiotic that is returned to the plasma. Compounds that are ionized and polar are poorly reabsorbed and thus remain in the urine and are excreted. Proximal tubules carry on an active energy-dependent secretion of some xenobiotics.

2. **Clearance** is the amount (volume) of plasma cleared of a specific xenobiotic each minute. It only defines the amount of xenobiotic eliminated, but does not define the extent to which plasma concentration is decreased by renal excretion.
   a. Clearance is calculated as follows:

   $$\text{Clearance} = \frac{\text{urinary drug concentration (mg/ml)} \times \text{urine flow rate (ml/min)}}{\text{plasma drug concentration (mg/ml)}}$$

   b. For example,

   $$\text{Clearance} = \frac{0.25 \text{ mg/ml}}{0.01 \text{ mg/ml}} \times \frac{50 \text{ ml}}{5 \text{ min}} = 250 \text{ ml/min}$$

3. **Rate of elimination.** Elimination of chemicals from the blood or plasma is usually **exponential** and is called "first-order" elimination (Figure 1-5). As time passes, the amount of chemical excreted becomes progressively less.
   a. Twenty half-life periods will virtually eliminate chemical residues from the body.
   b. **Half-life** is the term used to define the time needed for one-half of a chemical to be eliminated from the body.
      (1) The half-life for first-order elimination is defined by the formula:

      $$Cr = Cie^{-kt}$$

      where Cr = concentration remaining; Ci is the initial concentration; e = 2.72 (base of the natural log); k is the elimination rate constant for a tissue, toxicant, and species; and t is time in hours or days.
      (2) Using experimental data on initial and remaining concentrations, the rate constant can be calculated and that value used to calculate a half-life.
      (3) In clinical situations, the actual elimination may be defined by a multicompartment model that accounts for storage in more than one tissue or organ. For example:

      $$C = Ae^{-k_1 t} + Be^{-k_2 t}$$

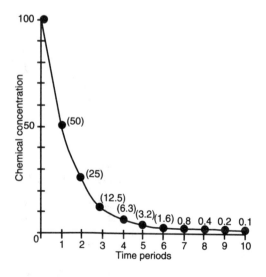

FIGURE 1-5. Half-life is a common expression for elimination of chemicals to one-half of the prior concentration within a specified time period. Notice that initial excretion is rapid, but it becomes progressively less with each successive half-life period.

DIRECTIONS: Each of the numbered items or incomplete statements in this section is followed by answers or by completions of the statement. Select the **one** numbered answer or completion that is **best** in each case.

1. The dosage of a poison received by an animal:

(1) is the total amount of poison received.
(2) is expressed as an amount of poison per unit of animal weight.
(3) has no relationship to the dose received by the animal.
(4) is determined by the route of administration of the poison.
(5) is necessary for calculating an LD_{50}.

2. If the LD_{50} of a drug is 100 mg/kg of body weight and the ED_{50} is 20 mg/kg of body weight, what expression of relative safety of the drug can be calculated?

(1) The LD_{99}
(2) The toxic dose–low
(3) The highest nontoxic dose (HNTD)
(4) The median lethal dose (MLD)
(5) The therapeutic index (TI)

3. The slope of a dose–response curve is important because:

(1) it shows the number of animals needed for future studies.
(2) the slope is used to calculate the therapeutic index (TI).
(3) the slope shows the range of toxic doses in a group of animals.
(4) it is used to calculate potency of the poison.
(5) it is an initial guide to the potential for chronic toxicity.

4. Toxicosis is *most accurately* described as:

(1) the amount of a poison that will cause detrimental effects under specified conditions of exposure.
(2) the threshold dose at which measurable toxic effects occur.
(3) the observed rate of deaths produced by a specific dosage of poison.
(4) the disease condition that results from exposure to a poison.
(5) the degree of hazard produced by exposure to a poison.

5. A measure of the tendency for a poison to cause cumulative effects is shown by the ratio:

(1) acute LD_{50}/acute ED_{50}.
(2) acute LD_{99}/acute LD_1.
(3) acute LD_{50}/90-day LD_{50}.
(4) 90-day LD_{50}/acute LD_{50}.
(5) 90-day ED_{50}/90-day LD_{50}.

6. One nanogram per gram (1 ng/g) is equivalent to:

(1) 1 part per trillion (ppt).
(2) 10 ppt.
(3) 100 ppt.
(4) 1000 ppt.
(5) 1,000,000 ppt.

7. An analytical result expressed as 8.7 µg/g is equivalent to what percentage value?

(1) 0.0000087%
(2) 0.00087%
(3) 0.0087%
(4) 0.087%
(5) 0.87%

8. A swine ration contains 500 g of a feed additive per ton. What is the approximate daily dosage of the additive to pigs weighing 110 lbs and consuming 2 kg of the feed daily?

(1) 2 mg/kg
(2) 20 mg/kg
(3) 100 mg/kg
(4) 200 mg/kg
(5) 400 mg/kg

9. A field of alfalfa is accidentally sprayed with 2,4-dichlorophenoxyacetic acid (2,4-D) herbicide at the rate of 1 gal of spray containing 20% 2,4-D per acre. (One acre is 43,560 sq ft.) The field is estimated to yield 4 tons of forage per acre and is ready to cut for dairy cows. The average weight of the cows is 1540 lbs, and each will be fed approximately 30 lbs of alfalfa daily. What is the estimated dosage per cow on a body weight basis, assuming all spray stays on the alfalfa?

(1) 0.5 mg/kg
(2) 4 mg/kg
(3) 10 mg/kg
(4) 21 mg/kg
(5) 84 mg/kg

10. The *most common* means of toxicant transport is:

(1) active transport.
(2) passive diffusion.
(3) facilitated diffusion.
(4) endocytosis.
(5) carrier-mediated transport.

11. Which statement is true about a chemical that is a weak acid, with a pK_a of 3.0, present in the stomach of a dog?

(1) Conditions in the stomach will not affect ionization and absorption.
(2) The chemical will become mainly ionized and less polar, promoting absorption from the stomach.
(3) The chemical will be largely un-ionized and may be absorbed from the stomach.
(4) The chemical will become protonated, which will give it a positive charge and prevent its absorption.
(5) The chemical will lose a proton, giving it a negative charge and preventing its absorption.

12. If half-life is the loss of 50% of a chemical from the body, how many half-lives would reduce residues to less than 1% of the original value?

(1) 3
(2) 7
(3) 10
(4) 16
(5) 20

ANSWERS AND EXPLANATIONS

1. The answer is 2 *[I C 2]*. Dosage is the amount of toxicant per unit of body weight or any other defined unit. Dose is the total amount per animal. The distinction between dosage and dose is important when reading toxicology literature or when evaluating exposure. Dosage is the common denominator that allows expression of toxicity across many different sizes of organisms.

2. The answer is 5 *[I D 1]*. The therapeutic index (TI), which equals the LD_{50}/ED_{50}, is the only product that can be calculated from the information given. The LD_{99}, toxic dose–low, highest nontoxic dose (HNTD), and median lethal dose (MLD) are doses or dosages defined by experimental procedures.

3. The answer is 3 *[I F 1 b (6)]*. The slope of the LD_{50} curve shows the range between no effect and maximal effect (LD_{100}) and is thus a measure of the probability of surviving a lethal dose (i.e., a lethal dose is likely to kill most of a population exposed). For example, a compound with a steep LD_{50} curve would make an effective rodenticide because the lethal dose range is narrow and survivors are unlikely.

4. The answer is 4 *[I B 4]*. The appropriate term for the condition of being poisoned is "toxicosis." Many people misuse the term toxicity to describe the pathology caused by poisoning; however, toxicity is the amount of chemical needed to produce toxicosis.

5. The answer is 3 *[I F 4 c]*. The ratio of the acute LD_{50} to the 90-day LD_{50} is known as the chronicity factor, and it is used as a general indicator of the cumulative nature of a toxicant.

6. The answer is 4 *[II B 1 b]*. One nanogram per gram (1 ng/g) is one part per billion (ppb). Given that one part per trillion (ppt) is 1000 times less than 1 ppb, 1000 ppt are equal to one ppb.

7. The answer is 2 *[II B 1 c (2) (c)]*. At 8.7 μg/g the concentration is the same as 8.7 parts per million (ppm). Moving the decimal four places to the left converts to the percentage 0.00087%.

8. The answer is 2 *[II B 2 b (5)]*. Given that 1 g of feed additive per ton is 1.1 parts per million (ppm), the concentration of 500 g of feed additive per ton is 550 ppm. The milligrams of feed additive per kilogram of body weight (110 lbs, or 50 kg) equal the feed level in ppm times the percentage of body weight eaten as feed. The percentage of body weight eaten is 2 kg/50 kg, or 0.04 (4%). In pigs, the daily dosage of additive is 550 ppm × 0.04, or 22 mg/kg.

9. The answer is 2 *[II C 1 b, D 2 b; Table 1-4]*. This problem involves a chain of conversions, which, if followed closely, lead to the answer. The 2,4-dichlorophenoxyacetic acid (2,4-D) was sprayed at a rate of 1 gal/acre.

1 gal = 3.8 L = 3.8 kg
3.8 kg × 0.2 active ingredient = 0.76 kg/A
.76 kg = 760 g = 760,000 mg/A
4 tons/A = 3666 kg/A
760,000 mg/A ÷ 3666 kg/A = 206 mg/kg forage
30 lb forage = 13.7 kg × 206 mg/kg = 2822 mg
2822 mg ÷ 700 kg = 4 mg/kg

10. The answer is 2 *[III B 1]*. Passive diffusion (or simple diffusion) is the most common means of chemical transport. Chemicals move along a concentration gradient in proportion to differences in concentration. Small molecular weight toxicants with little charge and high lipid solubility are transported by this principal mode of toxicant absorption.

11. The answer is 3 *[III B 1 c (1)]*. Acids do not lose protons (i.e., they remain protonated) in an acid medium such as the stomach. Protonated acids are un-ionized. Using the Henderson-Hasselbalch equation, it can be shown that low pH and low pK_a favor a high proportion of un-ionized compound.

12. The answer is 2 *[III D 3]*. The first half-life depletes residue from 100% to 50%, the second to 25%, and so on. By following this principle, the residue will be under 1% within seven half-lives.

Chapter 2
The Action of Poisons

I. CELLULAR BASIS FOR TOXIC INJURY

A. **Cellular damage is the basis for most toxicologic injury,** and the toxic response to any specific chemical is the result of dysfunction of relatively few basic biologic processes.

B. **Toxic injury involves quantitative differences in the function of cells, tissues, and organs.**

   1. The interactions of cells within tissues and the effects of organs on one another and on the entire organism account for the complexity of the toxic response in vivo.

   2. Normal processes can be suppressed or stopped completely, or they can be enhanced beyond normal physiologic limits and, in turn, affect other systems dependent on their controlled function.

C. **Cellular response of chemical toxicants occurs through both structural and metabolic mechanisms in the cell.**

   1. **Altered membrane integrity** can interfere with fluid and electrolyte movement.

   2. **Cell volume regulation can be altered** as a result of direct membrane damage or from loss of metabolic energy. An **alteration in energy metabolism** can reduce the energy available to drive active transport and the synthesis of macromolecules and to maintain osmotic balance.

   3. **Abnormal accumulation of lipids and pigments** can occur as a result of metabolic defects.

   4. **Protein synthesis may be altered** when nucleic acid control is disturbed and enzymes or structural proteins are denatured (altered).

   5. **Growth regulation may be disturbed** (causing, for example, hyperplasia or carcinogenesis) as a result of DNA damage that either is not properly repaired or that exceeds homeostatic control.

D. **Foreign compounds (xenobiotics) are biotransformed to electrophilic (electron-attracting) intermediates by the microsomal mixed function oxidases (MFOs).**

   1. MFOs are a family of nonspecific enzymes that act primarily in the endoplasmic reticulum to promote phase I metabolism (i.e., the oxidation of lipophilic xenobiotics), which prepares the xenobiotics for conjugation and excretion (see also Chapter 3 III A 1).

   2. Electrophilic intermediates are believed to bind covalently to important cellular macromolecules.
      a. These macromolecules (e.g., lipids, proteins, DNA) may be denatured by the binding.
      b. Electrophiles also bind to reduced glutathione (GSH), which is considered to be a protective mechanism in the cell.

   3. Covalent binding to macromolecules has a high correlation with cellular damage, carcinogenesis, or both, although a causal role for covalent binding has not been proven experimentally.

E. Cellular macromolecules may be damaged by free radicals.

1. **A free radical** is a compound with an unpaired electron, a result of an enzyme-catalyzed addition of electrons to a carbon bond, with subsequent cleavage.

2. **Superoxide** is formed when some compounds are oxidized by MFOs to free radicals, with electrons transferred to oxygen (e.g., paraquat herbicides).
   a. **Active oxygen (superoxide)** reacts with polyunsaturated lipids, initiating an auto-catalytic chain reaction, leading to lipid-free radicals and then lipid peroxidation (see I E 3 a).
   b. **GSH** can be depleted, which enhances oxidative damage and leads to cell death. Agents that deplete GSH increase cell susceptibility to lipid peroxidation.

3. **Several major effects are initiated after free radical formation** (Figure 2-1).
   a. **Lipid peroxidation** occurs because hydrogen from an unsaturated lipid is available to quench the radical.
      (1) The lipid radical reacts with oxygen to form a peroxyl radical.
      (2) Autocatalytic reactions continue: Lipid molecules reacting with free radicals themselves become free radicals and propagate a chain reaction of damage.
      (3) Peroxidation damages organelle and cellular membranes, reducing their structural integrity and control of selective absorption and active transport.

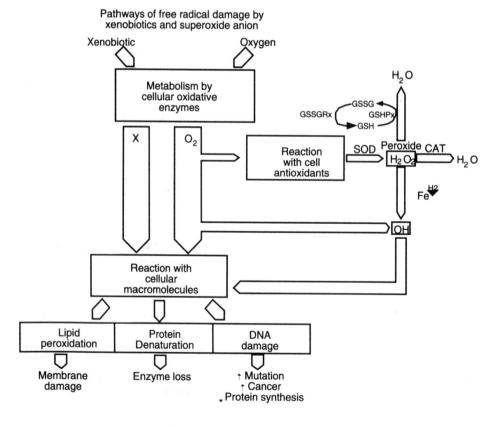

FIGURE 2-1. Pathways of free radical damage by xenobiotics and superoxide anion. CAT = catalase; GSH = reduced glutathione; $GSHPx$ = glutathione peroxidase; $GSHRx$ = glutathione reductase; $GSSG$ = oxidized glutathione; $OH^{\bullet}$ = hydroxyl radical; $O_2^{\top}$ = superoxide free radical; SOD = superoxide dismutase; $X^{\bullet}$ = chemical free radical.

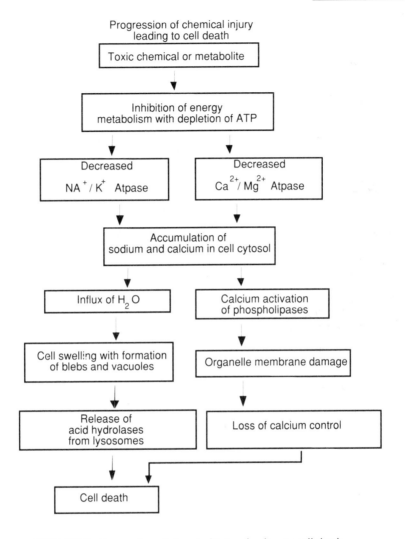

FIGURE 2-2. Progression of chemical injury leading to cell death.

(4) As membranes are damaged, there is loss of calcium sequestration in the organelles, leading to a marked increase in cytosolic calcium.

(5) Loss of calcium homeostasis leads to activation of phospholipases, auto-digestion of membranes, loss of membrane function, swelling of cells, and eventual irreversible cell injury progressing to necrosis (Figure 2-2).

b. **Naturally occurring protein thiol groups (e.g., glutathione) in cells may also be depleted** by free radicals or oxidative damage, leaving essential cell macromolecules at even higher risk.

c. **Defenses against free radicals are built into cells as antioxidants,** including:

(1) **Superoxide dismutase,** a copper- and zinc-dependent enzyme that catalyzes the reduction of superoxide anion to hydrogen peroxide

(2) **Catalase,** which is highly concentrated in peroxisomes of cells and catalyzes the conversion of hydrogen peroxide to water and oxygen

(3) **Glutathione peroxidase,** a selenium-dependent enzyme that catalyzes the GSH-mediated conversion of hydroperoxides to water or alcohol

(4) **Vitamin E,** which acts as a biologic antioxidant with a hydroxyl group on the benzene ring that acts to reduce free radicals

II. SPECIFIC MECHANISMS OF INTOXICATION

A. Chemical injury

1. Direct chemical injury to tissues alters the membrane-dependent homeostatic control of cell functions.
2. Damage occurs when cell membranes contact strong **corrosives** (acids), **caustics** (bases), or **compounds that coagulate proteins or damage lipids** in the cell membrane.
   a. The most susceptible areas are the skin, eyes, upper respiratory tract, and oral cavity.
   b. Damage is usually immediate (i.e., there is no latent period), localized, and nonspecific.
   c. Agents commonly involved are acids, bases, phenols, aldehydes, alcohols, petroleum distillates, and some salts of heavy metals.

B. Necrosis of epithelial cells.
Systemic toxins can cause epithelial necrosis throughout the body. Damage is most common in cells with high metabolic activity and cellular replication, including cells of the renal tubules, hepatocytes, bone marrow, and intestinal epithelium. Toxicants affect key enzymes or metabolic intermediates in these cells.

1. An **energy deficit** [i.e., loss of adenosine triphosphate (ATP) production] reduces active transport and control of cell electrolytes and water. Synthesis of enzymes or structural proteins may be reduced.
2. **Ischemia** (reduced blood flow) due to toxicants can result in damage to metabolically active cells by causing cellular anoxia, which leads to an energy deficit.

C. Inhibition of or competition with enzymes.
Enzymes normally allow cell reactions to proceed within restricted temperature and concentration ranges.

1. **Enzymes can be inactivated or denatured by direct chemical interaction with toxicants.**
   a. This can include alteration of spatial relationships and the tertiary or quaternary structure of the enzyme.
   b. If alternative pathways are not available, the inhibition affects survival.
   c. The severity and duration of poisoning can be influenced by the strength of the toxin–enzyme interaction.
2. **Competitive inhibition** is a common means of toxicant interference with enzyme action.
   a. Inhibition is maximal when the competing material is structurally very similar to the substrate.
   b. The enzyme-inhibitor complex formed is reversible, and the inhibitor molecule is not changed by the reaction.
   c. Examples in toxicology include:
      (1) Oxalic acid (plant toxin) and fluoroacetate (rodenticide), which inhibit succinic dehydrogenase and aconitase, respectively, in the tricarboxylic acid (TCA) cycle
      (2) Organophosphate and carbamate insecticides, which inhibit cholinesterase

D. Interference with body metabolism or synthesis
causes loss of products used for energy, structure components, or growth.

1. **Uncoupling of oxidative phosphorylation.** The release of energy in the electron transport chain becomes uncoupled from the formation of energy by the phosphorylation of adenosine diphosphate (ADP) to ATP.
   a. Uncoupling agents increase oxygen utilization, but energy is dissipated as heat rather than stored in high-energy phosphate bonds. Thus, body temperature rises.
   b. Dinitrophenol and chlorophenol fungicides and arsenates are examples of oxidative uncouplers.

2. **Inhibition of oxidative phosphorylation** (e.g., by trisubstituted tin fungicides) results in limited oxygen uptake with lower ATP formation. The effects of **fatigue and weakness** are similar to the effects of oxidative uncouplers, but there is no fever.

3. **Inhibition of nucleic acid and protein synthesis** can be initiated by toxicants that injure DNA or that bind to ribosomes during transcription or translation.
   a. Many inhibitors combine with small or large ribosomal subunits. Some toxins alkylate DNA, inhibiting its replication or transcription.
   b. A delay, or latent period, is common with this mechanism, since existing structural or enzyme proteins must be depleted before clinical effects appear.
   c. Examples include aflatoxin, organomercurials, and amantine (i.e., *Amanita phalloides* mushroom toxin).

4. **Interference with fat mobilization** occurs when toxins affect the rough endoplasmic reticulum. Results of this mechanism include:
   a. Reduced synthesis of lipid acceptor protein
   b. Reduced incorporation of phospholipids and triglycerides into transport lipoproteins, leading to accumulation of fat in the cell

E. Functional effects on the nervous system result from exposure to a wide range of toxicants.

1. **Normal reflexes may be enhanced** by blocking the inhibitory neurotransmitters of the reflex arc. This results in uncontrolled reflexes ending as tetanic seizures. A common example of this mechanism is caused by strychnine, which blocks glycine in the spinal reflex system.

2. **Toxicants can change the permeability of nerve cell membranes to ions.** Sodium and potassium currents are altered by poisons such as DDT and pyrethrins, changing the threshold for action potentials at the membrane.

3. **Inhibition of enzymes** essential to balanced synaptic function changes the characteristics of synaptic transmission (e.g., acetylcholinesterase inhibition by organophosphate insecticides).

F. Lesions of the central nervous system (CNS) or peripheral nervous system affect neuronal function or axonal transmission. They are often chronic and can be permanent.

1. **Neuronal necrosis** can occur either from direct or indirect toxic effects on neurons.
   a. **Direct effect.** Organomercurials impair essential neuronal protein synthesis.
   b. **Indirect effect.** Anoxia induced by carbon monoxide or cyanide causes secondary neuronal damage.

2. **Demyelination** affects nerve transmission by altering the spread of the action potential along the axon.

3. **Impaired transport within the axon itself** results in slow, progressive impairment of axonal transmission.

G. Injury to the blood and vascular system

1. **Hypoplasia or aplasia of cellular components** of blood may result from direct toxic effects on bone marrow precursor cells.

2. **Hemoglobin** may be affected by several mechanisms.
   a. **Synthesis may be reduced,** with resultant anemia or elevated amounts of hemoglobin precursors, or both, resulting in **porphyria**.
   b. **The iron in hemoglobin may be oxidized from the ferrous to the ferric valence,** forming **methemoglobin,** which cannot carry oxygen. (Nitrite poisoning is a toxicosis that produces methemoglobin.)
   c. **Oxidative denaturation of hemoglobin** with formation of Heinz bodies (denatured hemoglobin) increases both erythrophagocytosis and spontaneous hemolysis. (Cat hemoglobin is highly sensitive to Heinz body formation.)

d. Carbon monoxide, which has high affinity for hemoglobin, may **bind with hemoglobin to form carboxyhemoglobin,** which cannot carry oxygen.

3. **Coagulopathy** from toxic interference with vitamin K results in spontaneous hemorrhages. Rodenticides, such as warfarin and brodifacoum, prevent the reactivation of vitamin K needed to finalize the synthesis of prothrombin and factors VII, IX, and X.

H. | **Exposure to agents with action similar to normal metabolites or nutrients**

1. **Hormonal effects from exogenous estrogens** can mimic excessive activity of normal endogenous hormones. Estrogenic mycotoxins, plants, and feed additives may alter reproductive cycles.

2. **Excessive levels of nutrients,** such as vitamin D, selenium, and iodine, produce toxicosis in the same organs affected by deficiencies.

I. | **Immunosuppression** is an increasingly recognized response to industrial and natural toxicants.

1. **Toxicants affect both humoral and cell-mediated immunity.** Reduced antibody synthesis, interference with complement, changes in delayed-type hypersensitivity, altered neutrophil function, and reduced lymphoblastogenesis are all toxic effects.

2. **Examples of immunotoxicants** include heavy metals, dioxins, and mycotoxins.

J. | **Developmental defects** occur primarily in utero as a result of toxicants affecting susceptible cells during organogenesis.

1. **Toxicant exposure in the first trimester** of pregnancy results in severe effects that threaten survival of the fetus. Most teratogenic effects altering the morphology of the fetus occur in the first trimester of pregnancy.

2. **Toxicant exposure in the third trimester** results in reduced growth of a fetus that is already morphologically developed.

K. | **Carcinogenesis is a delayed effect of DNA damage.**

1. **The initiation phase** of carcinogenesis is associated with excessive damage to DNA or defective repair of DNA damage.

2. **Promotion** of carcinogenesis is caused by chemicals that produce tissue irritation or damage to macromolecules, resulting in expression of the cancer process initiated by DNA damage.

DIRECTIONS: Each of the numbered items or incomplete statements in this section is followed by answers or by completions of the statement. Select the **one** numbered answer or completion that is **best** in each case.

1. Which statement about free radicals in toxicology is true?

(1) They are compounds with shared electrons.
(2) They interact with calcium, increasing free calcium concentration in the cytosol.
(3) They initiate lipid peroxidation by the addition of hydrogen from the free radical to lipids.
(4) Lipid peroxidation occurs when hydrogen is removed from the lipids to quench the free radical.
(5) They damage membranes by sequestering calcium in the bimolecular layer of the cell membrane.

2. Which enzyme involved in protection against oxidative damage is selenium-dependent?

(1) Superoxide dismutase
(2) Catalase
(3) Glutathione peroxidase
(4) Phospholipase A
(5) Succinate dehydrogenase

3. Which statement is true about competitive inhibition?

(1) Inhibition is maximal when competing material is structurally similar to the normal substrate.
(2) The enzyme-inhibitor complex formed is irreversible.
(3) The enzyme-inhibiting molecule is chemically altered by the reaction with the enzyme.
(4) It is a relatively uncommon form of toxicant action on enzymes.
(5) Enzyme-inhibitor complexes stimulate cell reactions to proceed more readily than under normal conditions.

4. Toxicants such as DDT and pyrethrins alter the action potential of nerves because they:

(1) inhibit cholinesterase, thus reducing acetylcholine (ACh) stimulation of postsynaptic receptors.
(2) block γ-aminobutyric acid (GABA) at the synaptic cleft.
(3) inhibit the release of ACh from nerve cell endings.
(4) block axonal transport.
(5) alter sodium and potassium currents across neuronal membranes.

5. Porphyria is a syndrome that results from:

(1) increased destruction of denatured hemoglobin, which binds to the erythrocyte membrane.
(2) reduced synthesis of the erythrocytic cell series in the bone marrow, resulting in aplastic anemia.
(3) oxidation of iron in hemoglobin, interfering with oxygenation of hemoglobin in blood.
(4) impaired synthesis of hemoglobin pigments, releasing hemoglobin precursors into the blood.
(5) abnormal sensitivity to oxidative agents in animals with congenital glucose-6-phosphate dehydrogenase (G6PD) deficiency.

6. The promotion phase of carcinogenesis is associated with chemicals that:

(1) cause DNA damage.
(2) covalently bind with cellular macromolecules.
(3) produce tissue irritation or damage.
(4) accumulate in the nucleus.
(5) enhance DNA repair.

7. Epithelial cell necrosis that is caused by chemicals:

(1) is most common in cells with low metabolic activity.
(2) is reversible.
(3) occurs only where chemicals are applied directly to tissues.
(4) occurs immediately after exposure to the chemical.
(5) can be produced by both metabolic inhibitors and ischemia.

ANSWERS AND EXPLANATIONS

1. The answer is 4 *[I E 3]*. Free radicals have an unpaired electron, which is quenched by the hydrogen that can be extracted from cellular lipids. This initiates an autocatalytic chain reaction in which cells and organelle membrane lipids can become free radicals (peroxyl radicals). The result is a loss of cellular homeostasis, terminating eventually in cell dysfunction or death.

2. The answer is 3 *[I E 3 c]*. Glutathione peroxidase is the only one of the three major antioxidant enzymes (the others are superoxide dismutase and catalase) that is dependent on selenium to maintain its activity. Vitamin E, although not an enzyme, serves as an antioxidant to reduce free radicals and can partially compensate for a lack of selenium and glutathione peroxidase.

3. The answer is 1 *[II C 2]*. Competitive inhibition is a reversible process that is maximal when the competing material is structurally similar to the usual substrate. The inhibitor is not changed by the interaction, and the enzyme-inhibitor complexes slow or stop enzyme activity, thus inhibiting the normal cellular reactions.

4. The answer is 5 *[II E 2]*. The action potential of nerve cell membranes is dependent on the instantaneous influx of sodium and efflux of potassium to initiate nerve conduction. All other mechanisms offered as possible answers involve synaptic transmission or axonal transport but are not directly involved in generating the action potential.

5. The answer is 4 *[II G 1, 2]*. Porphyria is a term that means porphyrins in the blood. Porphyrins are intermediates in the synthesis of the iron-containing porphyrin ring known as hemoglobin. The other choices offered involve either cellular proliferation or destruction of blood components already formed.

6. The answer is 3 *[II K]*. Promotion is the process of enhancing or expressing carcinogenesis after DNA damage occurs during the initiation phase. Promoting agents are typically strong tissue irritants.

7. The answer is 5 *[II B 1, 2]*. One mechanism of epithelial cell necrosis is interference with energy metabolism, which reduces adenosine triphosphate (ATP)-dependent Na^+-K^+-ATPase activity. Energy deficit (i.e., a loss of ATP production) reduces active transport and control of cell electrolytes and water. Loss of control of the calcium level within the cell can trigger the release of degradative enzymes, which damage the cell and organelle membranes and cause coagulative necrosis.

Chapter 3
Factors Influencing Toxicity

I. **INTRODUCTION.** For a toxic effect to occur, the toxic agent or its metabolites must reach an appropriate site of action at a sufficiently high concentration and for sufficient time to initiate a toxic change.

A. **Interacting factors may change response to toxicants** and substantially influence dose–response assessment and diagnostic decisions. Although reaction to any individual factor may be small, the composite effect of several factors can be significant. Factors that affect toxicity include:

1. **Factors in the toxicant** that influence how it interacts with receptors or the cell membrane

2. **Factors in the host animal** that change its ability to activate, detoxify, or adapt to the toxicant

3. **Factors in the environment** that affect either the toxicant or the host animal

B. **Variations of the expected response to toxicants** are defined according to the response.

1. **Allergic effects** are immunologically mediated and result from previous sensitization to a chemical. They are also termed **hypersensitivity reactions**.
   a. An allergic reaction is likely to be characteristic for a species, and it is often not obviously dose related.
   b. Many chemicals can elicit a similar reaction.
   c. The lungs, eyes, gastrointestinal tract, cardiovascular system, and skin are frequently involved in an allergic reaction.
   d. Low doses can induce a severe allergic reaction in sensitized animals, and there is likely some degree of dose–response relationship.

2. **Idiosyncratic reactions** are genetically based. The cause is often an abnormal pattern of metabolism or detoxification resulting in an abnormal, usually excessive, reaction to a chemical.
   a. The reaction **is usually qualitatively similar to that in normal animals** but occurs at very low dosages.
   b. Conversely, and much less common, are responses in animals that are unusually reactive to a specific chemical.
   c. Idiosyncratic reactions are at each end of the Gaussian distribution of dose and response.

3. **Delayed toxicity** is a response that may not be manifest for days, months, or even years (e.g., carcinogenesis, neurotoxic effects from some organic chemicals). Delayed reactions can occur long after exposure stops.

4. **Synergism** occurs when the combined effects of two or more chemicals are greater than the sum of the individual effects. This could occur, for example, if one chemical affects the solubility, binding, metabolism, or excretion of the other.

5. **Potentiation** occurs when one chemical enhances the toxicity of another, even though the toxicity of the potentiator is minor or nonexistent.

6. **Antagonism** occurs when two chemicals administered together interfere with one another's action.
   a. Antagonism can be **physiologic,** as when epinephrine antagonizes the hypotensive effects of phenobarbital.

b. It can be **chemical,** as when the chelator ethylenediaminetetraacetic acid (EDTA) complexes with lead, which reduces its toxicity.

c. It can be **metabolic,** as when ethyl alcohol competes with ethylene glycol in antifreeze to prevent activation to toxic metabolites.

II. FACTORS IN THE TOXICANT

A. Composition of the sample

1. **Impurities** may change the apparent toxicity of commercial products. Agent Orange was hazardous because of contamination by dioxin produced during the manufacture of the main ingredient, 2,4,5-T.

2. **Modification of the basic active molecule** may change chemical properties and response of receptors. Examples include the exchange of anions to form different salts (e.g., copper sulfate to copper oxide) and chelation of metals to enhance absorption.

3. **Instability of the toxicant under conditions of use** may affect the toxicity. Thus, the organophosphate insecticide coumaphos may decompose in dipping vats to form potosan, which has increased toxicity to cattle.

B. Solubility, polarity, and ionization

1. **Chemicals with high lipid solubility** are more readily absorbed through the lipid-protein matrix of the cell membrane than those without.

2. **Nonpolar compounds of low molecular weight** are more readily absorbed than large complex molecules.

3. **Compounds containing groups ionized at physiologic pH** are usually more water soluble and less likely to absorb across membranes. These include amines, carboxyls, phosphates, and sulfates.

4. Binding of toxicant to physiologic proteins (e.g., albumin) can restrict the availability of active drug by limiting its passage across membranes. Such binding may also retard excretion by reducing the glomerular filtration of the toxicant.

C. Formulation and vehicle effects

1. The **vehicle,** a medium for diluting and carrying a chemical or drug, can include water, propylene glycol, organic solvents, and natural or synthetic gums or colloids.
   a. Vehicles that are nonpolar and lipid soluble can carry solubilized chemicals across most biologic membranes.
   b. **Active ingredients** in suspensions or emulsions may have different levels of toxicity than if they are soluble in the vehicle.
   c. Vehicles (sometimes called **inert ingredients**) can be toxic. For example, some animals may be affected by hydrocarbon carriers of pesticides. Use of unapproved vehicles (such as kerosene) can cause toxicosis.

2. **Formulations** of wettable powders, suspensions, and emulsions can affect the retention rate on hair and skin or the absorption rate from the intestine.
   a. Plant pesticide formulations may be dangerous if used on animals because of the retention properties of the pesticide, which allow excessive pesticide accumulation on animal hair or skin.
   b. Uneven mixing or settling, or both, of powders and emulsions may change the concentration of active ingredient in a vehicle. Thus, part of the mixture is at low concentration, and part is at high concentration.

D. Direct chemical interactions

1. Direct chemical combinations can result in formation of insoluble precipitates, thereby reducing either toxicity or efficacy.

2. Chemical interactions that change chemical composition can change apparent toxicity. For example:

a. Exchange of anions in salts (e.g., from copper sulfate to copper oxide) can change the degree of copper toxicity to sheep.

b. Hydrolysis of ester groups of organic molecules, such as organophosphate insecticides, can alter toxicity.

III. FACTORS IN THE HOST ANIMAL

A. Biotransformation and bioactivation

1. Mechanisms of biotransformation. Foreign compounds are commonly metabolized to different chemical forms by a complex system of enzymes known as the **mixed function oxidases (MFOs)**. The smooth endoplasmic reticulum is a major site of MFO activity, especially in the **liver,** where a substantial increase in enzyme activity is apparent within several days of exposure. **Cytochrome P-450** is a specific key component of biotransformation processes and is active in the metabolism of many xenobiotics.

a. Phase I metabolism. The MFO system acts primarily on nonpolar lipophilic compounds. MFOs add functional groups that are polar and less lipophilic. This process is known as phase I metabolism, and it **prepares the xenobiotic for phase II metabolism.**

(1) Phase I reactions can be **enhanced** by enzyme induction. The MFO system is stimulated to increased activity by previous exposure to the same or to a similar foreign compound, which in turn generally increases the biotransformation of these compounds. Barbiturates, halogenated hydrocarbons, and endogenous steroids are examples of MFO enzyme inducers.

(2) Phase I biotransformation can be **inhibited** (e.g., by piperonyl butoxide, which is used to increase pyrethrin toxicity in insects).

(3) Phase I **reactions** include oxidation (e.g., hydroxylation, sulfoxide formation), reduction, and hydrolysis.

b. Phase II metabolism is a series of **conjugation reactions** involving xenobiotics modified in phase I to combine with endogenous agents.

(1) Conjugation produces a compound that is less lipophilic and more water soluble than the parent compound.

(2) Conjugated products are excreted more readily in urine and are often less toxic than the parent compound or the phase I intermediates.

(3) Common conjugating agents include glucuronic acid, amino acids, acetates, sulfates, and glutathione.

2. Circumstances that alter biotransformation and affect toxicity

a. Liver disease may reduce the activity of MFOs.

(1) Quantitatively, the liver is the most important biotransformation organ in the body.

(2) Regeneration of liver tissue after hepatic injury may actually increase biotransformation.

(3) Diseases that reduce hepatic biotransformation, in order of greatest to least effect, are cirrhosis, liver toxicosis, carcinoma, and cholestasis.

b. Localization of toxicant in tissues with little MFO activity may affect biotransformation. Agents that partition strongly in lipid, bone, or brain tissue may be largely unavailable for biotransformation.

c. Age can have an effect. Newborn and very old animals may lack enzymes needed for biotransformation.

d. Nutrient deficiencies can limit the chemicals necessary for the synthesis of enzymes or conjugating agents [e.g., deficiencies of minerals (calcium, copper, iron, magnesium, zinc), vitamins (E, C, B complex), and proteins].

e. Different species, breeds, or strains may have different phase I or phase II enzyme activities (e.g., guinea pigs have compromised N-demethylation activity compared with other animals).

    f. Sex differences can affect biotransformation. Males often have higher MFO activity related to endogenous steroids such as testosterone.

    g. Route of exposure to a xenobiotic can have an influence. Oral exposure allows the substance a first pass through the liver before systemic involvement, increasing the probability of biotransformation.

    h. Decreased body temperature may decrease activity of microsomal enzymes.

    i. Diurnal variations in cytochrome P-450 and reduced glutathione (GSH) are associated with altered biotransformation that correlates with the variations in those components.

B. **Morphologic characteristics** can account for species differences pertaining to toxicity.

    1. Ruminants store large volumes of ingesta, potentially prolonging absorption of toxicant.

    2. Microbial action in the rumen can reduce toxicity by metabolizing the poison.

    3. Ruminal metabolism can enhance toxicity by activating the toxic agent (e.g., when nitrate is converted to nitrite).

    4. Anatomic or physiologic inability to vomit (e.g., in the horse, rat, or rabbit) can increase the adverse effects of poisons that are emetic in nature.

    5. The blood–brain barrier is an anatomic region of cellular tight junctions that help exclude chemicals from the brain. In some animals, a poorly developed blood–brain barrier permits the passage of certain chemicals, leading to toxicosis (e.g., ivermectin poisoning in collies).

C. **Metabolic characteristics** account for most of the known genetic and species differences associated with a toxic reaction to a specific chemical.

    1. Bioactivation of compounds (i.e., phase I metabolism) to more toxic forms (sometimes called **lethal synthesis**) varies among species. Dogs rapidly metabolize the rodenticide fluoroacetate to fluorocitrate, and its toxicity is six to eight times greater for dogs than rats. Mice and sheep form only limited amounts of bioactivated aflatoxin and are relatively resistant compared to other species.

    2. Differences in phase II biotransformation (i.e., conjugation) are observed among several species, resulting in delayed conversion and excretion of toxicants. Examples of differences are:

        a. Glucuronide formation is reduced in the cat and the Gunn rat, and, therefore, these animals are highly susceptible to poisoning by substances such as phenols.

        b. Sulfate conjugation is defective in swine.

        c. Mercapturic acids are poorly formed in guinea pigs.

        d. Acetylation of aromatic amino compounds is deficient in dogs.

D. **Distribution and excretion**

    1. Distribution and storage affect retention of xenobiotics and may enhance or reduce their concentration at susceptible receptors.

        a. High lipid solubility may cause accumulation in specific organs (e.g., concentration of DDT insecticide in nervous tissue).

        b. Binding to endogenous molecules, such as plasma protein or metallothionein, may increase retention of a xenobiotic in the body, but it can limit toxicity.

        c. Liver disease with bile retention prevents excretion, allowing some toxicants to accumulate in blood. Photosensitization results when plant pigments that are normally excreted in bile are retained in blood and transported to skin, where sunlight causes them to become photodynamic.

    2. Xenobiotics can compete with one another for plasma protein binding sites.

        a. Binding limits the available free drug that can cross membranes or attach to receptors, or both.

        b. One relatively nontoxic agent can displace a toxicant bound to plasma protein. The results may be complex and variable.

(1) Displaced toxicant is free, and its effect may be enhanced. A well-known example is the ability of phenylbutazone to displace plasma-bound warfarin, thereby increasing its toxicity.

(2) Conversely, an agent displaced from protein binding may be excreted more readily, reducing its toxicity.

3. Differences in active transport of organic acids or bases in the kidney can affect toxicant excretion (e.g., dogs excrete 2,4-dichlorophenoxyacetic herbicides poorly because of a poorly developed organic acid transport system).

E. Sex and hormone differences

1. Sex differences in susceptibility to chemicals is related to the status of the reproductive organs.

a. Sex differences in reaction to xenobiotics are minimal in prepubertal animals.

b. There is minimal difference between castrated and ovariectomized animals in susceptibility to toxicants.

2. Hormone differences

a. The high, constant levels of testosterone in males is associated with greater xenobiotic biotransformation by males compared to females.

b. Toxicants with hormone-like effects (e.g., the mycotoxin zearalenone, which is a physiologic estrogen) are most likely to affect animals of the sex that is dependent on that hormone.

3. Pregnancy and lactation cause marked hormone and metabolic changes.

a. Organs such as the liver, adrenals, ovaries, and uterus increase markedly in size and in protein content during pregnancy. Some of the additional protein may be microsomal protein, which enhances biotransformation.

b. Development of the placenta enhances the metabolism of some xenobiotics.

c. Lactation may enhance the excretion of some lipophilic toxicants [e.g., DDT, polychlorinated biphenyls (PCBs)].

d. Lactation increases the size and weight of the gastrointestinal tract, allowing for some dilution of orally ingested toxicants.

F. Age, maturity, and metabolic activity

1. Age

a. Age affects absorption or passage across biologic membranes.

(1) The gastrointestinal mucosa and blood–brain barrier in young animals are less well developed than in older animals.

(2) Active transport systems may be less effective in neonates.

b. Young animals generally have less active xenobiotic-metabolizing enzymes. This deficiency usually disappears by adolescence in most species.

2. General metabolic activity is usually greater in smaller or younger animals.

a. True metabolic body weight (mbw) is sometimes defined by animal surface area and is related to actual body weight (bw) by the equation

$$mbw = bw^{2/3}$$

b. By this approach, larger animals have a lower metabolic body weight and, therefore, likely have lower rates of biotransformation.

3. Changes in body composition may affect distribution and storage of toxicants. Newborns have high body water and low body fat, while old animals lose structural proteins, but have increased stores of collagen and body fat.

G. Pathologic conditions

1. Liver disease can cause reduced synthesis of protective binding macromolecules, allowing increased effects of toxicants. Glutathione, ligandin, and metallothionein are examples of binding agents synthesized by the liver.

2. **Filtration and reabsorption by the kidney** may be altered by disease, which may affect the excretion or secretion of xenobiotics.

3. **Gastrointestinal irritants,** by reducing transit time and absorption, can reduce the toxic reaction to oral poisons. Conversely, if gastroenteritis or ulcers are present, toxicant absorption may be enhanced.

IV. ENVIRONMENTAL (EXTERNAL) FACTORS

A. Volume and concentration of the toxicant

1. **Volume and concentration of the toxicant affect exposure (dosage) and the rate of exposure.** A bolus (i.e., one large dose by gavage) may produce poisoning with a much lower dosage than if the toxicant was diluted in an entire day's food supply and obtained by voluntary consumption.

2. **This volume and concentration principle affects the evaluation of toxicity from natural exposures.**
   a. For example, the dosage of nitrate toxic by gavage is 200 mg/kg body weight for cattle, but it is 1000–2000 mg/kg body weight if distributed naturally in hay.
   b. In addition, a type of dilution by time, or a reduction in the rate of dosage, can be illustrated by the time required for a toxicant to be released via digestion of food.

B. Route and site of administration

1. **The region and the type of tissue involved in absorption can influence toxicity from parenteral exposure.**
   a. Deposition in connective tissue and fat depots may retard absorption.
   b. Injection into highly vascular areas may accelerate absorption.
   c. Dermal absorption varies with body location. For example, thin-skinned vascular areas, such as the inguinal region, are more absorptive than thicker or more keratinized regions.

2. **Route of administration may affect biotransformation** since oral and intraperitoneal routes pass initially through the liver, while inhaled toxicants may access the lungs first.

3. **Fractionation of daily dosage generally reduces toxicity for acute toxicants** that are rapidly metabolized and excreted. If the agent is a toxicant with cumulative, chronic effects, fractionation of dosage is less likely to affect toxicity.

C. Environmental temperature

1. **Low environmental temperatures enhance biotransformation** of xenobiotics, possibly because metabolic activity increases to keep the animal warm.

2. **Temperature may influence the amount and pattern of food intake,** thereby altering exposure to toxicants in the food.

3. **High environmental temperatures increase water intake,** increasing exposure to water-borne toxicants. When water has been withheld, thirsty animals may drink rapidly and obtain a bolus dosage of water-borne toxicants.

4. **High environmental temperatures increase susceptibility to poisons that alter metabolism or thermal regulation.**
   a. **Oxidative uncouplers** increase body temperature, and their toxic effect is increased in hot weather.
   b. Dermal toxicosis of insecticides may be greater in hot weather when animals divert more blood to the skin to effect cooling, making more blood available for rapid insecticide absorption.

D. **Atmospheric pressure**

1. Changes in response to toxicants are generally associated with **changes in environmental oxygen tension**.

2. **Hyperbaric oxygen exposure** has been used to treat poisoning by carbon monoxide, barbiturates, and cyanide.

E. **Nutritional and dietary factors**

1. **Inactivation of chemicals by dietary components** can occur via intake of either natural food components or therapeutic agents.
   a. Phytic acid (inositol hexaphosphate) in plants can chelate metals and minerals, reducing their absorption.
   b. Dietary calcium and zinc influence the absorption of lead, which competes for the same divalent cation transport system.
   c. Dietary tannins and proteins can complex with toxicants and reduce their absorption.

2. **Palatability** may increase voluntary intake. For example, flavored and paraffin-embedded rodenticides are used to enhance palatability, and thus increase dosage, to rodents.

3. **Nutrient deficiencies and excesses** affecting toxicants are part of a large and complex group of interactions. Interactions commonly involve energy, proteins, vitamins, and minerals. Common examples are:
   a. Energy deficits induced by fasting, with reduced blood glucose, decrease the activity of drug metabolizing enzymes.
   b. Protein malnutrition impairs enzyme synthesis, MFO activity, and hepatic glutathione concentration.
   c. Vitamin deficiency, especially the antioxidants vitamin C and vitamin E, can result in increased damage from free radical formation.

STUDY QUESTIONS

1. All of the following are characteristic of an allergic response *except*:

(1) previous exposure or sensitization is required.
(2) clinical reaction is often typical for a species.
(3) response is stereotyped and similar for many different chemicals.
(4) high doses of the allergen are required for clinical response.
(5) organs commonly involved include the lungs, eyes, and skin.

2. The enhanced clinical effect from the interaction of two chemicals is called:

(1) idiosyncratic response.
(2) antagonism.
(3) synergism.
(4) bioactivation.
(5) additivity.

3. Biotransformation of foreign compounds (xenobiotics) could produce all of the following effects *except*:

(1) compounds that are more readily excreted in the urine.
(2) compounds with toxicity different from the parent compound.
(3) increases in the mixed function oxidase (MFO) activity of cells.
(4) hepatic lipid accumulation in the smooth endoplasmic reticulum.
(5) increase in liver size.

4. Which of the following statements regarding biotransformation related to age is correct?

(1) Xenobiotic-metabolizing enzymes are more active in newborn animals than in adults.
(2) Sexual maturity has more effect on the biotransformation capabilities of males than females.
(3) Newborn animals have higher body fat depots, which can sequester xenobiotics and prevent biotransformation, than adults.
(4) General metabolic activity of younger or smaller animals is less than that of older or larger animals respectively.
(5) The blood–brain barrier enhances the metabolism of foreign compounds by allowing access of chemicals to cerebral metabolism.

5. Lethal synthesis is a term used to describe:

(1) production of chemicals designed as pesticides.
(2) a genetic defect where body metabolism produces toxic by-products.
(3) conjugation of foreign compounds with endogenous nutrients.
(4) biotransformation of chemicals to a more toxic form.
(5) unusual susceptibility to poisoning that is not dose related.

6. Idiosyncratic reactions to drugs or chemicals are characterized by all of the following *except*:

(1) susceptibility to the chemical is often genetically based.
(2) response to the chemical occurs at very low dosages.
(3) reactions usually have an abnormal pattern of metabolism or detoxification.
(4) prior exposure to the chemical is required for the idiosyncrasy to develop.
(5) reactions are usually qualitatively similar to normal toxic response.

ANSWERS AND EXPLANATIONS

1. The answer is 4 *[I B 1]*. An allergic response is a specialized form of response to chemicals. Prior sensitization is a prerequisite for an allergic response to a chemical, which is true regarding responses to other antigens. The responses are stereotyped and are similar for many chemicals, but they are specific within a species. However, once sensitization has occurred, the dose required to initiate the response is small, and there may be no apparent dose–response relationship.

2. The answer is 3 *[I B 4]*. Synergism is the enhanced response to two chemicals given together; the total response is greater than the sum of the individual responses. Interactions that affect response can occur because of changes in solubility, binding, metabolism, or excretion.

3. The answer is 4 *[III A 1]*. Foreign compounds (xenobiotics) are modified in phase I of biotransformation and are combined with endogenous molecules in phase II in a process known as conjugation. Conjugated products are usually less polar, less lipophilic, and more readily excreted in urine than the parent compound. Biotransformation can increase or decrease the toxicity of a compound. During biotransformation by the mixed function oxidases (MFOs), the activity of these enzymes is increased, or induced, so that other similar foreign chemicals are also more readily metabolized. This process occurs mainly in the liver and causes an increase in liver size and proliferation of the smooth endoplasmic reticulum.

4. The answer is 2 *[III E 2]*. Young animals have fewer or less active mixed function oxidases (MFOs) than adults. In addition, fat depots and the blood–brain barrier are poorly developed in neonates, generally increasing their susceptibility to toxicants. Sexual maturity has more effect on the biotransformation capabilities of males than females, and males, with high testosterone levels, are more likely to have highly active biotransformation enzymes.

5. The answer is 4 *[III C 1]*. Lethal synthesis is a term that suggests adverse consequences of biotransformation (i.e., activation to a more toxic product). Many chemicals metabolized by phase I metabolism become more toxic and may bind to essential cell macromolecules or initiate lipid peroxidation before conjugation, or other detoxication reactions can occur. The concept is important since metabolism of foreign chemicals can be harmful as well as helpful.

6. The answer is 4 *[I B 2]*. Idiosyncratic reactions are unexpected responses because they generally do not demonstrate an obvious dose–response relationship and often cannot be predicted by toxicologic testing. The unusual susceptibility is often due to lack of mechanisms for metabolism or detoxification.

Chapter 4
Diagnostic Toxicology

I. **DIAGNOSIS** is the evaluation of a patient and the signs and symptoms of a disease or dysfunction to arrive at a cause. It allows application of specific measures to correct the effects of poisoning.

A. **Clinical diagnosis** may be used initially to determine the organ systems affected (e.g., systemic shock, grand mal seizures, respiratory arrest) and the disturbances that must be controlled to save the animal's life.

B. **Lesion diagnosis** is used to describe the changes that occur in tissue (e.g., acute multiple focal hepatic necrosis).

C. **Etiologic diagnosis** (the determination of the cause or source of the disease or dysfunction) is the most important diagnosis because it enables specific therapy and preventive measures to proceed.

1. **Specific antidotes** should not be used without an etiologic diagnosis.

2. **Protection of public health** from residues entering the food chain is promoted through confirmation of specific toxicosis.

3. **Determination of liability and damages** is difficult without a specific etiologic diagnosis.

II. **GATHERING IMPORTANT INFORMATION.** The role of the veterinary clinician is to elicit as much diagnostic information as is practicable using the approaches described.

A. **History and circumstances of exposure**

1. **It must be determined if exposure to a known or suspected toxicant has occurred.**
   a. The owner (client) should be questioned about changes in location, food source, recent chemical applications (e.g., spraying for insects, lawn or pasture fertilization, treatment of the animal with drugs), and other practices that may contribute to poisoning (Table 4-1).
   b. The premises where the animal is kept should be examined, if necessary.

2. **The presence of a toxicant in the environment,** or even consumption of a toxicant, does not confirm poisoning but **only suggests avenues of further investigation.** These include:
   a. Confirmation that **sufficient exposure occurred** to cause poisoning
   b. Documentation of **clinical, metabolic, and tissue effects** typical of the suspected poison
   c. Determination of a **toxic level** of the suspected poison in an appropriate organ or tissue

B. **Clinical signs and effects.** Clinical signs are often the only information available and must be used to initiate a search for poisons.

1. **Clinical signs alone are often insufficient** to confirm a diagnosis of poisoning.
   a. Thousands of different chemicals can cause similar effects in a limited number of body organs (i.e., organs and tissues respond similarly to many different chemicals).
   b. Many of the signs of poisoning (e.g., vomiting, seizures) can also be caused by infectious diseases or metabolic and endocrine disorders.

TABLE 4-1. Checklist for Evaluation of History and Circumstances of Animal Poisoning

---

Owner Data
Date:
Owner's name:
Address:
Phone number:

Patient Data
Species:
Breed:
Sex:
Weight:
Age:

Health History
Illness in the past 6 months:
Exposure to other animals in the past 30 days:
Vaccination history:
Medications, sprays, dips, wormers, etc. in the past 6 months:
Last examination by a veterinarian:

Current Clinical History
For herds/flocks, what is the size of the group:
Are animals purchased or home raised:
For herds/flocks, what is the morbidity: _____ mortality: _____
First observed sick:
For herds/flocks, how long has problem been present in the group:
If animal(s) found dead, how long since seen alive and healthy?

Environmental Data
  Large animals/livestock
    Location of animal (e.g., pasture, woods, drylot, feedlot, near river or pond; housed in confinement, in closed building with mechanical ventilation; held on slatted floors over manure pit; near roadway, near industrial site; access to trash)
    Changes in exposure (e.g., recently moved; pesticide spraying in area, use of rodenticides; new construction, renovation of old buildings; manure removal)

  Small animals
    Location of animal (e.g., housebound, outdoors in fenced yard, outdoors in kennel; roams free in neighborhood; access to businesses or industry)
    Changes in exposure (e.g., spraying for insects; lawn-care treatment; access to cleaning agents, over-the-counter medications, prescription medications, automotive products, outdoor or indoor plants)

Dietary Data
Type of diet:
Recent changes in diet (specific times in relation to observed illness):
Change in method of feeding (e.g., limited to free choice):
Presence of spoiled or moldy feed/food:
Source of drinking water:
Change in water supply:

Clinical Signs

Ataxia	Vomiting	Icterus
Salivation	Diarrhea	Bleeding
Blindness/vision	Melena	Hemoglobinuria
Depression	Polyphagia	Hematuria
Excitement	Polydipsia	Straining
Seizures	Polyuria	Fever
Dysphonia	Dyspnea	Weakness
Other (describe)		

Postmortem Findings (Describe in detail)

2. **Accurate definition of which organs, tissues, and metabolic processes are most affected** is an important factor in the diagnostic procedure.
   a. The type of change must be characterized in affected organs or in the entire animal (e.g., acute epileptiform seizures versus depression and ataxia).
   b. The organ system characterization should be used to develop a list of differential diagnoses compatible with the clinical signs.

3. **Chronology and progression** of the clinical signs have diagnostic value.
   a. The clinician may see only **one phase of the progression** of the disease. The owner should be asked if she has seen other signs.
   b. **Speed of onset and duration** of signs may identify some toxicants and rule out others.
   c. **Morbidity and mortality rates** may be clues to the type of toxicant, availability of the toxicant, and the available dosage of the toxicant.

4. **Other factors** may influence the susceptibility of an animal to poisoning with suspected toxicants. These include:
   a. Species of the animal
   b. Sex of the animal
   c. Interaction with nutrients, other drugs, or chemicals
   d. Previous stress or organ damage

C. **Clinical tests.** Different toxicants may cause characteristic changes in organs or metabolic pathways. Clinical laboratory tests that can confirm and quantify toxicologic damage to organs include:

1. **Serum enzyme profiles** for liver or kidney damage

2. **Coagulation tests** [e.g., prothrombin time (PT), activated partial thromboplastin time (PTT)]

3. **Urinalysis** (for blood, bilirubin, hemoglobin, casts, oxalates)

4. **Complete blood count** for anemia (including aplastic anemia), basophilic stippling, and platelet deficiency

5. **Electrolyte** (e.g., calcium, magnesium, potassium, sodium) **analyses**

6. **Blood pH, bicarbonate, osmolality, anion gap**

D. **Animal and environmental samples** (Table 4-2)

1. **Animal samples**
   a. **Blood** is the major vehicle for body transport of toxicants.
   b. **Vomitus or feces** provide evidence of recent oral exposure; some toxicants are eliminated in feces via excretion in bile.
   c. **Urine** is the major route of excretion for many toxicants.
   d. **Hair** provides evidence of chronic accumulation of metals and some organic toxicants.

2. **Environmental samples.** These do not confirm diagnosis but serve to establish a **source of poison** or suggest **a probable means of exposure**. Samples should include:
   a. Recent samples of **food, feed, forages, and water**. Multiple samples may be necessary to obtain a representative sample.
   b. Suspected **poisonous plants,** which should be examined for evidence of consumption by the poisoned animal
   c. **Baits,** which are concentrated sources of toxicants
   d. **Chemicals, pesticides, household products, solvents,** and objects that the animal may have come into contact with
   e. **Drugs and medications** available to poisoned animals or recently used in therapy

E. **Necropsy and examination of lesions.** If the animal dies, a thorough necropsy should be performed and appropriate specimens collected (see Table 4-2).

TABLE 4-2. Specimens and Samples for Diagnostic Toxicology

Sample or Specimen	Amount	Comments
Antemortem		
Blood	5–10 ml	Useful for detecting exposure to most metals, trace elements, cholinesterase, pesticides, and ethylene glycol, and for evaluating erythrocyte and leukocyte morphology
Serum	5–10 ml	Useful for evaluation of electrolytes, urea nitrogen, ammonia nitrogen, and organ function; exposure to metals, drugs (e.g., antibiotics), and vitamins
		Serum should be removed from clotted blood, taking care to avoid hemolysis
Urine	50 ml	Useful for detecting exposure to alkaloids, metals, electrolytes, antibiotics, drugs, sulfonamides, and oxalates
Feces	250 g	Useful for detecting recent oral exposures or drugs or toxicants excreted primarily in bile
Vomitus	250 g	Useful for detecting ingested poisons of all types, especially those that cannot be measured in tissue (e.g., organophosphates, ionophores)
		Indicator of recent oral exposure
Hair	5–10 g	Useful for detecting dermal exposure to pesticides; chronic accumulation of some metals (e.g., arsenic, selenium)
		Must be interpreted based on time of year, area of body where sampled, and external contamination
Postmortem		
Liver	100 g	Major organ of biotransformation
		Accumulates metals, pesticides, alkaloids, phenols, and some mycotoxins; bile may be useful for detecting toxicants concentrated by bile (e.g., lead)
		Usually frozen until analysis
Kidney	100 g	Major organ of excretion for antibiotics and other drugs, metabolized toxicants, alkaloids, herbicides, some metals, phenolic compounds, oxalates
Stomach contents	500 g	Confirmation of recent oral toxicant exposure; see also "vomitus"

Sample	Amount	Comments
Rumen contents	500 g	Confirmation of oral toxicant exposure Rumen may degrade some toxicants (e.g., nitrates, mycotoxins) Quantitative analysis is difficult as a result of variability of concentrations and lack of correlation with toxic levels in tissues Samples should be collected from several locations in the rumen and kept frozen until analysis
Fat	250 g	Useful for detection of cumulative fat-soluble toxicants (e.g., chlorinated pesticides, dioxins)
Ocular fluids	Entire eye	Useful for evaluating electrolytes (e.g., sodium, calcium, potassium, magnesium), ammonia nitrogen, nitrates, and urea nitrogen; ocular potassium and urea have been used to estimate time since death Both aqueous and vitreous humor are useful, but should be collected separately
Brain	Entire brain	Useful for detecting some neurotoxicants (e.g., chlorinated pesticides, pyrethrins, sodium, mercury) Brain should be separated by midline sagittal section, and the caudate nucleus collected for cholinesterase determination Half of brain should be frozen, half fixed in 10% buffered formalin
Environmental		
Feeds	2 kg	Multiple representative samples should be taken and then either combined and mixed for a composite sample or retained as individual samples (to detect variability in the source), or both
Forages (e.g., pasture, hay, silage)	5 kg	Samples should be taken from multiple locations in a pasture or storage facility, using a forage (core) sampler for baled hay or stacks Silage should be frozen to prevent mold and deterioration
Baits	All	Entire suspect bait and label should be submitted if available
Water	0.5–1 L	Useful for detection of nitrates, sulfates, total solids, metals, algae, and pesticides Water should be allowed to run to clear pipes before collecting from well or storage tank Bodies of water from the probable site of exposure should be sampled Water should be kept refrigerated until analysis
Soil	1 kg	Soil should be collected from root zone depth if plant contamination is suspected Sampling from multiple sites may be appropriate A soil scientist or agronomist may be of assistance

1. **Lesions, or lack of lesions, should be observed.**
   a. Common lesions for toxicants include gastroenteritis, fatty liver, centrilobular hepatic necrosis, pale swollen (necrotic) renal cortex, hemoglobinuria, cardiac dilatation, cardiac necrosis, hydrothorax and pulmonary edema, and ocular irritation.
   b. Many toxicants characteristically cause neither gross nor microscopic lesions.

2. **Stomach and intestinal contents should be examined** for abnormal color and the presence of plant material, foreign objects, tablets, or capsules.

3. **Appropriate organs and tissues should be saved** in 10% neutral buffered formalin for microscopic examination by a pathologist.
   a. Formalin volume should be 10 times the tissue volume.
   b. Tissues should be cut in thin sections (one-eighth inch or 3 mm) to ensure adequate penetration of formalin.
   c. Some poisonings can be confirmed by microscopic examination (e.g., renal oxalate crystals appear in ethylene glycol antifreeze poisoning; hepatic lipidosis and bile duct proliferation occur with aflatoxicosis).

4. Alternatively, an **entire representative animal** may be submitted for necropsy by a pathologist or toxicologist.

F. **Chemical analysis**

1. The concentration of a toxic chemical or its metabolites in tissues or organs is often the strongest evidence to confirm toxicosis.

2. Chemical analysis for toxicants generally should not be used alone to make a diagnosis.
   a. The concentration of chemical should be consistent with the poisoning; however, some chemicals produce toxicosis but are present at very low levels (below detection limits) in tissue.
   b. Some chemicals (e.g., organophosphates) can cause poisoning without being detectable in tissues by usual analytic procedures.
   c. Some chemicals can accumulate to high levels in certain tissues without causing toxicosis (e.g., chlorinated hydrocarbon residues in body fat).
   d. Interactions with other agents or nutrients can inactivate a toxicant stored in tissue (e.g., mercury can form a complex with selenium and protein, resulting in a nontoxic storage form).

G. **Experimental evidence**

1. **Experimental feeding of suspected baits or foods** may be useful when other approaches are inadequate, and it has been used diagnostically.
   a. This diagnostic application is limited because of the relatively high uncertainty of reproducing field conditions and to avoid unnecessary suffering of laboratory animals.
   b. One useful application is the test feeding of diets suspected of causing poor performance or reduced feed consumption.

2. **Response to a test dose of specific antidote** in a poisoned animal may help confirm a clinical diagnosis. For example, clinical improvement (reduced salivation and vomiting) after administration of atropine is presumptive experimental evidence of organophosphate toxicosis.

III. SPECIMEN COLLECTION TO SUPPORT CHEMICAL ANALYSIS

A. **Principles of good specimen collection**

1. **The correct sample** must be provided for the analysis required.
   a. The **liver** is the major organ for toxicant metabolism and excretion.

b. The **kidney** is the principal route of excretion for many toxicants.

c. **Stomach and intestinal contents** reflect recent oral exposure but may not be representative for toxicants with delayed or chronic effects.

d. **Skin and hair** are important for suspected dermal exposures.

e. **Feed, water, and forages** consumed by the animal are needed to identify potential sources of poisoning. It is important to remember that the food that caused the problem may no longer be available.

f. **Sprays, dips, baits, plants, soil, and other suspect objects** from the environment of the poisoned animal may be useful in finding potential sources of poisoning.

2. **Sample size must be adequate** to conduct the tests required. While modern analytical methods *may* use very small samples, preferred amounts of samples are:

   a. Serum or blood: 5–10 ml

   b. Urine: 50 ml

   c. Organs or tissues: 200 g each

   d. Stomach or rumen contents: 500 g

   e. Feed or forage: 2-kg minimum

3. **Adequate preservation** of the sample is essential to prevent loss of toxicant from leaching or decomposition.

B. **Maintaining the quality and integrity of samples for toxicologic diagnosis**

1. **The toxic agents to be tested must be determined** and the samples needed to support a diagnosis confirmed.

   a. It is necessary to keep a list of samples needed for routine toxicologic analyses at the laboratories used for analysis. Most laboratories publish a list of client services and specimens needed for specific analyses.

   b. For unusual analyses or if there is doubt about samples needed, the laboratory should be called for information.

2. **The history, clinical findings, and necropsy results should be recorded** and accompany the laboratory submission. As much information as possible should be obtained (see Table 4-1).

   a. Specific analyses may be requested of the laboratory.

   b. If specific analyses are not requested, the history and other findings assist the diagnostician in selecting appropriate specimens and tests.

   c. A written record of history and examinations is very important if insurance or liability claims are likely.

3. **Consistent sampling procedures** are important for quality specimen collection.

   a. Samples should be kept clean and free from contamination by dirt, debris, hair, and other environmental influences.

   b. Each sample must be sealed in a clean, individual container.

   (1) Clean glass or plastic containers are sufficient for most samples.

   (2) For pesticide residue analysis or other low-level organic contaminants, containers should be glass rather than plastic.

   (3) Organic contaminants in clean glass jars can generally be eliminated by one cycle through a self-cleaning oven.

   c. Preservatives must not be added to samples unless laboratory instructions specifically recommend them.

4. **Sample preservation is essential to adequate chemical analysis.**

   a. Most samples should be frozen unless specific analyses require other treatment.

   (1) Freezing prevents loss of volatile agents (e.g., ammonia or cyanide) and generally prevents enzyme or bacterial activity that could inactivate toxicants.

   (2) Conversely, freezing can inactivate some sensitive tests involving enzyme activity. The toxicologist or analytic laboratory should be consulted if doubt exists about the recommended preservation.

b. **Serum should be separated from the clot** because interpretation of serum results may be affected by leaching of materials from the erythrocytes.

c. For some trace elements, special **element-free tubes may be necessary**.

d. Feed and forage **samples that are high in moisture** (>15%) **should be dried or refrigerated** to retard mold growth.

e. **Adequate coolant must be used.** At least a 4:1 ratio of coolant to specimens is recommended.

f. **Biologic specimens should be double-bagged and sealed** to prevent leakage of blood and tissue fluids.

g. Applicable **rules** of the United States Postal Service or commercial carriers **regarding transportation** of biologic and infectious or toxic materials should be followed.

5. **Recommendations of the Federal Bureau of Investigation (FBI) for proper sealing and transmittal of evidence should be followed.** Sample integrity and chain of custody may be important for cases involving insurance claims or litigation.

a. Evidence must be **packed securely** in a box.

b. The box must be **sealed and marked** as "evidence."

c. A copy of the **transmittal letter** should be placed in an envelope and marked "invoice."

d. The **envelope must be affixed to the outside** of the sealed box.

e. The **box must be wrapped and sealed** with tape or gummed paper.

f. The **mailing label is attached** and is directed preferably to a specific person who has been notified in advance.

IV. SELECTING A LABORATORY

A. **A laboratory should be selected based on assurances of quality and service.** Characteristics of a good laboratory include:

1. **A written schedule of fees and services**

2. **Quality control programs and accreditation with recognized certifying agencies**

3. **Information about the qualifications of the staff**

4. **Use of modern analytic equipment**
   a. **Major instrumentation** should include ultraviolet and visible spectrophotometers, atomic absorption spectrophotometers, gas liquid chromatographs, high-performance liquid chromatographs, and fluorometers.
   b. **Additional desirable capabilities** are inductively coupled plasma element analysis, immunoassay, nuclear magnetic resonance, and mass spectrometry.

5. **Instructions in collection and preservation of samples** and interpretation of the results in the context of the samples being analyzed and the source of the specimens

6. **Availability of a veterinary diagnostician** for consultation and interpretation of results

7. **Documentation of normal or expected values** for the tests performed

B. **Good communication with the laboratory should be regularly maintained.**

1. The laboratory should be contacted for a listing of fees and services.

2. Policies for emergency after-hours service, security of samples, and reporting of results should be discussed.

3. The names of persons who can consult on chemical analysis and veterinary interpretation of results should be determined.

STUDY QUESTIONS

DIRECTIONS: Each of the numbered items or incomplete statements in this section is followed by answers or by completions of the statement. Select the **one** lettered answer or completion that is **best** in each case.

1. Which of the following actions should be delayed until an etiologic diagnosis is reached?

(1) A search of the premises to find potential sources of poisons
(2) Evaluation of the patient's vital signs
(3) Application of lifesaving emergency and supportive therapy
(4) Use of specific antidotes against specific toxicants
(5) Chemical analysis of blood and urine from affected animals

2. The type of evidence or information *most often* initially available to a clinician during the diagnostic process is:

(1) exposure to a poison in the absence of clinical signs.
(2) exposure to a poison associated with a sick animal.
(3) a sick animal with no known exposure to a poison.
(4) the client's recollection of previous clinical signs.
(5) product labels from the suspected toxicant.

3. Use of vomitus for chemical analysis when poisoning is suspected:

(1) is the best sample because the toxicant is most concentrated.
(2) reflects the total toxicant intake of the animal.
(3) can be correlated with concentration of toxicants in tissues.
(4) reflects recent exposure to a poison.
(5) confirms toxicosis if the sample is positive.

4. Which statement about lesions associated with toxicosis is correct?

(1) Many toxicoses present no gross lesions at necropsy.
(2) Most toxicoses can be diagnosed from the presence of microscopic lesions in formalin-fixed tissues.
(3) Cellular inflammatory reaction is a common microscopic response to intoxication.
(4) Lesions are the best single indicator of toxicologic damage.

5. Which of the following situations is *least likely* to invalidate chemical analysis to confirm poisoning?

(1) The chemical is metabolized to another form in the target organ.
(2) The chemical is excreted to undetectable levels before sampling.
(3) The chemical has accumulated in a tissue that is not a target site for toxicosis.
(4) The chemical has formed a complex with other agents, resulting in a nontoxic storage form.
(5) The chemical is toxic at concentrations that are below detection limits for the methodology available.

6. What type of preservation is *most* applicable to a wide variety of chemical analyses for toxicants?

(1) Refrigeration
(2) Freezing
(3) Drying
(4) Formalin fixation
(5) Heat fixation

ANSWERS AND EXPLANATIONS

1. The answer is 4 *[I C 1–3]*. The most important aspect of the etiologic diagnosis is that it allows application of specific countermeasures and preventive approaches that cannot be logically used without knowing the specific cause. Antidotes are powerful drugs that act against specific toxicants. Their use in animals in which that toxicant is not present (to balance their physiologic effect or complex with the antidote) leaves the animal susceptible to the pharmacologic and toxicologic effects of the antidote. For example, use of atropine at the high dosages needed for organophosphate toxicosis can cause atropine toxicosis if the cholinesterase-inhibiting organophosphates are not present.

2. The answer is 3 *[II B 3–4]*. Most often when an animal is acutely ill, the client submits the animal to a veterinarian or calls to describe general clinical signs. The first response for the clinician must be to associate specific clinical signs or combinations of clinical signs with a list of tentative diagnoses that may include toxicoses. Usually some questioning by the clinician will help the client to recall potential exposures that are compatible with the clinical signs expressed. Therefore, although clinical signs are rarely used to confirm a diagnosis, they are the principal entry point for the diagnostic process. A less common but still frequent scenario is the discovery by the client that an animal has been exposed to a toxicant, but is not yet exhibiting clinical signs. This leads the clinician to consider the potential dose received and whether or not preventive detoxification procedures are needed.

3. The answer is 4 *[II D 1 b; Table 4-2]*. Vomitus from a live animal or the stomach contents of a dead animal is invaluable evidence of recent oral exposure to a toxicant. The clinician must remember that this sample reflects only what has been ingested in the previous 1–6 hours. In some rare cases involving basic drugs (e.g., strychnine alkaloid) a small portion of the toxicant in blood may partition back into the stomach. However, for the many toxicants that have a delayed onset or whose effects occur only after many days' exposure, the most recent ingestion may not represent a known toxic dose or may not contain any of the significant toxicant. For this reason, stom-ach contents should be only one of multiple samples collected for toxicologic analysis.

4. The answer is 1 *[II E 1 b]*. Unfortunately, many important toxicants provide no gross lesions as clues to their presence. Furthermore, many toxicants produce only minimal or no microscopic lesions. For those toxicants that produce lesions, many are nonspecific and could be attributed to other causes. The number of specific, pathognomonic lesions of toxicosis is few. Detailed pathologic examination is important both to detect those toxicants that may cause lesions and to suggest other diagnoses (e.g., infectious, metabolic, or degenerative disease) that may be recognized from the lesions produced.

5. The answer is 1 *[II F 1–2]*. For most of the common toxicants, analysts can detect the chemical or its major metabolites in the body. Analyses are less useful, or even misleading, when the tissue stores the toxicant but is not indicative of poisoning, when the agent suspected has formed a complex with other agents and is stored in a nontoxic form, or when the agent is so toxic that it occurs at concentrations below the detection limit of routinely available analytic methods.

6. The answer is 2 *[III B 4 a]*. Freezing is usually the safest form for preservation unless the samples contain sensitive agents (e.g., enzymes) that are damaged by freezing. Freezing prevents volatilization losses and slows enzyme activity and bacterial proliferation, which could inactivate toxicants of interest. However, many toxicants are stable in refrigerator temperatures. The important issue is that chemical preservatives should not be added, nor drying or autolysis allowed, because these change the water content, can inactivate some toxicants, and allow leaching of tissue fluids, which can change the analytic results.

Chapter 5
Therapy and Management of Toxicoses

I. **INTRODUCTION.** A logical and planned approach is the most effective way to deal with acute poisonings. Toxicoses occur infrequently, but they are often life-threatening, so a well-organized response to decontamination and emergency supportive therapy is essential to survival in the first few hours of an acute intoxication. Determining the cause of the toxicosis (etiologic diagnosis; see Chapter 4) is essential to a rational approach to management. In addition, supportive therapy and convalescent care are key factors in recovery of altered metabolism and damaged organs. The overall approach emphasizes the well-known phrase: "Treat the patient, not the poison."

II. **EXPOSURE TO THE TOXICANT: REDUCTION OR ELIMINATION**

A. **Removal from the toxic environment**

  1. **Telephone instructions.** This information may aid the owner in first aid to the animal and removal from toxic exposure.
     a. **Serious illness.** If the animal appears to be seriously ill (e.g., recumbent, comatose, seizuring), the owner should be advised to take the animal to a veterinary facility immediately.
     b. **Toxicant label.** If the animal has been exposed to a suspect toxicant and if a label for the toxicant lists ingredients and antidotes, the amount (dosage) of toxicant can be estimated. Sometimes exposure is below the likely toxic dosage and treatment may be unnecessary.
     c. **Time of exposure.** The client is asked to estimate when the animal ingested the suspect toxicant. If exposure is recent, this information aids in attempts at intervention by removal from the toxicant.
     d. **Vomiting.** If the animal has not yet vomited, emetics administered at home may be useful.

  2. **Physical removal or separation from the toxicant.** When toxicosis has occurred or is occurring, further exposure to the toxicant should be avoided.
     a. **Livestock.** Changing pastures or feedlots may prevent further exposure.
     b. **Pets.** Changing the location from the yard to the house or from the basement to another area may be helpful.
     c. **Feed and water.** Changing the feed and water source is a general but rational action to prevent further potential ingestion of toxicants.
     d. **Mild or moderate poisoning.** Changing the environment may be the only action that is needed, since natural processes, such as vomiting and glomerular filtration, may lead to recovery.
     e. **New locations.** Animals placed in new locations may encounter other hazardous materials.
     f. **Owner exposure.** Toxic exposure can occur when the owner handles poisoned animals (e.g., when buildings are contaminated by toxic gases or animals are dermally contaminated by pesticides).

B. **Absorption of ingested toxicants.** Removing poison from the stomach is most effective in the first 2 hours after ingestion and is of limited benefit more than 4 hours after ingestion. Dosages for emetics and other emergency decontamination procedures are summarized in Table 5-1.

TABLE 5-1. Dosages of Therapeutic Agents for Acute Toxicosis

Emesis: first aid by owner
   Ipecac syrup
   A centrally acting emetic given orally to small animals. Dosage for dogs: 1–2 ml/kg. Dosage for cats: 3 ml/kg. Vomiting expected in 15–20 minutes; one repeat dose may be given. Bitter taste may make this drug difficult for owner to administer. May cause excessive vomiting or CNS depression.
   Hydrogen peroxide (3%)
   Given orally at 1–5 ml/kg, preferably after a moistened meal. Dosage not to exceed 50-ml total dose in dogs or 10-ml total in cats.
   Liquid dishwashing detergent
   A mixture of 3 T in 8 oz of water is given at 10 ml/kg. Laundry and electric dishwasher detergents should never be used.

Emesis: veterinary use in dogs
   Apomorphine
   Given at 0.04 mg/kg IV or IM, 0.08 mg/kg SQ, or SC instillation of 0.25 mg in saline. Vomiting may be excessive, and CNS depression can occur. Not recommended for cats.

Emesis: veterinary use in cats
   Xylazine
   1.1 mg/kg IM is effective in most cats. Respiratory depression may occur but can be reversed with yohimbine (0.1 mg/kg IV).

Gastric lavage
   Water or saline used initially at 10 ml/kg in a large-bore stomach tube with fenestrated tip. Lavage fluid should be tepid. Administration must be gentle, preferably by gravity flow, to avoid potential injury to the stomach. Process is repeated 15–25 times or until lavage fluid is clear.

Adsorption therapy
   Activated charcoal is the most effective adsorbent for a wide variety of toxicants. Administered in a water slurry of 1 g/5 ml water at 2–5 g charcoal per kg body weight. Not to be given concurrently with other orally administered drugs. May be followed with an osmotic cathartic.

Osmotic catharsis (with or without use of activated charcoal)
   Sodium sulfate: 250 mg/kg orally.
   Sorbitol: (70%) 3 ml/kg orally.
   Either cathartic may be given 30 minutes after administration of activated charcoal. Not to be used if animal has diarrhea.

Cleansing of skin or hair
   Animal should be washed several times using **mild shampoo or liquid dishwashing detergent.** Water should flow over the animal so it does not remain in contaminated rinse water. Persons washing animals should wear gloves and other protective garments.
   Long or matted hair may be clipped if necessary for complete removal of toxicant residues.

Cleansing of eyes
   The eyes are flushed numerous times with **water** or **saline.**

Respiratory stimulation
   Doxapram: 1–10 mg/kg.
   Care is necessary because excessive dosage can cause seizures. Relapses to depressed status may occur after effect diminishes.

Reversal of respiratory depression due to opiates
   Naloxone: 0.04 mg/kg in dogs IV, IM, or SC.

Cardiac arrhythmias: See Table 5-2.

Seizure control
   Diazepam
   Used for initial treatment at 0.5 mg/kg IV. May be repeated if needed every 20 minutes up to three times.
   Phenobarbital
   If diazepam fails, phenobarbital can be used at 6 mg/kg IV.
   Pentobarbital
   If phenobarbital fails, pentobarbital can be given as needed to control seizures. Anesthesia should be as light as possible.

TABLE 5-1. Continued

Histamine blocking
   Cimetidine is given for gastric irritation and vomiting. Dosage for dogs: 5–10 mg/kg orally.
Metabolic acidosis
   Sodium bicarbonate
   Given at 0.5–2.0 mEq/kg every 4 hours IV. Blood pH, bicarbonate, and other indicators of acid–base status should be monitored.
   Sodium lactate
   0.17 molar concentration is given at 16–32 mg/kg IV.
Ion trapping of basic drugs
   Urinary acidifier: ammonium chloride
   Dosage for dogs: 100 mg/kg orally; dosage for cats: 20 mg/kg orally. Given daily in divided doses. Ammonia toxicosis is reported to occur from overdosing.
Ion trapping of acidic drugs
   Urinary alkalinizer: sodium bicarbonate
   0.5–2.0 mEq/kg every 4 hours IV.
Diuresis
   Maintaining urine flow: mannitol: 1 g/kg IV.
   Reducing cerebral edema: mannitol: 2 g/kg IV.
   Relieving heart failure: furosemide: 2–4 mg/kg IV or IM twice daily.
   Reducing ascites from liver failure: furosemide: 1–2 mg/kg orally or SQ twice daily.
   Correcting pulmonary edema: furosemide: 2–4 mg/kg IV or IM two to four times daily.
   Combating acute renal failure: furosemide: 5–20 mg/kg IV as needed.

CNS = central nervous system; IM = intramuscular(ly); IV = intravenous(ly); SC = subconjunctival(ly); SQ = subcutaneous(ly).

1. **Emesis.** Induction of emesis is the most effective means of emptying the stomach in those animals that can vomit readily. Early emesis may remove as much as 80% of ingested material.
   a. **Contraindications.** Emetics are not recommended for rodents, rabbits, horses, or ruminants because they cannot vomit safely or effectively. Emetics are contraindicated when:
      (1) The animal is **unconscious** or **very depressed** because aspiration of vomitus may occur
      (2) The animal is in **seizure** or is susceptible to spontaneous seizures
      (3) The animal has ingested **corrosive or caustic materials** (e.g., acids, lye), so the damaged stomach wall could rupture and damaging materials may regain access to the esophagus and pharynx
      (4) **Petroleum distillates or other volatile materials** (e.g., gasoline) were ingested and the animal is at risk of aspiration pneumonia
   b. **Emetics administered by the owner.** Emetics that the owner administers as first aid are often not effective. Dangerous emetics include table salt and copper sulfate. If emesis is attempted at home, the following approaches are acceptable.
      (1) **Ipecac syrup,** available from pharmacies for emergency emesis in children, has been used orally in dogs, 1 to 2 ml/kg body weight, and in cats, 3 ml/kg body weight.
         (a) If vomiting has not occurred in 15 minutes, one repeat dose may be given. Ipecac is ineffective in approximately half of all dogs treated.
         (b) Ipecac may cause excessive vomiting or depression of the central nervous system (CNS).
         (c) Ipecac can be inactivated by concurrent administration of activated charcoal.
      (2) **Hydrogen peroxide (3%),** given orally at 2 to 5 ml/kg body weight, is most effective if it follows a moistened meal or if the stomach contains ingesta. Dosage should not exceed 40 to 50 ml total.

(3) Liquid dishwashing detergent (3 T in 8 oz water), given at 10 ml/kg body weight, should produce vomiting within 20 minutes.
(a) Phosphate-containing detergents are most effective.
(b) Laundry detergents and detergents for dishwashing machines are highly irritating and thus should be avoided.

c. Emetics recommended for veterinary use
(1) Dogs. Apomorphine is given by intravenous or intramuscular routes (0.04 mg/kg); by subcutaneous injection (0.08 mg/kg); or by subconjunctival instillation (0.25 mg total dissolved in saline) if the dog can vomit effectively. (It is not readily available through veterinary pharmaceutical sources.)
(a) CNS depression may limit its use if the animal is already depressed.
(b) Naloxone (0.04 mg/kg intravenously) should be available as a narcotic antagonist if apomorphine causes excessive CNS or respiratory depression.
(2) Cats. Xylazine (1.1 mg/kg intramuscularly) may be a useful emetic, although it is not universally effective. Respiratory depression from xylazine may be reversed with **yohimbine** (0.1 mg/kg intravenously).

2. Gastric lavage is an alternative means of gastrointestinal decontamination. It can be used when emesis is ineffective or contraindicated. Lavage must be performed in an unconscious or anesthetized animal.
a. An **endotracheal tube** must be in place to prevent aspiration of stomach contents.
(1) The stomach tube should be as large as possible, with one or two openings laterally near the tip. This helps to avoid plugging during aspiration of contents.
(2) The tube should be inserted no further than the distance from the tip of the nose to the xiphoid cartilage.
(3) The anesthetized animal should be on its back, with the head inclined ventrally at a 20° to 30° angle.
(4) Lavage fluid (water or saline) is administered gently by gravity flow at 10 ml/kg body weight. (Warm or tepid lavage fluids promote gastric emptying.) Stomach contents and fluid are aspirated after a few minutes.
(a) The procedure can be repeated 15 to 25 times or until the lavage fluid is clear.
(b) Excessive pressure should be avoided because it could damage a weakened stomach wall.
b. Enterogastric lavage (also called a "through and through enema") is the combination of gastric lavage and a retrograde high enema given with the gastric tube and endotracheal tube still in place. Enema fluid is administered gently until fluids flow from the gastric tube, indicating nearly complete evacuation of the gastrointestinal tract. As enema fluids reach the upper intestines, spontaneous vomiting may occur.
c. For ruminants, a large hose inserted in the rumen is used to introduce water gently until the abdomen expands slightly.
(1) The stomach tube is then lowered and allowed to discharge as much as possible.
(2) This can be repeated multiple times if the net retention of water is not excessive.

3. Adsorption therapy with activated charcoal. Adsorption is the physical binding of a toxicant to an unabsorbable carrier, which is eliminated in the feces.
a. Activated charcoal has gained almost universal acceptance as the adsorbent of choice for many toxicoses.
(1) It is most effective for large, nonpolar molecules.
(2) Ionized agents are less strongly adsorbed than neutral compounds.
(3) Activated charcoal is relatively ineffective against ammonia and cyanide.
b. Drugs and treatments administered in the presence of activated charcoal are likely to be adsorbed and reduced in efficacy.
c. Activated charcoal can be given following emesis or gastric lavage or administered when these procedures are contraindicated and ingesta must remain in the stomach or rumen.
(1) Dosage is 2 to 5 g/kg body weight in a water slurry in which 1 g is suspended in 5 ml of water.

(2) Charcoal is usually administered with a cathartic such as sodium sulfate (250 mg/kg body weight orally) or 70% sorbitol (3 ml/kg body weight orally). This combination hastens removal of the toxicant–charcoal complex and helps prevent the constipation that can occur from the charcoal.

4. **Gastrotomy or rumenotomy** may be necessary in situations that are refractory to emesis, lavage, or activated charcoal.
   a. **Foreign bodies,** especially those containing toxic metals such as lead or zinc, are indications for surgical intervention. An abdominal radiograph may be useful in detecting retained toxic metals.
   b. **Persistent materials,** such as toxic oils, tars, or agents that reduce rumen motility, may require surgical evacuation.

5. **Reducing dermal and ocular exposure**
   a. Exposed animals should be washed with warm water and a soap or mild detergent, and the process repeated as needed.
   b. Long-haired animals may require clipping to remove toxic residues.
   c. For toxic ocular exposures, immediate flushing with water is recommended. This should be repeated many times, up to 20 to 30 minutes to enhance the decontamination.

III. EMERGENCY INTERVENTION

A. **Appropriate emergency supportive and symptomatic treatment** is often the most valuable part of early treatment for toxicoses. The suggestions that follow are not comprehensive therapeutic regimens but are summaries of essential supportive care that must be considered in effective toxicology therapy. Resources in internal medicine or veterinary critical care provide details.

B. **Major life-threatening effects** of toxicants need to be assessed. Early in the course of toxicologic management, the following should be evaluated and treated appropriately.

1. **Respiratory depression or failure**
   a. **A patent airway** should be established with a cuffed endotracheal tube to prevent aspiration of vomitus in a comatose or anesthetized animal.
   b. **Mechanical ventilation** or oxygen should be used if needed for apnea, anoxia, or severe anemia.
   c. **Centrally acting respiratory stimulants** should be used only if necessary. Their use is controversial, and response is difficult to predict.
      (1) **Doxapram,** 1 to 10 mg/kg intravenously, is most commonly recommended for respiratory depression. Excessive dosage may cause seizures, or the animal may relapse to a comatose state.
      (2) **Naloxone,** 0.04 mg/kg intravenously, intramuscularly, or subcutaneously, may be used to treat dogs with respiratory depression from opiate exposure.

2. **Cardiac arrhythmias** of several types may occur in toxicoses. Table 5-2 lists major expected cardiac arrhythmias, toxicants, and recommended treatments.

3. **Shock** may be a sequela to toxicants that cause fluid loss, vomiting, diarrhea, blood loss, or cardiomyopathy.
   a. Recommended **monitoring procedures** for shock include hemoglobin, packed cell volume, arteriovenous blood gases, arterial oxygen saturation, central venous pressure (CVP), and blood lactate.
   b. Fluid loss may initially be treated with **lactated Ringer's solution** (40 to 50 mg/kg intravenously or subcutaneously) or **plasma expanders**. CVP must be monitored to avoid cardiac overload.
   c. The need for whole blood is evaluated, and up to 10 to 20 mg/kg cross-matched blood is administered as needed.

TABLE 5-2. Cardiac Arrhythmias, Toxicants, and Treatment

Arrhythmia	Toxicant	Treatment
Sinus bradycardia (regular sinus rhythm, slowed heart rate)	Organophosphates Carbamates β-blockers Calcium blockers Phenothiazines Digitalis	Atropine (0.01–0.2 mg/kg IV or IM) Glycopyrrolate (0.005–0.01 mg/kg IV or IM)
AV block	Digitalis	Atropine (0.01–0.2 mg/kg IV or IM) Dopamine (3–5 mg/kg/min) Isoproterenol (0.01 mg/kg/min by IV drip)
Atrial standstill (emergency state)	Hyperkalemia Potassium-sparing diuretics NSAIDs	Saline IV Sodium bicarbonate Insulin with dextrose
Ventricular tachycardia		In dogs: lidocaine hydrochloride (2–3 mg/kg IV slowly); no epinephrine In cats: no lidocaine; may be neurotoxic.

AV = atrioventricular; IM = intramuscular(ly); IV = intravenous(ly); NSAIDs = nonsteroidal anti-inflammatory drugs.

4. **CNS dysfunction,** whether seizures or CNS depression, is a common result of toxicoses. Seizures may be associated with hypoxia, vomiting, hyperthermia, and acidosis, or they may be due to disturbances in brain neurochemistry. Seizure control may be needed before the specific cause is known.
   a. **Diazepam** (0.5 mg/kg intravenously) is the treatment of choice for acute seizures of unknown etiology. Diazepam has a short (2-hour) half-life and must be readministered every 10 to 20 minutes for up to several treatments.
   b. **Phenobarbital** (6 mg/kg intravenously) may be used if diazepam is ineffective or prolonged seizure control is needed.
   c. **Pentobarbital** can be used carefully to induce light anesthesia for seizures refractory to phenobarbital. Excessive or prolonged use may cause respiratory depression.
   d. **Analeptics,** such as **doxapram,** have been used to treat CNS depression, especially when respiratory depression is of concern [see III B 1 c (1)]. **Naloxone** can be used when depression is due to opiates [see III B 1 c (2)].
   e. **Phenothiazine tranquilizers are not recommended for seizure control.** They are relatively ineffective, generally are considered to lower the seizure threshold, and may induce seizures in some patients.

5. **Prolonged vomiting or diarrhea** of toxicologic origin may be due to either CNS causes (e.g., organophosphate toxicosis) or local irritation.
   a. **Gastrointestinal hyperactivity** initially helps to eliminate ingested toxicants but can result in dehydration, acid–base disturbances, and electrolyte losses. If these conditions are serious, they must be controlled.
   b. **Histamine-2 (H_2) receptor blockers** (e.g., cimetidine in dogs, 5 to 10 mg/kg orally) may result in clinical improvement of simple gastritis due to local irritation.

6. **Acid–base disturbances and electrolyte imbalances** should be monitored by evaluation of packed cell volume, blood gas analysis, bicarbonate status, and electrolyte profiles followed by appropriate fluid and electrolyte therapy.
   a. **Metabolic acidosis** is the most common toxicant-associated acid–base disturbance; it can initially be treated with either sodium bicarbonate (0.5 to 2.0 mEq/kg every 4 hours) or sodium lactate 0.17 molar concentration (16 to 32 ml/kg).

b. Patients should be monitored to prevent **alkalosis** from excessive administration of alkalinizing agents.

7. Hypothermia or hyperthermia may occur during toxicosis. Seizures may be accompanied by hyperthermia, whereas the anesthesia used to control seizures can promote hypothermia.

    a. Hyperthermia is treated with cold baths, ice packs, or cooled intravenous fluids. Dehydration as a result of hyperthermia should be controlled with fluid therapy.

    b. Hypothermia may be prevented through the use of blankets, warm water bottles, and heating pads. Warming the surroundings of the animal is considered safer than directly applying heat to the body.

IV. ANTIDOTES

A. **Known toxicosis.** On initial presentation, often the specific toxicosis is unknown, and specific antidotes will not be indicated.

    1. In some cases, use of a specific antidote when the toxicant is unknown can lead to adverse effects from the antidote.

    2. When clinical signs and history clearly indicate the use of a specific antidote, an initial test dose should be administered while continuing to monitor the response of the animal.

B. **Specific antidote therapy** is discussed in Chapter 6.

V. DECONTAMINATION

A. **Diuresis**

    1. Diuresis to promote rapid renal filtration of toxicants may be of limited value.

        a. Toxicants must be at high concentration in an unbound form.

        b. Often a substantial portion of filtered toxicants is resorbed by the renal tubules.

        c. Forced diuresis with excessive fluid administration may result in complications, including cerebral edema, pulmonary edema, and disturbances in acid–base or electrolyte status.

    2. Diuretics may be useful in **edema** due to complications of poisoning.

        a. Mannitol is an osmotic diuretic given intravenously as a 5% to 25% solution at 1 g/kg to maintain urine flow. For cerebral edema, the dosage may be raised to 2 g/kg as a slowly administered intravenous solution.

        b. Furosemide can be used for toxicant-related complications, according to the following schedule:

            (1) Heart failure: 2 to 4 mg/kg intravenously or intramuscularly twice daily

            (2) Ascites from liver failure: 1 to 2 mg/kg orally twice daily

            (3) Pulmonary edema: 2 to 4 mg/kg intravenously, intramuscularly, or orally twice to four times daily

            (4) Acute renal failure: 5 to 20 mg/kg intravenously as needed

B. **Ion trapping** can be effective for acidic or basic compounds by blocking reabsorption of toxicants in the gastrointestinal tract or kidney tubules.

    1. The **Henderson-Hasselbalch equation** provides the basis for ion trapping of ionized drugs (see Chapter 1 III B 1 c). In essence, chemicals filtered in the urine can avoid tubular resorption (trapping) when they are ionized.

    2. Generally, **acidic drugs** are more effectively ionized and excreted in **alkaline urine,** whereas basic drugs are more effectively ionized and more readily excreted in **acidified urine.**

3. Examples of acidic and basic drugs
   a. Acidic agents include aspirin, acetaminophen, barbiturates, and phenoxy herbicides.
   b. Basic drugs include amphetamines and most alkaloids.

4. Agents used to change the pH of urine
   a. Acid urine is promoted by ammonium chloride (for dogs: 100 mg/kg every 12 hours orally; for cats: 20 to 40 mg/kg every 12 hours orally) or ethylenediamine dihydrochloride (1 to 2 tablets daily).
   b. Alkaline urine is promoted by sodium bicarbonate at 1 to 2 mEq/kg every 4 hours intravenously or 50 mg/kg every 8 hours orally.

C. **Peritoneal dialysis** has limited value for the management of some poisonings.

   1. Peritoneal dialysis is most useful in situations of renal failure or anuria.

   2. Peritoneal dialysis methods involve ion-trapping principles.

   3. Dialysis fluids may need frequent change and attention to prevent infection.

D. **Activated charcoal** and other adsorbents can help interrupt the enterohepatic cycling of toxicants.

E. **Stimulation of hepatic microsomal enzymes** is a theoretical means of improving excretion of toxicants.

   1. Stimulation of phase I metabolism can lead to increased conjugation and excretion in the urine.

   2. Application of this approach on a practical basis is relatively limited in veterinary medicine.

VI. MONITORING THE CLINICAL STATUS

A. Metabolized toxicants may become more or less toxic than the toxic compound ingested.

B. Secondary changes or sequelae to the original insult may induce organ damage that must be managed in addition to the initial effects of the toxicant.

VII. SUPPORTIVE MEASURES DURING THERAPY AND CONVALESCENCE

A. Gastrointestinal or organ damage may require special diets or fluids while damaged epithelial cells and organs are regenerating and regaining function.

B. Metabolism and excretion of chemicals or drugs may be impaired during convalescence, so drug therapy should be chosen carefully.

VIII. OWNER EDUCATION can reduce the incidence of toxicosis. Therapy and management should include changing the care, supervision, and environment of the animal to prevent further occurrences of poisoning.

DIRECTIONS: Each of the numbered items or incomplete statements in this section is followed by answers or by completions of the statement. Select the **one** numbered answer or completion that is **best** in each case.

1. How long after ingestion does physical removal of ingested toxicants from the stomach become generally ineffective?

(1) 30 minutes
(2) 1 hour
(3) 3 hours
(4) 8 hours
(5) 24 hours

2. Which agent is recommended for animal owners inducing emesis at home?

(1) Copper sulfate
(2) Liquid dishwashing detergent
(3) Hydrogen peroxide
(4) Table salt
(5) Xylazine

3. Which drug or agent is administered in combination with activated charcoal as treatment for an ingested poison?

(1) Atropine
(2) Cimetidine
(3) Phenobarbital
(4) Sodium lactate
(5) Sorbitol

4. The treatment of choice for toxicant-induced sinus bradycardia is:

(1) atropine.
(2) digitalis.
(3) dopamine.
(4) isoproterenol.
(5) lidocaine.

5. When the toxicant responsible for seizures is unknown, the *initial* treatment of choice for seizure control is:

(1) acepromazine.
(2) diazepam.
(3) pentobarbital.
(4) phenobarbital.
(5) xylazine.

6. Aid in treatment of aspirin toxicosis should:

(1) promote diuresis with intravenous fluids.
(2) acidify the urine.
(3) alkalinize the urine.
(4) both (1) and (2).
(5) both (1) and (3).

7. One disadvantage of diazepam in treating toxicant-induced seizures is:

(1) lowered seizure threshold for toxicants.
(2) prolonged central nervous system (CNS) depression.
(3) short half-life.
(4) gastrointestinal stasis.
(5) cardiac arrhythmias.

8. All of the following antiarrhythmic agents can be used in cats *except:*

(1) atropine.
(2) glycopyrrolate.
(3) isoproterenol.
(4) lidocaine.
(5) saline.

ANSWERS AND EXPLANATIONS

1. The answer is 3 *[II B]*. Rapid removal from the stomach is essential. Gastric emptying begins within 30 minutes and may be nearly completed after 4 hours, depending on the nature of the food ingested and the effects of the toxicant on gastric motility. Ingestion of poisons along with food usually delays absorption, but the stimulation of a full stomach may initiate gastric emptying more rapidly.

2. The answer is 3 *[II B 1 b; Table 5-1]*. Of the agents listed, only hydrogen peroxide is considered safe enough for home use by animal owners. Copper sulfate can induce copper toxicosis and may be damaging to the gastric mucosa. Table salt in excess can induce hypernatremia and osmosis-related cerebral edema. Dishwashing detergents are alkaline and strong irritants, which may further injure a toxicant-damaged stomach. Xylazine is not available to pet owners and should be used only when there is access to yohimbine, which can reverse the occasional depressant effects and cardiac arrhythmias associated with xylazine.

3. The answer is 5 *[II B 3 c (2)]*. Sorbitol acts as an osmotic cathartic by attracting water to the intestinal lumen. Overuse may result in excessive intestinal fluids and diarrhea. The use of sorbitol speeds the passage of gastrointestinal contents and toxicants adsorbed to charcoal, thus removing them from the intestine rapidly and helping to prevent the constipation that may be caused by oral charcoal.

4. The answer is 1 *[Table 5-2]*. Atropine has anticholinergic effects on the heart, generally counteracting the sinus bradycardia caused by toxicants such as organophosphate cholinesterase inhibitors, calcium channel blockers, and digitalis. Use of atropine is recommended to reverse sinus bradycardia and return the heart to a normal rate and rhythm. Glycopyrrolate is also effective for this use and its likelihood of causing central nervous system (CNS) effects is lower than that of atropine.

5. The answer is 2 *[III B 4 a]*. Diazepam is the treatment of choice for most toxicant-induced seizures of small animals. It is safe and has a short half-life so prolonged depression is not likely. In some cases, diazepam may not suppress seizures, and phenobarbital or pentobarbital may be needed. In large animals, diazepam is usually cost-prohibitive, so pentobarbital is often used carefully to effect, with close attention to avoiding central nervous system (CNS) depression and the accompanying possibility of respiratory depression. Chlorpromazine tranquilizers are not recommended for seizure disorders as they are largely ineffective and may potentiate seizures by lowering the seizure threshold in animals.

6. The answer is 5 *[V A 1, B]*. Aspirin is an acidic drug that is largely ionized in a basic environment where the acidic drug loses protons and becomes charged; thus, it is less likely to be reabsorbed by the renal tubules. Diuresis without ionization of the drug is likely to result in glomerular filtration, but the toxicant will be reabsorbed again in the tubules. This clinical application of the Henderson-Hasselbalch equation defines the quantitative behavior of acidic and basic drugs.

7. The answer is 3 *[III B 4 a]*. While the short half-life of diazepam reduces the probability of an adverse effect such as prolonged depression, the drug may need to be administered at intervals of 20 to 30 minutes to maintain seizure control. Thus, patients need consistent supervision so that no unattended seizures recur.

8. The answer is 4 *[Table 5-2]*. The use of lidocaine in the cat is somewhat controversial. Some authorities suggest that lidocaine is neurotoxic in the cat and may cause tremors, seizures, or both; it is not recommended for arrhythmias in cats. In the dog, the dosage is 2 to 4 mg/kg intravenously.

Chapter 6

Antidotes

I. INTRODUCTION

A. **Definition.** Antidotes are agents with a specific action against the activity or effect of a poison.

B. **Principles of antidotal therapy**

1. **Applications.** Antidotes are generally administered after exposure to a toxicant and often in response to clinical toxicosis.

2. **Dosage considerations**
   a. Dosages given may be based on trials in experimental animals or on human experience.
   b. Antidote duration of effectiveness may be different from the duration of action of the poison. This difference must be considered when establishing the dosing schedule.
   c. Some antidotes may be toxic if used excessively or for too long during therapy.
   d. Adverse effects of antidotes may be more likely if administered in the absence of the toxicant; thus, correct diagnosis is important prior to the use of antidotes.

3. **Limitations to antidote effectiveness**
   a. Antidotes may be ineffective or inadequate if general decontamination of the animal is not carried out first.
   b. Some animals may be less tolerant than others to certain antidotes because of species or age.

II. MECHANISM OF ACTION

A. **Chemical antidotes** specifically interact with or neutralize the toxicant. Relatively few antidotes act in this manner.

1. **Complex formation.** Antidotes can complex with (i.e., bind to) the toxicant, making it unavailable to cross cell membranes or to interact with susceptible receptors. To be effective, the complex must be both inactive and stable until excreted.
   a. Dimercaprol and dimercaptosuccinic acid (DMSA) are sulfhydryl compounds that bind metals such as arsenic or lead, making them unavailable to susceptible receptors.
   b. Specific binding agents against toxic divalent cations [e.g., calcium disodium ethylenediaminetetraacetic acid (EDTA), deferoxamine, and D-penicillamine] act by chelation of the metal, forming a more water-soluble complex that is readily excreted in the urine.
   c. Antivenins against snake venoms and antibodies against digitoxin are immunologically generated agents that bind specifically to the venom or toxin.

2. **Metabolic conversion.** Some antidotes enhance metabolic conversion (i.e., detoxification of the toxicant to a less toxic product).
   a. Nitrite interacts with hemoglobin and cyanide to form cyanmethemoglobin, which is less toxic than cyanide and interferes with cyanide access to the cytochrome oxidase system.

    b. Thiosulfate provides sulfur, which interacts with cyanide to form thiocyanate. Thiocyanate is readily excreted in the urine.

B. **Pharmacologic antidotes** produce an effect that neutralizes or antagonizes the effect of the toxicant.

  1. Prevention of toxic metabolite formation. Antidotes in this class are most effective when given shortly after exposure to the toxicant and before significant metabolic activation has occurred.

    a. Mechanism of action. These antidotes prevent biotransformation to a more toxic metabolite from the original toxicant.

    b. Examples include **ethanol** and **4-methylpyrazole (4-MP),** which compete with alcohol dehydrogenase to prevent the formation of toxic acidic intermediates from ethylene glycol (antifreeze).

  2. Enhancement of toxicant excretion. Antidotes in this category facilitate more rapid or complete excretion of the toxicant.

    a. Mechanism of action. The antidote may change the physicochemical nature of the toxicant, allowing better glomerular filtration or reduced tubular resorption.

    b. Examples include **molybdenum** and **sulfate,** which form a water-soluble complex with copper that is readily excreted in urine.

  3. Competition for receptor sites

    a. Mechanism of action. In **competitive antagonism,** the relative amounts or potency of toxin versus antidote determine which effect predominates.

    b. Example. Naloxone blocks the action of opioids by competing for the same opioid receptor sites.

  4. Blockade of receptors responsible for the toxic effect

    a. Mechanism of action. In this scenario, the physiologic effect induced by a toxin is prevented by the antidote, although the toxicant involved is unchanged and may still be active.

    b. Examples include **atropine,** which blocks the physiologic effect of acetylcholine (ACh) at cholinergic synapses and neuromuscular junctions.

  5. Restoration of normal function

    a. Mechanism of action. The antidote promotes return to normal function by repairing a defect or enhancing a function that corrects the effects of the poison.

    b. Examples

      (1) In nitrite poisoning, **methylene blue** interacts with reduced nicotinamide adenine dinucleotide (NADPH) to reduce the ferric iron of methemoglobin back to ferrous ion in hemoglobin, which can again transport oxygen.

      (2) Acetylcysteine supplies the precursor amino acids for glutathione, which serves as a biologic antioxidant against acetaminophen toxicosis.

III. **COMMON ANTIDOTES IN VETERINARY MEDICINE.** Relatively few antidotes are cleared for veterinary use, and, in fact, antidotes are used relatively infrequently in veterinary practice. Table 6-1 summarizes the most common toxicoses for which antidotal therapy is appropriate.

A. **Acetylcysteine** is a reducing agent that counteracts **acetaminophen toxicosis.**

  1. Storage. Stability of acetylcysteine is moderate, and opened vials should be refrigerated and used within 96 hours.

  2. Absorption, metabolism, and excretion. Acetylcysteine is **most effective** if given within 8–16 hours of ingestion of the toxicant.

    a. Maximum plasma concentrations are reached within 2–3 hours after oral dosing, and detectable levels remain for 4–6 hours after dosing.

b. Metabolites include cysteine, cystine, glutathione, and sulfate.

3. Effects from overdosage are unlikely, except for possible anaphylactic reactions, nausea, or vomiting. The oral median lethal dose (LD_{50}) in dogs is greater than 1000 mg/kg.

B. **Ammonium molybdate** and **ammonium tetrathiomolybdate.** The accumulation, followed by the sudden release, of copper from the liver causes an acute hemolytic crisis in sheep. Molybdate treatments, which currently are not approved by the Food and Drug Administration (FDA), **promote excretion of copper in sheep.**

C. **Antivenins** act against **crotalid snake venoms.**

1. Storage. Stability may be reduced if stored at temperatures above 37 °C. Reconstituted product should be used within 48 hours.

2. Adverse effects. Because this product is derived from equine serum, hypersensitivity or anaphylaxis can occur. Animals should be skin-tested for potential reactions before administration, and epinephrine or diphenhydramine should be available to counteract possible anaphylactic reactions.

D. **Ascorbic acid** reverses **methemoglobinemia in cats.**

1. Storage. Ascorbic acid is unstable in air and alkaline conditions.

2. Absorption, metabolism, and excretion. The drug is rapidly absorbed and distributed throughout the body, including in milk of lactating females.

3. Adverse effects
   a. Ascorbic acid acidifies the urine, which may affect disposition of other drugs used concurrently.
   b. Ascorbic acid is reported to interfere with the oral absorption of iron.

E. **Atropine sulfate** counteracts **anticholinesterase poisoning.**

1. Storage. Atropine is mildly unstable to light and it should be stored protected from light and air.

2. Absorption, metabolism, and excretion. Atropine's half-life is short (approximately 3 hours); therefore, dosage may need to be repeated.

3. Effects of overdosage. The drug crosses the blood–brain barrier, and overdose can result in central nervous system (CNS) disturbances (e.g., depression, disorientation), dry mucous membranes, and gastrointestinal hypomotility.

F. **Calcium disodium EDTA** is used in chelation therapy of **lead and zinc toxicoses.**

1. Absorption, metabolism, and excretion. EDTA is rapidly excreted in urine, with up to 95% found in urine within 24 hours after dosing.

2. Adverse effects. EDTA may chelate other essential divalent cations such as calcium, magnesium, and copper, but affinity for these is less than for lead.

G. **Dimercaprol [British antilewisite (BAL)]** is the classic antidote for **arsenic poisoning,** and may also be used in mercury, antimony, and lead toxicosis. Dimercaprol has limited efficacy in animals with clinical signs.

H. **Ethanol (20%)** alleviates the effects of **ethylene glycol** ingestion and toxicosis by preventing its metabolism to acidic intermediates. CNS depression caused by ethylene glycol and its resultant acidosis may initially be increased by the alcohol, which is also a depressant.

1. Absorption, metabolism, and excretion. Ethanol is rapidly metabolized and must be repeatedly administered. It is most effective if given within 4 hours of ethylene glycol ingestion.

2. Adverse effects. Ethanol acts as a diuretic and increases fluid replacement needs.

TABLE 6-1. Antidotal Therapy of Common Veterinary Toxicoses

Toxicosis	Antidote	Dosage	Route	Contraindications
Acetaminophen	Acetylcysteine	Loading dose: 140 mg/kg, 70 mg/kg every 6 hours, for up to seven treatments	Oral	Incompatible with oxidizing agents, amphotericin B, tetracyclines, erythromycin, ampicillin, hydrogen peroxide
Anticholinesterase poisoning	Atropine sulfate	0.2 mg/kg	IV-1/4 SQ-3/4	Sodium bicarbonate injections
Antifreeze (ethylene glycol)	Ethanol (20%)	Dogs: 5.5 ml/kg every 4 hours for five treatments, then every 6 hours for four treatments	IV	. . .
		Cats: 5 ml/kg every 6 hours for five treatments, then every 8 hours for four treatments	IV	
	4-Methylpyrazole	Initial dose: 20 mg/kg in a 5% solution 15 mg/kg at 12 and 24 hours 5 mg/kg at 36 hours	IV	Not recommended for cats Not FDA-approved for animals
Arsenic	Dimercaprol (BAL)	Preclinical exposure: 3 mg/kg every 8 hours Clinical disease: 6 mg/kg every 8 hours for 3–5 days; renal function must be monitored during therapy	IM	Not FDA-approved for animals
	DL-6, 8–Thioctic acid	50 mg/kg every 8 hours at two to three injection sites	IM	Not FDA-approved for animals
Copper toxicosis in dogs (hepatotoxicity)	Ascorbic acid	500–1000 mg daily	Oral	. . .
	D-Penicillamine*	10–15 mg/kg twice daily	Oral	Not FDA-approved for animals
Copper toxicosis in sheep	Ammonium molybdate	200 mg/day for 3 weeks	Oral	Not FDA-approved for animals
	Ammonium tetrathiomolybdate (for acute toxicosis)	1.7–3.4 mg/day; three treatments on alternate days	IV or SQ	Not FDA-approved for animals

Toxicant	Antidote	Dosage	Route	Comments
Coumarin and indanedione anticoagulants	Vitamin K₁ (phytonadione)	2–5 mg/kg/day in divided doses twice daily, then 2–3 mg/kg/day in divided doses three times daily for 1 week If second-generation rodenticides are suspected, administer 1–2 mg/kg/day in divided doses three times daily for up to 6 weeks	Oral or SQ Oral Oral	...
Cyanide	Sodium nitrite	22 mg/kg	IV	...
	Sodium thiosulfate	660 mg/kg	IV	...
Lead	Calcium disodium EDTA†	110 mg/kg/day in three to four divided doses; dilute to 1 g/ml in 5% dextrose‡	IV-initial dose SQ thereafter	Not FDA-approved for food animals
	D-Penicillamine	110 mg/kg for 1–2 weeks; re-evaluate animal 1 week after initial course of therapy	Oral	...
	Ascorbic acid	30 mg/kg 4 times daily	Oral	...
Methemoglobinemia in cats	Methylene blue (1%)	4–15 mg/kg; may be repeated in 6–8 hours	IV	May induce methemoglobinemia or Heinz-body anemia in cats; incompatible with alkaline materials and oxidizing or reducing substances Not FDA-approved for food animals
Nitrate, nitrite, or chlorate toxicosis in large animals				
Organophosphate insecticides	Pralidoxime chloride (2-PAM)	10–15 mg/kg two to three times daily until recovery	IV or SQ	Not FDA-approved for animals
Snake (crotalid) venom	Antivenins	1 vial, administered slowly	IV	...
Zinc	Calcium disodium EDTA	see "Lead"		...

BAL = British antilewisite; EDTA = ethylenediaminetetraacetic acid; FDA = Food and Drug Administration; IM = intramuscularly; IV = intravenously; SQ = subcutaneously.
*Long-term therapy for the chronic familial accumulation of copper that occurs in Bedlington terriers and some other breeds.
†Some evidence supports the use of calcium disodium EDTA with dimercaprol when clinical signs of lead poisoning are present or blood lead levels are high. The combination appears to reduce the toxic effect of high blood levels that may accompany EDTA therapy.
‡Stop therapy and evaluate animal after 2–5 days' therapy to avoid potential nephrotoxicity.

I. **Methylene blue** is a reducing agent that corrects **methemoglobinemia from nitrate, nitrite, or chlorate toxicosis** in large animals.

1. Methylene blue is currently not approved by FDA for use as an antidote.

2. **Absorption, metabolism, and excretion.** Urinary excretion is the main route of elimination, and the drug colors the urine blue or green as the oxidation product (methylene blue sulfone) is formed.

J. **4-MP** is an alternative therapy for **ethylene glycol toxicosis**.

1. **Absorption, metabolism, and excretion.** 4-MP is most effective when given soon after exposure to ethylene glycol, preferably within 3–8 hours postingestion. In cats, it does not effectively inhibit ethylene glycol metabolism unless given concurrently with the ethylene glycol.

2. Use of 4-MP is not approved by the FDA; an investigational new drug application (INDA) must be obtained. Therefore, a commercial dosage form of 4-MP currently is not available.
   a. The antidote can be prepared by adding 5 g of 4-MP to 50 ml of polyethylene glycol and 46 ml of bacteriostatic water to make 100 ml.
   b. The solution is then filter sterilized through a 0.22 μm filter.

K. D-**Penicillamine** is effective against **copper and lead toxicoses**.

1. **Absorption, metabolism, and excretion**
   a. Penicillamine is ß,ß-dimethylcysteine, a monothiol chelating agent with affinity for copper, lead, and mercury.
   b. A major portion of penicillamine is believed to be excreted in the urine.

2. **Adverse effects.** Penicillamine is reported to cause a variety of adverse reactions in humans, including allergic reactions, moderate proteinuria, leukopenia, and vomiting. Incidence of these problems in dogs is not reported.

L. **Phytonadione (vitamin K$_1$)** reverses the effects of **coumarin anticoagulants**.

1. **Storage.** Phytonadione, the synthetic form of vitamin K$_1$, is a fat-soluble naphthoquinone that is photosensitive and therefore should be protected from light.

2. **Absorption, metabolism, and excretion.** Absorption is enhanced by the presence of bile salts or administration with a high-fat meal.

3. **Adverse effects.** Intravenous administration of phytonadione may cause anaphylactic reactions, and therefore, is not recommended. In addition, animals may bleed from the injection site.

M. **Pralidoxime chloride (2-PAM)** is a reversal agent against **organophosphate insecticides**.

1. **Storage.** Reconstituted pralidoxime is considered stable up to 2 weeks if refrigerated and protected from light.

2. **Absorption, metabolism, and excretion.** Treatment is **most effective** if given within 24 hours after exposure to organophosphates, because of "aging" (i.e., irreversible binding of the organophosphate to receptor sites). In some cases of prolonged toxicosis resulting from delayed dermal absorption, 2-PAM may be helpful for more than 24 hours after exposure.

N. **Sodium nitrite** and **sodium thiosulfate** are used in the treatment of **cyanide poisoning**. Evidence shows that large doses of thiosulfate without the use of nitrites are also effective. Improvement occurs within minutes after treatment, and repeated treatment may not be necessary.

BIBLIOGRAPHY

Bailey E, Garland T: Toxicologic emergencies. In *Veterinary Emergency and Critical Care Yearbook.* St. Louis, Mosby, 1992, pp 427–452.

Goldstein A, Aronow L, Kalman S: *Principles of Drug Action: The Basis of Pharmacology,* 2nd ed. New York, John Wiley, 1974, pp 394–428.

McEvoy G (ed): *AHFS Drug Information.* American Society of Hospital Pharmacists, 1993.

Morgan R: *American Animal Hospital Association Formulary.* American Animal Hospital Association, Denver, Colorado, 1991, pp 1–67.

Osweiler G, Carson T, Buck W, Van Gelder G: *Clinical and Diagnostic Toxicology,* 3rd ed. Dubuque, IA, Kendall Hunt, 1985, pp 52–66.

DIRECTIONS: Each of the numbered items or incomplete statements in this section is followed by answers or by completions of the statement. Select the **one** numbered answer or completion that is **best** in each case.

1. Which antidote acts by a mechanism that does not involve forming a complex with the toxicant to inactivate it?

(1) Antivenin
(2) Atropine
(3) Calcium disodium ethylenediaminetetra-acetic acid (EDTA)
(4) Dimercaprol
(5) D-Penicillamine

2. Which pair of antidotes has identical mechanisms of action against the same toxicant?

(1) Ammonium molybdate and atropine
(2) Penicillamine and ascorbic acid
(3) Ethanol and 4-methylpyrazole (4-MP)
(4) Methylene blue and acetylcysteine
(5) Thiosulfate and cyanide

3. Which agent is currently considered ineffective as an antidote in cats?

(1) 4-Methylpyrazole (4-MP)
(2) Ascorbic acid
(3) Calcium disodium ethylenediaminetetra-acetic acid (EDTA)
(4) Ethanol
(5) Vitamin K_1

4. Which agent is most effective for long-term oral therapy to reduce hepatic copper stores in dogs?

(1) Calcium disodium ethylenediaminetetra-acetic acid (EDTA)
(2) D-Penicillamine
(3) Deferoxamine
(4) Dimercaprol
(5) Ammonium molybdate

5. Which of the following agents is *not* recommended for intravenous use because of the high potential for anaphylaxis?

(1) Antivenin
(2) Dimercaprol
(3) Calcium disodium ethylenediaminetetra-acetic acid (EDTA)
(4) Phytonadione
(5) Sodium nitrite and sodium thiosulfate

1. The answer is 2 *[II A 1 b, B 2, 4]*. Atropine acts by blocking a receptor site that is affected by acetylcholine (ACh); however, atropine does not interact directly with the organophosphate insecticide or other agents that inhibit cholinesterase and allow the accumulation of ACh. All other choices are agents that bind directly by chelation [calcium disodium ethylenediaminetetraacetic acid (EDTA)] or sulfhydryl–metal interaction (dimercaprol, penicillamine), or by an antigen–antibody reaction (antivenin).

2. The answer is 3 *[II B 1 b]*. Ethanol and 4-methylpyrazole (4-MP) both prevent the metabolism of ethylene glycol to acidic intermediates, and, ultimately, to calcium oxalate, thus preventing generation of the toxic metabolites. Ammonium molybdate promotes copper excretion in sheep, whereas atropine counteracts the effects of anticholinesterase poisoning. Ascorbic acid reverses methemoglobinemia in cats, while penicillamine is used to treat copper and lead poisoning. Although both acetylcysteine and methylene blue are reducing agents, acetylcysteine is used in acetaminophen toxicosis and methylene blue is used to treat methemoglobinemia from nitrate, nitrite, or chlorate toxicosis in large animals. Thiosulfate is used in the treatment of cyanide poisoning; cyanide is a toxicant, not an antidote.

3. The answer is 1 *[III J 1]*. 4-Methylpyrazole (4-MP) is an effective alternative therapy for ethylene glycol toxicosis in dogs, but not in cats. Even when treated with 4-MP shortly after ingestion of ethylene glycol, cats continue to metabolize the ethylene glycol to the toxic acid intermediates. Ascorbic acid is used to treat methemoglobinemia in cats and hepatotoxicity from copper toxicosis in dogs. Calcium disodium ethylenediaminetetraacetic acid (EDTA), ethanol, and vitamin K_1 are all effective for cats.

4. The answer is 2 *[Table 6-1]*. D-Penicillamine is an oral product with high affinity for copper in dogs. Calcium disodium ethylenediaminetetraacetic acid (EDTA) is not absorbed orally and is a less effective chelator of copper than is penicillamine. Ammonium molybdate is effective for copper removal in sheep, but evidence for its efficacy in dogs is not available. Deferoxamine has affinity for iron, and dimercaprol has affinity for arsenic and mercury.

5. The answer is 4 *[III L 3; Table 6-1]*. Although phytonadione is effective intravenously against coumarin anticoagulants, a high incidence of anaphylactic reactions occurs when it is used intravenously. Recent evidence shows that in animals, dosing with phytonadione in conjunction with a high-fat meal stimulates rapid absorption and activation of phytonadione and is nearly equally effective as intravenous administration without the risk of anaphylaxis. Antivenin, calcium disodium ethylenediaminetetraacetic acid (EDTA), sodium nitrite, and sodium thiosulfate are all administered intravenously. Dimercaprol is in an oil carrier and is administered by intramuscular injection.

Part II

CLINICAL TOXICOLOGY
OF BODY SYSTEMS AND ORGANS

Chapter 7

Neurotoxicology

I. INTRODUCTION

A. Nervous system

1. **Divisions.** The nervous system can be broadly divided into the **central nervous system (CNS)** and the **peripheral nervous system (PNS)**.

   a. The **CNS** is comprised of the **brain, brain stem,** and **spinal cord,** which consist primarily of **neurons** and their supporting cells (**astrocytes** and **glial cells**).

   b. The **PNS** is comprised of the nerves and ganglia outside of the brain and spinal cord.

2. **Function.** The nervous system is involved in the **transfer of information**. Transfer of electrical stimulation from the axon of one neuron to the dendrite of the next is mediated by a variety of chemicals collectively known as **neurotransmitters**.

   a. Information that controls the actions and functions of the animal is transmitted from **cerebral neurons** via **axons,** which transfer electrical signals that activate neurons in the ventral root of the spinal cord.

   b. **Spinal neurons** transfer electrical signals to effector organs or neuromuscular junctions.

3. **Functional design**

   a. **Neurons** are the controlling cells of the nervous system (Figure 7-1).

   (1) The **cell body** is the site for **protein synthesis**.

   (2) The **plasma membrane, cell body,** and **dendrites** are **transducers of synaptic input**.

   (3) The **axons** and **axoplasm** are **conduits** for synthesized material.

   (4) The **axolemma** and **nodes of Ranvier** generate and propagate **action potentials**.

   (5) The **synaptic (nerve) terminals** and **postsynaptic receptors** handle **chemical communication** from nerve to nerve and nerve to muscle.

   b. **The blood–brain barrier.** The blood–brain barrier prevents many foreign chemicals from gaining access to the CNS.

   (1) **Tight junctions** between endothelial cells form physical barriers that limit the passage of toxicants.

   (a) Molecules must pass directly through the endothelial cell membrane to gain access to the nervous system.

   (b) Compounds of small molecular size that are non-ionized, nonpolar, and lipophilic are most likely to enter the nervous system. Certain molecules, such as glucose and amino acids, are actively transported into the CNS by specific and bidirectional carrier systems.

   (2) The blood–brain barrier in **neonatal animals** is not fully developed, so neonates are more at risk than mature animals to some toxicants.

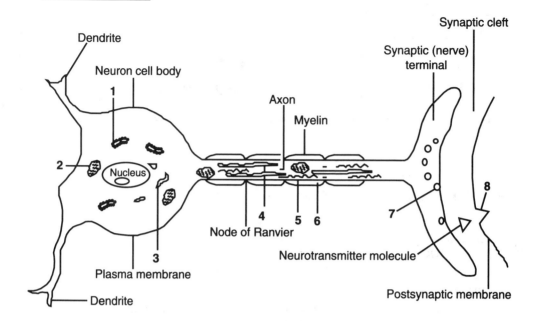

FIGURE 7-1. Major structural and functional components of neuronal and synaptic activity. (*1*) Rough endoplasmic reticulum (rER) is the site of protein synthesis and carbohydrate metabolism. (*2*) Mitochondria provide energy metabolism for cell maintenance and neurotransmitter synthesis. (*3*) Smooth endoplasmic reticulum (sER) transfers synthesized materials to the axolemma and nerve terminals. (*4*) Neurofilaments, microfilaments, and microtubules provide anterograde and retrograde transport of nutrients and messenger materials in the neuron. (*5*) Axonal membrane (i.e., the axolemma) propagates the action potential, which is generated in the axon. (*6*) Myelin, which is produced by Schwann cells, maintains the axon and enhances electrical conduction at the axolemma. (*7*) Synaptic vesicles are involved in the synthesis, storage, release, and reuptake of neurotransmitters. Neurotransmitter molecules in the synaptic cleft transfer specific information to postsynaptic receptors. (*8*) Postsynaptic receptors receive chemical information (i.e., the neurotransmitter) and begin the conformational and electrical changes necessary to initiate a postsynaptic action potential.

B. **Neurotoxins** act by altering the ability of the CNS to generate or transfer information to the PNS.

   1. Interference with the **metabolic processes** of the neuron affects the cell's ability to provide nutrients for the synthesis of neurotransmitters and cellular components.

   2. Changes in **axonal membranes** or **membrane ion channels** interfere with generation or transmission of the axon potential, which is necessary to stimulate neurotransmitter release.

   3. Alterations in the **release, inactivation,** or **uptake of neurotransmitters at the synaptic cleft** can impair transfer of information to postsynaptic neurons.

II. **EFFECTS OF TOXICANTS ON THE FUNCTIONS OF THE NERVOUS SYSTEM**
(Table 7-1)

A. **Functions of the neuron cell body.** Neurons do not regenerate, so irreversible damage to the cell body from anoxia or toxicosis produces **permanent loss of neuronal function**.

   1. **Metabolism.** The metabolic requirements of neurons depend heavily on the oxidation of glucose. **Anoxia or ischemia** quickly and severely inhibits neuronal function, so toxicants (e.g., **cyanide, carbon monoxide**) that cause anoxia or ischemia are indirect sources of neurologic damage.

TABLE 7-1. Toxicants Affecting Nervous System Function

Function	Toxicant
Metabolism and protein synthesis	Fluoroacetate (rare), cyanide, ammonia, nitrofurans, bromethalin, mercury
Generation and transmission of action potentials	DDT, pyrethrins, tetrodotoxin
Axonal transport	Tri-ortho-cresyl phosphate, carbon disulfide, colchicine, lead, some organophosphates
Myelin formation	Phenylarsonic feed additives, triethylin (a fungicide), hexachlorophene, arsanilic acid, *Coyotillo* plants, diphtheria toxin, lead (experimental)
Synaptic transmission	
Synaptic vesicle formation	4-Aminopyridine, botulinus toxin, black widow spider toxin, cocaine
Neurotransmitter formation	
Inhibitory neurotransmitters	Metaldehyde, lead, ivermectin, ryegrass, strychnine
Excitatory neurotransmitters	4-Aminopyridine, botulinus toxin, atropine, curare
Neurotransmitter activation	Organophosphate insecticides
Neurotransmitter access to receptor	Curare, atropine
Neurotransmitter imitators	Muscarine, nicotine

    a. Effects of anoxia on neurons. Glucose is catabolized by glycolysis and the **tricarboxylic acid (TCA) cycle. Glycogen content of the brain** is only enough to sustain metabolism for a short time. Effects of anoxia include:

      (1) Decreased adenosine triphosphate (ATP) levels and reduced ATP synthesis

      (2) Increased glycolysis and decreased glycogen

      (3) Loss of the energy-dependent sodium pump

      (4) Neuronal swelling due to imbibition of water

      (5) Increased cellular lactate and acidosis

      (6) Swelling and loss of organelles

    b. Relative sensitivity

      (1) Gray matter has a **higher oxygen consumption than white matter,** possibly because of the numerous synapses that require metabolic energy.

      (2) The cells of the CNS, ordered according to sensitivity to anoxia, are: neuron, oligodendrocyte, astrocyte, microglia, and capillary endothelium.

  2. Protein synthesis is the primary synthetic function of neurons. **Toxic agents that interrupt essential protein synthesis** (e.g., **mercury**) often cause a **slowly developing neurotoxicosis** as essential proteins are catabolized without being replaced.

    a. Nearly all **organelles and membranes** originate from the neuron cell body, and **axons and nerve terminals** depend on the cell body for a continual supply of these components.

    b. Protein synthesis begins in the **rough endoplasmic reticulum (rER)** but shifts to the **smooth endoplasmic reticulum (sER)** to facilitate **axoplasmic transport** (see II C). Proteins also may be formed on free ribosomes.

B. **Generation of action potentials and nerve impulses**

  1. The **action potential,** which is an electrical vehicle for communication between cells, is a **regenerative electrical impulse** conducted rapidly over the length of the axonal membrane.

a. The **sudden, explosive event** has a distinct **threshold** and is initiated by rapid changes in the intracellular and extracellular concentrations of sodium and potassium. Chloride is involved in maintaining the resting membrane potential.

   (1) Sodium. Changes in sodium channels initiate a **rapid influx** of sodium into the axon, initiating the action potential and producing the **upstroke**.

   (2) Potassium. The somewhat slower flow of potassium out of the cell balances the sodium flow, and represents the action potential.

b. Each action potential is followed by a **refractory period** when the membrane is insensitive to stimulation.

c. Calcium influences the action potential by stabilizing the membrane and maintaining a margin between the resting potential and the threshold potential. In addition, calcium ions reduce the ionic current produced by depolarization (i.e., the influx of sodium).

2. Toxicants that affect sodium or potassium flux (e.g., DDT, pyrethrins) often cause **sudden and dramatic clinical signs** characterized by changes in nerve electrical activity.

C. **Axonal transport** is a specialized form of **cytoplasmic streaming** that occurs in the axon and functions to deliver proteins and other materials to and from the neuron cell body.

1. Classification. Axonal transport is classified based on **rate** and **direction of movement**.

   a. Fast anterograde transport carries proteins that are encapsulated in vesicles from synthetic sites in the cell body at the rate of 400 mm/day.

      (1) Specific proteins such as **acetylcholinesterase** and **dopamine ß-hydroxylase** are conveyed in this manner.

      (2) Interference with fast anterograde transport depresses synaptic transmission.

   b. Intermediate anterograde transport moves materials distally at a rate of approximately 50 mm/day and is associated with **replacement of organelles within the axon**.

   c. Slow anterograde transport occurs at a rate of 1 mm/day and is associated with structural components known as **microtubules** and **neurofilaments**. Constriction of the axon results in accumulation of these components and swelling of the axon anterior to the constriction.

   d. Retrograde transport can carry both endogenous and exogenous substances from distal sites at a rate of approximately 100 mm/day.

      (1) Transport is associated with **vesicles composed of sER**.

      (2) Retrograde transport may serve as a signal system from remote parts of the neuron, and to recycle endogenous materials.

2. Effects of toxicants. Toxicants that interfere with axonal transport cause toxic **axonopathies**, sometimes called **"dying back" neuropathy**.

   a. Mechanism. Distal parts of larger, longer axons in the CNS and PNS are affected first. "Dying back" neuropathy may include **swelling, accumulation of tubulovesicular material,** or both, proximal to the degenerating axon (Figure 7-2).

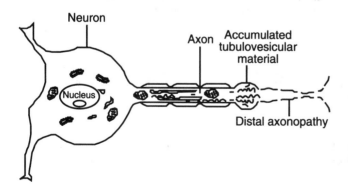

FIGURE 7-2. Axonopathy of the peripheral nerves results in "dying back" of the distal nerve, with accumulation of tubulovesicular material proximal to the damaged axon.

b. Clinical effects, which are generally slow to develop and may be irreversible, include a **slowly ascending symmetrical paresis, paralysis,** and **loss of sensation,** first in the rear limbs and eventually in the forelimbs; therefore, the animal becomes quadriplegic. If recovery occurs, there may be **residual spasticity** and **ataxia.**

D. **Myelin formation**

1. **Formation and composition.** Myelin is formed by **oligodendrocytes** in the CNS and **Schwann cells** in the PNS. It is rich in **specialized proteins and lipids.**

2. **Function.** Myelin serves as an **electrical insulator;** therefore, myelinated nerves **conduct nerve impulses faster** than nonmyelinated nerves.

3. **Effects of toxicants. Demyelination** slows nerve conduction velocity. **Segmental demyelination** is severe myelin loss at intervals along the axon.
   a. Mechanism. Demyelination can result from separation of myelin lamellae, known as intramyelinic edema, or from failure of the Schwann cells or oligodendrocytes to synthesize or maintain myelin.
   b. Recovery. Remyelinization of nerves brings marked improvement in conduction and is more likely in the PNS than in the CNS.

E. **Synaptic transmission** (Figure 7-3)

1. Synaptic transmission depends on **neurotransmitters,** chemicals that are released at the synapse (junction) between two nerve cells as a result of the action potential, which has traveled down the axon.
   a. Mechanism. The neurotransmitter passes across the **synaptic cleft** and interacts with specific chemoreceptors, which alter membrane permeability and initiate an action potential in the **postsynaptic neuron.**
      (1) Initiation. Neurotransmitters are released in discrete amounts from individual vesicles in the nerve terminals. Neurotransmitter release depends on the presence of ionized calcium.
      (2) Termination. Neurotransmitter action may be terminated via two mechanisms:
         (a) Recycling from the synaptic cleft, with uptake of the neurotransmitter by the presynaptic terminal and storage in vesicles
         (b) Degradation of the neurotransmitter (e.g., enzymatic hydrolysis of acetylcholine)
   b. Well-known neurotransmitters include norepinephrine, dopamine, 5-hydroxytryptamine (5-HT, serotonin), acetylcholine, γ-aminobutyric acid (GABA), glycine, histamine, ʟ-aspartic acid, ʟ-glutamic acid, endorphins and enkephalins, and substance P. Some neurotransmitters are classified as **excitatory** or **inhibitory** to postsynaptic

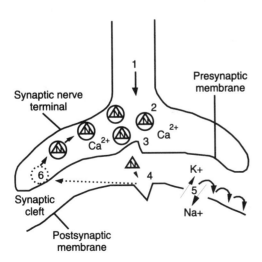

FIGURE 7-3. Action of neurotransmitters in synaptic transmission. (*1*) Neurotransmitters are synthesized in the neuron or axon and (*2*) carried to the nerve terminal in vesicles. (*3*) The vesicles move to the presynaptic membrane and, influenced by calcium (Ca^{2+}), are released into the synaptic cleft. (*4*) Neurotransmitters then interact with receptors to induce conformational and electrical changes that (*5*) initiate the action potential in the postsynaptic membrane. (*6*) Neurotransmitters are eventually inactivated and may be lost or resynthesized and reused via endocytosis in vesicles at the presynaptic nerve terminal membrane. K^+ = potassium; Na^+ = sodium; N = neurotransmitter.

TABLE 7-2. Seizure-Inducing Toxicants

Toxicant	Mechanism of Action	Seizure Characteristics/General Comments
Ammonia/urea	Ammonia or other nitrogenous products in blood may stimulate CNS; inhibits TCA cycle causing cerebral energy deficit	Seizures often accompanied by excitement, belligerence, tremors; urination and bloat occur in cattle; most commonly affects ruminants
Amphetamines	Promote catecholamine release from CNS and adrenals	Seizures accompanied by stimulation of respiratory center, cerebral cortex, reticular activating system; excitement, hyperreflexia, and tremors predominate
4-Aminopyridine	Increases acetylcholine release and inhibits repolarization by potassium current	Seizures accompanied by hyperexcitability, tremors, tachycardia, arrhythmia; used as an avicide
Bromethalin	Uncouples oxidative phosphorylation in the CNS, leading to loss of energy metabolism and decreasing the activity of the sodium pump, causing cerebral edema	Dose-dependent; low dosages cause depression, tremors, posterior weakness, ataxia; high dosages may cause seizures, tremors, occasional paralysis
Caffeine	Inhibits adenosine receptors and phosphodiesterase, increasing cAMP production; enhances catecholamine release and effects	Excitement and hyperreflexia predominate; accompanied by tachycardia, cardiac arrhythmia, hyperthermia
Cocaine	Inhibits reuptake of catecholamines at nerve terminal, enhancing sympathetic stimulation	CNS signs range from excitement to depression; often accompanied by vomiting, salivation, tachycardia
Crimidine	Vitamin B_6 antagonist primarily affecting CNS; occasionally used as a rodenticide	Acute, convulsive seizures
Cyanide	Inhibits cytochrome oxidase in electron transport system, leading to cerebral energy deficit	Generalized seizures and hyperpnea followed initially by weakness
Ergot	Lysergic acid diethylamide (LSD-type alkaloids)	Excitement and hallucinations accompanied by tremors
Fluoroacetate	Inhibits aconitate hydratase in TCA cycle, causing cerebral energy deficit and accumulation of citrate and lactate	Clonic seizures accompanied by wild running, barking, urination, defecation; very rare
Hexachlorophene	Uncouples oxidative phosphorylation, leading to cerebral edema	Seizures accompanied by excitement, tremors, hypermetria; response to lower dosages or chronic exposure include blindness, posterior ataxia
Lead	Not well-characterized; inhibits several enzymes; causes cerebral edema and neuronal degeneration; inhibits the inhibitory neurotransmitter GABA	CNS signs highly variable; they include tremors, excitability, hysteria (in dogs) accompanied by anorexia, gastrointestinal stasis, mild anemia with regenerative response

Agent	Mechanism	Clinical signs
Metaldehyde	Metabolized to acetaldehyde; toxicosis is correlated with decreases in 5-hydroxytryptamine (5-HT, serotonin) and GABA in the brain	Continuous seizures; include prominent muscle tremors and incoordination, salivation, tachycardia; not induced by stimuli
4-Methyl imidazole (4-MI)	Directly toxic to CNS; mechanism unclear	Excitement, tremors, running (cattle)
Nitrofurazone	Inhibits oxidative phosphorylation and energy metabolism in the brain; calves highly susceptible	Acute seizures, facial tremors, hyperexcitability, paddling
Organochlorine insecticides	Diphenyl aliphatics (e.g., DDT, methoxychlor) inhibits both the "turning off" of the inward sodium current and the "turning on" of the outward potassium current, decreasing the action potential threshold and stimulating nervous activity	Hypersensitivity; moderate excitement
	Cyclodiene insecticides (e.g., aldrin, chlordane endrin, heptachlor, toxaphene) inhibit receptor binding of the inhibitor for GABA, promoting excitatory transmission in the CNS	Grand mal seizures, accompanied by paddling, chewing, opisthotonos, refractory interictal phase, hyperthermia
Pyrethrins	Prolong sodium influx and reduce potassium efflux, enhancing the action potential and promoting repetitive discharge	Hyperexcitability and tremors dominate; actual seizures are less common
Sodium ion toxicosis	Interferes with aerobic glycolysis, reducing the activity of the sodium pump and resulting in sodium-related accumulation of water, cerebral edema, and seizures	Stereotypical of cranial to caudal clonic seizures; blindness and cerebral malacia occur as sequelae to acute seizures; often associated with water deprivation
Strychnine	Inhibits the action of the inhibitory amino acid glycine in the CNS, preventing the action of inhibitory interneurons in the spinal cord	Acute hyperesthesia, hyperreflexia, tetanic seizures; severe extensor rigidity
Water hemlock (Cicuta, cicutoxin)	Mechanism is not characterized	Violent acute tetanic seizures, muscle twitching, extensor rigidity
Zinc phosphide	Phosphine (PH₃) is released in stomach and presumably absorbed; mechanisms related to CNS effects are unclear	Clonic spasm of the head and neck, paddling, generalized tremors; animals are not hyperesthetic; vomiting, acidosis, liver damage often occur

cAMP = cyclic adenosine monophosphate; CNS = central nervous system; GABA = γ-aminobutyric acid; LSD = lysergic acid diethylamide; TCA = tricarboxylic acid cycle.

TABLE 7-3. Toxicants Inducing Depression or Coma

Toxicant	Mechanism of Action	Characteristic Response/General Comments
Alcohols*	Mechanism not clarified and likely to be complex; alcohols may interact with the phospholipid bilayer of membranes, increasing their fluidity	. . .
Alpha chloralose*	Selectively depresses neurons of the ascending reticular formation, suppressing normal arousal response; used as a rodenticide	Small doses increase motor activity; toxic doses induce profound depression and general anesthesia
Aspirin*	. . .	Severe acidosis in advanced poisoning leads to depression and coma; occasional seizures and tremors from cerebral edema
Avocado (Persea)*	Unknown	Depression or mild tremors associated with depression and other systemic signs
Barbiturates	γ-Aminobutyric acid (GABA)-like action results in inhibition of neurotransmission	CNS depression, general anesthesia, slowed respiratory rate, coma
Boric acid	Unclear	Seizures, tremors, depression
Bracken fern*	Thiaminase principle induces thiamine deficiency in Equidae	Peripheral neuropathy with progressive posterior weakness, incoordination, ataxia
Bromethalin	Uncouples oxidative phosphorylation in the CNS, leading to loss of energy metabolism and decreasing the activity of the sodium pump and causing cerebral edema	Dose-dependent; low dosages cause depression, tremors, posterior weakness, ataxia; high dosages may cause seizures, tremors, occasional paralysis
Carbon disulfide	Forms dithiocarbamates with pyridoxine and tryptophan, resulting in interference with pyridine-dependent enzymes and destruction of biogenic amines	Ranges from depression and somnolence to tremors and depression
Carbon monoxide*	Forms carboxyhemoglobin, leading to severe anoxia, which causes anoxic degeneration and necrosis of neurons	. . .
Citrus oils (e.g., d-Limonene)*	Unknown; possibly related to inability of cats to metabolize ingredients via glucuronide conjugation	Severe CNS depression in cats
Fumonisin*	Inhibits the enzymatic conversion of sphinganine to sphingosine; this mechanism is not proven in horses	In horses, leukoencephalomacia (fumonisin toxicosis) produces CNS signs of severe depression, paralysis of the tongue and facial muscles, blindness, prostration, and death

Substance	Mechanism	Clinical Signs
Hydrogen sulfide*	Inhibits cytochrome *c* oxidase and electron transport; rapidly affects respiratory center	Respiratory paralysis, acute CNS depression, loss of consciousness
Ivermectin*	Stimulates presynaptic release and postsynaptic binding of GABA, enhancing the inhibitory effects of GABA in the CNS; primarily affects collie breeds because the drug crosses the blood–brain barrier in these breeds	Depression, ataxia, blindness, coma; signs in non-collie breeds occur only at excessive dosages
Lead*	Not well-characterized; inhibits several enzymes; causes cerebral edema and neuronal degeneration; inhibits the inhibitory neurotransmitter GABA	May be dose dependent; depression, coma, and blindness occur intermittently with excitement or seizures; see also Table 7-2
Lysergic acid diethylamide (LSD)	. . .	Excitement and hallucinations accompanied by tremors; see also Table 7-8
Mercury (alkyl form)*	Interrupts sulfhydryl enzymes of protein synthesis in the cerebral cortex, and possibly, the cerebellum; causes fibrinoid degeneration of medial layer of cerebral arteries	Severe depression, coma, tremors, hypermetria, abnormal postures, blindness
Methionine	. . .	Hepatic encephalopathy secondary to liver damage; in small animals, primary signs are depression, disorientation, mild tremors
Opiates (e.g., morphine, codeine)*	Interact directly with a variety of receptors in the CNS	Primary responses to overdose include CNS depression, coma, respiratory depression
Phenothiazine tranquilizers	. . .	Clinical depression, lethargy; may lower seizure threshold and potentiate seizures
Snake venoms*	. . .	Cobra and coral snake venoms induce rapid depression, incoordination, tremors, paresis
Vacor	Antagonizes nicotinamide, reducing nicotinamide-adenine dinucleotide (NAD) synthesis	Range from tremors, ataxia, and peripheral neuropathy to paresis and blindness; formerly used as a rodenticide
Yellow star thistle (*Centaurea*)	Unknown toxin causes nigropallidal encephalomalacia, with possible release of CNS from inhibitory control of brain nuclei	Mild tremors of face and lips; paralysis of tongue in horses

*These substances induce depression or coma via CNS mechanisms.
CNS = central nervous system; GABA = γ-aminobutyric acid.

neurons. The response depends on the type of ionic channels that open on the post-synaptic membrane.

   (1) Excitatory neurotransmitters include **norepinephrine, dopamine, acetylcholine, L-glutamic acid,** and **L-aspartic acid.**

   (2) Inhibitory neurotransmitters include **γ-aminobutyric acid** and **glycine;** these neurotransmitters are affected by many common toxicants.

   2. **Effects of toxicants.** Synaptic transmission becomes abnormal through an increase or decrease in:
   a. Biosynthesis or release of the neurotransmitter
   b. Metabolic degradation of the neurotransmitter
   c. Uptake or reutilization of the neurotransmitter by the presynaptic terminal

III. CLINICAL MANIFESTATION OF NEUROTOXICOSIS

A. **Seizures** (Table 7-2) result from **excessive uncontrolled electrical activity** originating generally in the gray matter anterior to the midbrain.

   1. **General characteristics of seizures**
   a. Seizures can extend **throughout the nervous system,** affecting either part or all of the body.
   b. Seizures occur in **four phases.**
      (1) The **prodromal stage** includes subtle behavioral changes.
      (2) The **aura,** or beginning of the seizure, may be localized.
      (3) The seizure, or **ictus,** recognized by most animal owners usually involves symmetrical and dramatic motor activity.
      (4) The **postictal phase** is a return to the normal state.

   2. **Toxicologic seizures**
   a. **Identification of toxicant.** Many toxicants cause seizure activity, so **accurate association of seizures with potential toxicoses** requires attention to the specific characteristics of the seizures.
   b. **General characteristics.** Toxicologic seizures are often **acute, generalized, symmetrical,** and **severe** (e.g., **status epilepticus**); animals may progress quickly into the ictal phase without a recognized aura.
      (1) Animals may be **unconscious,** but their **eyes are open.**
      (2) Extensor rigidity and **opisthotonos** are prominent.
      (3) Chewing movements are common.
      (4) Running or paddling motions of the limbs may be continuous or intermittent.
      (5) Autonomic signs (e.g., **salivation, vomiting, diarrhea**) and **hyperthermia** as high as 106°F–108°F may accompany toxicologic seizures.
      (6) Animals may be **depressed** and appear **exhausted** in the postictal phase.

B. **Depression or coma** (Table 7-3) result from toxicants (e.g., **narcotics, depressants**) that interfere with the **synthetic or neurotransmitter functions** of the brain and its neurons. Toxicants that induce severe **acidosis** may also cause depression or coma.

C. **Tremors, tetany, and myoclonia** (Table 7-4) can originate at many sites in the CNS, PNS, or muscles.

   1. **Identification.** Because animal owners often classify any violent motor activity as a "seizure" or "convulsion," tremors or tetany must be **differentiated from true seizures** for accurate clinical diagnosis. **Anamnesis** and **clinical examination** must be careful, thorough, and critical or clinical diagnosis can be erroneous.

   2. **Tremors and tetany** that result from toxicosis are usually **symmetrical** and **generalized,** and **may be secondary to toxicants that cause metabolic or electrolyte dysfunctions:**
   a. **Hypocalcemia** from oxalate toxicosis

TABLE 7-4. Tremor-Inducing Toxicants*

Toxicant	Mechanism of Action	Characteristic Response
Bermuda grass (*Cynodon dactylon*)	Toxic principle is not described	No distinguishing lesions; signs include tremors and stiff-legged gait, which exercise may worsen
Dallis grass (*Claviceps paspali*)	Sclerotia (i.e., fungal growth in the grass ovary) produces alkaloids similar to lysergic acid	Continuous tremors that lessen at rest and are exacerbated by exercise or excitement; staggers
Locoweed (*Astragalus*)	Toxic principle is swainsonine; inhibits α-mannosidase, resulting in mannose-containing vacuoles in CNS neurons, especially cerebellar neurons	Tremors, ataxia, proprioceptive deficits
Organophosphate and carbamate insecticides	Acute nicotinic effects of cholinesterase inhibition allow acetylcholine excess at neurons	Muscle fasciculations and tremors leading to paralysis at high dosages
Rayless goldenrod (*Haplopappus*)	Unknown	Similar to white snakeroot, below
Ryegrass (*Lolium perenne*)	An endophytic fungus in the grass produces the toxin lolitrem B, which is associated with changes in GABA neurotransmitter	Tremors and ataxia ("staggers"), weakness in cattle, sheep, and horses
Tremorgenic mycotoxins	Penitrem A, produced by several *Penicillium* species, facilitates impulse transmission at motor endplates by increasing the resting potential, endplate potential, and the length of depolarization phase; inhibitory neurotransmitters (e.g., GABA, glycine) may be inhibited	Muscle tremors, ataxia, incoordination, weakness; may progress to death
White snakeroot (*Eupatorium*)	Unknown	Tremetone (formerly called tremetol) and its dihydro- and hydroxy-analogs cause ataxia, weakness, and continuous tremors, which may worsen when the animal is exercised or excited; cattle exhibit primarily the neurologic syndrome, but horses develop cardiac damage and arrhythmias as well

*Seizures, depression, or both are minimal in these toxicoses.
CNS = central nervous system; GABA = γ-aminobutyric acid.

TABLE 7-5. Toxicants Affecting the Autonomic Nervous System

Toxicant	Mechanism of Action	Characteristic Response/General Comments
Parasympatholytics		
Amanita muscaria, A. pantherina	Contain ibotenic acid and muscimol, which compete with the inhibitory neurotransmitter GABA	Seizures, opisthotonos, anticholinergic signs similar to those seen with atropine (see below)
Atropine, atropine-like plants (e.g., *Datura, Hyoscyamus, Jessamine, Physalis*)	Competitive antagonism of acetylcholine receptors at parasympathetic postganglionic nerve terminals	Tachycardia, gastrointestinal atony, mydriasis, hyposalivation, disturbed vision, hallucinations
Glycopyrrolate	Drug action similar to that of atropine but does not cross blood–brain barrier; therefore, no CNS effects	. . .
Scopolamine	Competitive antagonism of acetylcholine receptors at parasympathetic postganglionic nerve terminals	Tachycardia, gastrointestinal atony, mydriasis, hyposalivation, disturbed vision, hallucinations
Parasympathomimetics		
Muscarinics		
Arecoline	Alkaloid from *Areca catechu* (betel nut)	Primarily affects postganglionic parasympathetic effector organs (e.g., heart, smooth muscle, salivary glands)
Carbachol	Similar to acetylcholine	Salivation, vomiting, diarrhea, miosis, bradycardia
Muscarine	Stimulates muscarinic receptors of the postganglionic parasympathetic effector organs; mushroom genera (e.g., *Inocybe, Boletus, Clitocybe*) contain muscarine or other cholinergic toxins that cause acute onset of cholinergic signs; blood–brain barrier prevents access to CNS	Salivation, vomiting, diarrhea, miosis, bradycardia
Cholinesterase inhibitors	This group of compounds stimulates pre- and post-ganglionic parasympathetic nerves by interacting with acetylcholinesterase and preventing the enzymatic degradation of acetylcholine, allowing excessive action and duration of parasympathetic stimulation	Salivation, lacrimation, gastrointestinal motility, bronchoconstriction, bradycardia
Organophosphates	Cause prolonged inhibition of cholinesterase ("aging")	

Carbamate insecticides*	Cholinesterase–carbamate bond is rapidly cleaved with rapid reversal of cholinesterase inhibition	
Blue-green algae (anatoxin A)	Unlike the cholinesterase-inhibiting insecticides, anatoxin A does not cross the blood–brain barrier	
Solanum (nightshade)	Several of the Solanaceae family reported as exhibiting cholinesterase-inhibiting activity	Cholinesterase inhibition is not clearly linked to poisoning by these plants
Nicotinics		
Blue-green algae (anatoxin A)	Contains the alkaloid depolarizing neurotoxin, "fast death factor"	Rapid onset of tremors and muscle rigidity followed by paralysis
Cholinesterase inhibitors	Nicotinic effects of acetylcholine are stimulation of post-ganglionic neuromuscular junctions	Muscle fasciculations followed by weakness, paralysis
Nicotine	Stimulates acetylcholine receptors at sympathetic and parasympathetic ganglia and neuromuscular junctions	Tremors, excitement, and some parasympathetic signs occur at low dosages or early in the course of the poisoning, progressing rapidly to complete paralysis
Plants with nicotine-like effects	. . .	Similar to those of nicotine; include rapid onset of tremors, excitement, and ataxia followed by weakness, paralysis, or both; often causes death within minutes to hours after ingestion; parasympathetic signs often present as well
Lobelia	Contains alkaloids lobeline, lobelidine	
Conium	Toxic principle is coniine and related alkaloids	
Gymnocladus	Contains the quinolizidine alkaloid cytisine	
Laburnum	Contains cytisine, similar to Gymnocladus	
Lupinus	Contains multiple alkaloids of the quinolizidine and piperidine class	

*Cholinesterase–carbamate bond is rapidly cleaved with rapid reversal of cholinesterase inhibition.
CNS = central nervous system; GABA = γ-aminobutyric acid.

TABLE 7-6. Toxicants Inducing Muscle Weakness or Paralysis*

Toxicant	Mechanism of Action	Characteristic Response
Acacia berlandieri	N-methyl-β-phenethylamine	Chronic ataxia and paresis known as "limberleg" or "Guajillo wobbles"; worsens with exercise
Botulinum toxin (*Clostridium botulinum*)	Prevents release of acetylcholine from vesicles at the nerve terminal	Flaccid paresis and paralysis, which may include facial muscles and tongue
Black widow spider (*Latrodectus*)	Venom contains α-latrotoxin, which stimulates release and depletion of acetylcholine and norepinephrine from postganglionic sympathetic synapses	Neurologic effects include difficult deglutition, loss of tendon reflexes, paresis, paralysis
Curare	Neuromuscular blocking agent that acts by competing with acetylcholine for cholinergic receptor sites at neuromuscular junctions	Nondepolarizing paralysis of skeletal muscles
Furazolidone	Inhibits thiamine and monoamine oxidase in CNS; affects peripheral nerves in swine and poultry	Ataxia, hypermetria, paresis, paralysis; similar to signs of phenylarsonic feed additive toxicosis (see below)
Karwinskia	Plant contains C-15 polyphenol, which is only suspected as a toxic agent	Bilateral, symmetrical ascending neuropathy with lesions of segmental demyelination and axonopathy, eventually resulting in paralysis
Lathyrus	Contains β-amino-propionitrile, which directly affects peripheral nerves	Initial muscle rigidity followed by weakness, ataxia, paralysis
Phenylarsonics	Unknown, but may involve interference with B-complex vitamins	Segmental demyelination (primarily of peripheral nerves) resulting in ataxia, weakness, hypermetria, incoordination, paresis, paralysis
Selenium	Attacks motor neurons of the ventral horn of the spinal cord in swine	Poliomyelomalacia, especially of the cervical and thoracic regions, causing weakness that progresses to irreversible quadriplegia
Sorghum species	Unknown; postulated to be a chronic cyanide toxicosis or a lathyrogenic effect from β-cyanoalanine	Sorghum cystitis (ataxia syndrome) affects horses; they are ataxic, weak, and develop flaccid posterior paralysis combined with cystitis
Tick paralysis	Unknown toxin appears to inhibit depolarization of lower motor neurons, with associated slowed synaptic transmission and reduced nerve conduction velocity	Posterior incoordination and paresis progressing to ascending paralysis terminating in quadriplegia; dyspnea and difficulty swallowing; death may occur from respiratory paralysis

Triaryl phosphates, some organic phosphates	Inhibit neurotoxic esterase and interfere with axoplasmic transport, reducing nutritional and trophic influences in the axon and leading to axonopathy	Ascending flaccid paresis; permanent paralysis
Zootoxins		
Ciguatera toxin	Present in a number of reef-dwelling fish (e.g., amber-jack, barracuda, grouper, parrot fish, surgeon fish, emperor fish, red snapper); lipophilic toxin increases sodium permeability at the nerve membrane, lowering the action potential threshold	Acute paresthesia, paralysis
Saxitoxin	Found in several shellfish of the US West Coast; associated with the "red tide" or marine algae blooms of *Gonyaulax*; blocks sodium channels in nerve and muscle membranes	Paralysis
Tetrodotoxin	Produced in several organs (e.g., liver, ovaries, intestines) of the puffer (Fugu) fish in Pacific Rim areas; similar mechanism to that of saxitoxin (see above)	Rapid and often fatal paresthesia followed by paralysis

*These toxicoses are unrelated to cholinergic or nicotinic mechanisms.
CNS = central nervous system.

TABLE 7-7. Toxicants Inducing Incoordination and Cerebellar or Vestibular Effects

Toxicant	Mechanism of Action	Characteristic Response
Aminoglycoside antibiotics	May cause postsynaptic receptor blockade or suppression of acetylcholine release at synapse	Ataxia, nystagmus, incoordination
Ohio buckeye (*Aesculus*)	Aesculin, a glycoside toxin, probably involved; mechanism not yet clarified	Incoordination, ataxia, trembling, weakness, paralysis
Dutchman's breeches (*Dicentra*)	Isoquinoline alkaloids; mechanism unknown	Trembling, staggering, ataxia
Locoweed (*Astragalus*)	Toxic principle is swainsonine; inhibits α-mannosidase, resulting in mannose-containing vacuoles in CNS neurons especially cerebellar neurons	CNS-related signs are incoordination, hypermetria, proprioceptive deficits, and habituation to the plant; systemic signs are related to teratogenic effects or selenium toxicosis, or both
Mercury	Interrupts sulfhydryl enzymes of protein synthesis in the cerebral cortex, and possibly, the cerebellum; causes fibrinoid degeneration of medial layer of cerebral arteries	Cerebellar signs may be prominent, but are usually associated with other severe CNS changes (see also Table 7-3)
Metaldehyde	Metabolized to acetaldehyde; toxicosis is correlated with decreases in 5-hydroxytryptamine (5-HT, serotonin) and GABA in the brain	Severe tremors and hypermetria are part of the neurologic syndrome that may include seizures and salivation (see also Table 7-2)

CNS = central nervous system; GABA = γ-aminobutyric acid.

TABLE 7-8. Toxicants Affecting Behavior

Toxicant	Mechanism of Action	Characteristic Response
Belladonna alkaloids	Block action of acetylcholine at postsynaptic receptors	Disorientation, delirium, agitation, occasional seizures
Ergot alkaloids (*Claviceps*)	Act either as agonists or antagonists of adrenergic, dopaminergic, or serotonin receptors; behavioral signs may relate to the lysergic acid principle in ergot sclerotia	Ataxia, depression, disorientation, and incoordination may occur intermittently with excitement or seizures
Lead	Mechanism unclear	Depression, mania, hysteria, or other forms of behavioral change in several domestic species (dog, cat, horse, cow); systemic clinical toxicosis
Lysergic acid (LSD)	Inhibitory effects of 5-hydroxytryptamine (5-HT) on neurons; changes in intracellular serotonin	Hallucinations
Marijuana (*Cannabis*)	Tetrahydrocannabinol and analogs may affect action of major neurotransmitters	Significance of the mechanism to behavioral changes not fully known; major signs in animals are mydriasis, ataxia, nystagmus, tremors, excitement
Morning glory (*Convolvulus*)	LSD-like toxic principle	. . .
Nutmeg (*Myristica*)	Myristicin, a major toxin, inhibits monoamine oxidase	Variable excitation or depression, dizziness, anxiety
Periwinkle (*Vinca*)	Toxins are vincristine and vinblastine, which inhibit microtubule formation during mitosis and are associated with disrupted axoplasmic transport in neurons	Hallucinations can occur, but possibly not as a result of this mechanism

    b. Hepatic encephalopathy and **hyperammonemia**

    c. Alkalosis, which lowers the threshold for seizures from other causes

    d. Uremia, resulting from toxic renal tubular damage

    e. Hypoxia, which results from methemoglobinemia, hemolytic anemia, or cyanide toxicosis

  3. Myoclonia is the localized contraction or trembling of muscle fibers or groups. It is not generalized or symmetrical, and it is not usually associated with toxicosis.

D. **Autonomic signs relating to the parasympathetic nervous system** are indicators of toxicosis by synthetic and natural toxins (Table 7-5).

  1. Parasympatholytic effects are caused by **agents that block the action of acetylcholine** at the nerve terminal.

  2. Parasympathomimetic effects can be caused by **muscarine** (an agent that mimics the action of acetylcholine) or **anticholinesterase** (an agent that inhibits the termination of acetylcholine action).

E. **Paresis or paralysis** (Table 7-6) may result from damage to lower motor neurons or from axonal damage or demyelination. Paraplegia or quadriplegia may occur.

F. **Ataxia** (Table 7-7) may result from a combination of weakness, loss of central control (cerebral, cerebellar, and vestibular), and peripheral nerve damage.

  1. Cerebellar or vestibular signs are apparent as head tilt, circling, nystagmus, and incoordination.

  2. Relatively few toxicants produce primary cerebellar or vestibular signs. One group of vestibular toxicants important in veterinary medicine are the **aminoglycoside antibiotics**.

G. **Behavioral changes** (Table 7-8)

  1. The summation, or endpoint, of functional integration in the nervous system includes sensory, motor, and cognitive signs.

  2. Behavioral changes induced by toxicants are documented in veterinary medicine, but have not been thoroughly studied.

BIBLIOGRAPHY

Anthony DC, Doyle GG: Toxic responses of the nervous system. In: *Casarett and Doull's Toxicology: The Basic Science of Poisons,* 4th ed. Edited by Amdur MO, Doull J, Klassen CD. New York, Pergamon, 1991, pp 402–426.

Bloom FE: Drugs acting on the central nervous system. In *Goodman and Gilman's The Pharmacological Basis of Therapeutics,* 8th ed. Edited by Goodman Gilman A, Rall TW, Nies AS, Taylor P. New York, Pergamon, 1990, pp 244–268.

Beasley VR, Dorman DC, Fikes JD: A systems affected approach to veterinary toxicology. Reference notes for Toxicology VB 320. University of Illinois, Urbana, IL, 1990.

Cheek PR, Shull LR: Natural Toxicants in Feeds and Poisonous Plants. Westport, CT, AVI Publishing Company, 1985.

Chrisman CL: *Problems in Small Animal Neurology,* 2nd ed. Philadelphia, Lea & Febiger, 1991.

Jacob LS: *The National Medical Series for Independent Study: Pharmacology,* 2nd ed. Media, PA, Harwal, 1987, pp 27–76.

Nicholson SS: Tremorgenic syndromes in livestock. *Vet Clin North Am: Food Animal Practice.* 5:291–300, 1989.

Spencer PS, Schaumburg MD: *Experimental and Clinical Neurotoxicology: Section A—Targets and Classification of Neurotoxic Substances.* Baltimore, Williams & Wilkins, 1980, pp 2–101.

STUDY QUESTIONS

DIRECTIONS: Each of the numbered items or incomplete statements in this section is followed by answers or by completions of the statement. Select the **one** numbered answer or completion that is **best** in each case.

1. In the nervous system, the cell body is the main site for:
(1) release of neurotransmitter chemicals.
(2) fast anterograde transport of materials for synaptic transmission.
(3) saltatory conduction.
(4) protein synthesis.
(5) synthesis of myelin.

2. Which statement about energy metabolism in the central nervous system (CNS) is true?
(1) The pentose phosphate pathway is the main source of energy for the neuron.
(2) Sensitivity to anoxia is higher for glial cells than for neurons.
(3) Glycogen content is higher in the brain than in other body tissues.
(4) Anoxia can lead to cerebral edema.
(5) Oxygen consumption is higher in white matter than in gray matter.

3. Which pair of ions is most important to generating an action potential?
(1) Calcium and magnesium
(2) Magnesium and potassium
(3) Potassium and sodium
(4) Sodium and magnesium
(5) Magnesium and chloride

4. Toxicants that lower the threshold for the action potential are most likely to cause:
(1) slow ascending paralysis due to "dying back" of the axon.
(2) reduced conduction velocity and slowed reflexes.
(3) flaccid paralysis, with loss of sensation in the limbs.
(4) hallucinations and abnormal behavior.
(5) muscle tremors, seizures, and increased reaction to stimuli.

5. Neurotransmitter release from vesicles depends on the presence of which ion?
(1) Sodium
(2) Chloride
(3) Potassium
(4) Calcium
(5) Magnesium

6. Which statement about the blood–brain barrier is true?
(1) Junctions between capillary endothelial cells are very tight compared with those in other areas of the body.
(2) Compounds that are polar and ionized are most likely to pass the blood–brain barrier.
(3) Glucose and amino acids diffuse passively across the blood–brain barrier.
(4) The blood–brain barrier of neonatal animals protects them from chemical exposures that would harm mature animals.
(5) Lipids are excluded from the brain by the blood–brain barrier.

7. The most active and obvious phase of a toxicant-induced seizure is the:
(1) aura.
(2) ictus.
(3) prodromal phase.
(4) postictal phase.
(5) refractory phase.

8. All of the following are characteristic of a toxicant-induced seizure *except*:
(1) It is bilateral and symmetrical.
(2) It is often accompanied by autonomic signs.
(3) If often has no recognized aura.
(4) Extensor rigidity and opisthotonos are common.
(5) The postictal phase usually includes excitement and hyperreflexia.

1. The answer is 4 *[I A 3 a (1); II A 2]*. Protein synthesis begins in the rough endoplasmic reticulum (rER) of the neuron cell body, and then shifts to the smooth endoplasmic reticulum (sER). Structural and functional proteins for the rest of the neuron are transported in an anterograde manner by the axon tubulovesicular system. Agents that interrupt protein synthesis (e.g., methyl mercury) usually cause slowly developing and often nearly irreversible lesions. Synaptic vesicles and the synaptic (nerve) terminal are involved in the release of neurotransmitters. Saltatory conduction of the action potential takes place along the axons of myelinated nerves. The myelin, which is produced by Schwann cells and oligodendrocytes, covers the axon and allows impulses to "jump" from one node of Ranvier to the next.

2. The answer is 4 *[II A 1 a–b]*. The main pathway of energy metabolism in the central nervous system (CNS) is the tricarboxylic acid (TCA) cycle, which depends heavily on aerobic conditions. Toxicants that cause acute or prolonged anoxia (e.g., cyanide, carbon monoxide) can deplete cellular energy and impair the sodium pump, allowing cellular influx of sodium ions. The resultant increased sodium content and osmotic pressure, when combined with the imbibition of water, lead to swelling in the brain. Gray matter has a higher oxygen consumption than white matter, and glial cells are less sensitive to oxygen deprivation than neurons. The glycogen content of the brain is only enough to sustain metabolism for a short period of time.

3. The answer is 3 *[II B 1 a]*. The action potential is dependent on an initial rapid influx of sodium, which produces an electrochemical gradient that is balanced more slowly by the movement of potassium out of the cell. Although chloride has a role in balancing the electrical charges at the membrane and calcium assists by stabilizing the membrane, the essential first event is the transmembrane movement of sodium and potassium.

4. The answer is 5 *[II B 1 a; III C 2]*. Muscle tremors, seizures, and increased reaction to stimuli can result from facilitation of the action potential, which is an acute and explosive event. Substances that lower the threshold enhance nerve conduction, resulting in increased neurologic activity. Toxicants that interfere with axonal transport cause "dying back" neuropathy, which can lead to slow ascending paralysis. Toxicants that interfere with the synthesis of myelin or degrade the myelin sheath that covers the axon reduce conduction velocity. Toxicants that interfere with the release of certain neurotransmitters (e.g., acetylcholine) can lead to flaccid paralysis. Toxicants that inhibit or otherwise affect normal neurotransmitter action can lead to hallucinations and abnormal behavior.

5. The answer is 4 *[II E 1 a (1); Figure 7-3]*. Neurotransmitter release from the nerve terminal membrane depends on the presence of ionized calcium. Calcium plays an essential role in the binding of vesicles to the presynaptic membrane prior to neurotransmitter release.

6. The answer is 1 *[I A 3 b]*. A major physical barrier in the central nervous system (CNS) is the blood–brain barrier, which is characterized by very tight junctions in the capillary endothelium. These tight junctions allow passage of chemicals only through the cell membrane itself, thereby limiting passage to chemicals that are of low lipid solubility and are generally small, non-ionized, and nonpolar. Neonates are more susceptible than adults to most xenobiotics, because the blood–brain barrier is not yet fully developed.

7. The answer is 2 *[III A 1 b]*. The ictus is the active motor phase of the seizure syndrome. Many toxicants induce seizures that progress rapidly to the ictal stage and thus appear clinically as acute, explosive episodes that involve violent motor activity and loss of consciousness accompanied by autonomic signs. The prodromal phase includes subtle behavior changes. The aura, the beginning of the seizure, may be localized and not readily apparent. The postictal phase is the return to the normal state. Seizures are not classified as having a refractory phase.

8. The answer is 5 *[III A 2 b; Table 7-2]*. The postictal phase following an acute toxicant-induced seizure is commonly characterized by exhaustion and depression; during this stage the animal may be depressed and refractory to seizures. Body temperature may be elevated, and lactic acidosis occurs after prolonged seizures. Although increased motor activity may occur in the postictal period, the most common response is exhaustion and depression.

Chapter 8

Toxicology of the Liver and Biliary System

I. INTRODUCTION

A. **Central role of the liver.** The role of the liver in the excretion of xenobiotics exposes it to high concentrations of toxicants and their metabolites.

1. Toxicants taken orally enter the liver directly via the portal circulation, exposing the liver cells to high concentrations of **unmetabolized toxicants.**

2. **Metabolic changes** to toxicants occur in the liver. These changes can increase or decrease the effect of the toxic agent. **Mixed function oxidases (MFOs;** e.g., cytochrome P-450) oxidize the toxicant and prepare it for conjugation and excretion; in the process, MFOs can produce toxic intermediates.

B. **Anatomy of the liver**

1. **Hepatic units** (Figure 8-1)
   a. **Hexagonal model.** Early descriptions divided the liver into hexagonal lobules 1–2 mm in diameter, oriented around a central vein, and bounded by portal triads (i.e., a hepatic artery, portal vein, and bile duct). In this model, blood flows from the portal triads to the central vein.
   b. **Acinar model.** Recent studies suggest that the newer acinar model is more appropriate for toxicologic considerations. The acinus is divided into three zones, designated 1, 2, and 3.
      (1) **Zone 1** is closest to the portal triad and receives the **highest exposure to toxicants in the blood. Enzymes of intermediary metabolism are prominent** in acinar zone 1.
      (2) **Zone 2**
      (3) **Zone 3** is farthest from the portal triad. This zone has the lowest oxygen tension and contains the greatest concentration of microsomal MFOs, which can alter the toxicity of xenobiotics.

2. **Implications**
   a. **Susceptibility of the liver to toxicants.** Different regions of the liver vary in their blood supply, complement of activating or detoxifying enzymes, and metabolic and synthetic activities that support body function.
   b. **"Zonal" (differential) response.** The presence of different anatomical and biochemical regions helps to explain the "zonal," or differential, response to toxicants in various parts of the liver.

C. **Range of liver damage.** Liver injury involves a broad spectrum of changes, from trivial cholestasis to acute fulminant hepatic necrosis. Different biochemical aberrations may produce similar clinical signs, because the clinical manifestations of liver injury are limited to a few characteristic changes.

1. **Exposure.** The lesions of toxic liver injury depend on the chemical agent and the duration of exposure. Dose–response relationships are not always apparent.
   a. **Acute exposure** can cause cellular lipid accumulation (fatty change), hepatocyte necrosis, or hepatobiliary dysfunction (cholestasis).
   b. **Chronic exposure** can cause fibrosis, which may advance to a progressive fibrosing condition known as cirrhosis.

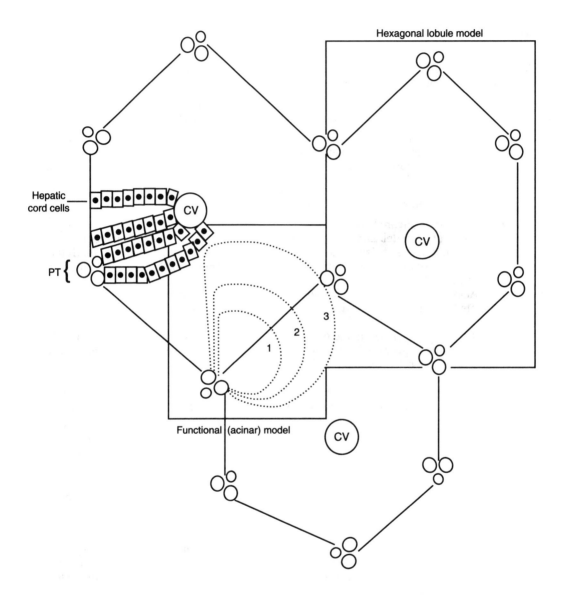

FIGURE 8-1. Comparative structural and functional features of the liver. In the hexagonal lobule model, the central vein (*CV*) receives blood from the portal vein via the hepatic sinusoids. Bile, on the other hand, flows from the central vein toward the portal triad (*PT*). The centrilobular area, where the central vein is located, is the least oxygenated area and contains the highest concentration of mixed function oxidases (MFOs). In the functional (acinar) model, the various zones (*1, 2,* and *3*) are characterized by different levels of blood flow, oxidative enzymes, and MFOs.

c. Prolonged or severe exposure with damage to nucleic acids can lead to neoplastic nodules or to hepatic carcinoma.

2. Severity. Some forms of injury are reversible; others may cause permanent damage.
   a. Mortality rates from liver toxicosis vary. Twenty percent of the liver parenchyma can perform enough detoxification and synthetic function to support life.
   b. If the animal survives, hepatic cells are readily regenerated and will resume normal function.

II. CHOLESTASIS is hepatic injury that is characterized by arrested bile flow accompanied by little or no overt parenchymal injury. It is relatively uncommon in domestic animals.

A. **Classification.** Different agents induce different forms of cholestasis.

   1. Hepatocellular cholestasis is caused by intrahepatic excretory defects that are associated with diffuse liver disease or toxicosis.

   2. Pure cholestasis is a defect in bile flow with no hepatocyte disease.

B. **Anatomy of the bile duct system**

   1. Direction of bile flow. In the bile canaliculi, bile flows from the central vein toward the portal triad; sinusoidal blood flow occurs from the portal vein to the central vein.

   2. The **bile canalicular membrane,** which is oriented opposite the sinusoid, comprises approximately 13% of the hepatocyte surface. In drug-induced cholestasis, the cytoskeleton (microfilament network) of the canalicular membrane undergoes changes in membrane fluidity (permeability). There is loss of tone, pulsatile function, or both.

C. **Mechanism of bile formation**

   1. Bile acids
      a. Primary bile acids [i.e., **cholic acid (trihydroxy)** and **chenodeoxycholic acid (dihydroxy)**] are synthesized from cholesterol in the liver.
      b. Secondary bile acids (e.g., **lithocholic acid**) are produced by bacterial reduction of primary bile acids in the intestine.

   2. Enterohepatic circulation enables the body to return bile acids from the small intestine to the liver, where they are resecreted.
      a. After the bile acids are returned to the liver, they are conjugated with taurine, ornithine, glycine, and other substances to form **bile salts**.
      b. Lithocholic acid is reabsorbed after enterohepatic cycling, detoxified by sulfate conjugation, and excreted in the feces. Excess lithocholic acid damages the canalicular membrane.
      c. After bile duct injury, bile salt resorption is increased, accompanied by the formation of intracanalicular precipitate known as **bile plugs**.

   3. Bile salts are secreted from the hepatocytes into the canaliculi.
      a. Bile salt–dependent flow. The accumulation of bile salts in the hepatocyte creates an osmotic pressure, which increases the driving force for the transport of bile salts out of the hepatocyte and drives bile flow.
      b. Bile salt–independent flow is poorly characterized but is not dependent on bile salt production. A sodium-potassium-adenosine triphosphatase (ATPase) pump may provide the energy that creates the osmotic gradient needed to drive bile flow.

D. **Cholestatic agents**

   1. Chlorpromazine is a tranquilizer that causes clinical jaundice in 1% of human users. It decreases sodium-potassium-ATPase and calcium-magnesium-ATPase activity, reducing actin polymerization and membrane fluidity.

2. **Cytochalasin B** (fungal toxin) and **phalloidin** (mushroom toxin) disrupt the microfibrillar system, causing canalicular paralysis and dilatation.

3. **Sporidesmin,** the fungal toxin of *Pithomyces chartarum,* causes facial eczema in sheep. Sporidesmin reacts with membrane sulfhydryls to produce deformation of the canalicular membrane. As a result, sheep cannot excrete photodynamic metabolites of chlorophyll. Thus, photosensitization, known as **hepatogenous photosensitization,** develops because the impaired liver cannot excrete the degradation products of normal plant pigments.

4. **C-17 anabolic steroids** are a common cause of cholestasis and hepatic dysfunction.

E. **Detection of cholestasis**

1. **Morphologic changes**
   a. **Bile plugs** appear as golden-brown pigment in bile ducts and canaliculi.
   b. **Bile canaliculi** are dilated as the result of bile-plugged ducts or loss of pulsatile tone.
   c. **Microvilli** are decreased in the canaliculi.

2. **Functional changes**
   a. **Clinical signs.** Bile flow is reduced, accompanied by **jaundice** and **bilirubinuria.**
   b. **Laboratory studies**
      (1) **Plasma bromsulphalein retention is increased.** This laboratory evaluation uses a dye to test a pathway similar to that of bile secretion.
      (2) **Plasma conjugated bilirubin** and **serum bile acids** are increased.
      (3) Specific **plasma enzymes** are elevated, especially **alkaline phosphatase (AP),** **5'-nucleotidase (5'N), γ-glutamyl transpeptidase (GGT),** and **leucine amino peptidase (LAP).**
         (a) AP and GGT are most commonly used in veterinary medicine. Both have estimated plasma half-lives of 48–72 hours in dogs.
         (b) Table 8-1 compares enzyme changes in cholestasis and hepatic cytotoxicity.

III. **CYTOTOXICITY** (Table 8-2)

A. **Classification**

1. **Type I (intrinsic, predictable) hepatotoxicosis**
   a. **Characteristics**
      (1) A **distinctive lesion** is produced, and **similar lesions occur across different species** exposed to the same toxicant.
      (2) The **severity of the response** is **dose-related**.
      (3) There is a **predictable, brief latent period** before clinical response.
      (4) Response to these hepatotoxins is **experimentally reproducible**.
   b. **Type I hepatotoxins**
      (1) **Direct hepatotoxins** usually injure a variety of tissues including the liver. They affect many organelles or membranes and act after a brief latent period.

TABLE 8-1. Enzyme Changes in Cholestasis and Hepatic Cytotoxicity

Type of Toxicity	ALT	Arginase	SDH	AP	GGT	Bilirubin
Cholestasis	1+	1+	1+	2+	3+	3+
Cytotoxicity	4+	3+	2+	1+	0	0

ALT = alanine aminotransferase; AP = alkaline phosphatase; GGT = γ-glutamyl transpeptidase; SDH = sorbitol dehydrogenase.

TABLE 8-2. Hepatotoxic Drugs, Chemicals, and Plants of Importance in Veterinary Medicine

Source	Toxicant	Use or Exposure	Species Most Commonly Affected
Drugs	Acetaminophen	Analgesic	Dogs, cats (rare)
	Copper	Supplement	Sheep, swine
	Iron dextran	Supplement	Swine
	Mebendazole	Anthelmintic	Dogs
	Thiacetarsamide	Filaricide	Dogs
	Toluene	Anthelmintic	Dogs, cats
	Vitamin A	Supplement	Dogs, cats
Chemicals	Carbon tetrachloride	Solvent	Rare, all animals
	Carbon disulfide	Fumigant	Cattle
	Coal tar, pitch		Swine, cattle
	Nitrosamines	Contaminant	Rare, all animals
	Phenols	Disinfectants	Cats, swine
	Phosphorus	Rodenticide	Dogs
Mycotoxins	Aflatoxin		Swine, poultry, dogs
	Fumonisins		Horses, swine
	Rubratoxin		Rare, all animals
	Sporidesmin		Sheep
	Sterigmatocystin		Rare, all animals
Plants (hepatotoxic)	*Amanita* mushrooms		Dogs
	Blue-green algae		Dogs, cattle
	Cocklebur (*Xanthium* species)		Swine, cattle
	Cycad palm (*Cycas* species)		Cattle, swine
	Gossypol		Swine, calves
	Helenium species (sneezeweeds)		Cattle, sheep
	Hymenoxys species (bitterweed)		Cattle, sheep
	Lantana (*Lantana camara*)		Cattle, sheep
	Pyrrolizidine alkaloids (*Amsinckia, Crotalaria, Cynoglossum, Heliotropium, Senecio, Trichoderma*)		Horses, cattle
Plants (hepatogenous sensitizers)	Alsike clover (*Trifolium* species)		Sheep, cattle
	Agave (*Agave lechiguilla*)		Sheep, cattle
	Blue-green algae (*Microcystis*)		Swine, cattle
	Horsebrush (*Tetradymia* species)		Sheep
	Kochia (*Kochia scoparia*)		Cattle, sheep
	Lantana (*Lantana camara*)		Cattle, sheep, horses
	Pyrrolizidine alkaloids		Horses, cattle, sheep
	Puncture vine (*Tribulus* species)		Sheep
	Rape (*Brassica* species)		Swine, cattle
	Sacahuiste (*Nolina texana*)		Sheep, cattle

     (2) Indirect hepatotoxins affect a specific metabolic pathway. They alter the metabolic organization of the cell and cause damage by producing a deficiency of a key enzyme or cofactor. The response to indirect hepatotoxins may be more focused and subtle than that to direct hepatotoxins.

  2. Type II (idiosyncratic, unpredictable, drug-related) hepatotoxicosis has the following characteristics:

    a. Lesions are more variable than those of type I hepatotoxicity and may be accompanied by an allergic reaction.

    b. Effects are not dose-related.

    c. There is **no distinct latent period between the time of exposure and the response.**

   d. Only a small fraction of the exposed population is susceptible, and the syndrome **cannot be reproduced experimentally**. This lack of reproducibility may be caused by immune mechanisms: alternatively, some animals may be unusually sensitive or lack a key detoxification enzyme.

B. **Mechanisms of toxicologic damage**

   1. Biochemical alterations
   a. Lipid peroxidation of cellular and organelle membranes is the first toxic effect of many hepatotoxins.
      (1) Formation of free radicals (i.e., any molecule with an odd or unpaired number of electrons) causes peroxidative damage to the polyenoic unsaturated fatty acids of organelle membranes and initiates a chain reaction of lipid peroxidation that causes loss of membrane structure and function.
      (2) The resultant lipid peroxidation and membrane damage can lead to loss of cell homeostasis and, eventually, to necrosis.
   b. Accumulation of lipid in hepatocytes (i.e., **fatty liver, hepatic lipidosis**). Although lipid accumulation is not always injurious to the liver, it is an indication that important mechanisms of protein synthesis have been impaired.
      (1) Cellular fat accumulates when secretion of hepatic triglyceride into plasma is blocked.
      (2) Lipid accumulation in the liver may occur when acceptor lipoproteins are reduced because of decreased synthesis of the protein moiety.
         (a) In normal cells, the lipid acceptor protein is synthesized in the rough endoplasmic reticulum (rER) and assembled in the smooth endoplasmic reticulum (sER).
         (b) Chemicals that reduce lipoprotein levels include carbon tetrachloride, ethionine, yellow phosphorus, and puromycin.
   c. Altered protein synthesis. Some toxicants [e.g., carbon tetrachloride (CCl_4)] cause irreversible damage to protein synthesis; others (e.g., ethionine) cause reversible damage. Mechanisms include:
      (1) Degranulation of the rER
      (2) Alteration of ribosome monomers
      (3) Reduced incorporation of amino acids into lipoprotein, as caused by CCl_4
      (4) Interference with the action of amino acids (e.g., ethionine inhibits protein synthesis by interfering with the action of methionine)
      (5) Decreased synthesis of ribonucleic acid (RNA), such as that caused by galactosamine, which reduces available uridine triphosphate (UTP)
      (6) Covalent binding of toxic intermediates to nucleic acids and proteins (e.g., as caused by aflatoxin and pyrrolizidine alkaloids)

   2. Bioactivation of xenobiotics in the liver. Chemically stable xenobiotics activate reactive intermediates during biotransformation.
   a. Often the toxic intermediates are transient and cannot be isolated.
   b. The formation of toxic intermediates is usually inferred by the ability of the liver to alkylate or arylate endogenous macromolecules (e.g., nucleic acids and proteins).
      (1) Alkylation or arylation forms a covalent bond between the electrophilic intermediate and nucleophilic sites on endogenous macromolecules.
      (2) Increases in covalent binding correlate with the severity of liver damage, but only a few reactive intermediates probably become covalently bound.
      (3) Bioactivation is measured by the formation of specific metabolites or the presence of structural changes.
         (a) Peroxidative metabolites reduce cellular glutathione content and induce lipoperoxidation, producing **increased amounts of conjugated diene and ethane**.
         (b) **Liver weight and liver microsomal protein levels are increased** when bioactivation occurs.
         (c) Bioactivation is accompanied by **proliferation of the sER**.

C. **Evaluation of injury**

1. **Clinical signs** are similar for a variety of hepatotoxins and other agents.
   a. **Acute liver necrosis or hepatic failure** causes **depression, anorexia, abdominal pain, and vomiting**.
      (1) **Icterus** and **hepatomegaly** may occur as the acute phase becomes more severe or advanced.
      (2) **Coagulopathy** may occur if coagulation factor synthesis is inhibited.
      (3) **Stupor** or **coma** may occur as the acute phase becomes more severe or advanced.
      (4) **Hepatic encephalopathy** may also occur.
         (a) Hepatic encephalopathy is associated with **hyperammonemia,** which occurs when the liver does not adequately metabolize the end products of nitrogen metabolism or ammonia that is generated by lower intestinal and colonic bacteria.
         (b) Ammonia concentrations are not directly correlated with clinical signs because other toxic metabolites (e.g., mercaptans, methionine, and short-chain fatty acids) may also contribute to hyperammonemia.
         (c) The toxicity of ammonia is enhanced when systemic alkalosis occurs, allowing un-ionized ammonia to cross the blood–brain barrier.
   b. **Subacute liver failure** is an extension of acute liver failure. It usually occurs when exposure to the toxicant is minimal or when animals survive the acute phase. Clinical signs include:
      (1) **Vomiting, anorexia, and weight loss**
      (2) **Depression**
      (3) **Icterus;** possibly **changes in fecal color** as well
      (4) **Dull coat**
      (5) **Coagulopathy**
   c. **Chronic liver toxicosis** can occur after recovery from acute or subacute liver damage. Prolonged exposure to toxicants at lower dosages may also cause chronic liver toxicosis.
      (1) **Weight loss, anorexia,** and **reduced milk production** are common.
      (2) **Vomiting, nausea,** and **pale fecal material** occur intermittently.
      (3) **Icterus** occurs in some animals.
      (4) The **liver** is **usually not enlarged or palpable,** and it may become smaller and fibrotic. True cirrhosis (i.e., the destruction of normal hepatic architecture by fibrous septa that encompasses the regenerative nodules of hepatocytes) is rare in domestic animals with chronic hepatotoxicosis. Most chronic liver failure from acute or chronic toxicosis in animals is characterized by marked fibrosis, but does not involve regenerative nodules.
      (5) Grazing animals may develop **secondary photosensitization** because they cannot excrete chlorophyll metabolites.
      (6) Animals with hepatic damage **may be more susceptible to a variety of other drugs and toxicants.**

2. **Laboratory studies**
   a. **Serum enzyme activity.** The release of an enzyme through damaged plasma membranes increases levels of that enzyme in the systemic circulation.
      (1) Changes in serum enzyme activity are most useful for the detection of acute liver damage, but not for the detection of chronic liver damage or fatty change.
      (2) Increased serum enzyme activity correlates with increased hepatocyte damage.
      (3) The sensitivity and duration of elevation vary for each hepatic enzyme.
      (4) Changes in the activity of major groups of hepatic enzymes indicate different types of hepatic injury.
         (a) Elevation of levels of **group I enzymes** reflects cholestatic injury [see II E 2 b (3)].

(b) Elevation of levels of **group II enzymes** reflects nonspecific cytotoxic damage. Enzymes in this group include aspartate aminotransferase (AST), lactate dehydrogenase (LDH), and malate dehydrogenase (MDH).

(i) **Group IIB enzymes** are concentrated in the liver of most animals and include alanine aminotransferase [ALT, formerly known as glutamic pyruvic transaminase (GPT)] and isocitrate dehydrogenase (ICD). ALT has a half-life in dogs of approximately 60 hours. Levels may be elevated for 1–3 weeks after liver toxicosis occurs.

(ii) **Group IIC enzymes** are specific for the liver. They include ornithine carbamyl transferase (OCT), sorbitol dehydrogenase (SDH), and LDH isoenzymes. SDH is sensitive to hepatotoxicosis, but has a short half-life. SDH levels may return to normal within 1–2 days after hepatotoxicosis occurs.

(5) Activity of some enzymes (e.g., cholinesterase) is depressed by liver injury.

b. Excretion studies. Hepatic excretory function can be evaluated by measuring the disappearance of compounds that are actively secreted from plasma to bile.

(1) Excretion studies are time-related. Animals are administered a marker dye, blood is sampled at specified times, and disappearance of the dye from the blood is analyzed.

(a) Bromsulphalein, indocyanine green, and rose bengal are commonly used marker dyes. Availability of bromsulphalein has become increasingly limited.

(b) The proper dosage, which varies with species and the dye used, is important for accurate evaluation.

(2) Excretion of dye is limited by hepatic perfusion. Thus, excretion does not measure hepatocellular function, but indicates total liver function.

c. Serum bile acids are used to evaluate hepatobiliary function. After feeding the animal a small meal, serum bile acid levels are determined. Increased postprandial release of bile acids into the blood indicates impaired hepatobiliary function.

d. Biopsy or necropsy can be used to evaluate change in hepatic constituents.

(1) **Hepatic triglyceride** is increased by agents that alter protein synthesis.

(2) **Glucose-6-phosphatase** activity is a general indicator of damage to the endoplasmic reticulum (ER).

(3) **Microsomal protein synthesis** may be increased or reduced.

e. Drug metabolism. Depression of drug metabolizing ability is a measure of hepatic function.

(1) **Activity of cytochrome P-450 products** (e.g., metabolites of specified drugs) is depressed when the ER is damaged.

(2) **Lipid peroxidation products** (e.g., malondialdehyde, pentane, ethane, and thiobarbituric acid-reactive substances) are research tools that can be used to estimate peroxidative damage.

(3) **Covalent binding** often correlates with liver damage in experimentally induced hepatic toxicosis.

(4) **Glutathione status** parallels susceptibility to oxidative stress, and can be measured in a clinical laboratory.

(5) **Altered pharmacologic effects of drugs** indicate the ability of the animal to metabolize or excrete drugs.

f. Extrahepatic components may indicate impaired synthetic ability of the liver during subacute or chronic toxicosis. The liver synthesizes:

(1) **Blood coagulation factors**

(2) **Plasma proteins** (e.g., **albumin, complement**)

g. Light microscopy can confirm the nature and degree of hepatic damage in animals that die of liver toxicosis.

(1) Descriptive morphology often correlates with functional changes.

(2) Lesion descriptions are of limited use in determining the cause of toxicity because many chemicals cause similar biochemical and morphologic abnormalities.

(3) Histopathologic examination is helpful in estimating the extent of injury.

D. **Therapy and management.** Causes of death from acute toxic liver failure include toxemia from reduced detoxication of normal metabolic products, hypoglycemia, coagulopathy, shock, and disseminated intravascular coagulation (DIC).

1. **Exposure** to the responsible toxic agent **must be discontinued**.

2. **Treatment of emesis and dehydration** are important supportive measures.

3. **Nutritional considerations.** The diet should be high in carbohydrates, low in fat, and supplemented with limited amounts of high-quality proteins that reduce the need for waste nitrogen metabolism. Use of drugs or supplements that require liver metabolism should be avoided.

4. **Oral antibiotics** should be administered to control the generation of ammonia by intestinal and colonic bacteria.

5. The veterinarian should **monitor the animal for signs of coagulopathy or chronic damage that could influence subsequent health.**

BIBLIOGRAPHY

Cornelius CE: Liver function. In *Clinical Biochemistry of Domestic Animals,* 4th ed. Edited by Kaneko JJ. San Diego, Academic Press, 1989, pp 364–397.

Hardy RM: Hepatic encephalopathy. In *Current Veterinary Therapy,* vol 11. *Small Animal Practice.* Edited by Kirk RW, Hardy RM. Philadelphia, WB Saunders, 1992, pp 639–645.

Hoffmann WE: A review of hepatic enzymes of diagnostic importance. In *Proceedings of the 1992 Annual C.L. Davis Pathology Symposium: Diagnostic Toxicologic Pathology.* Urbana, IL, University of Illinois, 1992, pp 125–136.

Plaa G: Toxic responses of the liver. In *Casarett and Doull's Toxicology: The Science of Poisons,* 4th ed. Edited by Amdur MO, Doull J, Klassen CD. New York, Pergamon, 1991, pp 334–353.

Popp JA, Cattley RC: Hepatobiliary system. In *Handbook of Toxicologic Pathology.* Edited by Haschek WM, Rousseaux CG. San Diego, Academic Press, 1991, pp 279–314.

Rubin E, Farber JL: The liver and biliary system. In *Pathology.* Edited by Rubin E, Farber JL. Philadelphia, JB Lippincott, 1988, pp 723–786.

DIRECTIONS: Each of the numbered items or incomplete statements in this section is followed by answers or by completions of the statement. Select the **one** numbered answer or completion that is **best** in each case.

1. Which statement is correct regarding toxicant-induced hepatic lipidosis?

(1) Hepatic lipidosis is an indication of serious liver toxicosis.
(2) Hepatic lipidosis produces a permanent morphologic change.
(3) Increased synthesis of lipid acceptor proteins is part of the mechanism of fat accumulation in the hepatocyte.
(4) The organelle most closely involved in hepatic lipidosis is the ribosome.
(5) Visible fat accumulates as very low-density lipoprotein (VLDL).

2. Which bile component is toxic to bile canalicular membranes and dependent on enterohepatic recycling for its formation?

(1) Chenodeoxycholic acid
(2) Cholesterol
(3) Cholic acid
(4) Lithocholic acid
(5) Sulfocholic acid

3. Which group of three serum components provides the best indication of cholestatic damage?

(1) Alanine aminotransferase (ALT), arginase, and alkaline phosphatase (AP)
(2) ALT, blood ammonia, and arginase
(3) Aspartate aminotransferase (AST), ALT, and blood ammonia
(4) AST, ALT, and bilirubin
(5) AP, γ-glutamyl transpeptidase (GGT), and bilirubin

4. Which indicator would be expected to decrease in an animal with hepatic toxicosis?

(1) Ammonia
(2) Bilirubin
(3) Plasma proteins
(4) Prothrombin time
(5) Sorbitol dehydrogenase (SDH)

5. Which treatment measure would be most likely to aid in reducing the occurrence of hepatic encephalopathy?

(1) Intravenous sodium bicarbonate
(2) Administration of oral antibiotics
(3) Increasing the level of dietary protein
(4) Supplementation with vitamin A
(5) Administration of tranquilizers

6. All of the following statements regarding liver bioactivation of xenobiotics to a more toxic form are true *except*:

(1) Metabolites of the parent xenobiotic are chemically unstable and difficult to detect.
(2) Toxic or reactive xenobiotic metabolites are detected by measuring alkylation or covalent binding of endogenous macromolecules.
(3) Hepatic bioactivation of xenobiotics decreases liver microsomal proteins and reduces liver weight.
(4) Depletion of cellular glutathione is caused by the peroxidative metabolites of bioactivation.
(5) Conjugated dienes are characteristic end products of lipid peroxidation.

7. Acute onset of hepatic toxicosis with signs of depression, anorexia, and vomiting is likely to be accompanied by all of the following *except*:

(1) Coagulopathy
(2) Hepatomegaly
(3) Hypoglycemia
(4) Icterus
(5) Pale, clay-colored stools

ANSWERS AND EXPLANATIONS

1. The answer is 4 [*III B 1 b*]. Hepatic lipidosis induced by toxicants usually has a basis in protein synthesis. Formation of lipid acceptor protein is blocked by a variety of chemicals that degranulate the rough endoplasmic reticulum (rER) and alter ribosome monomers. Hepatic lipidosis is not considered a serious effect resulting in permanent morphologic change. It is, however, a signal that an important pathway of protein synthesis has been interrupted, and it can progress to hepatocyte degeneration or necrosis.

2. The answer is 4 [*II C 2 b*]. If it is not detoxified by sulfation, lithocholic acid can be toxic to the canalicular membrane. Bile acids are synthesized from cholesterol as trihydroxy and dihydroxy forms known as cholic acid and chenodeoxycholic acid, respectively. Chenodeoxycholic acid from biliary secretion is reduced by intestinal and colonic bacteria to form lithocholic acid, which is reabsorbed via enterohepatic recycling, detoxified, and excreted in the feces.

3. The answer is 5 [*II E 2 b; Table 8-1*]. In animals with cholestatic liver damage, several specific liver enzymes are released in the blood and may be detected in serum. These enzymes include alkaline phosphatase (AP), 5′-nucleotidase (5′N), γ-glutamyl transpeptidase (GGT), and leucine amino peptidase (LAP). In addition, bile stasis causes retention of bilirubin, which may also be reflected by elevated serum levels. Other hepatic enzymes [e.g., alanine aminotransferase (ALT), aspartate aminotransferase (AST), arginase] and ammonia in the serum indicate that the hepatocytes are damaged and cannot process ammonia through the urea cycle.

4. The answer is 3 [*III C 2 f; Table 8-1*]. Plasma proteins are manufactured in the liver and their serum levels are reduced when the ability of hepatocytes to synthesize proteins is impaired. The ammonia level rises when hepatocyte damage prevents biosynthesis of ammonia to urea. Bilirubin can increase as a result of either hepatocyte dysfunction or cholestasis. Prothrombin time increases because of the reduced availability of coagulation factors normally synthesized by hepatocytes. Sorbitol dehydrogenase (SDH) is a liver-specific enzyme that is released when hepatocyte membranes are damaged, releasing cellular enzymes into the blood.

5. The answer is 2 [*III C 1 a (4), D*]. Oral antibiotics decrease bacterial activity and the synthesis of ammonia, thus reducing the need for hepatic synthesis of urea from ammonia. If the conversion of ammonia to urea is impaired, the blood ammonia level increases. Hyperammonemia, which is associated with hepatic encephalopathy, may affect neurologic function. Administration of sodium bicarbonate is contraindicated in hepatic encephalopathy because alkalosis increases the amount of un-ionized ammonia in the blood and enhances its passage across the blood–brain barrier. Increasing the level of dietary protein increases the need for waste nitrogen metabolism; the animal's diet should be high in carbohydrates, low in fat, and supplemented with limited amounts of high-quality proteins. Use of supplements that require liver metabolism (e.g., vitamin A) should be avoided. Tranquilizers would exacerbate the effects of hepatic encephalopathy.

6. The answer is 3 [*III B 2 a–b*]. Liver size and weight increase when bioactivation occurs, because xenobiotic activation involves the endoplasmic reticulum (ER) and ribosomes. In protein synthesis, the size of the ER and microsomal protein levels increase, thus increasing the size and weight of the liver. Often toxic intermediates are transient and difficult to detect. Measuring alkylation (i.e., covalent binding) of endogenous macromolecules is one way of detecting toxic or reactive xenobiotic metabolites. Peroxidative metabolites reduce cellular glutathione content and induce lipoperoxidation, producing increased amounts of conjugated dienes and ethane.

7. The answer is 5 [*III C 1 a*]. Pale stools are an indicator of poor fat digestion resulting from reduced availability of bile salts. This symptom is not likely to occur until subacute or chronic damage depletes bile salt availability. Acute liver failure caused by hepatotoxins interferes with coagulation factor synthesis, and may induce shock and disseminated intravascular coagulation. Glucose metabolism is impaired, and icterus may develop because of acute cell swelling with retention of bile and hemoglobin degradation products.

Chapter 9
Renal Toxicology

I. INTRODUCTION

A. **Function.** As blood passes through the kidneys, the nephrons clear the plasma of some substances while retaining others. The kidneys maintain the constancy of the body's internal environment via three mechanisms: filtration, secretion, and absorption.

1. **Filtration** is the initial step in urine formation. Of the plasma reaching the kidney, 20% is filtered by the selectively permeable glomerular membrane. The resultant fluid is passed into Bowman's capsule.
   a. Filtration is **influenced by** the **glomerular hydrostatic pressure** and the **oncotic pressure of the filtrate**.
   b. Filtration is restricted at molecular weights above approximately 10,000 daltons. Thus, **proteins and protein-bound drugs are not filtered in the normal glomerulus**.
   c. **Charged molecules,** both anions and cations, **do not readily pass through the glomerular membrane**.

2. **Secretion** is the transport of solutes from the peritubular capillaries into the tubular lumen. It is the **addition of a substance to the filtrate**.

3. **Reabsorption** is the transport of substances from the tubular lumen into the peritubular capillaries. It is the **removal of a substance from the filtrate**. Reabsorption exerts significant control over tubular fluid volume and solute concentration.
   a. **Tubular fluid volume is reduced** by 99%, with approximately 80% of the reduction occurring in the proximal tubule.
      (1) Active reabsorption of water is mediated by energy-dependent sodium reabsorption in the proximal tubules.
      (2) Weak acids and bases absorb better if they are un-ionized.
   b. **Solute concentration of the filtrate is increased.**

B. **Exposure to toxicants.** The excretory function of the kidneys places them at high risk following exposure to toxicants.

1. **Cardiac output and total blood flow.** The kidneys receive a large portion of cardiac output and total blood flow, exposing them to circulating toxicants. **Renal blood flow** is 25% of cardiac output.
   a. **Biotransformation of xenobiotics to toxic intermediates** can occur in the renal tubular epithelium. Although the ability of the kidney to biotransform some drugs or chemicals is recognized experimentally, the contribution of this effect to clinical veterinary toxicology is not widely documented.
   b. **Endocytosis** or **pinocytosis** facilitates the uptake of small proteins in the proximal tubules; therefore, these mechanisms can concentrate toxicants in tubular cells. For example, cadmium is bound to metallothionein in the liver and cleared by glomerular filtration. Via endocytosis, the cadmium–metallothionein complex is concentrated in tubular cells. When the complex is metabolized, free cadmium, which is toxic to tubular cells, is released.

2. **Excretory mechanisms**
   a. **Tubular transport** (i.e., secretion and reabsorption) facilitates concentration of normal endogenous metabolites, as well as many toxicants, in renal proximal tubular cells.

(1) The glomerular filtrate is modified by active and passive processes.

   (a) Active transport in the tubules **affects xenobiotic elimination** by causing compounds to be excreted more quickly or more completely than by filtration alone, especially if the compounds are not filtered well.

   (b) Active transport **may perpetuate damage from toxicants.** For example, uranyl nitrate enters tubule cells with bicarbonate, where it is concentrated, causing cytotoxic injury.

(2) Renal clearance is the ratio of the renal excretion rate of a substance to its concentration in the blood plasma, expressed as fraction or multiple of the glomerular filtration rate (GFR). Both secretion and reabsorption can be measured indirectly using clearance calculations (see III A 1).

   (a) A clearance ratio equal to 1 indicates that on a net basis, the substance is neither reabsorbed nor secreted (i.e., it is only filtered).

   (b) A clearance ratio of less than 1 indicates that on a net basis, the substance undergoes reabsorption.

   (c) A clearance ratio greater than 1 indicates that on a net basis, the substance undergoes secretion.

b. Organic ion transport system. Two systems for transport exist primarily in the proximal tubules.

   (1) These systems, which **function to eliminate endogenous or exogenous compounds that may be toxic,** act on weak organic acids and bases that carry a charge at physiologic pH.

   (a) One system acts on **organic anions.** Para-aminohippuric acid (PAH) is used as a model for study.

   (b) The other system acts on **organic cations.** Tetraethylammonium is the model for study.

   (2) The organic ion transport system **may concentrate toxicants in tubular cells,** increasing the access of toxicants to susceptible areas in cells. The result is greater toxic effect. For example, dichloro-diphenylacetic acid (DDA, a DDT metabolite) and the herbicide 2,4-D accumulate in renal tubules at a concentration 20–40 times that of the plasma concentration. At high concentrations, these toxicants uncouple oxidative phosphorylation, leading to loss of energy that is needed for tubular transport and cellular viability.

C. **Renal toxicants.** Table 9-1 details toxicants that affect kidney function.

II. MECHANISMS OF ACUTE RENAL FAILURE.
Nephrotoxins may induce renal failure by interfering with glomerular or tubular function, or both.

A. **Filtration failure**

1. Diminished renal blood flow

a. Vasoconstriction. Nephrotoxins may induce renal vasoconstriction, reducing renal blood flow and causing tubular dysfunction secondary to ischemia and anoxia.

   (1) Both renal blood flow and GFR are reduced in many types of acute renal failure.

   (a) The GFR is maintained near the normal level until the renal blood flow decreases to less than one-third of the normal rate. The renin–angiotensin system, which uses biofeedback to elevate systemic blood pressure, is activated when GFR falls during acute renal failure.

   (b) Sufficient renal venous oxygen is maintained at a level adequate to prevent structural damage unless renal blood flow decreases to less than one-sixth of the normal rate.

   (2) Nephrotoxins that cause tubular necrosis may indirectly induce vasoconstriction and reduce renal blood flow. These changes may occur because altered delivery of solutes to the distal nephron affects the action of prostaglandins and the renin–angiotensin system.

b. Toxicoses that reduce systemic blood pressure and renal perfusion affect the GFR.

2. **Tubular obstruction.** The GFR can be diminished when obstructing **casts,** composed of hemoglobin or myoglobin pigments, necrotic tubule cells, and crystals, form in damaged renal tubules.

   a. The casts increase intratubular pressure, which counteracts the glomerular capillary hydrostatic pressure, thus reducing the GFR.

   b. Both hemoglobin from severe acute hemolysis or myoglobin from massive muscle necrosis or trauma (the **crush syndrome**) can form intratubular casts that affect nephron function.

   c. Cast formation may be a result of reduced GFR and renal tubular damage, rather than a cause of renal damage.

3. **Increased impedance of the membrane** or **decreased hydraulic pressure** may decrease ultrafiltration. This hypothesis has not been proven.

B. **Tubular cell injury.** Tubular destruction interferes with the passage of filtrate through the nephron.

1. **Leakage of filtrate** into the systemic circulation may occur across damaged tubules. Badly damaged tubules that leak are generally part of a nephron that is not forming filtrate; therefore, this hypothesis is not considered valid by all authorities.

2. **Direct toxic effects.** Nephrotoxins may render the tubular cells incapable of reabsorbing essential solutes and water.

III. EVALUATION OF RENAL DAMAGE

A. **Glomerular function**

1. **Clearance calculations** can be used to estimate the GFR. It is not necessary to anesthetize the animal in order to estimate clearance.

   a. A **test substance** is injected intravenously and then measured quantitatively in both blood and urine.

   b The **rate of urine formation** is measured.

   c. **Clearance is calculated** as follows:

$$C_x = \frac{U_x \times V}{P_x}, \text{ where}$$

C_x = clearance of the substance (ml/min)
U_x = concentration of the substance in urine (mg/ml)
P_x = concentration of the substance in plasma (mg/ml)
V = volume of urine output (ml/min)

   (1) Clearance is expressed as milliliters of plasma cleared completely per unit of time:

$$C_x = \frac{mg/ml \times ml/min}{mg/ml} = ml/min$$

   (2) The GFR is estimated using a marker that is **freely filtered** by glomeruli and not secreted or reabsorbed by tubules (e.g., **inulin, creatinine**).

   (a) **Inulin,** which must have an exogenous source, does not bind to plasma proteins. Therefore, it is an accurate measure of GFR, because clearance is affected when the substance binds to plasma proteins, reducing the availability of the substance for glomerular filtration.

   (b) **Creatinine,** which has an endogenous source, is used frequently in clinical practice to estimate GFR. Measurement of endogenous creatinine clearance is less accurate than estimations of clearance using exogenous substances.

TABLE 9-1. Important Toxicants that Affect Kidney Function

Agent or Toxicant Class	Mechanism of Action	Effects of Toxicant
Antimicrobials Aminoglycosides (gentamicin, neomycin) Oxytetracycline Polymyxins Sulfonamides	Active uptake by tubule cells, with possible inhibition of protein synthesis and Na^+-K^+-ATPase activity or lysosomal membrane damage and cellular necrosis Antianabolic effects may lead to azotemia Depressed GFR and tubular degeneration Crystalluria	Kidney maintains residue for extended periods; more toxic in animals that are older, dehydrated, or have existing renal disease; dogs appear most susceptible to tetracycline nephrotoxicosis
Antifungal agents Amphotericin B	Sterol interaction with tubule membranes leads to chloride leakage, reduced renal blood flow, and decreased GFR	Reversible renal damage occurs at recommended dosages, so use must be limited or intermittent
Anthelmintics Thiacetarsemide	See Metals	Some dogs react to arsenical therapy for heartworms with vomiting and hepatic and renal failure
Analgesics Acetaminophen Aspirin Ibuprofen and other non-steroidal anti-inflammatory drugs	Inhibit cyclooxygenase activity required for prostaglandin synthesis, leading to renal medullary necrosis	High dosages cause oliguria, azotemia, and hyperkalemia; additional effects are interstitial nephritis and retention of sodium and water
Cantharidin	Unclear; may be related to shock and reduced renal blood flow	Irritation of the gastrointestinal and urinary tracts
Ethylene glycol	Acute acidosis, with reduced renal blood flow and formation of calcium oxalate crystals in tubular lumen	Three phases of toxicosis: (1) ataxia and inebriation; (2) severe acidosis, shock, and coma; (3) oxalate nephrosis and renal failure
Fungicides Carbamate fungicides	Unknown	Renal and hepatic degeneration are mild to moderate and nonspecific
Herbicides Phenoxy herbicides Triclopyr herbicide	Unclear; renal damage is generally confined to swollen and vacuolated tubular cells	Vomiting and diarrhea; muscle stiffness (myotonia) or weakness may occur; renal damage may not account for serious signs or death
Metals/Boric acid Arsenic Cadmium Chromium Lead Mercury (inorganic)	Interfere with action of sulfhydryl enzymes in energy metabolism, causing necrosis in energy-dependent proximal tubules; most metals are concentrated in tubule cells during renal filtration and reabsorption	Most metals (e.g., lead, mercury) cause serious disturbances of many organ systems leading to vomiting, diarrhea, hepatic damage, hemolysis, and neurologic signs; renal damage may lead to secondary osteoporosis

Toxin	Mechanism	Clinical signs
Mycotoxins Citrinin Ochratoxin	Interfere with incorporation of amino acids into proteins; major target is renal proximal tubule cell	High levels may cause acute renal failure, but exposure to 3–10 ppm is associated with polyuria, polydipsia, and chronic nephrosis
Oxalates *Beta* (beets) *Chenopodium* (lamb's quarters) *Halogeton* (halogeton) *Kochia* (fireweed) *Rheum* (rhubarb) *Rumex* (curly dock) *Sarcobatus* (greasewood)	Soluble oxalates form calcium salts that precipitate as insoluble calcium oxalate in renal tubules	Acute hypocalcemia and acidosis may precede renal damage; damage occurs only after a latent period, when calcium oxalate precipitates form in the kidney
Plants (nonoxalate) *Amaranthus* (pigweed) *Lilium* (Easter lily) *Philodendron* (philodendron) *Quercus* (oaks) *Xanthium* (cocklebur)	Unknown; these agents cause coagulative necrosis of renal proximal tubules, with formation of casts and acute renal failure	Renal tubular necrosis is a prominent toxic effect of all plants, except cocklebur, for which liver damage is most evident; acute oliguric renal failure is typical of the syndrome described in IV A; cats appear especially sensitive to Easter lily
Solvents Carbon tetrachloride Chloroform and other halogenated hydrocarbons	Metabolic formation of active intermediates and free radicals that bind macromolecules and initiate lipid peroxidation of tubular cell membranes	May be acute or chronic, depending on dosage; additional prominent signs are central nervous system depression, ataxia, and hepatic failure
Vitamins Vitamin D$_3$ *Cestrum* (day-blooming jessamine) *Solanum malacoxylon* Cholecalciferol-based rodenticides	Direct tubular damage and glomerular degeneration by an unknown mechanism, in addition to calcification of tubular basement membranes	Early signs are nonspecific and may not suggest renal disease; signs progress over 1–3 days; hypercalcemia indicates grave prognosis
Vitamin K$_3$ (menadione) in horses	Not well established in the horse; may be related to a combination of auto-oxidation and hemoglobinuria in some species	Characteristic response is depression, colic, fever, and elevated blood urea nitrogen and creatinine levels

GFR = glomerular filtration rate; ppm = parts per million.

2. The **blood urea nitrogen (BUN) level** is a general indicator of GFR; however, it is elevated only after more than two-thirds of kidney function is lost. The BUN level also may be affected by other factors such as dietary protein intake, the postprandial sampling interval, and increases in protein catabolism.

3. The **serum creatinine level** has limitations similar to those encountered with BUN, but serum creatinine is less affected by extrarenal factors.

4. **PAH,** which is both filtered by glomeruli and secreted by the tubules, is used to measure renal blood flow.

5. Clinical signs
   a. **Acute renal failure. Nausea, vomiting, gastrointestinal bleeding, esophagitis, gastritis,** and **colitis** accompany the onset of **azotemia,** which leads to the clinical syndrome of **uremia**.
   b. **Chronic renal failure**
      (1) **Edema and hypertension.** A reduced GFR caused by a drop in renal perfusion stimulates the renin–angiotensin system, stimulating aldosterone secretion and leading to retention of sodium and water.
      (2) **Hypocalcemia, compensatory parathyroid activity, and osteodystrophy.** When the GFR is less than 25% of the normal rate, the serum phosphate level increases, stimulating bone calcium uptake and hypocalcemia.
         (a) In response to the hypocalcemia, parathyroid activity increases and osteodystrophy may occur.
         (b) Renal synthesis of active vitamin D may be impaired, reducing the absorption of calcium by the intestine and worsening the hypocalcemia.
      (3) **Decreased red blood cell count.** Damage to the epithelial cells of the renal cortical tubules and the juxtaglomerular cells around the glomerular arterioles interferes with the synthesis of erythropoietin, a hormone that stimulates the production of red blood cells by bone marrow.

B. **Tubular function.** Reabsorption of normal tubular solutes and water depends on proximal tubule function.

1. **Urinalysis**
   a. **Glucosuria** may occur when damage to the tubular epithelium impairs glucose absorption. Glucosuria may also be caused by hyperglycemia, in which the amount of glucose in the tubular filtrate exceeds the tubular capacity for reabsorption. Glucosuria caused by hyperglycemia is not an indication of renal failure.
   b. **Sodium concentration** in the urine may be increased.
   c. **Proteinuria**
   d. **Specific gravity**
   e. **Proteinaceous or granular casts**
   f. **Renal enzymes in the urine.** Enzymes may be inactivated in the collected urine sample, unless the sample is stored under refrigeration. Dialysis of the sample may be necessary prior to analysis of urinary enzymes.
      (1) **Maltase** and **alkaline phosphatase (AP)** may be released from the renal brush border as a result of renal damage.
      (2) **Lactate dehydrogenase (LDH)** and **AP** may be released from lysosomes in advanced or severe renal failure.

2. **Evaluation of urine concentrating ability.** Urine concentrating ability is determined using the **water deprivation test** or the **exogenous vasopressin test**.

3. **Evaluation of secretory activity.** The secretory activity of the renal tubules can be measured by determining the excretion of marker compounds (e.g., PAH) or dyes (e.g., Phenosulfophthalein). This approach is not often used in clinical evaluation of kidney function.

4. **Clinical signs**
   a. **Dehydration,** which is characterized by the voiding of large volumes (**polyuria**) of dilute urine (**hyposthenuria**), is caused by decreased urine concentrating ability.
   b. **Metabolic acidosis** resulting from reduced ammonia production reduces the buffering action of hydrogen ions in the urine. There are accompanying **decreases in the serum bicarbonate level** and **blood pH,** and **compensatory hyperventilation** occurs.

IV. **THERAPY AND MANAGEMENT.** Renal failure occurs in two distinct phases, the **oliguric/anuric phase** and the **diuretic phase**.

A. **Oliguric/anuric phase.** Rapid response is necessary to prevent acute life-threatening disturbances in fluid and electrolyte levels.

1. **Glomerular filtration and urine formation must be maintained.** An animal that fails to respond to diuretic and vasoactive therapy has a grave prognosis. Other therapeutic options include peritoneal dialysis or hemodialysis.
   a. **Catheterization.** The animal should be catheterized to empty the bladder and monitor urine output. Catheterization increases the risk of urinary tract infection.
   b. **Diuresis.** Urine output, which should begin within 15 minutes of initiating treatment, should be monitored continuously by catheterization.
      (1) **Balanced electrolyte solutions** are used to initiate diuresis. Because the administration of fluids may cause overhydration, the animal's central venous pressure should be monitored to avoid pulmonary edema.
      (2) **Mannitol** (0.5–1.0 g/kg in a 20% solution) is administered intravenously to inhibit water reabsorption and maintain an adequate flow of dilute urine. The dosage should not exceed 1.5 g/kg until after diuresis begins.
   c. **Vasoactive therapy. Dopamine** (1–3 µg/kg/min diluted in a 5% dextrose solution) administered intravenously enhances renal vasodilation and improves GFR.

2. **Acid–base dysfunction must be corrected. Acidosis** (i.e., the retention of hydrogen ions) is the most common acid–base abnormality associated with the oliguric/anuric phase. To correct acidosis, the bicarbonate need must be calculated, and then bicarbonate is administered.

3. **Hyperkalemia, if present, must be treated.**
   a. A **20% dextrose solution** given at 1 ml/kg intravenously **will aid the intracellular movement of potassium**. This effect is enhanced by administering insulin with the dextrose.
   b. **Hyperkalemic heart failure,** which is characterized by bradycardia, electrocardiogram (ECG) changes (i.e., a reduced P-wave amplitude, prolongation of the P-R interval and QRS interval), weakness, and depression, may be fatal.
      (1) **Calcium gluconate** (0.5–1.0 ml/kg in a 10% solution) should be administered slowly and intravenously to an animal with signs of hyperkalemic heart failure.
      (2) Cardiac function must be monitored during this process.

B. **Diuretic phase.** Recovering and regenerating tubular epithelium may be unable to concentrate urine and to control electrolyte losses.

1. **Fluid balance**
   a. Dehydration, packed cell volume, serum osmolality, and urine specific gravity must be monitored.
   b. Hydration must be maintained with a 5% dextrose solution or with balanced electrolyte solutions, or both.

2. **Electrolyte abnormalities**
   a. **Hypokalemia** may be treated with potassium, administered orally or intravenously, depending on the severity of potassium depletion.

    b. Hypernatremia can be controlled by alternately administering a 5% dextrose solution and a balanced electrolyte solution.

3. Sodium, potassium, BUN, and creatinine levels, and **acid–base status** should be monitored.

BIBLIOGRAPHY

Grauer GF: Toxicant-induced acute renal failure. In *Current Veterinary Therapy,* Vol 10. *Small Animal Practice.* Edited by Kirk RW. Philadelphia, WB Saunders, 1989, pp 126–130.

Hewitt WR, Goldstein RS, Hook JB: Toxic responses of the kidney. In *Casarett and Doull's Toxicology: The Basic Science of Poisons,* 4th ed. Edited by Amdur MO, Doull J, Klaassen CD. New York, Pergamon, 1991, pp 354–379.

Ross LA: Diseases of the Kidney. In *Handbook of Small Animal Practice,* 2nd ed. Edited by Morgan RV. New York, Churchill Livingstone, 1992, pp 559–583.

Thurau K, Mason J, Gstraunthaler G: Experimental acute renal failure. In *The Kidney: Physiology and Pathophysiology.* Edited by Seldin DW, Giebisch G. New York, Raven Press, 1985, pp 1885–1899.

DIRECTIONS: Each of the numbered items or incomplete statements in this section is followed by answers or by completions of the statement. Select the **one** numbered answer or completion that is **best** in each case.

1. Which type of toxicant would most likely be removed by glomerular filtration?

(1) An agent with a low molecular weight (i.e., less than 300 daltons) that is ionized and bound to plasma proteins

(2) An agent with a low molecular weight that is un-ionized and bound to plasma proteins

(3) An agent with a low molecular weight that is un-ionized and unbound to plasma proteins

(4) An agent with a high molecular weight (i.e., greater than 10,000 daltons) that is un-ionized and unbound to plasma proteins

(5) An agent with a high molecular weight that is lipophilic, un-ionized, and unbound to plasma proteins

2. Which one of the following statements regarding the role of vasoconstriction in toxicant-induced renal failure is true?

(1) Both renal blood flow and the glomerular filtration rate (GFR) are reduced in the initial stages of acute renal toxicosis.

(2) The renal venous oxygen level decreases rapidly in the early stages of reduced glomerular filtration.

(3) Glomerular filtration stops when renal blood flow is reduced by 25%.

(4) The renin–angiotensin system is not affected by changes that occur in GFR during acute renal failure.

(5) Renal tubular damage and renal blood flow are not related.

3. Which circumstance is most likely to cause nephrosis as a result of the sudden massive formation of casts in renal tubules?

(1) Acute ischemia caused by severe arterial vasoconstriction within the kidney

(2) Inhibition of prostaglandin synthesis by nonsteroidal anti-inflammatory drugs

(3) Tubular necrosis caused by the release of lysosomal acid hydrolases as a result of aminoglycoside antibiotic overdose

(4) Massive hemolysis and hemoglobinemia caused by drugs or chemicals

(5) Dehydration, with slowing or stopping of the flow of filtrate in the nephron

4. Inulin is injected intravenously in a dog with a measured rate of urine formation of 10 ml/min. Following the injection, inulin concentrations are analyzed in the blood and urine and found to be 5 mg/ml and 10 mg/ml, respectively. What is the glomerular filtration rate (GFR) in this animal?

(1) 5 ml/min
(2) 10 ml/min
(3) 15 ml/min
(4) 20 ml/min
(5) 25 ml/min

5. Which of these therapies would be contraindicated in treating acute oliguric renal failure?

(1) Initiating diuresis with multiple electrolyte solutions

(2) Administering dopamine intravenously

(3) Administering potassium

(4) Administering mannitol to maintain diuresis

(5) Providing bicarbonate in the intravenous fluids

6. All of the following are signs of acute toxicosis of the kidney *except:*

(1) elevated blood urea nitrogen (BUN) levels.
(2) elevated serum potassium.
(3) elevated serum phosphate.
(4) sodium and water retention.
(5) anemia.

ANSWERS AND EXPLANATIONS

1. The answer is 3 *[I A 1 b]*. Filtration in the glomerulus follows the rules for passive movement of chemicals across membranes. Selectivity of filtration depends on molecular size; molecules greater than 10,000 daltons are usually not filtered unless glomerular damage is present. In addition, binding of lower molecular-weight chemicals to plasma proteins limits their passage to the free, or unbound, portion of the chemical. Filtration is restricted further if the chemical is ionized (charged) at physiologic pH.

2. The answer is 1 *[II A 1 a (1)–(2)]*. Renal vasoconstriction is a common event in acute renal failure caused by either ischemia or exposure to various toxicants (many of which cause renal tubular damage). Renal vasoconstriction reduces renal blood flow, depressing the glomerular filtration rate (GFR) and causing ischemia that damages the oxygen-dependent proximal tubules. In the early stages of acute renal failure characterized by vasoconstriction, renal venous oxygen levels remain fairly steady; renal blood flow must decrease to less than one-sixth the normal rate before structural damage occurs. GFR is maintained near the normal level until the renal blood flow decreases to less than 33% of the normal rate. The renin–angiotensin system is activated when the GFR falls.

3. The answer is 4 *[II A 2]*. The "crush syndrome," which is often associated with severe muscle trauma and can be elicited experimentally by glycerol injection, is the massive destruction of muscle accompanied by the release of myoglobin. The myoglobin is believed to precipitate and form myoglobin casts in the renal tubules that are visible light microscopically. Hemolysis, such as that caused by acute copper toxicosis or zinc toxicosis, produces severe hemoglobinemia and hemoglobinuria, which can lead to blood pigment accumulation in the nephrons, causing "hemoglobinuric nephrosis." The formation of casts from necrotic tubule cells is not usually sudden or massive, as it is with hemolysis and hemoglobinemia. Aminoglycoside antibiotics interfere with tubular function and may cause tubular necrosis, but massive cast formation is not typical. Cast formation may result from vasoconstriction or dehydration, but this is rare because large molecules or cellular debris are usually not present in significant quanti-

ties. Impaired prostaglandin synthesis leads to medullary necrosis.

4. The answer is 4 *[III A 1]*. The dog's glomerular filtration rate (GFR) is 20 ml/min. Because inulin is freely filtered (i.e., not secreted or reabsorbed), its clearance is equivalent to the GFR. Inulin clearance can be calculated using the following equation:

$$C_{in} = \frac{U_{in} \times V}{P_{in}}, \text{ where}$$

C_{in} = inulin clearance (ml/min)
U_{in} = inulin concentration in urine (mg/ml)
P_{in} = inulin concentration in plasma (mg/ml)
V = volume of urine output (ml/min)

Substituting the values in the problem:

$$C_{in} = \frac{10 \times 10}{5} = 20 \text{ ml/min}$$

A simpler approach, often used in clinical situations, is to use this calculation and substitute endogenous creatinine measurements for the inulin value to estimate the GFR, thus eliminating the need to inject markers.

5. The answer is 3 *[IV A 3]*. Acute renal failure with oliguria or anuria can lead to the rapid development of hyperkalemia. Hyperkalemia has serious and potentially fatal consequences, such as hyperkalemic heart block. The administration of potassium to correct hypokalemia is often appropriate during the diuretic phase of renal failure, when the recovering tubules may have difficulty concentrating urine and electrolyte losses can result. The administration of multiple electrolyte solutions, dopamine, mannitol, and bicarbonate are all appropriate during the oliguric/anuric phase of renal failure.

6. The answer is 5 *[III A 2, 5 b (2)–(3); IV A 3]*. Anemia associated with renal failure is caused by reduced stimulation of erythropoietin secretion. Because there is a large functional reserve of mature and developing erythrocytes, anemia is usually a result of chronic renal insult. Acute renal failure with oliguria caused by a reduced glomerular filtration rate (GFR) and tubular swelling can result in rapid increases in blood urea nitrogen (BUN), potassium, and phosphate levels. Diminished sodium excretion leads to osmotic retention of water and, eventually, to edema.

Chapter 10
Toxicology of the Gastrointestinal Tract

I. INTRODUCTION

A. Exposure

1. **Ingestion.** The gastrointestinal system is a major portal of entry for toxicants.

2. **Biotransformation.** Significant biotransformation can occur in **intestinal epithelial cells;** however, some gastrointestinal toxicants act before typical phase I or phase II biotransformation occurs.

B. Clinical signs

1. Clinical signs may be **primary or secondary**.
   a. **Primary signs.** Table 10-1 lists toxicants that can cause primary signs of gastroenteritis in animals.
   b. **Secondary signs.** Examples of toxicoses that cause secondary gastrointestinal signs include:
      (1) Liver and kidney toxicoses, which induce metabolic disruptions (e.g., azotemia, hepatoencephalopathy) that may cause vomiting
      (2) Neurotoxicoses, which may affect neurogenic control of the stomach and intestines (e.g., organophosphate poisoning causes parasympathetic stimulation that results in vomiting and diarrhea)

2. The **severity of the gastrointestinal signs is not always correlated with the prognosis**, especially in acute toxicosis.

3. The most common clinical signs associated with gastrointestinal toxicoses (i.e., vomiting, diarrhea) are generally **manifestations of the body's attempt to eliminate or reduce exposure to the toxicant**.

II. UPPER ALIMENTARY TRACT

A. Exposure.
The upper alimentary tract (i.e., the mouth, pharynx, and esophagus) is directly exposed to chemical or physical agents, without dilution or metabolism. Liquids may cause more esophageal damage than solids because swallowing delivers them quickly to deeper regions of the upper alimentary tract. Healing of the damaged esophagus is slow because of its limited blood supply and relatively small amount of connective tissue.

1. **Cellular necrosis**
   a. **Causative agents** (Table 10-2)
      (1) Damage often occurs quickly after exposure to agents that are **corrosive (acids)** or **caustic (bases)**.
      (2) Agents that coagulate or denature proteins (e.g., **mercuric salts, phenols**) produce local irritation or necrosis.
   b. **Protection** from the direct effects of toxicants is provided by keratinized epithelium and a limited number of submucosal glands.

2. **Absorption of toxicants** directly from the upper alimentary tract is limited to low-molecular-weight compounds that are relatively nonpolar and highly lipophilic.

TABLE 10-1. Toxicants that Cause Primary Signs of Gastroenteritis

Inorganic/Synthetic	Natural	
	Species	**Common Name**
Ammonium salts	*Abrus* species*	Rosary pea
Antimony	*Amanita* species	Death angel mushroom
Arsenic	*Anemone* species	Windflower
Bismuth salts	Araceae family*	Dumbcane, philodendron
Calcium chloride	*Aspergillus* species	Cyclopiazonic acid mycotoxin
Cardioactive glycosides	*Brassica* species	Mustard
Chlorphenoxy herbicides	*Buxus* species*	Box
Cholinesterase inhibitor	*Clostridium* species	Enterotoxin
insecticides	*Colchicum* species*	Autumn crocus
Copper sulfate	*Daphne* species*	Spurge laurel
Crude oil	*Epicauta* species	Blister beetle
Fertilizers	*Euphorbia* species	Spurges
Fluoroacetate	*Fusarium* species	Trichothecene mycotoxin
Iron salts	Gram-negative bacteria	Endotoxin
Mercury, inorganic salts	*Helenium* species	Sneezeweed
Phosphorus, elemental	*Hyacinthus* species*	Hyacinth
Selenium	*Hymenoxys* species	Bitterweed
Thallium	*Ilex* species*	Holly
	Iris species*	Iris
	Kalmia species	Laurel
	Ligustrum species*	Privet
	Melia species	Chinaberry
	Narcissus species*	Daffodil
	Nerium species*	Oleander
	Phoradendron species	Mistletoe
	Phytolacca species	Pokeweed
	Pieris species	Andromeda, pieris
	Quercus species	Oak
	Ranunculus species	Buttercup
	Rhododendron species	Azalea, rhododendron
	Ricinus species*	Castor bean
	Robinia species	Black locust
	Saponaria species	Bouncing bet
	Sesbania species	Coffeeweed
	Solanum species	Nightshade
	Tulipa species	Tulip

*Cultivated plant

B. **Clinical signs of upper alimentary tract toxicosis**

1. **Salivation**

2. **Choking, gagging, and coughing**

3. **Dyspnea** caused by swelling of the pharynx or larynx

4. Labial and buccal **hyperemia**

5. **Vomiting**

C. **Mechanisms of toxicologic damage**

1. **Acute inflammation** begins almost immediately and persists for up to 48 hours.

2. **Necrosis** begins 24–48 hours after initial exposure and is characterized by the formation of dull, gray to white plaques on the mucosal surface and some sloughing of the superficial epithelium.

TABLE 10-2. Toxicants That Cause Primarily Direct Irritation of the Mouth, Pharynx, and Esophagus

Source or Substance	Alternate Names or Sources
Acids	Corrosives
Alkalies	Caustics
Araceae family plants	Dumbcane, philodendron, jack-in-the-pulpit, elephant's ear
Formaldehyde	Fixative
Hydrocarbons (e.g., solvent, fuel)	Gasoline, kerosene, ethanol, turpentine, methylene chloride
Hypochlorite	Liquid bleach
Phenols	Disinfectants
Plants that cause oral trauma	*Urtica* species (nettles), *Arctium* species (burdock), *Hordeum* species (wild barley), *Setaria* species (foxtail), *Cenchrus* species (sandbur), *Tribulus* species (goatheads), cacti

    a. Transmural necrosis may cause perforation of the esophagus. Esophagoscopy and oral intubation must be handled carefully because the mucosa and submucosa are susceptible to perforation.

    b. Constriction or scarring, or both, of the upper alimentary tract, especially the esophagus, is caused by fibroplasia and excessive formation of scar tissue. Constriction may interfere with deglutition.

D. Therapy and management of upper alimentary tract toxicosis

    1. Dilution of toxicant

        a. The toxicant can be diluted carefully with **milk or water,** either consumed voluntarily or given by gavage.

        b. Diluents should be used sparingly (i.e., no more than 10–100 ml of water or milk for small animals) to prevent vomiting, which can further damage the injured mucosa or muscularis.

    2. Contraindications

        a. Emetics and gastric lavage are contraindicated because of the risk of further damage to injured tissues.

        b. Neutralizing agents (i.e., acids or bases) are contraindicated because of the risk of exothermic burns from the reaction between acid and base.

    3. Glucocorticoids may be helpful in minimizing stricture formation; however, this application is somewhat controversial.

III. **STOMACH**

A. Functions

    1. Storage of food

    2. Initiation of digestion by maceration and by secretion of hydrochloric acid and pepsin

    3. Secretion of arachidonic acid metabolites (E series prostaglandins) to protect the gastric mucosa

        a. Prostaglandin inhibitors (e.g., aspirin, ibuprofen) reduce cytoprotective effects in the stomach.

        b. Inhibition of cyclooxygenase activity allows lipoxygenase metabolites to act without the protective action of prostaglandins. Lipoxygenase metabolites are strong vasoconstrictors that may produce ischemia in the gastric or intestinal mucosa.

4. **Secretion of mucus and bicarbonate to protect gastric mucosa from damage by enzymes and gastric acids**

5. **Synthesis, storage, and secretion of serotonin, histamine, glucagon, and gastrin** in response to autonomic and intraluminal stimuli

B. **Clinical signs of acute gastric toxicosis**

1. **Vomiting,** often preceded by hypersalivation, retching, and multiple contractions of the abdominal musculature
   a. **Medullary emetic (vomiting) center.** The medullary emetic center is stimulated by events such as irritation of the pharynx and stomach, distension of the stomach, and disequilibrium (Figure 10-1).
      (1) **Innervation.** The vomiting center is innervated by the cranial nerves, including the vagus, glossopharyngeal, facial, and vestibular nerves.
      (2) Neural connections allow for integration of impulses from the **chemoreceptor trigger zone,** which is located in the area postrema of the brain.
         (a) The chemoreceptor trigger zone is well-supplied with receptors for histamine, acetylcholine (ACh), and dopamine.
            (i) The chemoreceptor trigger zone is sensitive to apomorphine, ergot alkaloids, syrup of ipecac, apomorphine, and presumably many toxicants.
            (ii) Dopaminergic, muscarinic, and histamine 1 (H_1) antagonists are the basis for common antiemetic drugs.
         (b) Dopaminergic receptors in the stomach inhibit gastric motility during the early stages of the vomiting reflex, which can prolong the retention of ingesta that may be toxic.
   b. **Vomitus.** Examination of the vomitus may offer clues as to the toxicosis.
      (1) **Yellow- or green-stained vomitus** indicates reflux of bile from the intestines.
      (2) **Bright green or yellow vomitus** may indicate ingestion of dyed rodenticides or other toxicants.

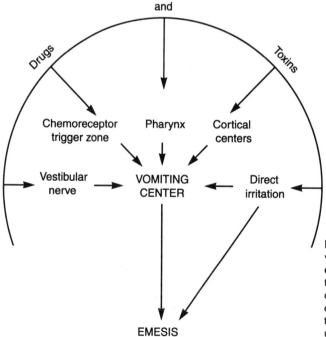

FIGURE 10-1. Routes to emesis. The vomiting center, which receives efferent impulses from several sites, controls and coordinates emesis. Irritation of the gastric mucosa and stimulation of the chemoreceptor trigger zone are the most common mechanisms of stimulating vomiting.

      (3) Bright red or dark, coffee-colored vomitus (hematemesis) indicates retention of blood in the stomach.

      (4) An **abnormal odor** (e.g., phosphine odor from zinc phosphide or garlic odor from arsenic or selenium) may lead to identification of the toxicant.

  2. Anorexia or pica

  3. Abdominal pain (colic), demonstrated by anxiety, stretching, rolling, and kicking at the abdomen

  4. Abdominal distension, resulting from gastric paralysis or gas

C. **Therapy and management of acute gastric toxicosis**

  1. Administration of antiemetics

    a. Indications. Antiemetics should be used only when necessary because they may block elimination of the toxicant and impair monitoring for improvement of clinical signs. Vomiting should not be prevented unless:

      (1) Vomiting is prolonged or severe and may lead to dehydration, loss of electrolytes (especially chloride and sodium), or metabolic acidosis (because of loss of duodenal bicarbonate along with gastric acids).

      (2) Aspiration is a threat (e.g., the animal is comatose or pharyngeal reflexes are absent).

      (3) The stomach is damaged and **perforation of the gastric wall may occur.**

      (4) Caustic, corrosive, or highly volatile toxicants have been ingested.

      (5) The **species is unable to vomit** without the risk of adverse effects (e.g., in horses vomiting may rupture the stomach).

    b. Agents. Antiemetics available, but with limited clinical application in veterinary medicine include:

      (1) Metoclopramide

        (a) Metoclopramide is a dopamine antagonist that blocks the chemoreceptor trigger zone and is used to prevent vomiting during cancer chemotherapy.

        (b) The usual dosage for dogs is 0.2–0.4 mg/kg intramuscularly or subcutaneously every 8 hours.

      (2) Phenothiazine tranquilizers (e.g., chlorpromazine)

        (a) Phenothiazine tranquilizers block both the chemoreceptor trigger zone and the medullary emesis center. However, these agents lower the seizure threshold and, because of their α-adrenergic blocking action, may promote dehydration as a result of vasodilation.

        (b) The recommended chlorpromazine dosage for dogs is 0.5 mg/kg intramuscularly or subcutaneously every 8 hours.

      (3) Antihistamines are most effective for damping input from the vestibular system. The usual canine dosage of diphenhydramine is 2–4 mg/kg orally every 8 hours.

  2. Correction of dehydration and acidosis

    a. Lactated Ringer's solution supplemented with potassium chloride may be used in most cases. In order to avoid cardiotoxic effects, potassium administration should not exceed 0.5 mEq/kg/hr.

    b. Body weight, capillary refill time, skin turgor, thoracic sounds, body temperature, and packed cell volume should be monitored. The central venous pressure should be monitored in serious cases of dehydration.

IV. **INTESTINAL TRACT**

A. **Functions.** Chyme is broken down by bile and enzymes secreted by the intestinal glands and pancreas, and absorption of nutrients, water, and electrolytes takes place. The colon and cecum play a major role in water absorption.

1. **Secretion.** Intestinal secretions play a significant role in digestion and maintenance of pH levels and acid–base balance. Secretion of intestinal fluids is a neurogenic response that may be initiated within the intestinal mucosa or from other areas.

2. **Motility** (i.e., contraction of the muscular wall of the intestine) helps to break down the chyme and move it through the intestinal tract. Motility of the intestine normally occurs in response to chyme entering a segment of the intestine.
   a. **Segmental motility** slows the movement of the chyme and allows better mixing and absorption.
   b. **Propulsive motility** increases the movement of the intestinal contents and assists in the excretion of wastes.

B. Mechanisms of toxicologic damage

1. **Disruption of intestinal epithelium.** Normally, the intestinal epithelium maintains an effective barrier against microorganisms while allowing absorption of nutrients and control of fluid and electrolytes.
   a. **Necrosis** interrupts the epithelial barrier when the rate at which cells are lost is greater than the replacement rate.
      (1) **Direct damage to epithelial membranes or interruption of essential metabolic pathways** that maintain cellular homeostasis by toxicants can lead to necrosis (see Chapter 2 II B).
      (2) **Ischemia** caused by toxicants that affect blood supply to the mucosa and submucosa can result in ischemic (anoxic) necrosis. For example, arsenic acts in part by affecting capillary circulation, which leads to submucosal edema and, eventually, cell death.
   b. **Suppression of mitotic activity.** Toxicants that suppress the mitotic activity of intestinal crypt cells reduce the replacement rate of intestinal epithelium.
      (1) Intestinal integrity is lost as aging epithelial cells die and are not replaced.
      (2) Radiation and cancer chemotherapy are potent inhibitors of epithelial regeneration. **Radiomimetic syndrome** is a clinical response to antimitotic activity that includes anemia, granulocytopenia, thrombocytopenia, diarrhea, and intestinal hemorrhaging.

2. **Interference with secretion**
   a. **Neural stimulation**
      (1) **Parasympathetic (muscarinic) agents** (e.g., organophosphates, carbamate insecticides, neostigmine) cause **hypersecretion and hypermotility,** leading to severe diarrhea.
      (2) **Parasympatholytic agents** (e.g., atropine, the belladonna alkaloids) cause **hyposecretion and hypomotility** (atony). These agents have been used to treat diarrhea.
   b. **Osmotic cathartics.** Strong osmotic effects of some toxicants can initiate diarrhea. Because water enters the intestinal lumen in response to hypertonic salts or hydrophilic colloids, high concentrations of sodium, sulfates, or nonabsorbable carbohydrates act as osmotic cathartics.
   c. **Endogenous chemicals** may cause diarrhea when stimulated by toxicants or when toxicants mimic the natural compound.
      (1) **Prostaglandins** increase mucus secretion and stimulate transfer of water and electrolytes into the intestinal lumen.
      (2) **Histamine** is a potent stimulator of gastric secretions and pancreatic juices.
   d. **Adenylate cyclase activation** by some toxicants (e.g., cholera toxin) stimulates secretion of large amounts of fluid in the small intestine. The ability of the large intestine to reabsorb these secreted fluids is overloaded, leading to potentially life-threatening diarrhea.

3. **Interference with motility**
   a. **Stimulation of propulsive motility**
      (1) **Cholinergic agents** (e.g., carbamylcholine, which mimics the action of ACh) stimulate propulsive motility.

      (2) Cholinesterase inhibitors allow the accumulation of natural ACh, thus stimulating propulsive motility.

      (3) Direct irritants (e.g., castor oil, aloe, cascara sagrada, histamine, and cardiac or saponin glycosides) stimulate smooth muscle in the intestinal wall and increase propulsive motility in an attempt to move irritants more quickly through the intestinal tract.

      (4) Osmotic cathartics increase fluid accumulation, stretching the intestinal wall and initiating reflex propulsive motility.

      (5) Hypersecretion. Intestinal distension from hypersecretion stimulates stretch receptors, which respond with increased intestinal motility. The combination of hypersecretion and hypermotility may result in severe and explosive diarrhea.

  b. Inhibition of propulsive motility. Parasympatholytic agents reduce or stop intestinal motility.

4. Interference with nutrient absorption

  a. Toxicants that interfere with **digestive secretions** reduce the absorption of nutrients.

    (1) Cholestatic liver damage reduces bile secretion and may interfere with absorption of lipids or fat-soluble vitamins.

    (2) Toxicants that effect **pancreatic lipase** action (e.g., aflatoxin) may cause lipid malabsorption.

  b. Chronic inflammation or epithelial damage may lead to hyperplasia of intestinal epithelium or granulomatous reactions that result in malabsorption and diarrhea.

5. Effects on bacteria in large intestine. The high population of microorganisms in the colon and cecum may be disturbed by drugs or toxicants. Species that depend on a large cecum (e.g., horses, guinea pigs, rabbits) are most susceptible.

  a. Antibiotics can **interfere with bacterial synthesis of essential vitamins** such as vitamin K.

  b. Antibiotic suppression of certain microorganisms may **allow proliferation of others with production of toxic products**. For example, in horses, rabbits, and guinea pigs, lincomycin and tetracycline are believed to allow clostridial proliferation that results in acute toxic colitis with diarrhea and severe colic. The extreme loss of fluids may lead to shock.

C. **Clinical signs of intestinal toxicosis**

  1. Abdominal pain (colic)

  2. Frequent defecation of soft or semiformed stools

  3. Watery diarrhea without significant straining (Figure 10-2)

  4. Melena (i.e., fresh or decomposed blood) in the stools

  5. Excessive flatulence with or without abdominal distension

  6. Intestinal tympany

  7. Dehydration

D. **Therapy and management of intestinal toxicoses.** Specific supportive and symptomatic therapy can be used according to the guidelines of internal medicine. (Treat the patient, not the poison.)

V. **RUMINANT FORESTOMACH**

A. **Function.** The ruminant forestomach (comprised of the rumen, reticulum, and omasum) is a modification of the esophagus. The rumen, an **anaerobic reducing environment** with high dependence on microbial activity and little secretory activity, has evolved to assist in digestion of complex carbohydrates high in cellulose.

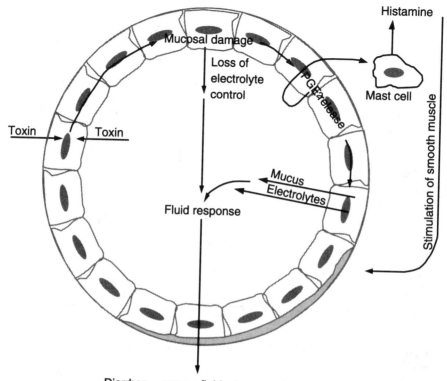

FIGURE 10-2. General pathogenesis of diarrhea caused by toxicants. Strong or persistent effects on motility and secretion upset homeostatic control, resulting in diarrhea, dehydration and, possibly, systemic acidosis or alkalosis. Toxins may reach the intestinal epithelium through either the intestinal lumen or the circulatory system. Toxic mucosal damage interferes with differential control of electrolytes and stimulates release of the prostaglandin PGE_2. PGE_2 activates mast cells, causing the release of histamine, which stimulates smooth muscle activity. Concurrently, PGE_2 induces the secretion of mucus and electrolytes. Electrolytes create an osmotic force for the influx of water into the lumen. The combination of excessive fluids and increased intestinal motility causes diarrhea.

B. **Principles of ruminant gastrointestinal toxicology**

1. The large size of the rumen affects response to oral toxicants. Initial exposure may result in dilution of toxicants and slowing of the rate of absorption.

2. A rumen that is filled with contaminated material is less readily detoxified by means used for monogastric animals.

3. Sampling for toxicologic analysis must consider the heterogeneity of rumen contents and the variable distribution of toxicant within the rumen.

C. **Mechanisms of toxicologic damage.** Toxicants that influence microbial activity or that are influenced by microbial activity are important in ruminant toxicology.

1. **Rumen microorganisms can detoxify some chemicals that are highly toxic to monogastric animals.**
   a. As a result of ruminal degradation, ruminants usually tolerate higher levels of mycotoxins than do nonruminants.
   b. Ruminants are less affected than nonruminants by oxalates in forage plants.
   c. Sheep detoxify pyrrolizidine alkaloids in the rumen more effectively than do cattle or horses.

    d. Phenolic compounds (e.g., gossypol) are better tolerated by ruminants than by monogastric animals.

2. **Rumen microorganisms can produce toxic effects from agents that are relatively nontoxic in monogastric animals.**
   a. Nitrates are reduced to toxic nitrites.
   b. Cyanide is released from cyanogenic glycosides.
   c. Lactic acid is produced by excessive levels of fermentable carbohydrates.
   d. Urea is hydrolyzed to ammonia and carbon dioxide, with a resultant potential for ammonia toxicosis.
   e. Tryptophan in forages is metabolized to 3-methyl indole, which can cause atypical bovine pulmonary emphysema.

BIBLIOGRAPHY

Beasley VR, Dorman DC, Fikes JD, Diana SG: A systems affected approach to small animal toxicology: reference notes for Toxicology VB 320. Urbana, IL, Val R. Beasley, 1993.

Bertram T: Gastrointestinal tract. In *Handbook of Toxicologic Pathology.* Edited by Haschek WM, Rosseaux CG. San Diego, Academic Press, 1991, pp 195–250.

Mozsik G, Snodgrass W: Clinical gastrointestinal toxicology. In *Gastrointestinal Toxicology.* Edited by Rozman K, Hanninen O. Amsterdam, Elsevier Science Publishers, 1986, pp 436–443.

Oehme FW, Barrett DS: Veterinary gastrointestinal toxicology. In *Gastrointestinal Toxicology.* Edited by Rozman K, Hanninen O. Amsterdam, Elsevier Science Publishers, 1986, pp 464–513.

Smith GS: Gastrointestinal toxifications and detoxifications in ruminants in relation to resource management. In *Gastrointestinal Toxicology.* Edited by Rozman K, Hanninen O. Amsterdam, Elsevier Science Publishers, 1986, pp 514–538.

DIRECTIONS: Each of the numbered items or incomplete statements in this section is followed by answers or by completions of the statement. Select the **one** numbered answer or completion that is **best** in each case.

1. A dog ingests liquid bleach. Which emergency treatment is most appropriate?

(1) Voluntary consumption of milk or water
(2) Emesis using apomorphine or dish detergent
(3) Gastric lavage with instillation of activated charcoal
(4) Oral administration of a neutralizing agent
(5) Ibuprofen or acetaminophen to control pain

2. Prostaglandins protect the gastric mucosa by:

(1) providing leukotrienes to repair damaged gastric mucosa.
(2) stimulating secretion of serotonin.
(3) counteracting the effect of lipoxygenase metabolites.
(4) complementing the action of cyclooxygenase inhibitors.
(5) interfering with the chemoreceptor trigger zone, thus preventing the reflux of gastric acids into the esophagus.

3. Castor oil, histamine, and some glycosides stimulate intestinal motility by what common mechanism?

(1) Stimulation of the chemoreceptor trigger zone
(2) Central stimulation of the vagus nerve
(3) Direct stimulation of smooth muscle in the intestine
(4) Release of prostaglandins, which promote inflammatory response
(5) Osmotic effects that attract fluids and stretch the intestine

4. Which one of the following animals is most likely to experience acute diarrhea and colic after administration of broad-spectrum oral antibiotics?

(1) Cat
(2) Dog
(3) Horse
(4) Pig
(5) Rat

5. All of the following substances are likely to induce vomiting *except:*

(1) apomorphine.
(2) ipecac.
(3) ergot alkaloids.
(4) histamine 1 (H_1) antagonists.
(5) cholinesterase inhibitors.

1. The answer is 1 *[II D 1 a]*. The dog should be allowed to consume small amounts of milk or water to dilute the toxicant at the damaged surface. Corrosives (acids, such as household bleach) and caustics (bases, such as oven cleaner) cause severe and direct damage to the pharyngeal and esophageal mucosa that may extend as far as the stomach. Emetics and gastric lavage are contraindicated because the violent contractions of vomiting and the physical trauma of the stomach tube may cause additional damage to the mucosa or even tear the submucosa and muscularis. The use of neutralizing agents (e.g., acids for bases) can produce an exothermic reaction. Neither ibuprofen or acetaminophen would be effective in this acute toxicosis. Measures should be taken to limit the effect of the toxicant.

2. The answer is 3 *[III A 3]*. Prostaglandins promote vasodilation and act to counterbalance the inhibitors of cyclooxygenase (e.g., aspirin, ibuprofen). Cyclooxygenase inhibitors allow lipoxygenase metabolites (e.g., the leukotrienes) to cause vasoconstriction, which leads to local gastric ischemia and subsequent gastric ulceration. Serotonin, which controls vascular dilation and development of edema, is secreted by the gastric mucosa, but not in response to prostaglandins. The chemoreceptor trigger zone, which is not influenced by prostaglandins, is involved with the vomiting reflex.

3. The answer is 3 *[IV B 3 a (3)]*. A variety of natural and endogenous compounds (e.g., castor oil, histamine, some glycosides) stimulate propulsive motility by directly irritating smooth muscle in the intestinal wall. This action initiates peristaltic waves that can speed the rate of chyme through the intestinal tract and may cause diarrhea. Castor oil, histamine, and cardiac or saponin glycosides are not osmotic cathartics (i.e., they do not induce fluid accumulation in the intestinal lumen). Prostaglandins, which increase mucus secretion and stimulate the transfer of water into the intestinal lumen, are endogenous chemicals that can cause diarrhea, but their release is not stimulated by castor oil, histamine, or glycosides. Stimulation of the chemoreceptor trigger zone or the vagal nerve can lead to vomiting.

4. The answer is 3 *[IV B 5]*. Horses and other species that depend heavily on cecal digestion (e.g., guinea pig, gerbil) appear to be more susceptible to the effects of oral antibiotics. Oral antibiotics can disturb the normal cecal or colonic flora and allow proliferation of toxin producers, such as clostridia. In horses, dosages of antibiotics such as tetracycline or lincomycin that are well-tolerated by other species can induce acute colic and diarrhea that may be fatal.

5. The answer is 4 *[III B 1 a (2) (a) (ii)]*. The chemoreceptor trigger zone is well supplied with receptors for acetylcholine (ACh), histamine 1 (H_1), and dopamine; therefore, H_1 antagonists would be least likely to induce vomiting. Cholinesterase inhibitors, which allow the excessive accumulation of ACh, stimulate vomiting. Apomorphine is a dopaminergic agonist and is an effective emetic. Ipecac stimulates vomiting by direct irritation of the stomach wall and stimulation of the chemoreceptor trigger zone. High dosages of ergot alkaloids directly stimulate the vomiting center in the central nervous system (CNS).

Chapter 11
Toxicology of the Respiratory System

I. INTRODUCTION

A. **Structure and function of the respiratory system.** The unique structure and function of the respiratory system render it susceptible to damage by toxicants (Figure 11-1).

1. **Structure**
   a. **Surface area.** The alveolar surface area can be as large as 1 m^2/kg body weight. It is the largest surface area of the body exposed to the environment, providing a substantial surface for toxicant contact and absorption.
   b. **Blood–gas barrier (alveolar–capillary membrane).** Respiratory airways and alveolar epithelium are in direct contact with environmental toxicants in air. Furthermore, in the lung, only the alveolar epithelium and capillary endothelium separate the blood from contaminated environmental air.
   c. **Cell types.** Five cell types are important in pulmonary toxicology (Figure 11-2).
      (1) **Type I alveolar cells** are squamous or membranous pneumocytes that are joined to one another by tight junctions known as zonula occludens. They resemble capillary endothelium.
         (a) **Function.** Type I alveolar cells, which line the alveolar spaces, are the only barrier between the ambient air and the capillary endothelium.
         (b) **Structure.** Type I alveolar cells have very little cytoplasm and few organelles. The large surface area and high membrane:cytoplasm ratio make them vulnerable to direct membrane damage.
      (2) **Type II alveolar cells** (known as large or granular pneumocytes) have a rough endoplasmic reticulum and many Golgi and multilamellar inclusions known as cytosomes.
         (a) **Functions**
            (i) Type II alveolar cells **synthesize surfactant,** which reduces surface active forces, stabilizes alveoli, and permits inflation of small alveoli at low pulmonary air pressures.
            (ii) Type II alveolar cells **act as stem cells** for type I alveolar epithelium. When type I cells are destroyed, type II cells, which are more resistant, proliferate to cover the alveolar surface. Approximately 2 days are required for replacement of type I cells with type II cells. Immature type II cells are cuboidal and transfer oxygen more slowly than type I cells.
            (iii) Type II alveolar cells **form part of the blood–gas barrier** in the alveoli.
         (b) **Structure.** Type II cells are attenuated in size. Although they constitute 60% of the cells in the alveoli, they are responsible for less than 10% of the surface area.
      (3) **Pulmonary alveolar macrophages** are phagocytic cells found throughout the alveoli.
         (a) **Function.** The primary function of macrophages is **particulate phagocytosis**.
         (b) When overloaded, these cells die and release acid hydrolases and phospholipases, which stimulate fibroblasts and lead to fibrosis in the lung.
      (4) **Clara cells** are nonciliated bronchiolar cells located only in small (terminal) bronchioles.
         (a) **Functions**
            (i) **Secretion,** although this function is not well documented

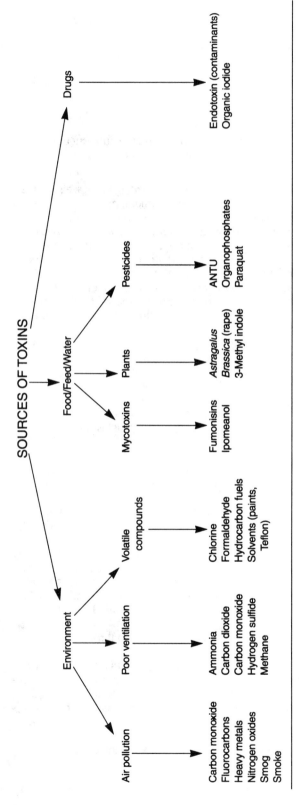

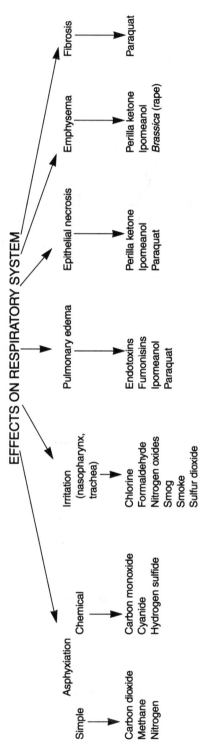

FIGURE 11-1. Overview of toxicants and their effects on the respiratory system. The respiratory system is prone to damage from toxicants because of the diverse functions it performs for the body.

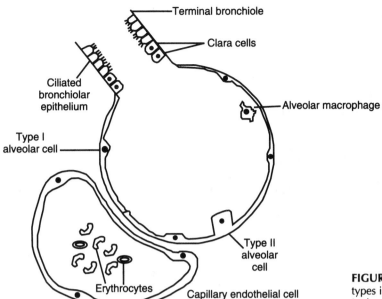

FIGURE 11-2. Major cellular types important to pulmonary toxicology.

(ii) **Xenobiotic metabolism** via cytochrome P-450, which is found in relatively high concentration in Clara cells

(b) Clara cells are **often a target cell for pulmonary toxicants**.

(5) **Endothelial cells** form the pulmonary capillaries. Functions include:

(a) Formation of a blood–gas diffusion barrier

(b) Maintenance of active transport systems

(c) Uptake and metabolism of pesticides (e.g., paraquat) and other xenobiotics

(d) Conversion of angiotensin I to angiotensin II (a potent vasoconstrictor) via enzymes

(e) Synthesis and metabolism of prostaglandins

2. **Functions**

a. **Gas exchange.** Respiration involves the transport of gas to and from the body cells.

(1) **Circulation.** The lung receives the entire cardiac output via the pulmonary artery; within 1 minute, the lung receives 1–5 times the body's circulating blood volume.

(a) **Toxicants from ambient air** are quickly absorbed from the lungs and cause systemic effects as well as local pulmonary effects.

(b) **Toxicants in the systemic circulation** reach the lungs quickly and in high concentration.

(2) **Excretion.** Because the lung functions as an excretory organ, volatile toxicants in the blood enter the alveoli. The lung rapidly clears nonionized compounds, especially those that are volatile and lipophilic (e.g., hydrocarbons such as gasoline).

b. **Movement of particulate materials** is enhanced by the cells and secretions of the respiratory tract.

(1) **Cilia** in the tracheobronchial region provide physical transport of particles back to the nasopharyngeal region.

(2) **Mucous secretions of goblet cells** in the trachea and nasopharynx provide a fluid medium for transport of particles.

(3) **Macrophages** phagocytose and immobilize particles, keeping them away from the respiratory epithelium.

(4) **Lymphatics** conduct particles away from the lung and into the systemic circulation.

    c. Regulatory functions of the lung may be affected by pulmonary damage. Lung damage that alters angiotensin, biogenic amines, and prostaglandin levels can cause inflammation within the lung and changes in pulmonary blood pressure, leading to ventilation–perfusion abnormalities and the loss of hemodynamic and electrolyte homeostasis.

B. **Important considerations in pulmonary toxicology**

    1. Type and amount of toxicant. The pulmonary response depends on the type and amount of toxicant.

    2. Form of toxicant. Exposure considerations are different for toxic vapors, as compared with particulates. The terms **"gas"** and **"vapor"** are often used interchangeably. Vapors normally exist in the liquid or solid phase at 20°C and normal atmospheric pressures, whereas a gas is not able to exist in the liquid phase at 20°C. Therefore, under normal conditions, "gases" are substances usually present in the gaseous phase, and "vapors" are the gaseous phase of a material more likely to exist in the liquid or solid phase.

II. **RESPIRATORY EXPOSURE TO TOXIC GASES AND VAPORS**

A. **Upper respiratory system (i.e., nasopharynx, larynx, trachea, bronchi)**

    1. Exposure. Goblet cells, which synthesize and secrete mucus, and **ciliated cells,** which assist in the movement of mucus toward the larynx, are found in the epithelial lining of the trachea, bronchi, and bronchioles. Although both cell types are affected by upper airway exposure to toxicants, ciliated cells are usually more sensitive than goblet cells.

    a. Ciliated cells. Compromised ciliary activity reduces the respiratory system's ability to clear bacteria and phagocytes from the lungs and may result in secondary infections.

        (1) Some gases inhibit ciliary action without causing cytotoxicity (e.g., cigarette smoke).

        (2) Ciliary action may be tested by measuring the clearance of nonpathogenic bacteria or iron particles from the lungs and tracheobronchial passages.

    b. Goblet cells. Mucous secretion may be influenced by extracellular factors; for example, vitamin A affects mucous epithelium activity, and cholinergic stimulation enhances mucus production.

    2. Clinical consequences. The upper respiratory tract is primarily affected by water-soluble irritants.

    a. Bronchoconstriction is a very common, acute response of the bronchial smooth muscle to irritant gases (e.g., sulfur dioxide, ammonia). It may also occur as an allergic response.

        (1) Reduced airway diameter increases resistance to airflow.

        (2) Atropine may be used to partially counteract bronchoconstriction.

    b. Watery eyes, upper respiratory inflammation, laryngospasm, sneezing, and **coughing** occur with upper respiratory irritants.

B. **Lower respiratory system (i.e., bronchioles, lungs)**

    1. Local implications. Relatively insoluble irritants reach the lung and induce inflammation, necrosis, or both in the bronchioles and alveoli.

    a. Exposure. In addition to inhalation, excretion of volatile compounds through the lung can be a route of pulmonary exposure to toxicants.

        (1) Volatile solvents (e.g., benzene, carbon tetrachloride) are excreted via the lung based on differential partial pressures between the capillary blood and the alveolar air.

        (2) Toxic intermediates (see also IV A–B). The lung, as well as the liver, may metabolize compounds to more active (i.e., toxic) intermediates via cytochrome

P-450 and other mixed function oxidases (MFOs). Toxic intermediates bind to pulmonary macromolecules, resulting in membrane damage or necrosis. For example, paraquat herbicide binds to lung tissue and generates active oxygen radicals.

b. Clinical consequences

(1) Distal airways. The transitional region between the bronchiole and alveolus is particularly **sensitive to oxidants** (e.g., ozone, nitrogen dioxide).

(2) Parenchyma. Direct irritation of air passages leads to acute inflammation, which either resolves or progresses to chronic inflammation with proliferation of macrophages and fibrosis. Severe damage to airway epithelium can result in epithelial necrosis, increased permeability, and intraluminal edema.

(a) Necrosis and the **replacement of type I alveolar cells with type II pneumocytes,** which are thicker and less effective for gas exchange, result from damage to alveolar epithelial cells.

(b) Emphysema (alveolar decompartmentalization) result from the destruction of elastin in alveolar walls. Neutrophils have elastase activity, which attacks alveolar walls and leads to alveolar rupture and decompartmentalization.

(c) Fibrosis, which is the production of collagenous connective tissue, occurs in response to inflammation or chronic irritation. Fibrosis leads to chronic constriction of the airways and loss of compliance in the lung parenchyma.

(d) Edema can result from damaged capillary endothelium with leakage of fluid to the lung interstitium. However, edema more often result from systemic exposure to an endothelial toxicant.

2. Systemic implications

a. Exposure. Diffusion is the dominant mechanism for the uptake of toxic gases by the bloodstream. The **concentration of gas** in the inspired air is the driving force for diffusion.

(1) Henry's law describes the transfer of a solute from a gas phase and states that "When a liquid and a gas remain in contact, the weight of the gas that dissolves in a given quantity of liquid is proportional to the pressure of the gas above the liquid."

(2) Permeability. The epithelial and endothelial cell membranes and the presence of mucus and surfactant affect the permeability of the alveolar–capillary membrane to gases and toxicants. If the toxicant does not initially damage the alveolar–capillary membrane, it is usually absorbed and transported via the blood to other locations.

(a) The **solubility of the gas in water** is often a dominant factor in toxicity.

(i) Organic cations and anions are absorbed primarily via aqueous channels (i.e., pores) by simple diffusion.

(ii) Diffusion of water-soluble neutral compounds is dependent on the molecular size of the compound and the pore size in membranes at the absorptive surface.

(b) Lipophilic compound absorption is influenced by the lipid solubility of the toxicant.

(i) Moderately lipid-soluble agents move rapidly to blood.

(ii) Highly lipid-soluble materials may dissolve in the lipid cell membrane and remain in the lung.

b. Clinical consequences. Asphyxiants deprive tissues of oxygen.

(1) Simple asphyxiants are physiologically inert, but crowd out oxygen. Twenty to thirty percent concentration in ambient air causes serious clinical effects.

(a) Common simple asphyxiants include nitrogen, hydrogen, methane, carbon dioxide, and helium.

(b) Clinical effects are hyperpnea, cyanosis, and excitement, followed by depression and death.

(2) Chemical asphyxiants interfere with oxygen transport or utilization.

(a) The mechanisms and lesions are not in the respiratory system, but the **route of exposure** is respiratory.

      (b) Clinical effects are seen primarily in the central nervous system (CNS) and the cardiovascular system.

      (c) Common chemical asphyxiants are carbon monoxide, cyanide, nitrogen dioxide, and hydrogen sulfide.

C. **Estimating exposure to toxic gases.** Calculation of the animal's exposure to volatile agents can be used to estimate the dosage received.

    1. Necessary data

      a. Vapor pressure of the agent (i.e., a measure of the tendency of a material to volatilize; usually given in mm Hg)

      b. Atmospheric pressure (760 mm Hg at sea level)

      c. Molecular weight (MW) of the agent

      d. Molar volume of the agent, which is the volume of air containing one mole of a compound at a specified temperature (e.g., 22.4 L at 0° C or 24.5 L at 25° C)

      e. Molar fraction, which equals the vapor pressure divided by the atmospheric pressure, multiplied by the molecular weight:

$$\text{Molar fraction} = \text{MW} \times \frac{\text{Vapor pressure}}{\text{Atmospheric pressure}}$$

    2. The **milligrams of agent/L of air (mg/L)** equals:

$$\text{mg/L} = \frac{\text{Molar fraction (gm)}}{\text{Molar volume (L)}} \times \frac{10^3 \text{ mg}}{\text{gm}}$$

    3. Mg/L must be converted to mg/m^3, which is a common expression of the concentration of toxic gases:

$$\text{mg/m}^3 = \text{mg/L} \times 10^3 \text{ L/m}^3$$

    4. To determine exposure, the **tidal volume** and **respiratory rate** for the species of interest are used to calculate the potential daily dosage received by the animal for a volatile compound present at a given concentration.

      a. For a 1200-lb (544-kg) cow, the tidal volume is 3.5 L and the respiratory rate is 20 respirations/min. Therefore, the 24-hour respiratory volume is 100,800 L, or 100.8 m^3 (3.5 L × 20 respirations/min x 60 min/hr × 24 hr/day).

      b. If the air concentration of the toxicant is 1.0 mg/m^3, then 1.0 mg/m^3 × 100.8 m^3 = 100.8 mg/cow/day. The dosage equals 100.8 mg/day divided by the weight of the cow (544 kg), or 0.185 mg/kg/day.

    5. Conversion of gas concentrations. In some cases, analytical data is given in one set of terminology and toxicologic data is given in another. To compare the two, conversion to common units must be made. To derive mg/L [parts per million (PPM)] from milligrams per cubic meter (mg/m^3), the following equation is used:

$$\text{PPM} = \frac{\text{mg/m}^3 \times \text{molar volume of the gas}}{\text{molecular weight of the gas}}$$

Rearranging the formula gives:

$$\text{mg/m}^3 = \frac{\text{PPM} \times \text{molecular weight of the gas}}{\text{molar volume of the gas}}$$

III. RESPIRATORY EXPOSURE TO PARTICULATES

A. **Forms of particulates.** Particulate materials are complex and may be heterogeneous mixtures.

1. **Aerosols** are relatively stable suspensions of solid particles or liquid droplets in a gaseous medium. Gases or vapors may adsorb to the surface of aerosol droplets.
   a. **Dust** is solid particles formed by grinding, milling, or blasting. Dusts are identical in composition to the parent material.
   b. **Fumes** are formed by combustion, sublimation, or condensation and often differ in chemical composition from the parent material.
      (1) Often fumes are metal oxides or hydrides; their toxic effects may differ from those of the parent metal.
      (2) Particulate size is small, ranging from 10 Å to 0.1 μm.
      (3) Fumes tend to aggregate and produce larger particles with age.
   c. **Smoke** is a combustion product of organic materials. Smoke particles are usually less than 0.5 μm in size and they do not settle readily.
   d. **Mist (fog)** is a liquid aerosol usually associated with particulate nuclei in air.

2. **Smog** is a complex mixture of particles and gases in the atmosphere, formed by irradiation of automobile exhaust and other combustion products including photochemical oxidants (e.g., nitrogen oxides, ozone).

B. **Deposition of particulates** in the respiratory tract is affected by the morphology and density of the particles, as well as patterns of airflow.

1. **Particle size**
   a. Particle size of a population of particles is usually described as the **median diameter** and its standard deviation.
   b. Particle size is **critical in determining regional deposition of particulates** in the respiratory tract (Figure 11-3). Inhaled particles under natural clinical and environmental circumstances are heterogeneous in size and occur in a nearly normal distribution.
      (1) Particles measuring **5–30 μm** in diameter deposit in the **nasopharynx** via **interception** and **impaction**.
         (a) **Interception** occurs when the trajectory of a particle allows the edge of the particle to contact the surface. Fibers such as asbestos are deposited by interception.

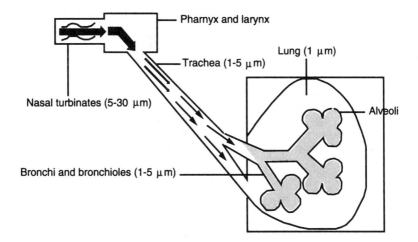

FIGURE 11-3. Schematic representation of particulate deposition in the respiratory tract. Large particles (as indicated by the *width of the arrows*) enter the nasal turbinates at high velocity. In the nasopharynx, the particles make an abrupt directional change. The size range for particles, which helps to determine where they are deposited in the lung, is indicated in *parentheses*. As air passes through the trachea to the lung, larger particles are arrested by interception or impaction. In the bronchi, bronchioles, and alveoli, smaller particles are stopped by sedimentation as the air velocity slows.

    (b) Impaction results from the inertia of large particles in a bending airstream. They travel in a nearly straight path until a bifurcation or other impediment is encountered.

    (2) Particles measuring **1–5 μm** in diameter deposit in the **trachea** and **bronchi** via **sedimentation (settling out)**. Sedimentation takes place primarily in the bronchi, bronchioles, and alveoli when gravity overcomes buoyancy and air resistance and when velocity is reduced in the lower airways.

    (3) Particles measuring less than 1 μm in diameter reach the **alveoli** and may be absorbed by diffusion following alveolar cell contact.

  2. Morphology. Nonspherical particles are affected by aerodynamic drag and deposit differentially in various parts of the respiratory tract.

  3. Airflow patterns. The direction and velocity of airflow in the respiratory tract influence the deposition of particles.

    a. Quiet breathing and a large anatomical dead space generally reduce deposition.

    b. Exercise, and the resultant high velocity of air movement, increase airway impaction and sedimentation.

    c. Breath holding increases sedimentation and diffusion.

C. **Clearance of particulates** occurs via physical and cellular mechanisms.

  1. Mucociliary transport, the primary form of particulate clearance in the upper respiratory tract, moves particles to the nasopharynx at rates of 7 mm/min in the nose and trachea and 1 mm/min in the upper bronchial tree.

    a. Retrograde mucociliary clearance from the bronchioles (i.e., the lower respiratory tract) occurs at a rate of 0.5 mm/min.

    b. Materials moved to the nasopharynx are either **swallowed or expectorated;** therefore, **respiratory exposure can result in oral exposure as well**.

  2. Phagocytosis of particles by macrophages takes place in the bronchi and alveoli.

    a. Macrophages migrate to the bronchi from the alveoli; after phagocytosing the foreign particles, they are cleared by mucociliary transport.

    b. In the alveoli, macrophages phagocytose particles. Clearance takes place via the lymphatics.

  3. Dissolution of particles and removal by blood or lymph occur in the lungs.

  4. Sequestration of particles involves the alveolar septal cells.

D. **Clinical consequences**

  1. Pneumoconiosis is the pathologic response of the lung to particulates. The lesion consists of **focal accumulations of macrophages** and, in severe cases, **fibrosis**.

    a. Activated macrophages are believed to **release cytokines** (e.g., IL-1) and other growth factors that attract fibroblasts, leading to **fibroplasia**.

    b. Fibrosis can occur when macrophages that have phagocytosed particles die, releasing acid hydrolases and phospholipids that damage cell membranes.

  2. Carcinogenesis is believed to be a response to chronic covalent binding and DNA damage in the lung.

IV. **METABOLIC BASIS FOR LUNG DAMAGE.** Like certain liver cells, certain lung cells have microsomal mixed function oxidases that can activate xenobiotics to toxic intermediates.

A. **Three models of bioactivation** have been described by Boyd:

  1. A toxin is activated in the liver, and then carried by the blood to the lung. For example, pyrrolizidine alkaloids are metabolized to reactive pyrrole metabolites in the liver; they then bind to both liver and lung cells.

2. Cyclic reduction and oxidation of compounds take place, leading to a high rate of consumption of cellular cofactors [e.g., reduced nicotinamide adenine dinucleotide (NADH), reduced nicotinamide adenine dinucleotide phosphate (NADPH)], depletion of reducing equivalents (e.g., glutathione), and generation of highly reactive oxygen radicals. The herbicide paraquat produces its toxic effects in this manner.

3. The ultimate active metabolite may be generated directly within the lung itself, and then covalent binding to lung microsomal proteins takes place. The toxin 4-ipomeanol, which is produced by *Fusarium solani* growing in molded sweet potatoes, is an example of a toxin that operates in this manner.

B. **Location.** Most lung bioactivation takes place in the Clara cells and some type II alveolar cells.

C. **Clinical consequences.** Chemical toxicants induce peroxidative membrane damage or covalent binding of pulmonary macromolecules. Principal effects are **acute pulmonary edema, proliferation of type II alveolar epithelium,** and **pulmonary fibrosis.**

V. EXAMPLES OF ACUTE PULMONARY TOXICANTS

A. **Perilla ketone,** produced by the purple mint plant (*Perilla frutescens*)

B. **Fumonisin B$_1$,** a mycotoxin produced by *Fusarium moniliforme* or *F. proliferatum,* which causes acute pulmonary edema in swine

C. **ANTU** (alpha naphthyl thio urea), an obsolete rodenticide

D. **Endotoxin** in some species, including pigs, ruminants, and horses

BIBLIOGRAPHY

Beasley VR, Dorman DC, Fikes JD: *A Systems Affected Approach to Veterinary Toxicology: Reference Notes for Toxicology VB 320.* Urbana, IL, Val R. Beasley, 1990, pp 731–756.

Boyd EH: *Environmental Health Perspectives* 55:47–51, 1984.

Gordon T, Amdur MO: Responses of the Respiratory System to Toxic Agents. In *Casarett and Doull's Toxicology: The Basic Science of Poisons,* 4th ed. Edited by Amdur MO, Doull J, Klaassen CD. New York, Pergamon Press, 1991, pp 383–406.

Osweiler GD, Carson TL, Buck WB, Van Gelder GA: *Clinical and Diagnostic Toxicology,* 3rd ed. Dubuque, IA, Kendall Hunt, 1985, pp 363–378.

STUDY QUESTIONS

DIRECTIONS: Each of the numbered items or incomplete statements in this section is followed by answers or by completions of the statement. Select the **one** numbered answer or completion that is **best** in each case.

1. How many cell layers continuously separate alveolar air from pulmonary capillary circulation?

(1) One: the alveolar epithelium
(2) Two: the alveolar epithelium and capillary endothelium
(3) Two: the alveolar epithelium and alveolar macrophages
(4) Three: the alveolar epithelium, alveolar macrophages, and capillary endothelium
(5) Three: the alveolar epithelium, fibroblasts, and capillary endothelium

2. Which mechanism is most essential to clearing particulate toxicants from the tracheobronchial tree?

(1) Ciliary action
(2) Pinocytosis
(3) Active transport
(4) Autophagy
(5) Mucus production

3. All of the following data are used to calculate an estimated concentration of volatile toxicant in the air *except* the:

(1) atmospheric pressure.
(2) lipid solubility of the toxicant.
(3) molecular weight (MW) of the toxicant.
(4) molar volume of the toxicant at the temperature of exposure.
(5) vapor pressure of the toxicant.

DIRECTIONS: Each group of items in this section consists of numbered options followed by a set of numbered items. For each item, select the **one** numbered option that is most closely associated with it. Each numbered option may be selected once, more than once, or not at all.

Questions 4–8

Match each function with the cell type that performs it.

(1) Type I pneumocyte
(2) Type II pneumocyte
(3) Clara cell
(4) Alveolar macrophage
(5) Capillary endothelium

4. Plays a major role in the removal of dusts and aerosols

5. Metabolizes foreign compounds delivered to the lung

6. Synthesizes surfactant

7. Forms over 90% of the alveolar epithelium

8. Acts as a precursor

ANSWERS AND EXPLANATIONS

1. The answer is 2 *[I A 1 b; Figure 11-1]*. At the alveolar level, inhaled gases are separated from pulmonary blood by only the capillary endothelium and the alveolar epithelium. The lack of connective tissue or significant interstitial tissue allows for relatively free exchange of gases by simple diffusion. The alveolar macrophages that may line the alveoli are mobile and are not a continuous barrier. Most of the alveolar surface is covered by type I epithelial cells, which have very little cytoplasm and few organelles and are joined to one another by tight junctions known as zonula occludens.

2. The answer is 1 *[II A 1]*. Both goblet cells, which produce mucus, and ciliated bronchiolar cells play a role in the clearance of particulates from the tracheobronchial tree; however, ciliary action is essential for facilitating the rapid movement of particles to proximal areas of the respiratory tract (i.e., the nasopharyngeal region) where they are swallowed or expectorated. Pinocytosis is the uptake of liquids by cells. Active transport functions in the endothelial lining of the pulmonary capillaries as a means of transferring substances from the capillaries to the alveoli. Autophagy is the consumption of damaged organelles within the cell.

3. The answer is 2 *[II C 1 a–d]*. It is not necessary to know the lipid solubility of the toxicant in order to estimate the concentration of a volatile toxicant in the air. The concentration of a volatile toxicant in air depends on the equilibrium between the agent and the surrounding air. The vapor pressure is a primary determinant of the tendency of the compound to volatilize. The ratio of the vapor pressure to the atmospheric pressure is multiplied by the molecular weight (MW) to determine the amount of a compound that is likely to be present as a gas (i.e., the molar fraction). The molar fraction represents a weight, which, when divided by the molar volume (i.e., the number of liters of air that contain a mole of gas), gives the grams of material per liter of air. This unit of measure is commonly converted to mg/L. Measuring or estimating the concentration of toxicant in the air is the first step in being able to estimate exposure to toxic gases.

4–8. The answers are 4-4 *[I A 1 c (3); III D 1]*, **5-3** *[I A 1 c (4)]*, **6-2** *[I A 1 c (2) (a) (i)]*, **7-1** *[I A 1 c (1)]*, **8-2** *[I A 1 c (2) (a) (ii)]*. Alveolar macrophages are phagocytic cells (i.e., they engulf foreign particles that reach the lungs). Large particles that reach the bronchioles or alveoli are phagocytosed and then delivered by migrating macrophages to the lymphatics, where they are physically removed from the lung. Active macrophages that are heavily loaded with particulates may die and release acid hydrolases and phospholipases, attracting fibroblasts and causing excessive fibroplasia in the lung. Fibroplasia may interfere with pulmonary compliance, compromising respiratory function.

Clara cells are nonciliated cells in the small bronchioles that contain a relatively high concentration of cytochrome P-450. Therefore, they are equipped to metabolize xenobiotics, and they may bioactivate chemicals to a more active or more toxic form. They are often a target for pulmonary toxicants.

Type II alveolar epithelial cells synthesize surfactant, which reduces surface tension, stabilizes the alveoli, and allows the inflation of small alveoli at low air pressures. In addition, type II alveolar cells act as stem cells (precursors) for type I alveolar cells, which are the primary cellular components of the alveolar epithelial lining.

Chapter 12

Toxicology of the Reproductive System

I. INTRODUCTION

A. Reproductive failure in veterinary medicine presents a significant **economic problem**. Animals are commonly culled from the herd because of poor reproductive performance.

B. **Suspected causes of reproductive failure** include infectious disease, poor nutrition, adverse weather, hormonal imbalances, stress, and exposure to toxicants. The complex relationships among these factors complicate clinical diagnosis and reproductive toxicology research.

II. MALE REPRODUCTIVE SYSTEM

A. Functions

1. **Spermatogenesis** takes place in the **testes**.
   a. **Spermatocytogenesis** is the process by which **spermatogonia** develop into **spermatocytes** and then into **spermatids**. During spermatocytogenesis, the spermatocytes undergo **meiosis,** a specialized cell division that produces spermatids containing a random sample of one-half the normal somatic complement of chromosomes.
   b. **Spermiogenesis** is the development of spermatids into **spermatozoa.**
      (1) A **tail** is added to facilitate movement in the female reproductive tract.
      (2) The **acrosome,** a specialized organelle, is added to assist in penetration of the oocyte.
      (3) **Mitochondria** develop in the spermatid to provide the energy that is needed to sustain life and complete fertilization.

2. **Fertilization.** During fertilization, the chromosomes of the spermatozoon combine with those of the oocyte to produce a full set of chromosomes.

3. **Synthesis**
   a. **Androgens.** The male reproductive system produces androgens, which promote masculinization. **Testosterone** is produced by **Leydig cells,** clustered epithelioid cells found in the testicular interstitium.
   b. **Proteins.** Sertoli cells, which line the seminiferous tubules, synthesize numerous proteins (e.g., androgen-binding proteins and others for which a function is not known).
   c. **Trophic substances.** Sertoli cells also produce large amounts of lactates, pyruvates, and α-keto acids that are used by spermatocytes.

B. Exposure to toxicants

1. **Biotransformation** of toxicants can interfere with both spermatogenesis and steroid production. However, cytochrome P-450, mixed function oxidases (MFOs), and epoxide-degrading enzymes are present in low levels in the seminiferous tubules.

2. **Blood–testis barrier.** The blood–testis barrier, which is formed by myoid cells and tight junctions between Sertoli cells, prevents free access of drugs and toxicants to the seminiferous tubules.

  a. The barrier is less developed in immature animals.
  b. Leydig cells are not part of the barrier and may be unprotected from toxicant exposure.

C. **Mechanisms of toxicologic damage.** Toxicants that impair spermatogenesis or the physical delivery of spermatozoa to the oocyte can interfere with reproduction (Table 12-1).

  1. Inhibition of cell division or differentiation
  a. Toxicants may affect stem cells or developing spermatogonia.
  b. Cell death or mutation (see IV) result.

  2. Inhibition of intermediary metabolism. Because spermatozoa are actively motile, they have high energy requirements, making them highly susceptible to inhibitors of intermediary metabolism.

  3. Interference with androgen production
  a. A reduced testosterone level **impairs the function of Sertoli cells,** which may in turn provide less nutrition and developmental support to the developing spermatocytes.
  b. Reduced testosterone production can **reduce secondary sexual characteristics and libido,** which are important factors in the behavioral aspect of male reproduction.

III. FEMALE REPRODUCTIVE SYSTEM

A. **Functions**

  1. Oogenesis (i.e., the formation of an oocyte with a haploid number of chromosomes) takes place in the ovary. **Ovarian follicles** contain oocytes in various stages of development surrounded by follicular epithelium. One or more of these follicles undergo changes that lead to **ovulation.**

  2. Implantation, placentation, and gestation. Cyclic endocrine function maintains a receptive environment for fertilization and implantation, and promotes placental development to supply nutrients and oxygen to the growing fetus.

  3. Birth and perinatal support through weaning. Hormonal preparation for birth and lactation (e.g., the release of relaxin and prolactin, respectively) takes place.

B. **Effects of toxicants on fertility** (see Table 12-1)

  1. Interference with normal ovarian function
  a. Impaired gonadotropin secretion interrupts the trophic and cyclic influences on normal ovarian function.
    (1) Food deprivation or starvation, which reduces energy levels, inhibits secretion of gonadotropins [e.g., luteinizing hormone (LH), follicle-stimulating hormone (FSH)].
    (2) Stress that leads to epinephrine secretion stimulates corticosteroid secretion, leading to reduced LH secretion.
    (3) Estrogens or estrogenic toxicants impair gonadotropin release and inhibit activity of the ovary.
      (a) In addition to suppressing ovulation, estrogens stimulate activity in the uterus and vagina. Estrogenic effects include uterine enlargement and edema, endometrial hyperplasia, increased myometrial activity, vaginal squamous metaplasia, and vaginal epithelial keratinization.
      (b) DDT and its metabolites cause eggshell thinning in raptors and have been associated with delayed estrus and fewer eggs laid.
  b. Impaired follicular development occurs when toxicants damage the oocyte or interfere with the ability of follicular (granulosa) cells to proliferate.

TABLE 12-1. Toxicants that Affect Reproduction in Animals

Affected Function	Toxicant
Male fertility	
Spermatogenesis	Antineoplastic drugs (alkylating agents)
	Chlorinated napthalenes
	Cottonseed (gossypol)
	Astragalus species (swainsonine, locoweed)
Testicular degeneration	Cadmium
Secondary sexual traits	Estrogens (estradiol, zearalenone)
Female fertility	
Oogenesis or estrus cycle suppression	Androgens (e.g., testosterone)
	Astragalus species
	Estrogens (benzene hexachloride, coumesterol, estradiol, o,p-DDT, zearalenone)
	Estrus-synchronizing drugs
	Progesterone
Early embryonic death or prevention of implantation	Ammonia nitrogen from high dietary nitrogen
	Astragalus species
	Estrogens (swine)
	Lead
	Veratrum californicum (false hellebore)
Abortion	*Astragalus* species
	Carbon monoxide
	Corticosteroids
	Dicumarol
	Fumonisins
	Gutierrezia species (broom snakeweed)
	Iva augustifolia (sumpweed)
	Lead
	Lupinus species (lupine, bluebonnet)
	Nitrate/nitrite
	Pinus ponderosa (ponderosa pine)
	Selenium
	Veratrum californicum (false hellebore)
Prolonged gestation	*Acremonium coenophialum* endophyte infection of fescue pastures
	Veratrum californicum (false hellebore)
Agalactia	*Acremonium coenophialum* infection of fescue pastures
	Claviceps species (ergot alkaloids)
Developmental or teratogenic effects	*Acremonium coenophialum* infection of fescue pastures
	Astragalus species
	Conium maculatum (poison hemlock)
	Halogenated dioxins
	Mercury (organic alkyl mercury)
	Nicotiana species (tobacco)
	Pinus ponderosa
	Selenium
	Veratrum californicum

2. **Interference with implantation.** Toxicants that alter uterine secretions may interfere with successful implantation of fertilized ova.

  a. **Zearalenone mycotoxins and other estrogens** may interrupt the necessary secretory responses that normally occur in the fallopian tubes and uterus just prior to implantation.

  b. **High protein diets for dairy cows** have been associated with reduced viability of fertilized embryos, apparently as a result of elevated ammonia levels in blood and uterine secretions.

3. **Stillbirth.** Toxicants that result in stillbirth (i.e., the antepartum death of an animal that is alive at the start of birth) are **rare**. Death often occurs during delivery as a result of fetal ischemia or anoxia.

4. **Extension of the postpartum interval.** Failure to return to estrus after the young are weaned is a form of reproductive failure that reduces the lifetime reproductive capacity of the dam. Common causes of increased postpartum interval include:
   a. **Abortion** (see III C 2 c (3)) with associated **uterine infection**
   b. **Extended lactation time**
   c. **Inadequate nutrition during lactation**
   d. **Ingestion of toxic plants,** including *Veratrum californicum* by sheep and *Lupinus* species by cattle
   e. **Zearalenone mycotoxin** and other estrogens in swine
   f. **Recombinant bovine somatotropin (rBST),** which has been associated with an increased postpartum nonpregnant period ("days open") in dairy cows with high milk production. The increase in days open may be caused by the increased milk production stimulated by rBST.
   g. **Hormonal implants, plant estrogens,** and **estrus-synchronizing agents** (e.g., the use of a thyroprotein feed additive during hot weather may cause infertility)

C. Effects of toxicants on embryonic and fetal development

1. **Exposure.** Toxicants that cross the placental barrier affect fetal growth or survival. Toxicant access to developing tissues depends on the nature of the chemical and the character of the maternal–fetal placenta. More complex placentas (e.g., the multilayered placenta of higher animals) make it more difficult for xenobiotics to gain access to the fetus.
   a. Except for radiation, maternal exposure to chemicals allows access to the fetus **through normal pathways** in the maternal body [e.g., orally ingested toxicants pass from the blood to the liver (metabolism) to the blood to the placenta to the fetus].
   b. **Placental barrier**
      (1) Chemicals are **absorbed across the cell membranes and intercellular junctions of the placenta** according to the common physical and chemical principles of absorption (e.g., molecular size, lipophilic nature, polarity, ionization).
      (2) **Xenobiotic metabolism** may occur in the placenta by mechanisms similar to those in the liver, but the amount of metabolic activity is usually less in the placenta.
   c. **Absence of toxic effects in the mother does not preclude toxic accumulation in the fetus.** For example, mercury exposure may not cause severe clinical signs in the mother, but mercury may accumulate in the fetus causing developmental defects because of the fetus' high requirement for protein synthesis.

2. **Outcomes**
   a. **Reduced fetal growth** may result from impaired fetal nutrition or from exposure to toxicants during the second and third trimester of gestation.
   b. **Teratogenesis** is the development of nonlethal structural or functional defects in the fetus. The typical dose–response curve for teratogens is very steep, presumably because the fetus has fewer detoxification mechanisms and less functional reserve than an adult.
      (1) **Morphologic changes**
         (a) During the stages of cleavage (blastocyst formation) and gastrulation, the probability of toxicants inducing morphologic changes is low. Toxicants usually cause death of the conceptus at this stage.
         (b) Susceptibility to morphologic alterations increases as germ layers begin to differentiate.
         (c) Morphologic changes are more likely to occur during early organogenesis (i.e., late in the first trimester) than when organs are fully differentiated. Each developing organ has a critical period during which it is most susceptible to specific teratogens.

(2) Functional changes affect metabolic or homeostatic processes (e.g., development and activation of a specific enzyme) and occur after organogenesis has taken place. Functional changes can occur without detectable morphologic changes.

    (a) Definitive organ function is usually not complete until after histogenesis (i.e., specific cell differentiation) is complete.

        (i) In the central nervous system (CNS), myelinization and glial proliferation continue after birth for several weeks to months depending on the species.

        (ii) Immunologic competence is not complete at birth. The neonate is dependent largely on maternal antibody obtained from the colostrum. Immunosuppressive chemical exposure late in gestation may reduce immunocompetence in the newborn.

    (b) Xenobiotic metabolism is not fully established at birth, but some capability exists in late gestation.

c. Fetal death

    (1) First trimester. Early fetal death causes delayed return to estrus and fetal resorption.

    (2) Second trimester. Death of more advanced fetuses may result in **mummification** of some or all of a litter. A mummy is the inspissated remains of a fetus after body fluids are resorbed by the uterus.

        (a) Mummification occurs after the beginning of skeletal calcification.

        (b) Few toxic causes of mummification are known, but **mycotoxins** such as zearalenone, ochratoxin, and trichothecenes are associated with increased mummification rates in swine.

    (3) Third trimester. Late fetal death causes **abortion** (i.e., the expulsion of a recognizable dead fetus). The cause of many abortions is unknown.

        (a) Toxicologic causes of abortion. Research involving toxicologic causes of abortion has been limited to a few well-defined agents, primarily **heavy metals** and **poisonous plants**. Known toxic causes of abortion are listed in Table 12-1.

        (b) Discovering the cause of abortion is complicated by several factors, such as:

            (i) Events leading to abortion often take place weeks or months prior to the expulsion of the fetus, and the agent may not be present or detectable in the conceptus at the time of abortion. For example, abortion from nitrites results from fetal anoxia secondary to methemoglobinemia. By the time the fetus is expelled from the uterus, the hemoglobin has returned to normal.

            (ii) Fetal death often precedes uterine expulsion by several days, and autolysis interferes with lesions or recovery of causative agents.

            (iii) Fetal membranes are often not available for examination.

            (iv) Few reliable diagnostic procedures are available to confirm the cause of abortions.

IV. MUTATION

A. **Gene mutations** are changes in the sequence of deoxyribonucleic acid (DNA) within a gene. In veterinary medicine, gene mutations resulting from chemical exposures are rare.

1. Changes are commonly associated with **electrophilic agents** that **covalently bind to DNA.**

2. Specific toxic agents may locate at specific positions on DNA. The type of mutation is determined by where the mutagen binds to the DNA, as well as by the alterations in DNA that the mutagen produces.

3. Gene mutations that occur in germinal cells may be **heritable** (i.e., capable of being passed on to the next generation).
   a. New dominant mutations are likely to be expressed in the next generation.
   b. Dominant mutations that are mild or expressed late in life are less likely to become established in the next generation.

B. **Chromosomal aberrations** are gross alterations of chromosome structure.

C. **Chromosomal numbers**

1. **Aneuploidy** is a deviation from an exact multiple of the haploid number of chromosomes. For example, if the normal diploid chromosome number is 46 (haploid = 23), then 47 chromosomes would be an aneuploid condition.

2. **Polyploidy** is an increase in a complete set of chromosomes (e.g., a change from a diploid to a triploid number of chromosomes).

BIBLIOGRAPHY

Dial GD, Marsh WE, Polson DD, Vaillancourt JP: Reproductive failure: differential diagnosis. In *Diseases of Swine,* 7th ed. Edited by Lehman AD. Ames, IA, Iowa State University Press, 1992, pp 88–137.

James LF, Panter KE, Nielsen DB, Molyneux RJ: The effect of natural toxins on reproduction in livestock. *J Anim Sci* 70:1573–1579, 1992.

Kirkbride CA: Diagnostic approach to abortion in cattle. *Compend Cont Ed Vet Pract* 4:S341–S346, 1982.

Scialli AR: *A Clinical Guide to Reproductive and Developmental Toxicology.* Boca Raton, FL, CRC Press, 1992.

Stabenfeldt GH, Edqvist L: Male reproductive processes. In *Duke's Physiology of Domestic Animals.* Edited by Swenson MJ, Reece WO. Ithaca, NY, Cornell University Press, 1993, pp 665–677.

Stabenfeldt GH, Edqvist L: Female reproductive processes. In *Duke's Physiology of Domestic Animals.* Ithaca, NY, Cornell University Press, 1993, pp 678–709.

STUDY QUESTIONS

DIRECTIONS: Each of the numbered items or incomplete statements in this section is followed by answers or by completions of the statement. Select the **one** numbered answer or completion that is **best** in each case.

1. Which statement about male reproductive function is true?

(1) Meiosis is specialized cell division that produces a random sampling of the normal somatic chromosome number in each spermatid.

(2) The acrosome of a spermatozoon promotes chromosomal rearrangement during meiosis.

(3) Spermatozoa are devoid of mitochondria and depend on metabolic activity from other sources to sustain life.

(4) The blood–testis barrier is a combination of myoid cells and tight junctions between Sertoli cells.

(5) Sertoli cells primarily synthesize steroids, which contribute to penetration of the ovum by the spermatozoa.

2. Which one of the following mycotoxins may increase the postpartum to estrus interval in swine?

(1) Aflatoxin
(2) Deoxynivalenol
(3) Fumonisin
(4) Ochratoxin
(5) Zearalenone

3. During which period of prenatal development is a teratogen most likely to cause a recognizable morphologic defect?

(1) At the blastula to gastrula stage
(2) Early organogenesis
(3) Late organogenesis
(4) During cellular differentiation within organs

4. All of the following effects are a result of estrogens or estrogenic toxicants *except:*

(1) enhanced gonadotropin release.
(2) uterine enlargement.
(3) uterine endometrial hyperplasia.
(4) vaginal squamous metaplasia.
(5) suppression of ovulation.

ANSWERS AND EXPLANATIONS

1. The answer is 4 *[II A 1 a, b (2)—(3), B 2]*. The blood–testis barrier, which prevents free access of drugs and toxicants to the seminiferous tubules, is formed by myoid cells in the basement membrane of seminiferous tubules and the tight junctions between the Sertoli cells. In addition to limiting the passage of xenobiotics into the testis, the blood–testis barrier prevents the leakage of spermatozoa into the testicular interstitium. Meiosis is specialized cell division that produces a random sampling of one-half the normal somatic complement of chromosomes in each spermatid. The acrosome facilitates penetration of the ovum by the spermatozoa. Mitochondria provide the spermatozoa with the energy they require to sustain life and complete fertilization. Sertoli cells synthesize proteins; Leydig cells synthesize steroids.

2. The answer is 5 *[III B 4 e; Table 12-1]*. Zearalenone is the only estrogenic mycotoxin among the choices given. As an estrogen, zearalenone can provide negative feedback to prevent the release of gonadotropin.

3. The answer is 2 *[III C 2 b (1) (c)]*. Developmental defects are most likely to occur as a result of chemical insult during the period of early organogenesis, when cells are relatively undifferentiated and full formation of organs and their characteristics is not complete. Early in gestation (i.e., at the blastula to gastrula stage), chemical toxicants usually interfere with implantation or kill the conceptus.

4. The answer is 1 *[III B 1 a (3)]*. Estrogens or estrogenic toxicants impair, rather than enhance, gonadotropin release. The release of gonadotropin is controlled in part by negative feedback from estrogen. As a result, the failure of gonadotropin-releasing hormone reduces the stimulus for follicle-stimulating hormone (FSH) and continuation of the cycle of ovulation. Uterine enlargement, uterine endometrial hyperplasia, and vaginal squamous metaplasia are classical effects of estrogens, both endogenous and exogenous, and estrogenic substances (e.g., the mycotoxin zearalenone).

Chapter 13
Ocular and Dermal Toxicology

I. INTRODUCTION

A. Both the eyes and the skin are exposed to the environment by direct contact through the air or direct chemical application.

B. Effects of toxic agents affecting the eyes or skin are most often local, but these agents can affect systemic health.

II. EYE

A. **Structure** (Figure 13-1)

1. **Protection and nourishment of the eye**
   a. **Bony orbit.** In most higher mammals, the eye is encased in a bony orbit that protects it from physical damage.
   b. **Sclera.** The sclera, a tough, fibrous covering, ensheathes the globe of the eye (i.e., the eyeball).
      (1) Ocular muscles that move the eye are attached to the sclera.
      (2) The sclera is transparent over the anterior part of the eyeball, allowing light to enter.
   c. **Cornea.** The cornea contributes to the optical capabilities of the eye (see II A 2 a) and is directly exposed to the environment. It is composed of five layers.
      (1) **Corneal epithelium** is flattened at the surface of the cornea, becoming more cuboidal toward the inner side. It is the principal protective layer of the cornea.
         (a) Corneal epithelium is highly impermeable to water-soluble substances.
         (b) Small lipophilic molecules that move via intracellular spaces are most likely to be absorbed by the corneal epithelium.
      (2) **Bowman's membrane** is an acellular layer of collagen and ground substance that interfaces between the epithelium and the stroma.
      (3) The **stroma** consists of collagenous material that is high in water content.
         (a) The stroma accounts for approximately 90% of the corneal thickness.
         (b) Corneal edema occurs in the stroma and produces cloudiness in the cornea.
      (4) **Descemet's membrane** is acellular elastic tissue that acts as a basement membrane for the corneal endothelium.
      (5) **Corneal endothelium** is a single cellular layer with high adenosine triphosphatase (ATPase) content. It supports active transport and the sodium pump that assists in proper hydration of the cornea.
   d. **Conjunctiva** is the membrane that extends from the cornea to the inner side of the eyelid.
      (1) Conjunctiva is squamous, nonkeratinized epithelium with numerous mucus-producing cells for lubrication of the eyelids and cornea.
      (2) **Lacrimal glands** in the conjunctiva contribute a tear film to the epithelial surface of the cornea.
         (a) Tears flush cellular debris and foreign materials from the eye and provide a nutrient and antibacterial medium for the corneal surface.

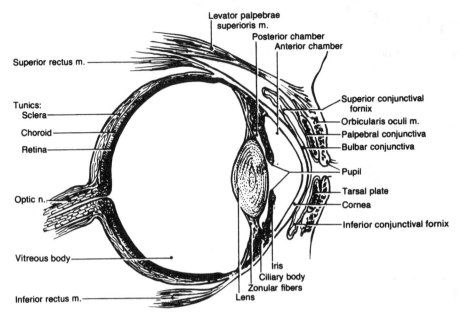

FIGURE 13-1. Anatomy of the eye. (Reprinted with permission from NMS *Anatomy,* 2e. Media, PA, Williams & Wilkins, 1990, p 466.)

        (b) The tear film enhances the optical uniformity of the cornea, which may lack structural uniformity.

    (3) Meibomian glands are specialized glands that secrete a sebaceous substance.

2. Vision
    a. Cornea. The cornea is a transparent refractive structure. Visual acuity depends on optimal tear flow, hydration, and blood supply.
        (1) Epithelial or endothelial damage, changes in ocular pressure, or interference with the sodium–potassium pump can cause corneal edema.
        (2) Changes in corneal curvature and thickness may change the optical properties of the cornea.
    b. Iris. The iris is a specialized, highly vascular, pigmented portion of the cornea that is interposed between the transparent cornea and the lens.
        (1) Aqueous humor surrounds the iris.
            (a) Aqueous humor is actively secreted into the posterior chamber and reaches the anterior chamber through the pupil.
            (b) Ocular pressure from aqueous humor is modulated by drainage through Schlemm's canal. Increased intraocular pressure (known as glaucoma) causes ischemic damage to the optic nerve and may lead to blindness.
        (2) The **pupil** is a variable opening in the iris that controls the amount of light that reaches the lens and the retina. Pupillary size is controlled by the **ciliary muscles** (see II A 2 c).
        (3) Damage to the iris is evident as hyperemia, edema, aqueous flare (i.e., a cloudy appearance caused by protein leakage into aqueous humor), and gross lesions.
    c. Ciliary body and ciliary muscle. The ciliary body and ciliary muscle act in opposition to one another to allow for accommodation of the lens.
        (1) Parasympathomimetic agents reduce the tension on the ciliary body and allow the lens to become more ovoid, thus increasing accommodation.
        (2) Parasympatholytic agents inhibit the action of ciliary muscle and allow the ciliary body to flatten the lens, thus reducing accommodation.
    d. Lens. The lens is an avascular multilamellar transparent body.

(1) The lens is composed primarily of water and protein contained by a collagenous elastic capsule that allows for changes in shape.

(2) Cellular organelles and active transport maintain a high potassium-to-sodium ratio.

e. Vitreous humor is a transparent gelatinous material that fills the eye posterior to the lens.

(1) The vitreous body aids in maintaining the shape and turgor of the eye.

(2) Electrolytes and metabolites (e.g., urea nitrogen) occur in the vitreous humor in characteristic ratios to the serum; therefore, altered serum chemistry may be reflected in the vitreous humor.

f. Retina. The retina is a complex layer of specialized receptor cells (i.e., rods and cones) that contain photosensitive pigments.

(1) Receptor cells synapse with ganglion cells deeper in the retina.

(2) Ganglion cells are the cell bodies of neurons. The axons of the ganglion cells form the optic nerve, which synapses in the lateral geniculate body of the mid-brain.

(3) The retina and optic nerve are differentially affected by a variety of chemicals. For example, the central retina and papillomacular bundle appear resistant to some toxicants that affect peripheral fibers of the optic nerve.

B. **Response to toxicants**

1. Irritation, necrosis, and corneal opacity. Direct irritants primarily affect the conjunctiva and cornea. These agents include acids, alkalies, organic solvents, detergents, lacrimators (e.g., Mace, pepper), and smog.

a. Acids

(1) The ability of acids to damage corneal tissue depends on both their pH and the ability of their anions to combine with corneal tissue. For example, sulfuric acid appears more dangerous than hydrochloric acid at the same pH.

(2) Effects

(a) Prolonged exposure (more than a few minutes) stimulates vascularization and scar tissue formation, which can interfere with sight.

(b) Ocular discomfort begins at a pH of approximately 4.5.

(c) Corneal epithelium is physically damaged at a pH of 3.5 or lower.

(3) Therapy. Generous flushing of the eye with water within 15 minutes of exposure is recommended to counteract ocular acid burns.

b. Alkalies commonly cause burns that result in effects or sequelae more serious than the immediate lesion. Ammonium ion penetrates corneal tissue more quickly and deeply than other alkali materials.

(1) Effects

(a) Late effects include delayed tissue repair, increased intraocular pressure, and the release of collagenase from neutrophils.

(b) Calcium hydroxide causes **lime plaques** that are difficult to remove.

(2) Therapy

(a) Irrigation, mild debridement, and chelation with ethylenediaminetetraacetic acid (EDTA) may aid in treatment of lime burns.

(b) Ascorbate and citrate show promise in the treatment of ocular alkali burns and corneal ulcers.

c. Organic solvents are lipophilic and penetrate corneal tissue, causing pain and multiple foci of corneal damage. Sequelae of organic solvent irritation are usually less severe and of shorter duration than those of acids and alkalies.

d. Detergents can cause immediate pain that is followed by the prolonged effects of vascularization and permanent scarring. Cationic substances are more damaging than anionic substances, which, in turn, are more damaging than neutral substances.

e. Photosensitization from plants and drugs can damage the cornea and result in photophobia and corneal opacity that leads to blindness.

2. **Cataracts** result from changes in lenticular metabolism or morphology that disturb the highly organized structure of the lens. Changes in the refractive index of different cell layers can lead to areas of varying opacity within the lens.
    a. **Chemicals that alter lenticular metabolism** and can lead to cataract formation include:
        (1) **2,4-Dinitrophenol** causes cataracts in humans, rabbits, and chicks; however, this effect is not necessarily related to its ability to uncouple oxidative phosphorylation.
        (2) **Corticosteroids** (e.g., cortisone, prednisone, dexamethasone) induce cataracts in humans and rabbits, possibly as a result of changes in sodium and potassium transport or synthesis of proteins in the lens.
        (3) **Cholinesterase inhibitors** (e.g., organophosphate and carbamate insecticides). Long-term inhibition of cholinesterase activity produces cataracts in humans and monkeys.
        (4) **Naphthalene** fed to rabbits is metabolized to 1,2-naphthoquinone, which is cataractogenic in rabbits.
    b. **Xenobiotic-induced cataracts.** The incidence of xenobiotic-induced cataracts in clinical veterinary medicine is not reported.

3. **Impaired pupillary response**
    a. Some drugs (e.g., morphine) constrict the pupil by central reinforcement of the pupillary light reflex.
    b. Visual disturbances from organophosphate and carbamate poisoning result from a combination of pupillary constriction and lack of accommodation of the lens.

4. **Lacrimation** results from stimulation of the corneal sensory nerves that produces reflex tearing.
    a. Lacrimators produce an **immediate response** upon exposure, and **signs rapidly regress when exposure to the lacrimator is discontinued**.
    b. **Photochemical smog** produces lacrimators to which animals may be exposed.
        (1) These lacrimators are formed by ultraviolet action on a mixture of oxygen and nitrogen oxide, and are associated with automobile-related air pollution.
        (2) Peroxyacetyl nitrates and other chemicals are lacrimators found in photochemical smog.

5. **Retinopathy.** Chemical-induced retinopathy is rare in veterinary medicine. Agents that are retinopathic to humans or experimental animals include:
    a. **Chloroquine,** an antimalarial agent that accumulates in the pigmented choroid and inhibits protein metabolism in the retinal pigment epithelium
    b. **Phenothiazine tranquilizers,** which cause diminished dark adaptation and reduced color vision by an unknown mechanism
    c. **Oxygen,** which at high concentrations damages the central retinal rods in rabbits and is toxic to the retinal vasculature of human infants
    d. **Methanol,** which is metabolized to formates that cause retinal edema and atrophy in humans, primates, and possibly, swine

6. **Neurologic blindness.** The optic nerve and central nervous system (CNS) control the transmission, processing, and interpretation of information from the eye.
    a. Systemic toxicants that affect the structure and function of the nervous system can cause blindness without detectable ocular lesions (i.e., **amaurosis**).
    b. **Common causes of neurologic blindness in veterinary medicine**
        (1) **Hexachlorophene** uncouples oxidative phosphorylation, causing demyelination and secondary axonal degeneration. Pupils are dilated and the pupillary light reflex is absent.
        (2) **Ivermectin** increases the activity of γ-aminobutyric acid (GABA) receptors, decreasing the menace response and causing reversible blindness in which the pupils respond to light. Ivermectin toxicosis primarily affects collies, shelties, and border collies.
        (3) **Lead poisoning** commonly causes blindness in cattle and horses, and sometimes in dogs. The mechanism of action is not clear, but lead interferes with CNS

neurotransmitters and may cause cortical degeneration and necrosis. Lesions in the eye are rare, but swelling of the optic disc and iridocyclitis are reported.

(4) Mercury interferes with protein synthesis in the CNS. Blindness is associated with neuronal necrosis in the calcarine sulci of the visual cortex.

(5) Phenylarsonic compounds are pentavalent organic arsenical feed additives that cause demyelination and secondary axonal degeneration of the optic nerves and other peripheral nerves.

III. SKIN

A. **Structure.** Skin is a water-resistant covering of multiple cell layers.

1. It has **two major divisions,** the epidermis and the dermis.
   a. The **epidermis** has four distinguishable layers, presented here in order from superficial to deep.
      (1) The **stratum corneum** is a highly cornified, water-resistant layer of cells with no metabolic activity. These cells are constantly being sloughed and replaced.
      (2) The **stratum granulosum** is located just below the stratum corneum and consists of differentiated viable cells.
      (3) The **stratum spinosum** is a distinctive layer of cells that is located just below the stratum granulosum.
      (4) The **stratum basale (germinativum)** is a metabolically active and rapidly dividing cell layer that serves as the source of the cells of the outer epidermis. **Melanocytes** are specialized neural cells located in the stratum basale. These cells produce the pigment **melanin,** which protects the animal against ultraviolet radiation and acts as a sunscreen.
   b. The **dermis,** which is interposed between the epidermis and underlying adipose and muscle tissues, is of mesodermal origin.
      (1) The dermis is supported by an extensive network of **loose connective tissue** containing reticulin, collagen, and elastin.
      (2) Vascularization. The dermis is richly supplied with blood vessels that are under active neurogenic control.

2. **Other components of the skin** include **hair follicles, sebaceous glands,** and **sweat glands;** these structures vary greatly among species.

B. **Function.** The skin forms a barrier against the changing external environment.

1. The skin modulates changes in temperature and humidity by varying blood flow and controlling piloerection.
2. It offers physical protection from pathogenic microorganisms.
3. It provides protection from ultraviolet radiation through stimulation of melanocytes and increasing pigmentation in the dermis.
4. The highly keratinized stratum corneum and the variable vascularization of the dermis modulate the exposure of the animal to toxic chemicals.

C. **Exposure to toxicants.** Skin, especially the stratum corneum of the epidermis, is relatively impermeable to water-soluble substances; however, **small nonpolar lipophilic toxicants readily penetrate the epidermis and are absorbed by the dermal vasculature.**

1. **Absorption** is enhanced by:
   a. **Anatomical location.** Chemical absorption through the skin varies with anatomical location.
      (1) Axillary, inguinal, mammary, and **scrotal skin** is highly permeable compared with skin in the dorsal and lateral body regions of most mammals.
      (2) Birds readily absorb toxicants through the **skin of their feet.**

b. Dermal hyperemia. Increases in environmental temperature may enhance absorption of chemicals. For example, in hot climates, dermal hyperemia may increase the toxicity of organophosphate insecticides to cattle.

c. Highly lipophilic substances or substances that contain surfactants or detergents

2. Biotransformation of xenobiotics

a. The deep layers of the epidermis have significant capability to metabolize foreign compounds. The dermis has no significant xenobiotic metabolizing activity.

b. Compounds that are biotransformed in other organs are delivered to the skin, where they exert toxic or photodynamic activity that damages the skin.

D. **Response to toxicants**

1. Irritation, degeneration, and necrosis (Table 13-1). Direct irritation of the skin by corrosive, caustic, or necrotizing chemicals (e.g., acids, alkalies, some metal salts) elicits an inflammatory response. Generally, materials with a pH of less than 2 or greater than 12 are strong irritants.

a. Agents that damage cell membranes result in irritation followed by the cardinal signs of inflammation (i.e., erythema, swelling, heat, and pain), leucocytosis, and increased vascular permeability.

b. Eschar formation, ulceration, and necrosis may permanently damage the skin.

2. Allergic contact dermatitis (Table 13-2)

a. Some chemicals act as antigens by combining with a carrier protein, eliciting a response from cellular components of the immune system.

b. Langerhans' cells or macrophages in the epidermis process the antigen and interact with appropriate T lymphocytes to form sensitized T lymphocytes.

c. Sensitized T lymphocytes react to later exposure to the antigen by producing a variety of cytokines. The cytokines initiate a series of changes that characterize the allergic response (i.e., erythema, edema, itching).

3. Photosensitization is an increase in susceptibility to ultraviolet light. Free radicals produced by photodynamic reactions can damage cell and lysosomal membranes (see Chapter 2 I E 3).

a. Conditions leading to photosensitization

(1) Photosensitization depends on the absorption of **ultraviolet light within a specific range of wavelengths (280–790 nm) and the presence of a photodynamic agent in the skin** (Table 13-3).

(a) Photodynamic agents form unstable high energy molecules when exposed to ultraviolet light.

(b) When the photodynamic agents return to the ground state, the energy released causes the molecule to fluoresce. The released energy damages epidermal cell membranes and forms free radicals that can initiate a chain reaction of membrane damage.

(2) Photosensitization is most prominent on areas of the body where protection from sunlight is least effective.

(a) Dorsal and lateral areas of the body

(b) Thin or unpigmented skin (e.g., the sclera, escutcheon, udder and teats, muzzle)

TABLE 13-1. Chemicals Commonly Associated With Dermal Irritation, Degeneration, and Necrosis

Acids	Hydrocarbon solvents (e.g., mineral
Alcohols	spirits, turpentine, kerosene)
Alkalies	Iodine
Arsenic	Mercuric salts
Detergents	Phenols
Formaldehyde	Thallium

TABLE 13-2. Plants Associated With Allergic Contact Dermatitis

Species	Common Name
Apium graveolens	Celery (rare in animals)
Pastinaca sativa	Parsnips (reported in swine)
Rhus toxicodendron	Poison oak
Toxicodendron radicans	Poison ivy (rare in animals)
Urtica urens, U. dioica	Nettles

   (3) Photosensitization is most likely to occur in sunny climates and during the spring and summer when sunlight is more intense or of longer duration each day.
  b. Clinical effects of photosensitization
   (1) Early signs are **erythema** and **edema.**
   (2) Pruritus, photophobia, and **hyperesthesia** follow.
   (3) Serious signs that occur later in the course of the disease include **exudation ("weeping") of serum, formation of vesicles, ulceration, exfoliation of damaged epidermis,** and, possibly, **blindness.**
      (a) In **sheep,** severe edema of the ears and face develops, resulting in a condition known as **"big head."**
      (b) Moderate to serious signs often are accompanied by **reduced feed intake** and **cessation of nursing and breeding.**
  c. Types of photosensitization
   (1) Primary photosensitization occurs when a photodynamic agent is directly ingested, absorbed through the skin, or injected, or when a chemical is biotransformed to a photodynamic metabolite.
      (a) The major effects of primary photosensitizers occur in the skin; other organs are usually spared.
      (b) Prompt removal of the photosensitizer and supportive treatment often results in recovery with few sequelae.
   (2) Secondary (hepatogenous) photosensitization occurs as a result of compromised liver function, which reduces the excretion of plant pigment metabolites from the body. Several toxic plants are known to cause hepatogenous photosensitization (see Table 13-3).
      (a) Normally, chlorophyll is metabolized to **phylloerythrin** by intestinal and colonic bacteria. Phylloerythrin reabsorbed from the gut is conjugated by the liver and excreted in the bile.

TABLE 13-3. Agents Associated with Photosensitization

Primary		Secondary	
Species	Common Name	Species	Common Name
Amni majus	Bishop's weed	*Agave lechiguilla*	Agave
Cymopteris watsonii	Spring parsley	*Brassica* species	Rape
Fagopyrum esculentum	Buckwheat	*Kochia scoparia*	Fireweed, kochia, burning bush
Hypericum perforatum	St.-John's-wort		
Phenothiazine anthelmintic		*Lantana camara*	Lantana
Sulfonamides		*Microcystis* species	Blue-green algae
Tetracyclines		*Nolina texana*	Sacahuiste, bunchgrass
		Panicum species	Panic grasses
		Pithomyces chartarum	Sporodesmin mycotoxin
		Senecio species	Senecio, groundsel
		Tetradymia glabrata	Horsebrush
		Tribulus terrestris	Puncture vine
		Trifolium hybridum	Alsike clover

TABLE 13-4. Plants That Cause Physical Injury

Species	Common Name
Cenchrus species	Sandbur
Setaria species	Foxtail
Stipa robusta	Sleepygrass, needle grass
Xanthium strumarium	Cocklebur

      (b) Failure of the liver to conjugate or excrete phylloerythrin allows it to accumulate in the dermal vasculature, where it is activated to a photodynamic state by ultraviolet light.

      (c) Liver damage and involvement of other organ systems may accompany the expected skin-related signs and lesions of photosensitization.

   d. Porphyria, which can cause photosensitization, is the presence of abnormal levels of porphyrins in the blood as a result of abnormal heme synthesis.

      (1) Congenital porphyria is an **inherited trait in cattle.** It must be differentiated from toxic causes of photosensitization.

      (2) In addition to photosensitization, porphyric animals have **brown teeth** and **urine that fluoresces.**

4. Trauma can occur from objects and plants grazed by large animals or encountered by small animals as they roam wild areas. Table 13-4 lists some common plants that cause physical injury to the muzzle, eyes, or skin.

5. Hyperkeratosis is the abnormal proliferation or keratinization of the superficial epidermis. Toxicants include highly chlorinated naphthalenes and hairy vetch (*Vicia villosa*).

6. Alopecia (hair loss) is associated with thallium, arsenic, and selenium toxicosis, chemotherapy with cytostatic drugs, and consumption of the leucaena plant (*Leucaena leucocephala*) by cattle.

7. Carcinogenesis of the skin is a common problem in small animals and some large animals. Skin cancer is usually not closely associated with chemical exposure in animals.

BIBLIOGRAPHY

Beasley VR, Diana SG, Dorman DC, et al: A systems affected approach to veterinary toxicology: reference notes for Toxicology VB 320. Urbana, IL, Val R. Beasley, 1990.

Emmet EA: Toxic responses of the skin. In *Casarett and Doull's Toxicology: The Science of Poisons.* Edited by Amdur MO, Doull J, Klaassen CD. New York, Pergamon, 1991, pp 463–483.

Potts AM: Toxic responses of the eye. In *Casarett and Doull's Toxicology: The Science of Poisons.* Edited by Amdur MO, Doull J, Klaassen CD. New York, Pergamon, 1991, pp 521–562.

Rowe LD, Johnson EA: Plants producing dermal injury. In *Current Veterinary Therapy 3: Food Animal Practice.* Edited by Howard JL. Philadelphia, WB Saunders, 1993, pp 361–364.

Directions: Each of the numbered items or incomplete statements in this section is followed by answers or by completions of the statement. Select the **one** numbered answer or completion that is **best** in each case.

1. Which agent is most likely to cause prolonged and advancing lesions of the cornea after initial exposure?

(1) Hydrochloric acid
(2) Ammonium hydroxide
(3) Organic solvents
(4) Phenylarsonic acid
(5) Photochemical smog

2. Which type of chemical is *least* likely to penetrate the stratum corneum?

(1) Highly lipophilic and nonpolar
(2) Long-chain fatty acids
(3) Hydrophobic, polar, and charged
(4) Hydrophilic and polar
(5) Strong surfactants and detergents

3. All of the following toxicants are likely to cause blindness by producing a physical lesion in the eye *except:*

(1) ammonium hydroxide.
(2) mercury.
(3) *Hypericum perforatum.*
(4) sulfuric acid.

Directions: The group of items in this section consists of numbered options followed by a set of numbered items. For each item, select the **one** numbered option that is most closely associated with it. Each numbered option may be selected once, more than once, or not at all.

Questions 4–5

For each of the following agents, select the ocular structure that it most affects.

(1) Cornea
(2) Iris
(3) Lens
(4) Retina
(5) Optic nerve

4. A parasympatholytic drug (e.g., atropine)

5. A metabolic inhibitor that reduces the activity of the sodium–potassium pump

ANSWERS AND EXPLANATIONS

1. The answer is 2 *[II B 1 b]*. Alkalies, such as ammonium hydroxide, have delayed effects that increase in severity following initial exposure; therefore, alkalies are perhaps the most dangerous type of corneal irritants. Acids cause severe burns and physical damage soon after exposure. Organic solvent irritation is short-lived and photochemical smog is classified as a lacrimator that directly stimulates tearing only while exposure continues. Phenylarsonic acids are feed additives that cause optic nerve demyelination and axonal degeneration.

2. The answer is 4 *[III A, C]*. The strateum corneum, which has a high concentration of keratin, is an effective barrier against water-soluble compounds, but more readily allows the passage of lipophilic molecules or those that have detergent or surfactant properties.

3. The answer is 2 *[II B 6 b (4)]*. Mercury causes blindness by preventing protein synthesis and neuronal necrosis in the calcarine sulci of the visual cortex; the eye itself is not affected. Acids and alkalies (e.g., sulfuric acid, ammonium hydroxide) can cause inflammation, ulceration, and scarring of the cornea. Photosensitization from plants (e.g., *Hypericum perforatum*) and drugs can cause corneal opacity that leads to blindness.

4–5. The answers are: 4-2 *[II A 2 b (2), c (2)]*, **5-3** *[II A 2 d]*. The iris is directly influenced by the autonomic nervous system, both sympathetic and parasympathetic. Stimulation of the parasympathetic nervous system causes miosis or pupillary constriction, whereas parasympatholytic drugs, such as atropine and the other belladonna alkaloids, block cholinergic receptors and dilate the pupil.

The transparency and optical properties of the lens are highly dependent on uniform microscopic morphologic features and degree of hydration. Actively metabolizing cells near the outer surface of the lens significantly affect the sodium-to-potassium ratio and, therefore, the hydration of the lens.

Chapter 14

Toxicology of the Musculoskeletal System

I. SKELETAL MUSCLE

A. Introduction

1. **Structure.** Skeletal muscle is a **syncytium** formed by embryonal fusion of many individual myoblasts.

2. **Muscle fiber types**
   a. **Type 1 (slow-twitch) fibers** are dark because of their **high myoglobin content**. They use **oxidative phosphorylation** rather than glycolysis as an energy source. They are **fatigue-resistant,** making them well-suited for sustained muscle action (e.g., posture or weight-bearing).
   b. **Type 2a (fast fatigue-resistant) fibers** also have a **high myoglobin content**. They rely on **glycolysis** as an energy source. Type 2a fibers respond quickly and contract rapidly.
   c. **Type 2b (fast-twitch) fibers** are pale because of their **low myoglobin content**. They rely on **glycolysis** as an energy source and **fatigue easily**. They generate large contractile forces and are capable of quick responses.

3. **Contraction**
   a. **Intracellular and extracellular calcium movement** is a major factor in the initiation and control of muscle contraction.
   b. **Cholinergic fibers** innervate skeletal muscle; contraction is usually **voluntary**. Excessive acetylcholine (ACh) stimulation (e.g., from organophosphate insecticides, heroin, amphetamines) causes sustained muscle contraction and may lead to muscle necrosis.

B. Mechanisms of toxicologic damage

1. **Peripheral motor neuropathy** from toxicants results in secondary muscle wasting. In veterinary medicine, triorthocresyl phosphate–delayed neuropathy, some forms of organophosphate toxicosis, arsanilic acid toxicosis, and selenium toxicosis (in swine) result in peripheral denervation with resultant **muscle atrophy**.

2. **Elicitation of an autoimmune response.** This mechanism is not well-studied in veterinary medicine. D-Penicillamine, sometimes used as a heavy metal antidote in animals, has been associated with an **inflammatory myopathy** that is considered to be the result of an autoimmune mechanism.

3. **Direct irritation.** Caustic or corrosive agents, hydrocarbon solvents, phenols, alcohol, injectable oxytetracycline, and some injectable iron preparations are examples of muscle-damaging agents.

4. **Interference with cell membrane function**
   a. **Ionophores** (e.g., monensin) alter the transport of sodium, potassium, or calcium, leading to mitochondrial calcium overload, impaired oxidative phosphorylation, and cellular necrosis.
   b. The **phenoxy herbicide 2,4-D** impairs the activity of glucose-6-phosphate dehydrogenase (G6PD) and alters membrane electrical activity, leading to **myotonia** in dogs.
   c. **Other agents** that interfere with cell membrane function include those that alter sodium–potassium–adenosine triphosphatase (ATPase) activity and free radicals, although neither mechanism is commonly associated with muscle damage.

5. **Damage to organelles or subcellular structures**
   a. **Sarcoplasmic reticulum**
      (1) Agents such as the anticancer drug **doxorubicin** are associated with cytoplasmic vacuolization and dilatation of the sarcoplasmic reticulum.
      (2) **Halothane** or **succinylcholine** can interfere with the sarcoplasmic reticulum's ability to take up calcium, triggering **malignant hyperthermia** in susceptible swine (**porcine stress syndrome**).
         (a) A defect in the uptake of calcium by the sarcoplasmic reticulum leads to a loss of calcium homeostasis, increased muscle contraction, and depletion of adenosine triphosphate (ATP) reserves.
         (b) Affected pigs develop muscle stiffness, acidosis, and hyperkalemia that can lead to cardiac failure.
   b. **Microtubules and myofilaments**
      (1) **Vincristine** and **colchicine** may damage microtubules, leading to muscle fiber necrosis.
      (2) **Emetine,** an alkaloidal constituent of ipecac, causes myofilament damage associated with a loss of oxidative enzyme activity. One of the effects of toxic levels of emetine is a loss of muscle cross-striations.
   c. **Lysosomes.** Agents that affect lysosomes (e.g., **chloroquine**) form stable complexes with lipids. These complexes accumulate in lysosomes and inhibit phospholipid-degrading lysosomal enzymes. Compounds causing damage to muscle lysosomes are not common in veterinary medicine.

6. **Interference with protein synthesis.** Prolonged use of fluorinated steroids can reduce protein synthesis in type 2 muscle fibers.

C. **Clinical effects.** The effects of toxicants on skeletal muscle are minimal and often generalized.

1. **Necrosis**
   a. **Causative agents** are described in Table 14-1.

TABLE 14-1. Agents that Cause Skeletal Muscle Necrosis

Agent	Effect	Affected Species
Corticosteroids	Reduced protein synthesis	Dogs, rabbits
Gossypol	Myocardial necrosis leads to cardiac failure	Swine, poultry, immature ruminants
Halothane	Precipitates malignant hyperthermia	Swine
Ionophores (monensin, lasalocid, narasin)	Accumulation of calcium in cells leads to necrosis	Most domestic livestock, especially horses
Iron dextran injectables	Direct irritation at injection site	Swine
Selenium	Acute overdose causes skeletal necrosis, but no cardiomyopathy	Lambs
Snake venom*	Swelling, edema, hemorrhage, necrosis in affected area	All species
Toxic plants		
Cassia species (cassia, senna)	Weakness, ataxia, tremors, recumbency, hemoglobinuria	Livestock—south central and southwestern United States
Eupatorium rugosum (white snakeroot)	Slow gait, stiffness, ataxia, weakness, myocardial necrosis	Livestock—eastern and midwestern United States
Karwinskia humboldtiana (coyotillo)	Weakness, tremors, incoordination, ataxia, recumbency	Livestock—south central and southwestern United States

*Those of the Crotalidae family (rattlesnake, cottonmouth, copperhead) are most common in the United States.

b. Diagnosis
   (1) Clinical signs. Affected animals have a stiff or rigid gait. They may collapse and be unable to rise.
   (2) Laboratory diagnosis
      (a) The **serum creatine kinase** level may be elevated five to ten times above the normal range.
      (b) Gross appearance. Necrotic muscle is characterized by longitudinal streaks of pale tan muscle with a cooked (boiled) appearance.
      (c) Microscopic changes usually include hyaline degeneration. Sarcoplasmic debris is removed by macrophages.
c. Prognosis. Damaged muscle tissue can regenerate. Satellite cells present at the sarcolemmal membrane serve as stem cells for myocyte regeneration.
   (1) Regeneration is most likely if the toxic insult is moderate and short-term.
   (2) Extensive necrosis with damage to endomysial connective tissues results in fibrosis of muscle tissue.

2. Neuromuscular blockade
a. Causative agents include those that exert a presynaptic local anesthetic-like action, block the postsynaptic receptors, interfere with ACh release, or impair muscle membrane conductance. For example, **aminoglycoside antibiotics** may cause neuromuscular blockade by preventing presynaptic release of ACh and reducing postsynaptic receptor receptivity.
b. Diagnosis. Neuromuscular function is impaired, but muscle lesions are not produced. Signs may range from trembling and weakness to complete collapse and flaccid paralysis.

3. Myotonia occurs when normal muscle contraction is not followed by full relaxation. Toxic dosages of the phenoxy herbicide 2,4-D causes myotonia in dogs.

II. CARTILAGE AND BONE

A. Introduction

1. Cartilage. Chondrocytes, the cells of cartilage, are surrounded by **chondromatrix** and occupy **lacunae.**
   a. Chondrocytes are derived from **chondroblasts.**
   b. The chondromatrix comprises fibers (mostly **collagen**) and fibrils embedded in an amorphous ground substance rich in glycosaminoglycans and proteoglycans.

2. Bone
a. Formation. Osteoblasts synthesize **osteoid** (i.e., the organic matrix composed of ground substance and collagen) and promote mineralization. When osteoblasts have surrounded themselves with matrix, they become **osteocytes,** which maintain the bone matrix.
   (1) Calcium is essential for mineralization. **Parathyroid hormone (PTH)** secretion increases as the plasma calcium concentration decreases.
      (a) PTH **increases renal tubular reabsorption of calcium** and **renal excretion of phosphate.**
      (b) PTH stimulates **osteolytic activity** in the osteocytes, making rapid movement of calcium from the bone to the extracellular compartment possible.
   (2) Vitamin D (calcitriol, 1,25-dihydroxy vitamin D_3) is essential for absorption of calcium. Synthesis of calcitriol depends on hydroxylation of vitamin D_3 in the liver, followed by additional hydroxylation in the renal tubular epithelium to form the dihydroxy metabolite.
   (3) Vitamin C is essential for collagen synthesis.
b. Resorption. Osteoclasts, which secrete enzymes that break down the bone matrix, mediate the resorption of bone to maintain serum calcium levels.

(1) Osteoclasts help to maintain bone thickness during growth and allow bone to respond to mechanical stress by changing shape during remodeling.

(2) Osteoclasts are stimulated under the synergistic influence of PTH and calcitriol.

B. **Mechanisms of toxicologic damage**

1. Primary

a. Interference with bone and cartilage formation

(1) **Excessive vitamin A** causes lysosomal instability and release of enzymes, which reduces the cartilage matrix and leads to chondromalacia.

(2) **Cadmium** inhibits chondroitin sulfate synthesis, which affects collagen synthesis and cross-linking.

(3) **Excessive zinc, copper, molybdenum,** or **beta-aminopropionitrile** (from *Lathyrus* species) inhibit the activity of lysyl oxidase, an enzyme integral to collagen formation.

(4) **Glucocorticoids** reduce protein synthesis and are associated with decreased formation of bone matrix.

(5) **Excessive dietary phosphorus** stimulates PTH and causes fibrous osteodystrophy.

(6) **Lead** accumulates in the metaphyses of growing bone, causing metaphyseal sclerosis and reducing the rate of linear growth.

b. Interference with calcium homeostasis and bone mineralization

(1) **Excessive calcitriol** [from rodenticides, plants (e.g., *Solanum malacoxylon, Cestrum diurnum*), or the diet] promotes excessive calcium absorption and causes soft tissue mineralization.

(2) **Excessive fluoride, prostaglandin E$_2$,** or **calcitriol** can all cause bone formation in excess of resorption, accompanied by impaired osteoid formation and reduced mineralization.

(3) **High dietary oxalates, phosphates,** or **zinc** diminish calcium absorption, leading to osteomalacia.

c. Teratogenic effects

(1) *Veratrum californicum* (false hellebore), which contains the alkaloids jervine and cyclopamine, causes **craniofacial malformations in sheep**.

(2) *Lupinus* species contain anagyrine, a quinolizidine alkaloid that causes arthrogryposis, torticollis, and cleft palate in cattle (**crooked calf syndrome**).

(3) **Piperidine alkaloids** found in *Conium maculatum* (poison hemlock) and *Nicotiana* species (tobacco, tree tobacco) cause **skeletal arthrogryposis**.

2. Secondary

a. Renal dysfunction

(1) Renal disease or toxicosis leading to increased serum phosphorus and low serum calcium levels stimulates secretion of PTH, leading to fibrous osteodystrophy.

(2) Damage to renal tubules can lead to loss of renal control of phosphate and calcium levels, diminishing calcium homeostasis and reducing control of bone formation or resorption.

(3) Cadmium toxicosis and other conditions that damage renal tubular epithelium can impair synthesis of calcitriol, leading to secondary osteomalacia.

b. Changes in blood flow and oxygen tension. Excessive prostaglandin E$_2$ or vagal stimulation may increase arterial blood pressure in the limbs, leading to periosteal edema and new bone formation.

C. **Factors influencing bone health**

1. Calcitonin, a hormone secreted by the thyroid gland in response to hypercalcemia, assists in calcium homeostasis by:

a. Inhibiting osteoclast activity, thus limiting calcium removal from bone

b. Decreasing intestinal absorption of calcium and phosphorus

c. Increasing renal excretion of calcium

2. **Insulin** regulates bone growth.

3. **Growth hormone** mediates changes in the production of **insulin-like growth factor (IGF),** which is a stimulator of bone growth.

4. **Estrogens** and **androgens** aid in skeletal maturation and reduce bone loss.

5. **Cytokines** may stimulate osteoclasts to enhance bone resorption.

BIBLIOGRAPHY

Van Vleet JF, Ferrans VJ, Herman E: Cardiovascular and skeletal muscle systems. In *Handbook of Toxicologic Pathology.* Edited by Haschek WM, Rousseaux CG. San Diego, Academic Press, 1991, pp 602–618.

Woodard JC, Webster WJ: Skeletal system. In *Handbook of Toxicologic Pathology.* Edited by Haschek WM, Rousseaux CG. San Diego, Academic Press, 1991, pp 489–534.

Directions: Each of the numbered items or incomplete statements in this section is followed by answers or by completions of the statement. Select the **one** numbered answer or completion that is **best** in each case.

1. The ability of an animal to react quickly to danger by rapid flight and evasive action would be most affected by a toxicant that:

(1) moderately increases intracellular calcium.
(2) moderately inhibits oxidative phosphorylation.
(3) moderately inhibits cytochrome P-450.
(4) mildly inhibits cholinesterase at the neuromuscular junction.
(5) causes mild hypocalcemia.

2. Which one of the following could be expected to increase the toxic effects of a continuing overdose of vitamin D?

(1) Excessive dietary phosphorus
(2) Excessive dietary zinc
(3) Chronic renal tubular disease
(4) A functional parathyroid adenoma
(5) Cadmium contamination of the water supply

3. Which biochemical event is *not* a significant consequence of overconsumption of monensin by cattle?

(1) Calcium accumulation in mitochondria
(2) Interference with normal sodium transport
(3) Impaired oxidative phosphorylation
(4) Increased serum creatine kinase
(5) Impaired glycogen synthesis

ANSWERS AND EXPLANATIONS

1. The answer is 2 *[I A 2]*. Muscle contraction is highly energy-dependent and relies on high energy phosphate bonds generated by oxidative phosphorylation. Mild to moderate increases in calcium could enhance muscle contraction. Cytochrome P-450 is a mixed function oxidase (MFO) that affects xenobiotic metabolism. Mild inhibition of cholinesterase enhances the availability of acetylcholine (ACh) and may increase muscle responsiveness. Mild hypocalcemia caused by stimulating the nervous system may enhance muscle stimulation.

2. The answer is 4 *[II A 2 a (1), B 1 b (1)]*. A functional parathyroid adenoma would produce excess parathyroid hormone (PTH). PTH stimulates osteoclastic activity and increases renal tubular calcium resorption, leading to hypercalcemia by increasing bone turnover. Vitamin D is metabolized to the active 1,25 dihydroxy form, which interacts with parathyroid hormone to produce hypercalcemia. Impaired renal tubular function in chronic renal disease (including cadmium toxicosis)

would likely reduce the metabolism of vitamin D and limit the production of active metabolites. In addition, the diseased kidney may not excrete phosphorus effectively, raising the serum phosphorus level. Increased serum phosphorus tends to lower serum calcium.

3. The answer is 5 *[I B 4 a]*. Monensin is an ionophore that facilitates sodium transport and interferes with the normal exchange of sodium and calcium, leading eventually to increased cellular calcium and calcium overload of the mitochondria. This early change is followed by impaired oxidative phosphorylation and cellular necrosis, which causes the release of creatine kinase from damaged muscle cells into the serum. Impaired glycogen synthesis is a minor and secondary feature of this toxicosis, because muscle function is dependent on calcium homeostasis and oxidative phosphorylation to supply high energy phosphate bonds to support contraction. The accumulation of calcium is eventually associated with irreversible cell degeneration and necrosis.

Chapter 15
Toxicology of the Cardiovascular System

I. INTRODUCTION

A. Normal cardiac function

1. **Energy sources**
   a. **Aerobic metabolism.** The tricarboxylic acid (TCA) cycle generates adenosine triphosphate (ATP), which provides the energy necessary for myocardial contraction.
      (1) **Free fatty acids** are catalyzed by **coenzyme A** to **acyl coenzyme A,** which undergoes β-oxidation to form **acetylcoenzyme A.** Acetylcoenzyme A is used in the TCA cycle.
      (2) Alternatively, cardiac muscle can use **lactate, pyruvate,** and **glucose** in the TCA cycle.
   b. **Glycogenolysis and lipolysis.** β-adrenergic stimulation activates cyclic adenosine monophosphate (cAMP), leading to glycogenolysis and lipolysis. The use of glycogen and triglycerides for energy is much less effective than aerobic metabolism.
   c. **Energy is stored** as the high-energy phosphates **ATP** and **creatine phosphate.**
      (1) Creatine phosphate is converted to ATP by reacting with adenosine diphosphate (ADP).
      (2) This reaction is catalyzed by creatine phosphokinase, which is abundant in cardiac muscle cells.

2. **Contraction**
   a. **Calcium release**
      (1) During an action potential, increased cytoplasmic calcium combines with **troponin,** the modulating myocardial protein. Troponin undergoes a conformational change that allows the myocardial contractile proteins, **actin** and **myosin,** to form a cross-bridge.
      (2) Calcium stimulates **myosin–adenosine triphosphatase (ATPase)** activity.
   b. **Cross-bridge cycling.** The activated contractile proteins use the **energy obtained by hydrolysis of ATP** to shorten and generate tension.

3. **Impulse formation and conduction**
   a. **Normal impulse formation** originates from spontaneous depolarization of the **sinoatrial node.**
      (1) The action potential is initially generated by the cellular **influx of sodium (fast current),** followed by a second phase of depolarization mediated by the **influx of calcium (slow current).**
      (2) **Neurogenic influences** can alter the rate of depolarization.
         (a) **Parasympathetic (vagal) stimulation** may slow or block sinoatrial activity.
         (b) **Sympathetic stimulation** increases sinoatrial activity.
   b. **Conduction of impulses** from the atria to the ventricles takes place at the **atrioventricular node,** which is the most common site for conduction disturbances.

B. **Cardiac function may be directly affected by a variety of toxicologic mechanisms** (Table 15-1).

TABLE 15-1. Veterinary Toxicants that Affect the Heart

Toxicant	Mechanism of Action	Physiologic or Clinical Effects
Cardioactive glycosides *Digitalis* species (digitalis, digitoxin) *Apocynum* species (dogbane) *Asclepias* species (milkweed) *Bufo* species (toads) *Convallaria* species (lily of the valley)	Interferes with Na^+/K^+–ATPase, decreasing intracellular potassium and leading to high-grade heart block and increased vagal tone	Initial signs are gastrointestinal upset with vomiting and diarrhea; cardiac arrhythmias are characterized by slowed atrioventricular conduction, dropped beats, S-T segment changes, and ventricular premature systoles or bigeminy
Andromedotoxin (grayanotoxin) *Kalmia* species (laurel) *Rhododendron* species (azalea) *Pieris* species (Japanese pieris)	Stabilizes voltage-sensitive sodium channels with action similar to that of digitalis	Vomiting and diarrhea, weakness, incoordination, paralysis, and coma
Cardiotoxic alkaloids *Aconitum* species (monkshood)	Alkaloid (aconite) causes hypotension, myocardial depression, and tachycardia	Vomiting, diarrhea, bloat, a rapid weak heartbeat, paresis, collapse, and death
Methylxanthines (caffeine, theobromine)	Stimulates catecholamine release and enhances calcium retention in the sarcoplasmic reticulum	Vomiting, excitement, hyperactivity, tachycardia, premature ventricular contractions, and hypertension
Taxus species (yew)	Inhibits conduction associated with depolarization within the heart	Sudden death, bradycardia and diastolic heart block, hypotension, and weakness
Miscellaneous natural toxicants *Cassia* species (senna, coffeeweed)	May block electron transport; hyperkalemia may be prominent; myocardial degeneration may occur	Tachycardia, altered QRS complex, displaced S-T segment, and tenting of T waves
Eupatorium species (white snakeroot)	Toxic ketones (tremetol) are formed, but specific mechanisms are not known	In horses, jugular pulse, tachycardia, ventricular premature beats, and S-T elevation
Gossypium species (cottonseed, source of gossypol)	Binds to free ε-amino groups of lysine; may also bind to phospholipids of the cell membrane, affecting potassium level in the cell	Increased amplitude of T wave and shortening of S-T segment similar to hyperkalemic heart failure
Persea americana (avocado)	Unknown	In caged birds, hydropericardium, congestion, and edema

Belladonna alkaloids	Atropine and related alkaloids exert parasympathetic effect on heart	Vagal block with ventricular arrhythmia, widened QRS complex, and prolonged Q-T segment
Feed additives		
Ionophores (monensin, lasalocid)	Facilitates sodium transport across membrane and alters the sodium-to-calcium ratio	Early effects may be anorexia and diarrhea; cardiac changes include S-T depression, atrial tachycardia and fibrillation, ventricular extrasystoles, cardiac necrosis, and fibrosis
Furazolidone	Inhibits enzymes of intermediary metabolism	In turkeys, cardiomyopathy ("round heart" disease)
Household products		
Fumes from overheating synthetic fluorine-containing resins (Teflon); chlorofluorocarbons; halogenated solvents	Sensitizes myocardium to sympathomimetic amines, especially in small caged birds, including finches, budgerigars, cockatiels, and parrots	Sudden death, dyspnea, convulsions, and collapse
Drugs		
Amphetamines	Stimulates catecholamine release and sympathetic nerve endings	Hypertension, tachycardia, and arrhythmias similar to those caused by methylxanthines
Cocaine	Inhibits reuptake of catecholamines, leading to sympathetic stimulation	Tachycardia; hypertension progressing to arrhythmias and hypotension
Tricyclic antidepressants	Inhibits uptake of serotonin and norepinephrine; quinidine-like cardiac effects	Tachycardia, hypotension, arrhythmia with prolonged QRS, P-R, and Q-T segments; ventricular tachyarrhythmias are common

Na^+-K^+-ATPase = sodium–potassium–adenosine triphosphatase.

II. **TOXICANTS AFFECTING AEROBIC METABOLISM.** The high energy demands of the heart make it susceptible to toxicants that interfere with oxygen availability, carbohydrate metabolism, or oxidative phosphorylation.

A. **Fluoroacetate** interferes with the TCA cycle.

B. **Dinitrophenols** and **pentachlorophenol** uncouple oxidative phosphorylation.

C. **Toxicants that cause anoxia, anemia,** or **ischemia** (e.g., **nitrite**) indirectly compromise cardiac function by limiting the availability of oxygen needed for aerobic metabolism.

III. **TOXICANTS THAT ALTER IMPULSE FORMATION OR CONDUCTION** cause arrhythmias.

A. **Toxicants that cause acidosis and hyperkalemia** (e.g., ethylene glycol) enhance slow current activity, increasing automaticity and promoting arrhythmia.

B. **Cardiotoxic divalent ions** (e.g., **barium, strontium**) replace calcium in slow-current channels and alter the efflux of potassium from myocardial cells, resulting in hypokalemia and arrhythmias followed by cardiac block.

C. **Halogenated hydrocarbons** (e.g., **chloroform, fluorocarbons**) suppress the sinoatrial node and sensitize the myocardium to the arrhythmogenic effects of sympathomimetic amines (catecholamines).

  1. The atrioventricular junction becomes the pacemaker region.

  2. Increased propagation of premature beats results when the refractory period of the Purkinje fibers is decreased.

D. **Digitalis glycosides**

  1. Digitalis glycosides **inhibit the sodium–potassium exchange mechanism,** decreasing intracellular potassium levels and increasing intracellular sodium levels. When intracellular potassium is depleted, digitalis glycosides increase myocardial sensitivity to catecholamines.

  2. Digitalis glycosides **increase the refractory period at the atrioventricular node**.

IV. **TOXICANTS THAT ALTER CELL MEMBRANE FUNCTION**

A. **Toxicants that alter cell membrane control of ion movement** affect the **rate and force of cardiac contraction**.

  1. Toxicants may alter **membrane-bound enzyme activity**.
     a. Toxicants affecting the **sodium–potassium–ATPase pump** affect the normal transmembrane gradients of sodium and potassium, which are necessary for initiation of the action potential.
     b. Toxicants affecting the **calcium–magnesium–ATPase pump,** located in the sarcoplasmic reticulum, alter cardiac contractility by affecting intracellular calcium levels.

  2. **Chemical ionophores** (e.g., **monensin**) facilitate the passage of sodium, potassium, or calcium and interfere with the normal transmembrane ionic balance.

    a. Monensin alters calcium and sodium transport, leading to increased intracellular calcium levels and **changes in myocardial contractility**.

    b. Excessive calcium accumulation impairs mitochondrial oxidative phosphorylation, leading to **myocardial necrosis**.

B. **Toxicants that bind to phospholipids** in the cell membrane (e.g., **gossypol**) **affect potassium transport**. The resultant hyperkalemia produces arrhythmias [visible on the electrocardiogram (EKG) as an increased T-wave amplitude and shortening of the S-T segment].

V. TOXICANTS THAT DIRECTLY DAMAGE MYOCARDIAL CELLS. Direct toxic effects on cardiac myocytes damage the pumping effectiveness of the heart by reducing the number of active myocytes.

A. **Mechanism of action.** Myocytes are susceptible to the same mechanisms of injury as other cells of the body.

    1. **Oxidative stress** and **lipid peroxidation** of cell and organelle membranes lead to cell swelling, altered calcium homeostasis, and irreversible myocyte injury.

    2. The **interaction of xenobiotics with enzymes or structural macromolecules** can cause cell degeneration and necrosis.

B. **Clinical response**

    1. **Early signs** include eosinophilia, loss of striations, granular cytoplasm, interstitial edema, and accumulations of inflammatory cells (e.g., lymphocytes, polymorphonuclear leukocytes, plasma cells).

    2. **Advanced changes** include myocytolysis, calcium deposition, proliferation of fibroblasts, and collagen deposition.

C. **Cardiac muscle cells do not regenerate.** Therefore, animals with necrotic cardiotoxic damage may have permanent cardiac insufficiency or exercise intolerance. Sudden death may occur.

VI. TOXICANTS THAT INDUCE VASCULAR CHANGES (Table 15-2)

A. **Changes in peripheral vascular resistance** alter blood and oxygen supply to the heart and may influence its ability to provide effective tissue perfusion.

    1. **Toxicants that stimulate α-adrenergic receptors** (e.g., amphetamines) increase vasoconstriction and peripheral vascular resistance.

    2. **Toxicants that stimulate β-adrenergic agonists** cause vasodilation, leading to reduced peripheral resistance and potential hypotension and tachycardia.

    3. **Toxicants that increase vomiting and diarrhea** (e.g., arsenic) may cause loss of body fluids, tachycardia, and hypotension as a secondary effect of the lesions in the gastrointestinal tract.

B. **Structural or morphologic changes in the peripheral vasculature**

    1. **Toxicants that alter the connective tissue of arterial vessels** (e.g., D-penicillamine, β-amino propionitrile) may lead to **aneurysms**.

TABLE 15-2. Vascular Toxicants of Veterinary Importance

Toxic Agent	Physiologic and Clinical Effects
Endotoxin	Activates arachidonic acid, leading to prostaglandin-associated vascular damage
Ergopeptide alkaloids from *Claviceps* species and endophyte-infected *Festuca* species (tall fescue)	Vasoconstriction and arterial medial smooth-muscle proliferation; dry gangrene of the extremities results in loss of tail, ears, and hooves
Lathyrus species (β-amino propionitrile)	Aneurysms as a result of altered arterial connective tissue
Metals (lead, mercury)	Fibrinoid necrosis of arterial media
Pyrrolizidine alkaloids (monocrotaline) from *Crotalaria* species	Medial hypertrophy of small arterioles; pulmonary arterial hypertension
Vitamin D	Medial calcification of arteries
Cholecalciferol rodenticides	
Solanum malacoxylon	
Cestrum diurnum	

   2. Toxicants that cause sudden or marked vasoconstriction may promote **thrombosis** or **embolism**.

   3. Toxicants that cause prolonged vasoconstriction (e.g., ergopeptide alkaloids) can lead to **proliferation of smooth muscle in small arteries**.

   4. Toxicants that directly irritate the vessels (e.g., some drugs when administered intravenously) may cause **phlebitis** or **endothelial damage,** leading to **local thrombosis**.

   5. Toxicants that cause endothelial damage (e.g., **endotoxin** in some species) cause extravasation of fluids, leading to **perivascular or interstitial edema**.

BIBLIOGRAPHY

Hanig JP, Herman EH: Toxic responses of the heart and vascular systems. In *Casarett and Doull's Toxicology: The Basic Science of Poisons,* 4th edition. Edited by Amdur MO, Doull J, Klaassen CD. New York, Pergamon Press, 1991, pp 430–462.

Moses BL: Cardiac arrhythmias and cardiopulmonary arrest. In *Handbook of Small Animal Practice,* 2nd edition. Edited by Morgan R. New York, Churchill Livingston, 1992, pp 71–91.

Van Vleet JF, Ferrans VJ, Herman E: Cardiovascular and skeletal muscle systems. In *Handbook of Toxicologic Pathology.* Edited by Haschek WM, Rousseaux CG. San Diego, Academic Press, 1991, pp 602–618.

DIRECTIONS: Each of the numbered items or incomplete statements in this section is followed by answers or by completions of the statement. Select the **one** numbered answer or completion that is **best** in each case.

1. An animal that is exposed to a halogenated hydrocarbon (e.g., chloroform) would be more sensitive to:

(1) yew plants.
(2) furazolidone.
(3) epinephrine.
(4) digitalis glycosides.
(5) monensin.

2. If an animal is suspected of being poisoned by a cardiotoxic dosage of barium chloride, which ion should be avoided during treatment of the affected animal?

(1) Calcium
(2) Carbonate
(3) Chloride
(4) Potassium
(5) Sodium

3. A feedlot steer that survived an overdose of monensin in the feed was found dead 3 weeks later. The most likely cause of death, if related to the monensin toxicosis, is:

(1) persistent depolarization and arrhythmia as a result of the sodium and calcium channel effects of monensin.
(2) pulmonary hypertension induced by the toxic cardiac changes caused by monensin.
(3) cardiac fibrosis and insufficiency as a result of cardiac muscle necrosis during acute monensin toxicosis.
(4) cardiac insufficiency because of monensin inhibition of sodium–potassium–adenosine triphosphatase (ATPase).
(5) reduced energy levels in cardiac muscle following inhibition of oxidative phosphorylation by monensin.

4. Which one of the following substances is least likely to cause clinical cardiac effects related to the activity of sympathomimetic amines?

(1) Amphetamines
(2) Caffeine
(3) Cocaine
(4) Fluoroacetate
(5) Tricyclic antidepressants

ANSWERS AND EXPLANATIONS

1. The answer is 3 *[II C; Table 15-1].* The halocarbon compounds (e.g., chloroform, halothane, freon) and the fumes from overheated synthetic fluorine-containing resin-coated (Teflon) cookware are indirectly cardiotoxic because they sensitize the heart to sympathomimetic amines such as epinephrine. Following exposure to these substances, even the release of endogenous epinephrine associated with stress can pose a hazard. Yew plants contain a cardioactive alkaloid that inhibits depolarization and produces bradycardia and diastolic heart block. Furazolidone interferes with intermediary metabolism, resulting in a lack of energy and a dilated, weak heart "round heart." Digitalis affects potassium content in the cell. Monensin is an ionophore that alters the sodium-to-calcium ratio and leads to cardiac necrosis.

2. The answer is 1 *[III B].* Barium replaces calcium in slow-current channels, promoting the slow phase of depolarization; therefore, calcium salts should be avoided. Potassium may be indicated because the affected animal would likely be hypokalemic. Carbonate and chloride anions are not involved in the depolarization of cardiac contractile cells.

3. The answer is 3 *[IV A 2].* Monensin, an ionophore, causes acute cardiac effects by interfering with calcium and sodium transport. Elevated intracellular calcium levels impair mitochondrial respiration, resulting in significant myocardial necrosis. The damaged myocardium is repaired by fibrosis, which leads to cardiac muscle insufficiency, exercise intolerance, and sometimes sudden death in survivors of acute monensin toxicosis.

4. The answer is 4 *[I 3 a (2) (b), II A; Table 15-1].* Amphetamines and caffeine (a methylxanthine alkaloid) stimulate catecholamine release, and tricyclic antidepressants and cocaine inhibit the uptake of released catecholamine neurotransmitters. Fluoroacetate is a metabolic inhibitor of aconitase in the tricarboxylic acid (TCA) cycle and its cardiac effects are the result of acute severe energy deficit in the myocardium.

Chapter 16

Toxicology of the Blood and Bone Marrow

A. **Exposure to toxicants.** Blood acts as a **transport medium (vehicle) for most toxicants**.

1. **Susceptibility to toxicosis.** Toxicants can affect:
   a. The production and maturation of blood cells (hematopoiesis)
   b. Hemoglobin synthesis or its ability to carry oxygen
   c. The longevity of erythrocytes
   d. Coagulation (hemostasis)

2. **Indications of exposure.** Exposure to toxicants may lead to:
   a. Hemoconcentration
   b. Morphologically altered erythrocytes or leukocytes
   c. Low oxygen tension
   d. Altered erythrocyte cholinesterase activity [from exposure to organophosphate (anticholinesterase) insecticides]
   e. Elevated levels of plasma enzymes released from the cells of damaged organs or tissues

B. **Cell types**

1. **Erythrocytes (red blood cells)** carry oxygen.

2. **Thrombocytes (platelets)** provide the basis for a stable hemostatic plug (clot).
   a. **Platelets reduce blood loss by adhering** almost instantly **to subendothelial surfaces that are exposed by trauma**.
   b. Adherence of platelets is followed by the **release of plasma factors** such as adenosine diphosphate (ADP). These factors stimulate additional platelets to aggregate, enhancing clot formation.
   c. Thrombocytes are also important in **syneresis (clot retraction)**. This process helps to form a stable clot. In a glass tube, platelet deficiency is seen as a failure of the erythrocytes in clotted blood to contract and separate from the serum.

3. **Leukocytes (white blood cells)** defend the body against foreign challenge, either by phagocytosis and killing, or by immunologic mechanisms. Leukocytes are either granulocytes or agranulocytes.
   a. **Granulocytes** comprise **neutrophils, eosinophils,** and **basophils**.
   b. **Agranulocytes** comprise **lymphocytes** and **monocytes**.

II. DISORDERS OF HEMATOPOIESIS

A. Introduction

1. The **pluripotent stem cell pool** in bone marrow gives rise to both lymphocytes and the myeloid precursors that differentiate into erythrocytes, thrombocytes, and several different granulocytes (Figure 16-1).

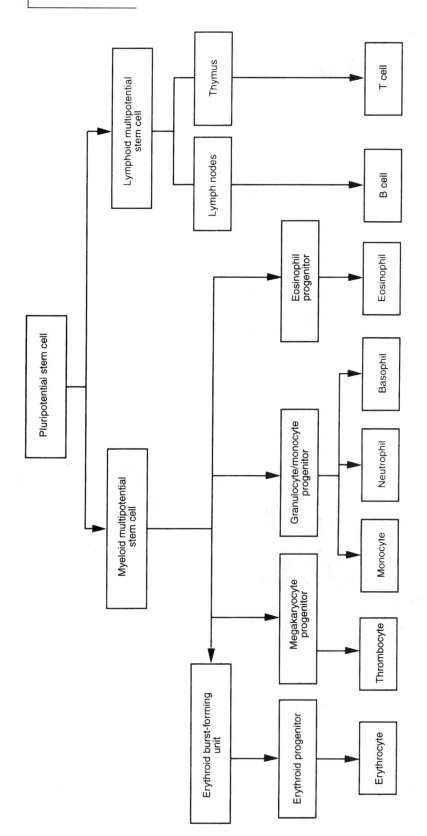

FIGURE 16-1. Steps in hematopoiesis. (Modified with permission from *NMS Hematology*. Baltimore, Williams & Wilkins, 1992, p 13.)

a. Prenatal hematopoiesis takes place in the **yolk sac, liver,** and **spleen.**
b. Postnatal hematopoiesis occurs primarily in the **bone marrow,** with some residual islands of hematopoiesis in the **liver.** Demands for increased oxygen transport (or reduced capability of the bone marrow) may stimulate postnatal hematopoiesis in the liver and spleen; however, these areas alone are not adequate to maintain the level of hematopoiesis needed to support life.

2. Erythropoiesis
a. Prenatal erythropoiesis
   (1) Erythrocytes containing **embryonic hemoglobin ($\alpha_2\epsilon_2$)** are replaced by erythrocytes containing **fetal hemoglobin ($\alpha_2\gamma_2$).**
   (2) Fetal hemoglobin endows fetal blood with a higher affinity for oxygen than adult blood.
b. Postnatal erythropoiesis
   (1) In humans, fetal hemoglobin is replaced with **adult hemoglobin ($\alpha_2\beta_2$)** by 4–6 months of age.
   (2) A **lowered blood oxygen tension serves as a stimulus** for erythropoiesis. Changes are detected by the kidney, which responds by releasing **erythropoietin,** a hormone that stimulates erythrocyte production.
c. Maturation of erythrocytes
   (1) **Immature red blood cells** contain a **nucleus** and **rough endoplasmic reticulum (rER).**
      (a) The nucleus and rER are **lost during the first 24–36 hours in circulation.**
      (b) Increased numbers of **nucleated erythrocytes and erythrocytes with retained rER (reticulocytes)** are evidence of the release of immature erythrocytes into the circulation.
         (i) This response in blood is called **reticulocytosis** and is recognized by a staining pattern known as **basophilic stippling.** Basophilic stippling is a characteristic sign of lead poisoning, which interferes with heme synthesis (see Chapter 17 V E 2 c).
         (ii) Reticulocytosis usually **indicates a proliferative response to an anemic stress** (e.g., intravascular hemolysis caused by chlorates, arsine, copper, or methylene blue).
   (2) The **erythrocyte mass** is maintained by adjustments in the rate of transformation of stem cells to nucleated red blood cells.

B. Anemias resulting from maturation defects

1. Microcytic (hypochromic) anemia often results from iron deficiency.
2. Macrocytic (megaloblastic) anemia is caused by defects in deoxyribonucleic acid (DNA) synthesis. These deficits are often the result of either folic acid or vitamin B_{12} deficiency; therefore, drugs that interfere with folic acid synthesis (e.g., methotrexate) can cause macrocytic anemia.

C. Aplastic anemia is caused by a decrease in the number and function of multipotential stem cells.

1. Effects include **reduced bone marrow volume** and, eventually, **pancytopenia.** The remaining active bone marrow locates in small, intensely active islands in an otherwise fatty bone marrow.
2. Characteristics
   a. Aplastic anemia is often **macrocytic.**
   b. **Reticulocytes are few in number,** but **relatively immature.** The presence of reticulocytes is indicative of an accelerated bone marrow transit time.
   c. Both **plasma iron** and **erythropoietin levels are high,** indicating reduced use by the diminished bone marrow mass.
   d. **Production of fetal hemoglobin is often increased,** especially in children.
   e. Advanced aplastic anemia is also accompanied by **granulocytopenia** and **thrombocytopenia.**

TABLE 16-1. Common Causes of Aplastic Anemia

Acetazolamide	Colchicine
Alkylating agents (e.g., cyclophos- phamide)	Estrogens
	Penicillin
Arsenicals	Phenylbutazone
Aspirin	Phenytoin
Benzene	Quinacrine
Bracken fern	Sulfisoxazole
Chloramphenicol	T-2 mycotoxin
Chlorpromazine	Toluene
Chlorthiazide	Trichloroethylene

3. **Causes.** Numerous drugs and toxins are associated with aplastic anemia (Table 16-1).
   a. **Chloramphenicol.** The use of this anti-infective agent is restricted because of the high incidence (1:10,000–20,000 cases) of fatal aplastic anemia.
      (1) **Effects.** Most animals treated with chloramphenicol experience mild, reversible depression of bone marrow activity, manifested as a reduced reticulocyte count, increased serum iron levels, and vacuolation of erythroid cells in the bone marrow.
      (2) **Mechanism of toxicity.** The mechanism of toxicity is still not completely known. Treated animals begin showing signs of bone marrow depression weeks to months after exposure to small amounts of the drug.
         (a) Normally, chloramphenicol suppresses ribosomal protein synthesis in bacteria, not in mammals.
         (b) It has been suggested that chloramphenicol causes inhibition of mitochondrial protein synthesis. Susceptibility to chloramphenicol toxicosis could be a genetic defect or an acquired hypersensitivity.
   b. **Chemotherapeutic alkylating agents** (e.g., **cyclophosphamide, chlorambucil**). Because rapidly proliferating cells are most affected by these agents, myelosuppression is a common side effect.
      (1) Alkylating agents interrupt the cell cycle at the G_2 (premitotic) stage.
      (2) Cells that accumulate behind the block at the G_2 stage have a double complement of DNA, indicating that the maturation of the precursor cells has been arrested.
      (3) Mitosis ceases within 6–8 hours of first exposure, leading to disintegration of formed elements in the bone marrow.

D. **Granulocytopenia** is a serious response to toxic agents that can lead to irreversible changes in the bone marrow. Often, the same agents that cause anemia cause granulocytopenia as well.

E. **Radiomimetic syndrome** is characterized by anemia, thrombocytopenia, and granulocytopenia. Radiomimetic syndrome can be induced by a variety of toxicants, including benzene, T-2 mycotoxin (a *Fusarium* mold metabolite), bracken fern (in cattle), alcohol, phenylbutazone, and anticancer drugs.

III. **DISORDERS AFFECTING HEMOGLOBIN**

A. **Introduction**

1. **Synthesis.** Hemoglobin synthesis occurs only in **erythroblasts, rubricytes** (i.e., developing erythrocytes), and, for 12–48 hours after the nucleus is lost, **reticulocytes.**

2. **Structure. Adult hemoglobin** is a tetrameric polypeptide of **four globin chains ($\alpha_2\beta_2$),** each with an **associated heme group** (Figure 16-2).

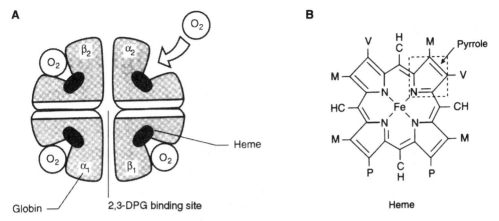

FIGURE 16-2. (*A*) Hemoglobin polypeptide. (*B*) Chemical structure of the heme group. *2,3-DPG* = 2,3-diphosphoglycerate; *Fe* = iron; *N* = nitrogen; *P* = propionyl side chain; *V* = vinyl. (Modified with permission from *NMS Hematology*. Baltimore, Williams & Wilkins, 1992, pp 60, 124.)

    a. Each porphyrinic **heme group** is composed of a **central iron atom** joined to **four nitrogens bound in a ring conformation**.

    b. Heme is **held in the pocket of each chain by hydrophobic forces** that link heme propionyl side chains to globin lysyl residues.

    c. In the **ferrous (2^+) state,** the iron of the heme group can **combine reversibly with oxygen,** or it can combine with oxygen in an oxidation–reduction reaction. Following an oxidation–reduction reaction, iron is converted to the **ferric (3^+) state,** forming **methemoglobin,** which is **incapable of reversible oxygenation**.

3. Hemoglobin–O_2 dissociation curve

    a. Cooperativity (i.e., interactions among the four subunits that alter the conformation of the hemoglobin, influencing its oxygenation) changes the characteristic sigmoid shape of the hemoglobin–O_2 dissociation curve.

        (1) The first of four oxygen molecules lost from the hemoglobin tetramer requires a drop in oxygen tension of approximately 60 mm Hg.

        (2) Because of cooperativity, the second oxygen molecule lost requires only a 15 mm Hg drop in oxygen tension.

        (3) Each successive oxygen molecule lost is unloaded with increasingly larger dissociation constants.

    b. Factors affecting the hemoglobin–O_2 dissociation curve

        (1) Hydrogen ion concentration. As the hydrogen ion concentration increases, the Bohr effect decreases the affinity of oxygen for hemoglobin because deoxyhemoglobin is a weaker acid than is hemoglobin.

        (2) 2,3-Diphosphoglycerate (2,3-DPG). After the erythrocyte has given up its oxygen, 2,3-DPG binds to the center of the hemoglobin polypeptide, decreasing its affinity for oxygen.

        (3) Carbon monoxide increases the affinity of hemoglobin for oxygen. That is, carboxyhemoglobin increases the affinity of the remaining deoxyhemoglobin for oxygen.

        (4) Methemoglobinemia reduces the oxygen tension, altering oxygen release by cooperativity.

B. **Porphyria** is an inherited or acquired block in the enzymatic steps that govern heme synthesis, resulting in overproduction of heme precursors above the block.

    1. Effects

        a. Hemolytic anemia with erythrocyte proliferative response

        b. Increased porphyrin content occurs because porphyrin is accumulated in the presence of reduced heme production. As porphyrin content increases, erythrocyte survival decreases.

      c. Reduced glutathione stability, which increases susceptibility to oxidative damage

      d. Increased reticulocyte maturation time. Heme synthesis controls the rate of reticulocyte maturation; therefore, in the presence of reduced heme synthesis, the maturation time increases from 3–10 hours to 50 hours.

2. Characteristics

      a. Hereditary porphyria is characterized by **increased urinary or fecal excretion of uroporphyrins or their precursors.**

      b. Acquired porphyria

        (1) Lead-induced porphyria is characterized by:

          (a) Increased levels of urinary aminolevulinic acid (ALA), erythrocyte protoporphyrin, and coproporphyrin III

          (b) Hypochromic and stippled erythrocytes

          (c) Lack of photosensitization. Because protoporphyrin is bound to zinc and hemoglobin it does not exit the erythrocyte. Therefore, it cannot pass into the skin where photoactivation and photosensitization could occur.

        (2) Hexachlorobenzene-induced porphyria is characterized by:

          (a) Increased levels of urinary uroporphyrin I and III and coproporphyrin I and III, which are not bound by zinc

          (b) Decreased levels of uroporphyrinogen decarboxylase

          (c) Reddish urine resulting from the presence of oxidized porphyrins

          (d) Photosensitivity

          (e) High serum and liver iron levels

C. **Carboxyhemoglobinemia.** Hemoglobin has no intrinsic mechanism to distinguish oxygen from carbon monoxide.

1. Mechanism of toxicity. Carbon monoxide competes reversibly with oxygen for ferrous heme binding. Carboxyhemoglobin affects the oxygen affinity of the remaining oxyhemoglobin, compounding the problem of anoxia.

      a. Affinity. In humans, the affinity of carbon monoxide for hemoglobin is 240 times that of oxygen. In canaries, the comparative affinity is only 110:1.

      b. Saturation. Blood is half-saturated at an ambient concentration of:

$$\frac{21 \text{ vol\% O}_2}{24} = 0.1 \text{ vol\% CO,}$$

      where O_2 = oxygen and CO = carbon monoxide.

      c. Half-life. The half-life of blood carboxyhemoglobin is 4 hours when breathing air at 1 atm, but breathing pure oxygen at 1 atm decreases the half-life of carboxyhemoglobin to 0.7 hour.

2. Clinical signs

      a. The characteristic **cherry-red color of the skin and mucous membranes** in carbon monoxide poisoning results from the color of carboxyhemoglobin, not oxyhemoglobin.

      b. Pregnant sows and ewes held in buildings with unvented fossil fuel heaters may develop levels of carboxyhemoglobin significant enough to cause **fetal anoxia,** leading to **near-term abortions** and **stillbirths.**

D. **Methemoglobinemia** occurs when oxidants [e.g., **nitrates** (in ruminants), **nitrites, copper, chlorates, acetaminophen** (in cats)] change ferrous hemoglobin to ferric hemoglobin, interfering with the ability of heme to accept oxygen.

1. Mechanism of toxicity. Methemoglobin lowers the oxygen content of the blood.

2. Clinical signs

      a. Methemoglobin causes the blood to take on a **dark brown hue.**

      b. Cyanosis and **dyspnea** are common.

      c. Weakness and **recumbency** occur in oxygen-deficient animals.

3. Reduction of methemoglobinemia
   a. Methemoglobin reductase is an enzyme found in erythrocytes that can slowly and spontaneously reduce methemoglobin iron to the ferrous state, using reduced nicotinamide adenine dinucleotide (NADPH) as a cofactor.
   (1) Some animals are born with a deficiency of methemoglobin reductase and may be chronically methemoglobinemic. These animals are also very sensitive to methemoglobin-generating chemicals.
   (2) Species differences in methemoglobin reductase activity exist.
      (a) Mice, rabbits, guinea pigs, and rats have high methemoglobin reductase activity.
      (b) Humans, pigs, dogs, cats, horses, and cows have low methemoglobin reductase activity.
   b. Methylene blue is used clinically to nonenzymatically reduce methemoglobin, after the methylene blue itself is reduced by an enzyme-catalyzed, NADPH-dependent reaction.

IV. DISORDERS INVOLVING DESTRUCTION OF ERYTHROCYTES

A. Introduction

1. Metabolism in erythrocytes
   a. Mechanism. Metabolism in erythrocytes is primarily via **anaerobic glycolysis** (65%) and the **pentose phosphate pathway**.
   (1) Erythrocytes lack nuclei, ribosomes, and a cytochrome system. Therefore, metabolism via the tricarboxylic acid (TCA) cycle, protein synthesis, and oxidative phosphorylation are impossible.
   (2) Insulin is not required for the entry of glucose into cells.
   b. Roles
   (1) Synthesis of a few simple compounds [e.g., ATP, nicotinamide adenine dinucleotide (NAD), reduced glutathione (GSH)]
   (2) Maintenance of the cell membrane and its deformability
   (3) Maintenance of critical ion concentrations via the sodium–potassium–adenosine triphosphatase (ATPase) pump
   (4) Maintenance of the active reducing potential via NADPH to protect hemoglobin and enzyme proteins from oxidative denaturation

2. Factors affecting susceptibility to hemolysis
   a. Cell age and hexokinase activity
   (1) The phosphorylation of hexose (catalyzed by hexokinase) is the rate-limiting step for erythrocyte glycolysis. This step is inhibited by oxidized glutathione (GSSG) and 2,3-DPG. In addition, hexokinase activity declines as the age of the erythrocyte increases.
   (2) The ability of the aging cell with limited hexokinase activity to generate NADPH is compromised. NADPH is necessary to regenerate GSSG to GSH, which protects against oxidative damage to the cell membrane.
   b. Prior exposure. After acute drug-induced hemolysis, the younger surviving population of erythrocytes is less susceptible to further oxidative damage.
   c. Glucose-6-phosphate dehydrogenase (G6PD). Sheep and goats have low G6PD activity; therefore, they are highly sensitive to copper-induced hemolysis.

B. Oxidative damage. Sulfhemoglobin formation, Heinz body formation, and hemolysis constitute a **triad of effects of oxidative damage**.

1. Sulfhemoglobin is most likely a mixture of oxidized and partially denatured hemoglobins. The toxicologic significance of sulfhemoglobin is not clear, except it appears to be an early change in the progression of oxidative damage to hemolysis.

2. **Heinz bodies** appear to be denatured hemoglobins covalently bound to the interior of the erythrocyte membrane.
   a. **Effect.** Heinz bodies reduce the flexibility and deformability of the erythrocyte membrane and increase phagocytosis of affected red blood cells in the reticuloendothelial system.
   b. **Causes**
      (1) Strong oxidant chemicals [e.g., **chlorates, nitrite, copper, naphthalene, N-propyl disulfide** (found in *Allium* species)] and **methylene blue overdose** produce Heinz bodies in normal erythrocytes.
      (2) Some agents (e.g., **fava beans, primaquine, aspirin**) produce Heinz bodies in G6PD-deficient cells. The incidence of this deficiency in animals is not well known.
      (3) The hemoglobin of cats is highly sensitive to auto-oxidation and Heinz body formation. This sensitivity is probably caused by different amino acid patterns or differences in the sulfhydryl content of the hemoglobin.

3. **Hemolytic anemia** may be induced in domestic animals by copper, zinc, phenothiazine, onions, *Acer rubrum* (red maple), *Brassica* species [rape (seed and forage), kale], saponin-containing plants, and rattlesnake or other pit viper venoms.

C. **Therapy.** The following substances can be used to offset erythrocyte degeneration and hemolysis by preventing oxidative damage to erythrocyte membranes.

1. **Glutathione peroxidase** catalyzes the reduction of lipid peroxidases (oxidants) to lipid alcohols.

2. **Superoxide dismutase** catalyzes the conversion of active oxygen to hydrogen peroxide.

3. **Catalase** aids conversion of hydrogen peroxide to water.

4. **Vitamin E (α-tocopherol)** acts as a scavenger of free radicals.

5. **G6PD** enhances the pentase phosphate pathway.

6. **NADPH** provides reducing capability to convert oxidized glutathione to reduced glutathione.

V. DISORDERS AFFECTING COAGULATION (HEMOSTASIS)

A. **Introduction**

1. The **coagulation cascade** is the serial activation of a set of coagulation factors that leads to the activation of fibrinogen and the formation of a stable fibrin clot.
   a. **Pathways.** The coagulation cascade can be initiated and proceed along either the **intrinsic pathway** or the **extrinsic pathway**. The two pathways converge and the final sequence of events, the **common pathway,** is the same for both systems.
      (1) In the common pathway, prothrombin is converted to thrombin, which converts fibrinogen to fibrin monomer.
      (2) The fibrin monomer polymerizes with calcium and factor XIII to form a stable, insoluble fibrin clot.
   b. Because the cascade is a series of sequential activating steps, interruption of one or more of these steps affects the full expression of the clot-forming process.

2. The **fibrinolytic system** comprises a group of zymogens and enzymes. This system aids in removing the clot as vessel healing and repair proceed.

B. **Coagulopathy from toxicants**

1. **Mechanism of toxicity.** Orally active coumarin derivatives interfere with the vitamin K–dependent hepatic synthesis of **factors II, VII, IX, X.**

TABLE 16-2. Half-lives of Coagulation Factors Affected by Oral Anticoagulants*

Factor	Half-life (hours)
II	60
VII	6
IX	24
X	40

*In dogs

    a. Precursors of the clotting factors undergo a final activation step to form active clotting factors.

    b. The vitamin K–sensitive step is a postribosomal carboxylation of 10 or more glutamic acid residues at the amino terminal end of the precursor protein to form a unique amino acid (γ-carboxyglutamate).

        (1) Oral anticoagulants interrupt the activity of the epoxide reductase enzyme. This enzyme is needed to regenerate the reduced (active) form of vitamin K that is used in the final carboxylation of clotting factors.

        (2) The formation of epoxide reductase is altered in rats with genetic resistance to warfarin; therefore, these rats also have higher vitamin K requirements than normal rats.

2. Exposure. Several commonly used **rodenticides** rely on anticoagulants (e.g., warfarin, coumarin) to exert their effects.

    a. Oral anticoagulants act only in vivo.

    b. A time lag between ingestion and the appearance of coagulation defects is caused by the persistence of existing coagulation factors. Table 16-2 lists the half-lives of the various factors that are inhibited.

    c. Large doses hasten onset only to a limited degree. A large loading dose prolongs the time that the plasma concentration remains at suppressive levels.

    d. A major difference in the ability of anticoagulants to produce and maintain hypoprothrombinemia is their half-life in the animal body. Anticoagulants with a long half-life include diphacinone, brodifacoum, and bromadiolone.

BIBLIOGRAPHY

Harvey JW: Erythrocyte metabolism. In *Clinical Biochemistry of Domestic Animals, 4th ed.* Edited by Kaneko JJ. San Diego, Academic Press, 1989, pp 185–234.

Kaneko JJ: Porphyrins and the porphyrias. In *Clinical Biochemistry of Domestic Animals, 4th ed.* Edited by Kaneko JJ. San Diego, Academic Press, 1989, pp 235–255.

Smith, RP: Toxic responses of the blood. In *Casarett and Doull's Toxicology: The Basic Science of Poisons,* 4th ed. Edited by Amdur MO, Doull J, Klaassen CD. New York, Pergamon Press, 1991, pp 257–281.

STUDY QUESTIONS

DIRECTIONS: Each of the numbered items or incomplete statements in this section is followed by answers or by completions of the statement. Select the **one** numbered answer or completion that is **best** in each case.

1. The fetus may be more susceptible to toxicants that affect the blood because:

(1) Hematopoiesis has not yet begun, so the blood cells available cannot be replaced before birth.
(2) The fetus contains a high population of erythroid cells that are susceptible to Heinz bodies because of increased sulfhydryl content in the membranes.
(3) The fetal concentration of 2,3 diphosphoglycerate (2,3-DPG) is elevated, and the susceptibility to oxygen loss is increased.
(4) Fetal hemoglobin has a different globin structure and a higher affinity for oxygen than adult hemoglobin.

2. Which statement about factors affecting the hemoglobin–O_2 dissociation curve is true?

(1) Increased hydrogen ion concentration in the erythrocyte increases the affinity of hemoglobin for oxygen.
(2) 2,3-Diphosphoglycerate (2,3-DPG) decreases the affinity of oxygen for hemoglobin.
(3) Carbon monoxide decreases the affinity of hemoglobin for oxygen.
(4) Adult hemoglobin has a higher affinity for oxygen than does fetal hemoglobin.

3. Which one of the following statements concerning methemoglobin is true?

(1) It imparts a brown color to blood.
(2) It is produced when the iron in heme is reduced to the divalent state.
(3) Methemoglobin oxidase reverses methemoglobinemia.
(4) Methemoglobin is produced with approximately equal probability in all animal species.
(5) Methemoglobin is most likely produced by chemicals that are strong reducing agents.

4. Which statement about carbon monoxide poisoning is *not* true?

(1) Carboxyhemoglobin increases the affinity of oxyhemoglobin for oxygen.
(2) The cherry-red color of the blood in carbon monoxide results from the high oxygen content.
(3) Treatment of carbon monoxide poisoning is enhanced by administration of hyperbaric oxygen.
(4) Hemoglobin has a much higher affinity for carbon monoxide than for oxygen.
(5) There is a natural low level of endogenous production of carboxyhemoglobin that results from the catabolism of heme.

5. Which statement about aplastic anemia is *not* true?

(1) Aplastic anemia often results in a macrocytic anemia with increased numbers of reticulocytes.
(2) Drug-induced anemia often results from drugs or chemicals that interfere with deoxyribonucleic acid (DNA)-controlled erythrocyte synthesis.
(3) Plasma iron and erythropoietin are reduced because of accelerated use by the bone marrow.
(4) Advanced aplastic anemia is usually characterized by reduced numbers of erythrocytes, leukocytes, and thrombocytes.
(5) Fetal hemoglobin concentrations may rise during aplastic anemia.

ANSWERS AND EXPLANATIONS

1. The answer is 4 *[II A 2 a (2)]*. Fetal hemoglobin has a demonstrated increased affinity for oxygen, which, under normal conditions, promotes the transfer of oxygen from the maternal circulation to the fetal circulation. Fetal hemoglobin is composed of two α and two γ globin chains, unlike adult hemoglobin, which has two α and two β chains. When oxygen tension is reduced, the kidney responds by releasing erythropoietin, a hormone that stimulates erythrocyte production. When oxygen tension is low, fetal hemoglobin retains higher amounts of oxygen, releasing less to the fetal tissues. Prenatal hematopoiesis takes place in the yolk sac, liver, and spleen. Fetal erythrocytes are not more susceptible to Heinz bodies than adult erythrocytes. Fetal blood does not contain more 2,3-diphosphoglycerate than adult blood.

2. The answer is 2 *[III A 3 b]*. The hemoglobin–O_2 dissociation curve is a sigmoid-shaped curve that represents the release of oxygen from hemoglobin. An increased 2,3-diphosphoglycerate (2,3-DPG) level favors placement of the 2,3-DPG molecule in the central cavity of deoxyhemoglobin. Because 2,3-DPG can be considered competitive with oxygen, it reduces the affinity of oxygen for the occupied hemoglobin. When the hydrogen ion concentration is increased, the Bohr effect decreases oxygen's affinity for hemoglobin because deoxyhemoglobin is a weaker acid than is hemoglobin. Carbon monoxide increases the affinity of hemoglobin for oxygen. Fetal hemoglobin has a higher affinity for oxygen than adult hemoglobin.

3. The answer is 1 *[III D]*. Methemoglobin is formed when the heme iron of hemoglobin is oxidized to the trivalent (ferric) state. This change interferes with hemoglobin's ability to bind oxygen and causes the blood to take on a dark chocolate-brown color. Methemoglobinemia is reversed by a natural body enzyme, methemoglobin reductase. Laboratory animals have high levels of this enzyme, but domestic animals, including ruminants, do not. Ruminants are also susceptible to methemoglobinemia because nitrates in plants are reduced to nitrites in the rumen. Nitrites and other strong oxidants produce methemoglobinemia.

4. The answer is 2 *[III C]*. The cherry-red color of carboxyhemoglobin results from the natural color of the chemical combination of carboxyhemoglobin. Formalin-fixed tissue that has a high carboxyhemoglobin content remains pink. During carbon monoxide poisoning, the remaining oxyhemoglobin has a high affinity for oxygen, but the total oxyhemoglobin level is decreased by the amount of carboxyhemoglobin present. Breathing 100% oxygen decreases the half-life of carboxyhemoglobin. Hemoglobin has a much higher affinity for carbon monoxide than oxygen (240:1 in humans). Healthy individuals have an endogenous carboxyhemoglobin level of approximately 1% from the catabolism of heme. This level is increased in the presence of hemolytic disease, burns, and pregnancy.

5. The answer is 3 *[II C]*. Plasma iron and erythropoietin levels are increased in aplastic anemia because the reduced bone marrow mass is unable to fully use these components in normal synthesis. Aplastic anemia usually is a result of reduced deoxyribonucleic acid (DNA)-controlled synthesis of pluripotent bone marrow precursors of erythrocytes, leukocytes, and thrombocytes. Fetal hemoglobin synthesis may increase in adults with aplastic anemia. Aplastic anemia is characterized by macrocytes and increased numbers of reticulocytes.

PART III

CLASSES OF TOXICANTS

Chapter 17
Metals and Minerals

I. **INTRODUCTION**

A. **General properties.** Metals are **intrinsic to nature**.

1. Environmental influences may alter the form or valence of a metal, but **as elements, metals cannot be destroyed**.

2. Metals **play an essential role in biologic processes**.
   a. They act as cofactors in enzyme systems.
   b. They are important for proper functioning of the nervous system.
   c. They play a role in oxidation and reduction.

3. At an appropriate dosage, **both essential and nonessential metals may be toxic**.
   a. **Redistribution of metals in the environment** (i.e., geochemical cycling) exposes humans and animals to toxic forms of metals that are not normally accessible (Figure 17-1).
      (1) **Industrial sources**
         (a) Mining produces dust, tailings, or contaminated water.
         (b) Processing by smelting or roasting releases fumes, particulates, and fugitive dusts into the environment.
         (c) Burning coal releases cadmium, mercury, and arsenic to the environment.
         (d) Sewage treatment plants contribute to the redistribution of industrial by-products in sewage sludge.
      (2) **Commercial sources.** Products (e.g., pesticides, medications, paints, automotive products) often contain concentrated amounts of metals as part of their active ingredients.
   b. **Changes in the chemical form of the metal**
      (1) **Oxidation–reduction reactions** result in valence changes that alter the chemical and toxicological properties of metals (see I B 2).
      (2) The formation of **carbon–metal bonds** (e.g., the conversion of metallic mercury to methyl mercury) influences the lipid solubility, toxicity, and environmental accumulation of metals.
      (3) Metals can **form complexes with** organic molecules known as **chelates (ligands)**.
         (a) Chelation is a reversible interaction between the metal and an anionic or neutral molecule that has at least one pair of nonbonded electrons.
         (b) Chelation can alter absorption, transport, and excretion of metals.
   c. **Interactions with other metals or nutrients.** Metal toxicity can be altered by nutrient deficiency or excess.
      (1) **Nutrient deficiencies** can enhance metal toxicity. For example, low dietary calcium, zinc, and iron enhance the absorption and toxicity of lead.
      (2) **Nutrient excess**
         (a) Excessive amounts of one metal can cause a secondary metal deficiency by antagonizing its absorption, transport, or retention (Table 17-1).

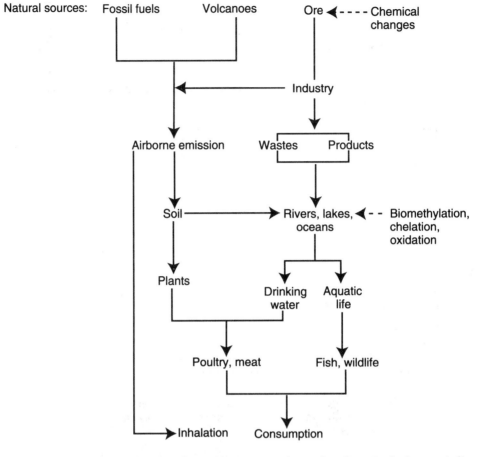

FIGURE 17-1. Redistribution of metals in the environment (geochemical cycling). *Dashed arrows* indicate the influence of processes that may affect the toxicity of the metal.

     (b) Conversely, high levels of some nutrient metals can antagonize the accumulation of metals or lessen the effect of specific metal toxicoses. For example:
        (i) High concentrations of selenium in marine environments favor a selenium–mercury–protein complex in tissues that reduces the toxic effects of mercury.
        (ii) Arsenic is reported to antagonize selenium toxicosis by promoting urinary excretion of selenium.
  d. The **route of exposure** and **potential for tissue accumulation** may influence the toxicologic effects of the metal.
    (1) Route of exposure
      (a) Oral route. Oral absorption of most metals is usually low (less than 10%) and is affected by many factors (e.g., the age of the animal, nutrient composition of foods, the presence of natural or commercial chelating agents).
      (b) Respiratory route. Exposure to metal fumes (hydrides of the original metal) or other volatile forms of metals results in rapid absorption of the metal.
    (2) Tissue accumulation. Metals may accumulate preferentially in specific tissue sites (e.g., lead in bone, methyl mercury in cerebral gray matter and the kidney, cadmium in the kidney).
      (a) Accumulation in susceptible tissues favors toxicosis of that organ or tissue [e.g., mercury accumulation in the central nervous system (CNS) results in neurotoxicosis].
      (b) Accumulation in some storage sites does not cause toxicosis (e.g., arsenic in hair).

TABLE 17-1. Secondary Deficiencies Caused by Nutrient or Metal Excess

Excessive Metal	Resultant Deficiency	Affected Species
Cadmium	Zinc	All
Molybdenum	Copper	Cattle
Potassium	Magnesium	Cattle
Iron	Phosphate	Swine
Calcium	Zinc	Swine

B. **Expression of toxicosis.** Toxicologic effects depend on the **chemical form** and **oxidation state (valence)** of the metal and can vary widely for a given metal. For example, inorganic forms of arsenic and mercury primarily affect the liver, kidney, and digestive tract; organic forms of these metals predominantly accumulate in and affect the nervous system.

1. **Chemical form.** Organometallic compounds more readily cross important biologic membranes, such as the blood–brain barrier and the placenta.

2. **Valence state.** The naturally occurring valence state of metals is often less toxic than metals developed for commercial use. For example:
   a. The natural form of arsenic (pentavalent arsenic) is less toxic than the salts commercially used as early pesticides (trivalent arsenic).
   b. Elemental mercury is less toxic than the mercuric salts used in early fungicides.
   c. Trivalent chromium is an essential trace element, but the hexavalent form, chromate, is highly toxic.

II. ARSENIC TOXICOSIS

A. **Sources**

1. **Environment**
   a. Ores (e.g., arsenopyrite, loellingite) are mined and then smelted to produce **elemental arsenic** and arsenic trioxide. Soils naturally contain low concentrations of elemental arsenic, but those near mining or smelting sites may be contaminated by mine tailings, smoke, fumes, and dust.
   b. Arsenic in the environment usually exists in the pentavalent form and may be methylated by microorganisms.

2. **Commercial forms**
   a. **Inorganic**
      (1) **Arsenic trioxide,** formerly used as a herbicide and currently used as a source for other arsenicals
      (2) **Pentavalent and trivalent forms** (**sodium, potassium,** and **calcium salts** of **arsenates** and **arsenites,** respectively), used as baits
   b. **Organic**
      (1) **Trivalent**
         (a) **Monosodium methanearsonate (MSMA)** and **disodium methanearsonate (DMSA),** used as herbicides
         (b) **Thiacetarsamide,** used for heartworm therapy in dogs
      (2) **Pentavalent arsenical feed additives** (e.g., **arsanilic acid, sodium arsanilate,** and **3-nitro, 4-hydroxyphenylarsonic acid**)

B. **Exposure.** Arsenic poisoning can result from:

1. Accidental exposure of livestock to **old pesticides** (e.g., lead arsenate, arsenic trioxide) that are improperly disposed of or stored

2. **Arsenic-contaminated soils or burn piles,** which are often licked by animals that crave salt or minerals

3. **Contaminated waters** in abandoned mining areas

4. **Ant baits** (e.g., **sodium or potassium arsenate**), which are attractive to small animals, especially cats

5. **Therapeutic use of thiacetarsamide** in some dogs

6. **Overdosage or extended use of organic arsenical feed additives in poultry or swine**

7. **Burning of wood products treated with arsenical preservatives**

C. **Toxicokinetics**

1. **Absorption.** Soluble arsenicals are readily absorbed from the gastrointestinal tract and through the skin.

2. **Metabolism.** Methylation of inorganic arsenicals occurs in vivo and may aid in detoxification. A small portion of pentavalent arsenic may be reduced by the kidneys to the more toxic trivalent form.

3. **Excretion.** Trivalent arsenic is excreted into the intestine via the bile, and pentavalent arsenic is excreted by the kidneys. Excretion is rapid in domestic animals and nearly complete within a few days.

D. **Mechanism of toxicologic damage**

1. **Trivalent arsenicals** (Figure 17-2)
   a. **Inhibition of cellular respiration.** Trivalent arsenicals bind to sulfhydryl compounds, especially lipoic acid and α-keto oxidases.
      (1) Lipoic acid, a tissue respiratory enzyme cofactor, plays an essential role in the tricarboxylic acid cycle (TCA).
      (2) Tissues with high oxidative energy requirements (e.g., actively dividing cells such as those of the intestinal epithelium, kidney, liver, skin, and lung) are most affected.
   b. **Capillary dilatation and degeneration.** Trivalent arsenic affects capillary integrity by an unknown mechanism. The gastrointestinal tract is most affected; capillary dilatation is followed by transudation of plasma into the gastrointestinal tract, resulting in submucosal congestion and edema.

2. **Pentavalent inorganic arsenicals** (i.e., arsenates) appear to substitute for phosphate in oxidative phosphorylation.
   a. Uncoupling of oxidative phosphorylation produces a **cellular energy deficit**.
   b. Elevated body temperature is not characteristic of pentavalent arsenical poisoning, as it is in poisonings by other oxidative uncouplers (e.g., nitrophenols).

3. **Pentavalent organic arsenicals** (i.e., feed additives) act by an unknown mechanism. Arsenical feed additive poisoning produces demyelination and eventual axonal degeneration, leading some researchers to believe that pentavalent organic arsenicals interfere with the B vitamins essential for maintenance of nervous tissue.

E. **Toxicity**

1. **Inorganic arsenicals.** Dosages to produce toxicosis depend on valence. **Trivalent forms are up to ten times more toxic than pentavalent forms.**
   a. **Acute toxicity.** For most species, the single dose lethal toxicity of inorganic trivalent arsenic ranges from 1–25 mg/kg body weight. Cats are most susceptible among the domestic animals, followed by horses, cattle and sheep, swine, and birds.
   b. **Subacute toxicity** occurs at lower dosages received over several days.
   c. **Chronic toxicity** from inorganic arsenicals is generally not described in domestic animals.

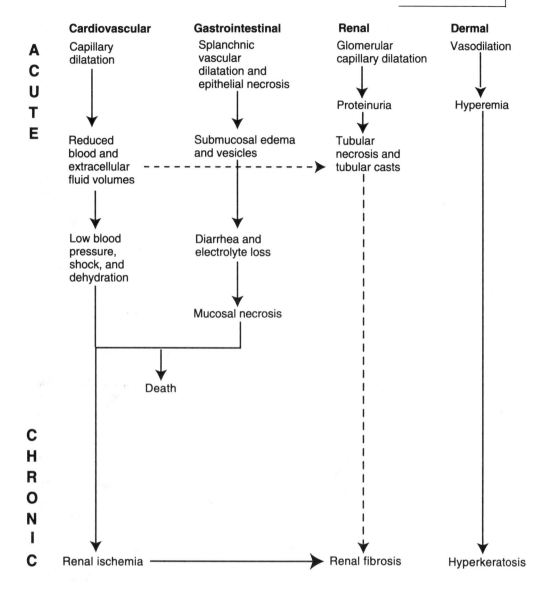

| | **Cardiovascular** | **Gastrointestinal** | **Renal** | **Dermal** |

FIGURE 17-2. Pathogenesis of toxicosis from trivalent arsenicals. These agents dilate the capillaries and cause necrosis of the intestinal epithelium, leading to diarrhea, shock, and acidosis. The decreased renal perfusion that occurs as a result of shock, along with necrosis of the renal tubules caused by the arsenical inhibition of energy metabolism, produces renal damage. *Dashed arrows* indicate indirect effects.

   2. Organic arsenicals
   a. Swine. Exposure to 500 ppm dietary arsanilic acid or 250 ppm 3-nitro, 4-hydroxy-phenylarsonic acid for 7–10 days produces arsenical feed additive toxicosis in swine.
   b. Poultry are affected by dietary exposure approximately twice that which affects swine.

F. **Diagnosis**

   1. Clinical signs
   a. Inorganic or organic trivalent arsenicals
      (1) Acute or peracute poisoning
         (a) Vomiting and intense abdominal pain
         (b) Weakness, staggering, ataxia, recumbency

        (c) Weak, rapid pulse with signs of shock (e.g., hypotension, dehydration, hemo-concentration, hypothermia)

        (d) Rapid onset of severe, watery diarrhea

        (e) Rumen and gastrointestinal atony

    (2) Subacute poisoning occurs when affected animals survive acute arsenic poisoning and live for three days or longer.

        (a) Watery diarrhea continues.

        (b) Oliguria and proteinuria, followed by polyuria with dilute urine (in longer-term survivors), are the manifestations of kidney damage.

        (c) Dehydration, acidosis, and azotemia may cause death.

  b. Organic pentavalent arsenical feed additives

    (1) Early signs, apparent after 2–4 days, include ataxia, incoordination, torticollis, and blindness. Furazolidone, another feed additive, enhances the nervous system effects of feed additive arsenicals.

    (2) Affected animals (most often swine) become weak, assume a sitting-dog posture, and eventually become paralyzed in lateral recumbency.

    (3) Appetite remains normal and affected animals are cognizant, except for some with blindness.

2. Lesions

  a. Gross lesions

    (1) Gastrointestinal irritation characterized by mucosal congestion, prominent submucosal edema, epithelial necrosis, and massive accumulation of fluids in a dilated atonic intestine

    (2) In subacute cases: pale swollen kidneys, pale liver, petechial hemorrhages of the intestinal serosa and mucosa

  b. Microscopic lesions include intestinal capillary dilatation, submucosal congestion and edema, intestinal epithelial necrosis, renal tubular necrosis, and hepatic fatty degeneration.

3. Laboratory diagnosis

  a. Packed cell volume increases.

  b. Blood urea nitrogen (BUN) increases.

  c. Urinalysis reveals proteinuria, increased specific gravity, and casts.

  d. Chemical residues in tissues or body fluids

    (1) Antemortem: urine, vomitus, feces, hair. During chronic poisoning, inorganic arsenic accumulates in the epidermis and hair and persists for weeks to months following exposure.

    (2) Postmortem: hepatic, renal, and nervous tissue

        (a) Inorganic arsenic toxicosis. During acute poisoning, inorganic arsenic concentrates in the liver and kidney, but it is rapidly excreted by animals that survive acute toxicosis.

        (b) Organic arsenic toxicosis. Organic pentavalent arsenicals accumulate in nervous tissue and may persist at elevated levels for several weeks after an acute poisoning. Formalin-fixed peripheral nerves are useful for microscopic evaluation of demyelination.

  e. Analysis of suspected baits, feed, plants, or soil

G. **Treatment and prognosis**

1. Treatment

  a. Early intervention comprising **gastrointestinal detoxification** and **supportive therapy** is essential.

    (1) Emergency and supportive therapy include correction of shock, acidosis, and dehydration. A blood transfusion may be necessary.

    (2) Emetics, activated charcoal, cathartic agents, or **gastric lavage** may be employed if ingestion is recent (see Chapter 5 II B).

(3) Antidotal therapy
  (a) Dimercaprol (British antilewisite, BAL) is the classic antidote for arsenic, but it is relatively ineffective unless given prior to onset of clinical signs. Table 6-1 gives dosage information.
  (b) Thioctic acid (see Table 6-1) is more effective than dimercaprol for arsenic-poisoned cattle; however, it is not available in a commercial dosage form and it is not currently approved for use in food animals.
  (c) Mesodimercaptosuccinic acid (MSMA) and **dimercaptosuccinic acid (DMSA)** are promising water-soluble analogs of dimercaprol, but these agents are not well tested or available in the United States.
    (i) Experimentally, MSMA and DMSA (30 mg/kg body weight) have been shown to be effective at preventing signs of arsenic toxicosis in rabbits.
    (ii) Higher dosages may cause necrotizing lesions at the site of administration, but MSMA and DMSA are less toxic than dimercaprol.
  b. Convalescent animals should receive bland diets containing reduced amounts of high-quality protein. Vitamin supplementation is recommended.

2. Prognosis
  a. Inorganic trivalent arsenicals. The mortality rate is high among acutely poisoned animals.
  b. Organic pentavalent arsenicals. There is a high morbidity rate but a low mortality rate associated with pentavalent arsenical feed additive toxicosis if good nursing and supportive care are employed. Recovery may require 2–4 weeks.

III. COPPER TOXICOSIS

A. **Acute copper toxicosis** occurs following ingestion or dosing of high concentrations of copper. Currently, acute copper toxicosis is not common in veterinary medicine.

1. Sources include copper sulfate foot baths, fungicides, and algicides.

2. Mechanism of toxicologic damage. Copper salts act as direct tissue irritants and oxidants and cause coagulative necrosis of the gastrointestinal mucosa.

3. Toxicity. The single oral toxic dosage is 25–50 mg/kg body weight.

4. Diagnosis is based on history, clinical signs and lesions, and confirmation of elevated copper levels in the gastrointestinal contents or kidney. Copper levels in the liver and blood are not usually increased.
  a. Clinical signs include the rapid onset of salivation, nausea, vomiting, colic, fluid or hemorrhagic diarrhea (sometimes green-tinged) with rapid dehydration, shock, and death.
  b. Lesions include severe gastroenteritis and congestion of the liver, kidneys, and spleen.
  c. Differential diagnoses include arsenic, mercury, or selenium toxicoses and infectious gastroenteritis (e.g., acute salmonellosis, canine parvovirus).

5. Therapy is nonspecific and directed at controlling dehydration, shock, and damage to the gastrointestinal tract.

B. **Chronic copper toxicosis in sheep**

1. Sources
  a. Feed additives (e.g., copper sulfate, copper oxide, copper chloride)
  b. Natural copper in soils and plants
  c. Soils contaminated by mining or smelting
  d. Soils and plants fertilized with used poultry litter or swine manure

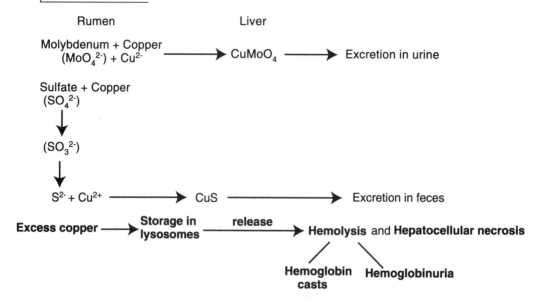

FIGURE 17-3. Hepatic copper accumulation in ruminants is associated with copper, molybdenum, and sulfate imbalances. Normally, molybdate ion (MoO_4^{2-}) binds with copper (Cu^{2+}) in the tissue in a molar ratio of 4:3, forming a copper–molybdate complex ($CuMoO_4$) that is readily excreted in urine, thus preventing hepatic accumulation. In addition, rumen sulfates and sulfites (SO_4^{2-}, SO_3^{2-}) are reduced to sulfides (S^{2-}) that bind with copper ion to reduce absorption of copper. *Bold type* indicates the consequences of insufficient molybdenum or sulfate or excessive copper.

    2. **Mechanism of toxicologic damage**
        a. **Accumulation** occurs in hepatic **mitochondria** and **lysosomes** and is demonstrable histologically with special stains (e.g., rubeanic acid). Copper accumulation in the liver causes **progressive hepatocyte organelle damage** and **cellular degeneration or necrosis**.
            (1) Hepatic copper accumulation in ruminants is associated with **copper, molybdenum, and sulfate imbalances** (Figure 17-3).*
            (2) **Liver damage from xenobiotics or toxic plants** (e.g., *Heliotropium*) may cause excess copper accumulation by hepatocytes [**hepatogenous (secondary) copper toxicosis**].
        b. **Acute hemolytic crisis.** Physiologic stress (e.g., starvation, transport stress, disease, hepatotoxins) may precipitate sudden loss of stored copper from the liver to the blood.
            (1) Excess copper in the blood oxidizes erythrocyte membranes, increasing their fragility and causing hemolysis.
            (2) Oxidation of hemoglobin by copper to form methemoglobin, which does not transport oxygen, may aggravate the acute hemolytic crisis.

    3. **Toxicity**
        a. Normal feed and forage copper levels (10–20 ppm) cause hepatic copper accumulation when molybdenum is deficient (less than 1–2 ppm) or sulfate is not available. Grains and forages often contain less than 1 ppm molybdenum.
        b. Two to ten weeks' exposure may be required for toxic accumulation in sheep.

    4. **Diagnosis**
        a. **Clinical signs of acute hemolytic crisis.** Acute anemia is responsible for most signs of acute copper toxicosis in sheep. Clinical signs include weakness, anorexia, fever, icterus, pale mucous membranes, and dyspnea.

---

*A dietary copper level that exceeds 250 ppm causes hepatic copper accumulation in swine that is apparently unrelated to dietary molybdenum.

b. Lesions of copper toxicosis in sheep are primarily in the liver, kidney, and spleen.
  (1) Gross lesions include hepatic icterus; an enlarged, pulpy spleen (indicative of hemolysis); and dark, bluish-black kidneys (known as **"gunmetal kidneys"**).
  (2) Microscopic lesions include swollen and necrotic hepatocytes, hepatocyte vacuolation, periportal fibrosis, occasional bile duct proliferation, renal tubular necrosis, hemoglobin casts in renal tubules, and excessive fragmented erythrocytes in the spleen.
c. Laboratory diagnosis
  (1) Changes in laboratory parameters include **elevated bilirubin levels, hemoglobinemia,** and **hemoglobinuria**.
  (2) Elevated levels of certain hepatic enzymes [e.g., aspartate aminotransferase (AST), lactate dehydrogenase (LDH), sorbitol dehydrogenase (SDH), and arginase] indicate hepatic necrosis [see Chapter 8 III C 2 a (4) (b), Table 8-1)]. Serum or plasma liver enzymes may be elevated 3–6 weeks before a hemolytic crisis and **may be used to predict animals at risk.**
  (3) Serum or whole blood copper levels are elevated, with values greater than 1.5 ppm copper considered diagnostic of copper toxicosis.
  (4) Liver and kidney copper levels greater than 150 ppm and 15 ppm, respectively, (wet-weight basis) are associated with copper toxicosis.
d. Differential diagnoses
  (1) Infectious diseases (e.g., leptospirosis, bacillary hemoglobinuria, babesiosis, anaplasmosis)
  (2) Plant toxicoses [e.g., onions, *Brassica,* red maple (*Acer rubrum*)]
  (3) Drug toxicoses (e.g., phenothiazine anthelmintic toxicosis)

5. Treatment and prevention
a. Treatment
  (1) Ammonium tetrathiomolybdate (see Table 6-1) aids in rapid binding and excretion of copper.
  (2) D-penicillamine (see Chapter 6 III K) is effective (50 mg/kg administered orally for up to 6 days), but it is expensive and not currently approved for use in food animals.
  (3) For less acute cases, molybdenized copper phosphate has been sprayed on pastures at a concentration of 4 ounces (120 g) per acre.
b. Prevention. Death may occur within 24–48 hours of an acute hemolytic crisis; **the mortality rate among affected animals is high.** Therefore, **emphasis should be placed on prevention of copper accumulation**.
  (1) Feeding rations blended for sheep ensures maintenance of the maximum copper:molybdenum ratio of 6:1.
  (2) Copper sulfate may be added to feed to correct a perceived deficiency.
  (3) Addition of molybdate to sheep rations (2–4 ppm) is an effective preventive measure, although federal regulatory guidelines for the addition of molybdenum to sheep feeds are not available.
  (4) Dosing with 50 mg ammonium molybdate and 0.3–1.0 g thiosulfate per day prevents copper toxicosis in individual animals.
  (5) Supplemental zinc (250 ppm) reduces hepatic copper accumulation.

C. **Chronic hepatic copper accumulation in dogs** is most common in Bedlington terriers, but has also been reported in West Highland white terriers, Doberman pinschers, and, occasionally, in other breeds.

1. **Etiology.** Chronic canine hepatic copper accumulation is inherited as an **autosomal recessive trait**. The disease usually **appears at 2–6 years of age,** with no remarkable prior signs.

2. **Mechanism of toxicologic damage.** Copper accumulates in the lysosomes of hepatocytes until their storage capacity is exceeded. The lysosomes then release the copper to the cytoplasm, where it causes necrosis and inflammation.

3. Diagnosis
   a. Clinical signs
      (1) Young dogs (i.e., less than 6 years of age) may exhibit an acute syndrome characterized by vomiting, anorexia, weakness, and dehydration.
      (2) Older dogs are more likely to develop anorexia, weight loss, icterus, ascites, and hepatic encephalopathy.
      (3) Occasionally, a hemolytic crisis may occur (see III B 4 a).
   b. Lesions
      (1) Gross lesions. The liver may range in appearance from large and necrotic to small and cirrhotic.
      (2) Microscopic lesions include focal hepatitis, chronic active hepatitis, and cirrhosis. Copper stains (e.g., rubeanic acid) show copper accumulation in hepatocytes.
   c. Laboratory diagnosis
      (1) Serum liver enzymes [e.g., alanine aminotransferase (ALT), alkaline phosphatase (AP)] and bilirubin levels are elevated.
      (2) Serum copper levels are normal, but the concentration of copper in the liver is usually greater than 1000 ppm (dry-weight basis). Hepatic biopsy confirms the presence of copper.
      (3) Plasma ceruloplasmin levels are normal. Ceruloplasmin is a copper-binding protein that is produced in the liver and released to the plasma to bind copper.

2. Treatment and prevention
   a. Treatment
      (1) Ongoing chelation therapy with D-penicillamine may be required for months, years, or a lifetime (see Table 6-1).
      (2) Adjunctive supportive therapy
         (a) Corticosteroids (0.5–1.0 mg/day) may be administered to stabilize hepatic lysosomal membranes.
         (b) Ascorbic acid (500–1000 mg/day) enhances copper excretion.
   b. Prevention. Copper intake should be limited. Normal dietary copper levels range from 5–10 ppm.

IV. IRON TOXICOSIS

A. Sources

1. Preparations for oral supplementation of iron, including powders, tablets, and premixes
   a. Ferrous fumarate
   b. Ferrous sulfate
   c. Ferric phosphate
   d. Ferrous carbonate

2. Injectable iron preparations for prevention of neonatal anemia or use as hematinics
   a. Ferric ammonium citrate
   b. Iron–dextran complexes

B. Exposure. Iron toxicity most often occurs as the result of accidental ingestion of oral supplements or overdosage.

C. Mechanism of toxicologic damage (Figure 17-4)

1. Normally, biologic levels of iron are maintained by **selective absorption using an energy-dependent carrier mechanism.**
   a. Absorbed ferrous iron is oxidized to ferric iron and **bound to transferrin,** a β-1 glycoprotein. In this form, iron is transported throughout the body.
   b. Iron is used primarily for oxygen transport by hemoglobin and myoglobin. Excess iron absorbed over a period of time is stored as hemosiderin or ferritin.

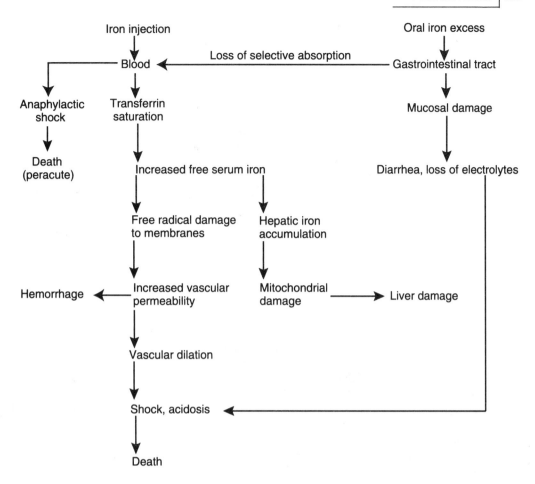

FIGURE 17-4. Pathophysiology of iron toxicosis. Excessive iron gains access to blood by oral or parenteral routes. Free serum iron that exceeds the transferrin-binding capacity initiates membrane damage that results in vascular and hepatic damage, shock, and death.

2. **An excessive single dose of iron** overwhelms the selective transport mechanism, causing the iron salts to be absorbed in a dose-dependent manner. Because the iron-binding capacity of transferrin is insufficient to handle the overload, excess iron circulates in the plasma as free iron.
   a. Unbound elemental iron is corrosive and a strong oxidant, causing **direct damage to epithelial cells** (e.g., the gastric mucosa).
   b. **Mitochondrial damage** causes **hepatic necrosis**.
   c. Increased capillary permeability and postarteriolar dilatation can lead to **cardiovascular collapse**.

D. **Toxicity.** Because most animals lack a mechanism for excreting iron, toxicity depends on the amount of iron already present in the body.

1. In general, toxicity is greater with injectable preparations than with oral preparations. Values for oral preparations are as follows:
   a. **Moderately toxic:** 20–60 mg/kg body weight
   b. **Severely toxic:** greater than 60 mg/kg body weight
   c. **Lethal:** greater than 200 mg/kg body weight

2. Diets containing more than 5000 ppm of iron interfere with phosphate absorption and can lead to retarded growth and rickets in piglets.

E. Diagnosis

1. Clinical signs
  a. Oral preparations
  (1) Early signs (appearing within 6 hours of ingestion) include drowsiness, depression, vomiting, and hemorrhagic diarrhea.
  (2) Apparent improvement may follow for 6–24 hours.
  (3) After 24 hours, the diarrhea returns, accompanied by dehydration, acute liver necrosis, shock, acidosis, and coma.
  (4) Occasionally, acute hemolytic anemia, icterus, hemoglobinemia, and coagulopathy occur as well.
  b. Injectable preparations can cause two distinct syndromes.
  (1) One syndrome is characterized by severe depression, shock, and acidosis resulting from the excessive circulating iron.
  (2) The other involves a peracute anaphylactic-like reaction that occurs almost immediately following the injection but may not be dosage related. This reaction appears to be related to histamine release.

2. Lesions
  a. Oral preparations
  (1) Mucosal necrosis, ulceration, or both
  (2) Enteritis, intestinal contents range from fluid to hemorrhagic
  (3) Congestion of splanchnic vessels, liver, and kidney
  (4) Liver necrosis, icterus, hemoglobinuria
  b. Injectable preparations. Yellowish-brown discoloration of tissues and edema at or near the injection site, and similar discoloration of the lymph nodes draining the area of the injection are characteristic.

3. Laboratory diagnosis
  a. Total serum iron levels are elevated. Concentrations 50%–100% above the normal range (normal: approximately 100–300 µg/dl) suggest toxicosis and the need for chelation therapy.
  b. Increased saturation of the serum total iron-binding capacity (TIBC) is expected, but correlates poorly with the severity of poisoning.
  c. Hemoconcentration, consistent with shock and dehydration, is evident.
  d. Acidosis is detectable.
  e. Serum hepatic enzymes and bilirubin levels are increased.
  f. Urinalysis reveals hemoglobinuria.
  g. Iron concentrations are elevated in the liver; however, interpretation of toxic values in the liver is difficult.
  (1) The normal range for neonatal animals varies widely.
    (a) Puppies may have liver iron values as high as 900 ppm (wet-weight basis).
    (b) Newborn piglets have liver iron values of 100–200 ppm; values normally increase to 600 ppm after parenteral injection with the recommended dose of 100 mg supplemental iron.
  (2) For most adult domestic animals, liver iron values below 400 ppm (wet-weight basis) are considered normal.
  h. Abdominal radiographs may reveal extent of ingestion of iron tablets.

F. Treatment

1. Decontamination of the gastrointestinal tract is recommended if ingestion is recent (less than 4 hours) and vomiting or diarrhea has not occurred (see Chapter 5 II B).
  a. Activated charcoal is not effective for adsorbing iron.
  b. Milk of magnesia administered orally will precipitate iron in the intestinal tract as insoluble iron hydroxide.

2. **Supportive measures to control shock, dehydration, and acidosis** are necessary.

3. **Chelation therapy** inactivates and removes excess iron. **Deferoxamine** given parenterally effectively chelates iron.
   a. **Dosages**
      (1) The **suggested deferoxamine dosage,** based on work in humans and experience in dogs, is intravenous infusion at a rate of 15 mg/kg/hr. Rapid administration may cause cardiac arrhythmia or enhance existing hypotension by promoting histamine release.
      (2) An **alternative dosage regimen** is 40 mg/kg at 4–6-hour intervals.
   b. **Oral ascorbic acid** administered concurrently with deferoxamine enhances excretion of iron.
   c. **Urine** is **reddish-brown** during the early stages of deferoxamine therapy because of the increased excretion of iron.
   d. **Serum iron levels** should be monitored until concentrations reach the normal range (i.e., 2–3 days).

4. **Convalescent care.** Survivors of acute iron toxicosis may have residual intestinal scarring and liver damage that require appropriate care.

V. LEAD TOXICOSIS

A. **Sources.** Because lead was widely used for commercial purposes in the past and is persistent in the environment, lead poisoning continues to occur in domestic animals. Sources include:

1. **Lead objects,** such as batteries, drapery weights, fishing sinkers, buckshot, and plumbing solder

2. **Paints and related products**
   a. Buildings constructed prior to 1950 may have been painted with lead-based paints.
   b. Certain automotive and metal primers contain lead; currently, availability is very limited.
   c. Caulking compounds containing lead are no longer commercially available, but they may remain in older buildings.
   d. Lead-containing pottery with poorly glazed surfaces may leach lead, especially if used for acidic foods or liquids.

3. **Farm machinery and automotive supplies**
   a. **Lubricants** (e.g., grease, used motor oils) from engines that burn leaded gas have been major sources of lead toxicosis. However, with the introduction of unleaded gas, used motor oil is no longer a source of lead, and currently available lubricants contain little or no lead.
   b. **Lead plates in automotive batteries**
   c. **Old automobile chassis and machinery** may be contaminated with lead-based lubricants or paints.

4. **Industry**
   a. **Lead mine tailings and dust** may contaminate pastures or hay crops.
   b. **Sewage sludge** often contains low levels of lead, but lead is poorly taken up by plants.
   c. **Smelters and battery reclamation plants**

5. **Pesticides.** Old orchard areas may be contaminated by previous use of lead arsenate.

B. **Exposure**

1. Cattle and horses are curious and lick or chew on batteries and peeling paint.

2. Puppies and young dogs chew on painted areas and ingest lead objects.

3. Cats have been poisoned by licking lead-contaminated dust from remodelling projects from their coats and paws.

4. Bottom-feeding waterfowl ingest lead shot, which is retained in the proventriculus (crop) or ventriculus (gizzard). Waterfowl may also ingest lead-contaminated mud in lakes or marshes. Recent restrictions on the use of lead shot have decreased the significance of this source.

5. Zoo animals and captive birds consume lead objects or lead-based paints used on cages.

C. Characteristics

1. Lead poisoning **may be seasonal,** with increased incidence in cattle and dogs during the spring and early summer.

2. Most cases of lead poisoning are **subacute.**
   a. Ingestion for several days or more may be necessary to achieve toxic concentrations.
   b. Lead objects persist in the gastrointestinal tract, providing a continuous source of exposure.

3. Young dogs (less than 1 year old) are most frequently affected.

D. Toxicokinetics

1. Absorption
   a. Oral absorption of lead salts and metallic lead is **slow and incomplete**. Only 2%–10% of ingested lead is absorbed, and the balance is excreted in feces.
      (1) Acidic diets may enhance absorption by promoting dissolution of the lead.
      (2) Diets deficient in calcium, zinc, or protein may enhance lead absorption.
   b. Absorbed lead is transported as lead proteinate on the erythrocyte membrane, with very low concentrations in serum.

2. Deposition
   a. Soft tissues. Lead is deposited briefly in soft tissues as diphosphate or triphosphate.
      (1) Nuclear inclusions in the **kidney,** visible by light microscopy, are a lead–proteinate complex.
      (2) Lead crosses the placenta and accumulates in the **fetus.**
         (a) Delayed neurologic developmental defects can occur.
         (b) Hyaline necrosis of uterine vasculature may cause abortion or stillbirth.
      (3) The immature blood–brain barrier of neonates may allow increased **CNS accumulation** of lead.
   b. Bone
      (1) Initial deposition in bone takes place preferentially at areas of active bone growth (e.g., the epiphyseal plate in growing animals).
      (2) Long-term bone deposition is in cancellous bone. Sixty percent of the total body burden is located in cancellous bone.
      (3) The presence of lead in bone marrow suppresses hematopoiesis.

3. Excretion
   a. Low blood levels of lead are excreted by active transport into bile.
   b. High blood levels result in urinary excretion.
   c. Limited evidence suggests that lead is excreted in milk in a ratio that equals approximately 5% of the blood concentration.

E. Mechanism of toxicologic damage

1. The exact mechanism of lead toxicosis at a molecular level is not fully known.
   a. Lead binds sulfhydryl groups and interferes with many sulfhydryl-containing enzymes.
   b. Lead may compete with or replace zinc in some enzymes.

2. Toxic or degenerative effects occur in the nervous system, gastrointestinal tract, and hematopoietic system.

    a. Neurotoxic mechanisms are not well documented, but may include:
      (1) Capillary damage and neuronal necrosis in the CNS
      (2) Demyelination and reduced conduction velocity in the peripheral nervous system (PNS)
      (3) Interference with the action of γ-aminobutyric acid (GABA)
      (4) Interference with cholinergic function in association with reduced extracellular calcium
      (5) Interference with dopamine uptake by synaptosomes
      (6) Possible interference with calcium needed to activate protein kinase C in brain capillaries
    b. Mechanisms of gastrointestinal toxicity. Specific mechanisms for the gastrointestinal effects of lead (e.g., anorexia, vomiting, colic) are not described, but could be secondary to neurologic mechanisms.
    c. Mechanisms of hematopoietic toxicity. The effects of lead on hematopoiesis are associated with inhibition of key enzymes in the pathway of heme synthesis (Figure 17-5).

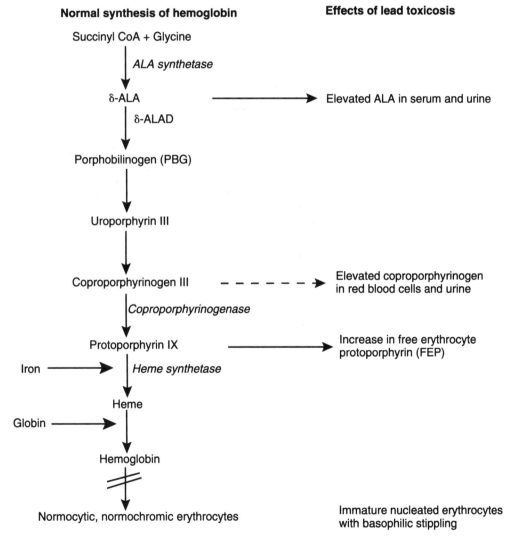

FIGURE 17-5. Effects of lead on heme synthesis. Enzymes inhibited by lead are in *italics*. *ALA* = aminolevulinic acid; δ-ALAD = δ-aminolevulinic acid dehydrase; *succinyl CoA* = succinyl coenzyme A.

    (1) Inhibition of the enzymes δ-aminolevulinic acid dehydrase (δ-ALAD), heme synthetase, and ferrochelatase reduces heme synthesis and causes accumulation of heme precursors (e.g., aminolevulinic acid, coproporphyrins, zinc protoporphyrin) in the blood.

    (2) Inhibition of the enzyme 5'-nucleotidase (5'N) allows retention of nucleic acid fragments and ribosomes, which results in basophilic stippling and increases the fragility of erythrocytes.

F. Diagnosis

1. Clinical signs

    a. General. Clinical signs common to all lead-poisoned animals include:

      (1) Some form of encephalopathy characterized by seizures, tremors, blindness, depression, or dementia

      (2) Anorexia and colic, often accompanied by vomiting and constipation

      (3) Anemia

      (4) Proteinuria

    b. Species-specific clinical signs are listed in Table 17-2.

2. Lesions

    a. Gross lesions in most species are mild and nonspecific.

      (1) Cattle may have pale musculature.

      (2) Lead objects, paint chips, or used motor oil may be visible in the gastrointestinal tract.

      (3) Plasma may fluoresce under ultraviolet light because of the presence of excess porphyrins. This change may not occur in acute cases.

    b. Microscopic lesions

      (1) Cerebral cortical necrosis and poliomalacia may occur in cattle. Neuronal necrosis and hyaline changes in arterioles are inconsistent lesions.

      (2) Renal tubular degeneration or necrosis may be mild to moderate, or absent.

      (3) Acid-fast nuclear inclusion bodies may be present in renal tubular epithelium and, rarely, in hepatocytes.

      (4) Rumen protozoa are reduced in number and often lack motility.

3. Laboratory diagnosis

    a. The **blood lead level** is elevated in all affected species.

      (1) Concentrations used to define toxicosis vary among species, but in general, a blood lead concentration **in excess of 0.4 ppm is abnormally high and associated with clinical signs**.

        (a) The normal background blood lead concentration is less than 0.1 ppm.

        (b) Concentrations between 0.1 ppm and 0.4 ppm suggest nontoxic or preclinical exposure.

      (2) Blood lead values should not be used to diagnose lead toxicosis in the absence of characteristic hematologic changes or clinical effects.

      (3) The blood lead level does not correlate well with the severity of clinical signs.

    b. Hematology

      (1) Increases in nucleated red blood cells in greater proportion than the degree of anemia warrants are indicative of lead toxicosis.

      (2) Basophilic stippling is an additional indicator of lead exposure, but is not consistent or prominent in all species. Dogs exhibit prominent basophilic stippling.

      (3) Zinc protoporphyrin levels increase, especially in dogs.

      (4) Plasma porphyrins and fluorescence under ultraviolet light are characteristic in cattle.

    c. Radiography

      (1) An abdominal radiograph in small animals may reveal radiodense particles or objects in the gastrointestinal tract.

      (2) Young animals (especially puppies and foals) show metaphyseal sclerosis as a result of chronic lead exposure.

TABLE 17-2. Species-specific Clinical Signs in Lead Poisoning

| Species | Neurologic | Clinical Signs | | |
		Gastrointestinal	Hematopoietic	Other
Cattle	Blindness; head-pressing (manifestation of cerebral edema); rhythmic twitching of ears and bobbing of head; ataxia; circling; stumbling; depression; severe, acute clonic–tonic seizures (rare)	Anorexia; rumen stasis; constipation	Elevated free erythrocyte porphyrins in plasma and urine; plasma fluoresces under ultraviolet light	Abortion (mid to late gestation)
Horses	Blindness; head-pressing; knuckling of fetlocks; "roaring" (stertorous sound caused by paralysis of recurrent laryngeal nerve)	Anorexia; mild to moderate colic		Epiphyseal enlargement in colts (lead-line)
Dogs	Range from depression and inactivity to hysteria, barking, seizures, and behavioral changes; signs are intermittent, with periods of nearly normal behavior	Vomiting, anorexia, colic, constipation appear early; abdominal pain is not increased by palpation	Mild anemia; basophilic stippling; nucleated red blood cells; elevated zinc protoporphyrin	
Cats	Depression; persistent meowing; seizures and hysteria are rare	Colic; vomiting		
Waterfowl	Paresis of wings ("wing drop")	Anorexia; weight loss; cachexia	Anemia	
Psittacine birds	Ataxia; blindness; torticollis; circling; seizures	Anorexia; regurgitation; diarrhea		

    d. Urinalysis
       (1) Urinary δ-ALAD levels increase.
       (2) Test-dosing with calcium disodium ethylenediaminetetraacetic acid (EDTA) may be performed if studies of blood lead and porphyrin levels are not conclusive.
          (a) A 24-hour urine sample is collected and tested for lead.
          (b) Calcium disodium EDTA is administered, and the urine is tested for lead 24 hours later.
          (c) A fourfold or greater increase in urinary lead levels following EDTA administration is indicative of lead accumulation and toxicosis.

G. | **Treatment**

    1. Chelation therapy
      a. Calcium disodium EDTA is the recommended chelating agent (see Chapter 6 III F).
        (1) Preparations
          (a) Currently, no product approved for veterinary use is commercially available, but the Food and Drug Administration (FDA) has allowed purchase of calcium disodium EDTA from chemical supply companies.
          (b) Calcium disodium EDTA preparations are available as a human product through pharmacies.

        (c) Tetrasodium EDTA should be avoided, because it may chelate calcium and cause hypocalcemia.

    (2) Dosage (see Table 6-1). Calcium EDTA is administered subcutaneously or intravenously.

    (3) Complications. Therapy is usually discontinued after 5 days to avoid complications or toxicosis from calcium EDTA therapy.

        (a) Side effects of excessive dosage or rate of administration are depression, anorexia, vomiting, and diarrhea. These effects are reportedly antagonized by zinc supplementation.

        (b) Prolonged therapy (longer than 5 days) may cause necrotizing proximal tubular toxicosis.

        (c) Calcium disodium EDTA occasionally increases signs of lead toxicosis, presumably by mobilizing more lead from inert storage (e.g., bone) without chelating lead in the CNS.

    (4) Administration of **dimercaprol** prior to initiation of calcium EDTA therapy may help alleviate acute neurologic signs, because it crosses the blood–brain barrier. In addition, lead excretion in both bile and urine is enhanced by dimercaprol.

  b. Dimercaptosuccinic acid (DMSA) is recommended for pet birds (25–35 mg/kg orally, twice daily for five days) because it is less toxic than calcium disodium EDTA for birds.

  c. D-Penicillamine is a sulfhydryl-containing, orally active, heavy metal chelator (see Chapter 6 III K, Table 6-1).

    (1) It is used for oral therapy of chronic toxicosis (8 mg/kg orally four times daily), or following parenteral calcium EDTA therapy.

    (2) Side effects are anorexia, listlessness, and vomiting, which are minimized if smaller doses are given more frequently, or if 5–7-day rest periods are alternated with 5–7-day treatment regimens. (The latter strategy is effective for calcium disodium EDTA therapy as well.)

2. Supplemental therapy

  a. Thiamine appears to promote recovery, especially in cattle.

    (1) The recommended dosage is 0.5–1.0 g/day.

    (2) Even without chelation therapy, some improvement is possible.

  b. Corticosteroids (e.g., dexamethasone) and an **osmotic diuretic** (e.g., mannitol) may reduce cerebral edema in cattle or horses.

  c. Zinc supplements may help alleviate the severity of epiphyseal enlargement in colts.

  d. Diazepam or barbiturates may be employed to control seizures.

3. Decontamination of the gastrointestinal tract

  a. An osmotic cathartic (e.g., sodium or magnesium sulfate) promotes gastrointestinal evacuation and precipitates lead to form an insoluble complex of lead sulfate.

  b. Surgical intervention

    (1) Ruminants with rumen stasis and heavy lead contamination may require rumenotomy.

    (2) Small animals or birds may require surgery or endoscopy to remove metallic lead or lead objects from the stomach or intestines.

4. Supportive and convalescent care

  a. Supplemental feeding and the administration of oral or parenteral fluids may be necessary to counteract anorexia, which may be prolonged.

  b. Reinoculation of the rumen with active ruminal contents or probiotics promotes return of normal rumen function.

H. | **Public health considerations**

1. Sources of lead are similar for humans and animals. Lead toxicosis in dogs or cats should call attention to review of potential lead exposure to children in a household.

2. Food animals that have recovered from lead poisoning store lead mainly in bone. Meat products containing scraps of bone or ground bone should be avoided.

3. Excretion of lead in milk of dairy cows contributes very small amounts of lead to the diet. However, individual cows recovered from lead toxicosis should be sampled for milk lead levels prior to entry into the herd.

4. Local and federal public health authorities should be contacted when herd outbreaks of lead poisoning occur in dairy or beef animals.

VI. MERCURY TOXICOSIS

A. **Chemical forms of mercury** are summarized in Table 17-3.

B. **Sources** (Table 17-4)

C. **Exposure.** Both acute and chronic clinical poisoning of animals is rare because of the limited availability of toxic amounts of mercury. When mercury poisoning does occur in domestic animals, it is most often related to the accidental consumption of obsolete mercurial products.

D. **Toxicokinetics**

 1. **Absorption**
 a. **Inorganic mercury**
 (1) **Inhalation.** Elemental mercury may be volatilized to mercury vapor, which is lipid-soluble and can be absorbed by inhalation.
 (2) **Ingestion.** Ingested elemental mercury and inorganic mercurial salts are absorbed very slowly from the gastrointestinal tract.

TABLE 17-3. Chemical Forms of Mercury

Form	Example	Characteristics	Pathologic Effects
Inorganic Elemental	Thermometers	Liquid at room temperature; metabolized slowly to divalent mercury in the body or to methyl mercury in the environment	Limited
Mercurial salts Mercuric (divalent) Mercurous (monovalent)	Preservatives, fixatives	Common form of inorganic mercury salts; can be reduced in lakes and other anaerobic-reducing environments to methyl mercury	Acute denaturation and coagulation of proteins, resulting in acute necrotizing gastroenteritis or acute renal tubular necrosis
Organic Alkyl mercurials Methyl mercury Ethyl mercury	Fungicides	Highly absorbable by the gastrointestinal mucosa	High lipid solubility leads to accumulation in the calcarine cerebral cortex of the brain, causing blindness, ataxia, paralysis, coma, and death
Aryl mercurials (e.g., phenyl mercuric acetate)	Anti-mildew paints	Specialized form bound to a phenyl ring; metabolized in the body to divalent mercury	Similar to inorganic divalent mercurial salts.

TABLE 17-4. Sources of Mercury

Mercury-containing products	Environmental
Thermometers	Fungicide-treated seeds*
Barometers	Mercury cathode use (chloralkali processing)*
Small storage batteries	Sewage sludge that contains industrial wastes
Mildew-proof paints*	Burning coal
Ointments (e.g., mercuric oxide)*	Mercury in marine fish[†]

*Of historical importance, but no longer a practical threat to animal health
[†]Transferred along the food chain with carbon–mercury bond intact; however, mercury accumulated in fish is bound to selenium, which reduces its availability and toxicity

    b. Organic methyl and ethyl mercury compounds are lipophilic and highly absorbed by the gastrointestinal mucosa.

  2. Distribution
    a. Inorganic mercurial salts are transported in erythrocytes and plasma. They **accumulate in the renal cortex** and localize in the lysosomes.
    b. Alkyl organic mercury compounds accumulate in the brain.
    c. All forms of mercury pass the placenta and accumulate in the fetus.

  3. Metabolism
    a. Elemental mercury is oxidized to divalent mercury by catalases in tissue.
    b. Aryl mercurials are rapidly metabolized to inorganic salts.
    c. Alkyl mercurials are slowly metabolized to divalent mercury.

  4. Excretion
    a. Inorganic mercury is excreted primarily in urine.
    b. Organic mercurials are excreted mainly in bile and feces.

E. **Mechanism of toxicologic damage**

  1. Inorganic mercurial salts cause direct tissue necrosis and renal tubular necrosis.
    a. Mercuric ion binds covalently with sulfur and inhibits sulfhydryl-containing enzymes in microsomes and mitochondria.
    b. Mercurial salts may also bind to proteins as mercaptides (binding to sulfhydryl groups of proteins).

  2. Organic alkyl mercurials interfere with metabolic activity and prevent synthesis of essential proteins, leading to cellular degeneration and necrosis. Their most important target organ is the brain.

F. **Toxicity** varies among different species and with different forms of mercury. Chronic methyl mercury toxicosis results from continued exposure to dosages of 0.2–5.0 mg/kg body weight.

G. **Diagnosis**

  1. Clinical signs
    a. Mercuric salts
      (1) Early signs of acute toxicosis include stomatitis, pharyngitis, vomiting, diarrhea, dehydration, and shock. Death may occur within hours.
      (2) Oliguria and azotemia, lasting for 1–2 days, follow in animals that survive acute mercuric ion toxicosis.
    b. Alkyl mercurials (e.g., methyl mercury dicyandiamide)
      (1) Clinical signs develop slowly over a period of 7–21 days.
        (a) Early signs are erythema of the skin, conjunctivitis, lacrimation, and stomatitis.
        (b) Intermediate signs
          (i) Neurologic signs include depression, ataxia, incoordination, paresis, and blindness.

         (ii) Dermatologic signs (e.g., dermatitis, pustules, ulcers) increase during the course of the disease.

         (iii) Other signs. Hematuria and melena occur in some animals, leading to anemia.

      (c) Advanced signs include proprioceptive defects, abnormal postures, complete blindness, total anorexia, paralysis, slowed respiration, coma, and death. The mortality rate among affected animals is very high.

2. Lesions

    a. Gross lesions

      (1) Gastrointestinal lesions include gastric ulcers, necrotic enteritis, and colitis.

      (2) Renal lesions include pale, swollen kidneys with renal tubular necrosis.

    b. Microscopic brain lesions (alkyl mercurials)

      (1) Fibrinoid degeneration of cerebral arterioles

      (2) Laminar necrosis of cerebral and calcarine cortices

      (3) Cerebellar hypoplasia in kittens born to cats exposed to mercury

3. Laboratory diagnosis

    a. In cases of acute exposure, concentrations of mercury in the blood or urine may be elevated.

    b. Concentrations of mercury may be elevated in the kidney (greater than 15 ppm), liver, and brain.

H. Treatment

1. Acute exposure to mercuric salts

    a. Inactivation

      (1) Egg white or **activated charcoal** may be administered to inactivate ingested mercury.

      (2) Oral sodium thiosulfate (0.5–1.0 g/kg body weight) also binds mercury.

    b. A **saline cathartic** or **sorbitol** promotes clearance from the intestinal tract.

    c. Oral D-penicillamine (15–50 mg/kg body weight daily) may be administered orally after the intestine is cleared of mercury.

    d. DMSA is effective for increasing urinary excretion of inorganic mercurials.

2. Alkyl mercurials. In most cases, by the time the toxicosis is apparent, substantive damage has already occurred. **Supplemental selenium and vitamin E are somewhat protective** against methyl mercury toxicosis.

I. Public health considerations. Alkyl mercurials can accumulate in edible organs and muscle; therefore, **mercury-intoxicated animals should never be used for food.**

VII.   **MOLYBDENUM TOXICOSIS.** Molybdenum is an essential trace element and a component of xanthine oxidase, which is utilized in purine metabolism.

A. Sources

1. Soil. Excess molybdenum may be found in soils, especially acidic, poorly drained soils or those contaminated with mining wastes. The major areas of contamination in the United States are Florida, California, Oregon, and Nevada.

2. Plants can absorb and accumulate water-soluble molybdates from contaminated soils. Molybdenum in herbage is minimal during the winter months, but begins to increase in the spring and reaches maximal concentrations in late summer or early autumn.

3. Industrial sources include **brick manufacturing plants** that use clay that is high in molybdenum, **steel mills,** and some **facilities that produce aluminum**.

4. Fertilizers

B. **Toxicokinetics.** Molybdenum is excreted in milk. Toxicosis may result in nursing calves when their dams are exposed to excess molybdenum.

C. **Mechanism of toxicologic damage**

1. **Cattle**
   a. Molybdenum **promotes hepatic copper excretion** by forming a copper–molybdate complex that is readily excreted in urine, **causing a clinical copper deficiency.**
      (1) Copper:molybdenum ratios of 2:1 or less promote excretion of copper, especially if high dietary sulfate levels are present.
      (2) Copper deficiency has the following effects:
         (a) The activity of lysyl oxidase (amine oxidase) is reduced. As a result, cross-linking is reduced, diminishing the stability and strength of collagen in bone and elastin in the major blood vessels.
         (b) Tyrosinase activity is reduced, interfering with melanin synthesis.
         (c) The integrity of red blood cells is diminished.
   b. Molybdenum may compete with phosphorus for mineralization of bone.

2. In **swine,** elevated molybdenum may promote **increased hepatic copper storage**.

D. **Toxicity**

1. **Cattle** are the most susceptible species to excess molybdenum. Young animals are more susceptible than adults.

2. Molybdenum toxicity is **increased by high levels of dietary sulfate** and **reduced by dietary copper**.

3. The **maximum tolerable dietary level** recommended by the National Research Council is **5–10 ppm,** depending on the level of dietary copper. Dietary copper levels of 8–10 ppm protect cattle against 5–6 ppm dietary molybdenum.

E. **Diagnosis**

1. **Clinical signs**
   a. **Diarrhea** occurs 8–10 days following access to pastures high in molybdenum. It is persistent and severe, characterized by its greenish color and fluid, bubbly nature.
   b. **Achromotrichia** (i.e., depigmentation of hair) occurs, especially around the eyes. In addition, the **hair coat** is **rough and dull**.
   c. **Milk production decreases.**
   d. **Reduced libido and infertility** occur in bulls and cows, respectively.
   e. **Joint pain, lameness, spontaneous fractures**
   f. **Anemia**
   g. **Pica**

2. **Lesions**
   a. Microcytic, hypochromic erythrocytes
   b. Enteritis with flaccid, fluid-filled intestines
   c. Bone rarefaction (e.g., osteoporosis) and exostosis
   d. Hemosiderosis

3. **Laboratory diagnosis**
   a. **Molybdenum levels** exceed 5 ppm (wet-weight basis) in the liver and 0.1 ppm in the blood.
   b. **Copper levels** are less than 10 ppm (wet-weight basis) in the liver and 0.6 ppm in the blood.

F. **Treatment**

1. For severe, subacute cases, **copper glycinate** may be injected subcutaneously (60 mg for calves; 120 mg for cattle).

2. Copper sulfate may be used to supplement the diet. To provide 1 g daily per adult cow, the following approaches may be taken:

   a. Copper sulfate (0.5 kg) may be mixed with 50 kg of salt and provided on an *ad lib* basis.

   b. Alternatively, 10 kg of copper sulfate may be added to each ton of grain and fed at a rate of 0.1 kg/cow/day.

VIII. SELENIUM TOXICOSIS

A. Chemical properties of selenium

1. Selenium is **similar to sulfur** and may replace sulfur in amino acids.

2. Elemental selenium is nearly **insoluble in water**.

3. Selenium exists in **several valence states**.

   a. Selenite (4^+) is extremely toxic.

   (1) It is reduced to elemental selenium under acid (reducing) conditions.

   (2) Damp, heavy soils favor reduction of selenite.

   b. Selenate (6^+) is both soluble and toxic.

   (1) Alkaline and oxidizing conditions (e.g., the arid, alkaline soils of the Great Plains) promote the formation of selenate.

   (2) Arid, alkaline soils maintain selenium near the surface, where it is available to plants.

B. Sources. The average selenium content of the earth's crust is 0.1 ppm, but content varies widely with geologic and climatic variation.

1. Plants have diverse tendencies to accumulate selenium.

   a. Obligate indicator plants require large amounts of selenium for growth and survival.

   (1) Plants in this category accumulate high concentrations of selenium as water-soluble amino acid analogs of cysteine and methionine.

   (2) Examples include *Astragalus* (locoweed), *Oonopsis* (goldenweed), *Stanleya* (prince's plume), and *Xylorrhiza* (woody aster).

   b. Facultative indicator plants absorb and tolerate large amounts of selenium if it is present in the soil, but they do not require selenium for growth.

   (1) Selenium may reach concentrations of 25–100 ppm in the tissues of facultative indicators.

   (2) Examples include *Atriplex* (saltbrush), *Machaeranthera*, and *Sideranthus*.

   c. Nonaccumulator plants include crop plants, which may accumulate 1–25 ppm of selenium if grown on seleniferous soils, especially soils where selenium has been brought to the soil surface, solubilized, and converted to organic selenium by the indicator plants.

2. Feed supplements containing 0.1–0.3 ppm selenium are used in selenium-deficient regions.

3. Injectable selenium supplements are available for calves, foals, lambs, and pigs.

4. Industrial and commercial sources include rectifiers, xerography, photoelectric cells, glass, and ceramics.

5. Seafood. Fish and shellfish normally accumulate selenium that exists naturally in the ocean, but usually not to toxic accumulations.

C. Exposure

1. Cattle, sheep, and horses may graze selenium-containing plants. Selenium-containing indicator plants have an unattractive odor that may deter animals from eating them; however, withered plants or those containing only moderate levels of selenium are not as offensive and therefore present a greater risk.

2. Swine and poultry may develop selenium toxicosis after consuming grain raised on seleniferous soil.

3. Waterfowl experience teratologic effects (e.g., underdeveloped feet and legs, malformed eyes and beak) when irrigation of crops causes leaching of selenium, which then concentrates in nearby bodies of water.

4. Erroneous use of feed or parenteral selenium supplements may cause toxicosis. Young or small animals are at high risk for overdosage resulting from the use of an inappropriate parenteral product.

D. Toxicokinetics

1. Absorption. At high concentrations, naturally occurring seleno-amino acids and soluble selenium salts are readily absorbed.
   a. Seleno-amino acids are more quickly absorbed than selenite and selenate, which are more quickly absorbed than the selenides and elemental selenium.
   b. The small intestine is the primary absorption site; no absorption takes place in the stomach or rumen.
   c. Absorbed selenium is transported by plasma proteins.

2. Metabolism
   a. Selenium is metabolized by both reduction and methylation.
   b. Selenium may form a complex with mercury and proteins that reduces the availability of the components of the complex. In marine environments, this phenomenon may be responsible for the reduced toxicity of accumulated mercury.

3. Deposition
   a. A selenium–protein–cadmium complex increases tissue deposition but reduces toxicity.
   b. Because of its ability to replace sulfur in amino acids, selenium has a high affinity for hair and epithelial structures (e.g., hooves, horns).

4. Excretion
   a. Urine is the major route of excretion in monogastric animals. Ruminants secrete significant amounts in the **feces** as well.
   b. Normally, very small amounts of selenium are excreted in **bile**. Arsenic enhances biliary excretion of selenium.
   c. Methylated selenium is volatile and may be excreted by the **lungs**.

E. Mechanisms of toxicologic damage

1. Glutathione depletion and lipid peroxidation are probable important factors in toxicosis.

2. Selenium replaces sulfur in amino acids, possibly affecting some essential proteins; however, this mechanism does not fully account for selenium toxicosis.

3. Chronic selenosis depresses adenosine triphosphate (ATP) formation.

4. Tissue ascorbic acid levels fall, possibly contributing to the vascular damage caused by selenosis.

F. Toxicity (Table 17-5)

G. Diagnosis

1. Clinical signs are described in Table 17-5.

2. Lesions
   a. Lesions of **acute toxicosis** include congestion of organs, gastroenteritis, renal necrosis and hemorrhages, hydrothorax, pulmonary edema, and pale cardiac muscle.

TABLE 17-5. Selenium Toxicosis: Toxicity and Clinical Signs

Type of Toxicosis	Species	Dosage	Clinical Signs
Acute			
Oral (selenites)	Horses	3.3 mg/kg	Behavioral: depression, anorexia
	Cattle	10 mg/kg	Respiratory: cyanosis, labored breathing, rales
	Swine	17 mg/kg	Gastrointestinal: colic, diarrhea
Parenteral	Horses, cattle, swine, sheep	0.2–0.4 mg/kg	Neurologic: trismus, mydriasis, incoordination
Subacute	Swine	20–50 ppm in diet for 3 days or more	Neurologic: incoordination, lameness, anterior paresis and paralysis followed by quadriplegia and permanent paralysis Other: Alopecia, swelling and separation of the coronary band, impaired hoof growth
Chronic (alkali disease)	Horses, cattle, swine	5–10 ppm in diets for several weeks or months	Rough hair coat, loss of hair from tail and mane, abnormal growth and structure of horn and hooves, stiffness, lameness, reduced activity, infertility

    b. Lesions of **subacute toxicosis** in swine include focal symmetrical poliomyelomalacia, which is most common in the cervical and thoracic spinal cord.

    c. Lesions of **chronic selenosis** include transverse lines of abnormal growth on the hooves, cardiomyopathy, and chronic hepatic fibrosis or cirrhosis.

3. Laboratory diagnosis

    a. Acute toxicosis. Blood, kidney, and liver selenium levels exceed 2 ppm.

    b. Chronic toxicosis. The selenium concentration in hair and hooves exceeds 5 ppm.

        (1) The hair and hooves must be washed prior to analysis to remove exogenous contaminating selenium.

        (2) In some species (e.g., swine) hair color may affect selenium content.

H. Treatment, prognosis, and prevention

1. Acute toxicosis. In advanced cases, treatment is of limited value. Recumbency and shock develop, and death usually occurs within a few days.

    a. Supportive treatment to combat gastroenteritis and shock is recommended.

    b. Acetylcysteine, a substitute for glutathione, may be effective. The initial dosage is 140 mg/kg of body weight administered intravenously, followed by 70 mg/kg of body weight daily in four divided doses.

2. Subacute toxicosis. Treatment is similar to that for chronic toxicosis (see VIII H 3). Death may result from complications of paralysis (e.g., malnutrition, pneumonia, trauma).

3. Chronic toxicosis

    a. Prevention. The addition of **copper** to the diet may help prevent selenosis. Soil and forages should be tested regularly in selenium-accumulating areas.

    b. The addition of **inorganic arsenicals** to the diet enhances biliary excretion of selenium.

    c. Increasing dietary levels of **sulfur-containing proteins** (e.g., methionine, cystine, cysteine) is beneficial.

IX. ZINC TOXICOSIS

A. Chemical properties of zinc

1. Zinc, a component of many metalloenzymes, is an essential element for mammals and birds; it is integral to growth, skeletal development, collagen formation, feathering, dermal health, wound healing, and reproduction.

2. Zinc has a valence of 2+, is generally soluble in acids and alkalies, and insoluble in water.

B. Sources

1. Zinc is used frequently in **alloys** (e.g., brass, bronze) and in **galvanized coatings** for iron and steel.

2. Zinc is found in automotive parts, electrical fuses, storage batteries, roofing materials, fungicides, and medications (e.g., zinc oxide). Pennies minted after 1983 contain more than 99% zinc.

C. Exposure

1. **Farm animals** and **zoo animals** obtain excessive zinc by chewing on galvanized bars, pipes, and wires. Excessive use of dietary zinc supplements can lead to toxicosis.

2. **Pet animals** may ingest objects containing zinc.

D. Toxicokinetics

1. **Absorption.** Approximately 25% of ingested zinc is absorbed primarily from the duodenum and intestine by a carrier-mediated mechanism that is enhanced by chelation.

2. **Deposition.** Absorbed zinc is initially bound to plasma albumin and β_2-macroglobulin. Most zinc is deposited in the liver, kidney, prostate, muscle, and pancreas, where it induces metallothionein synthesis in cells.

3. **Excretion.** Excretion of zinc is limited and takes place via the urine, saliva, intestinal tract, and bile.

E. Mechanisms of toxicologic damage

1. The exact toxicologic mechanism of zinc that produces the characteristic clinical signs is poorly defined.

2. High levels of dietary zinc interfere with hepatic copper storage and may compete with calcium for intestinal absorption. Diets high in either copper or calcium can induce zinc deficiency.

3. The antagonistic effects of zinc against copper and iron may result in suppression of hematopoiesis.

F. Toxicity

1. **Acute zinc toxicosis.** The median lethal dose (LD_{50}) of zinc salts (e.g., zinc chloride) is approximately 100 mg/kg body weight.

2. **Subacute zinc toxicosis.** Following ingestion of up to five pennies, dogs have developed subacute zinc toxicosis. The pennies remain in the stomach and slowly release metallic zinc.

3. **Chronic zinc toxicosis.** Dietary zinc levels that exceed 2000 ppm cause chronic zinc toxicosis in most domestic animals.

G. **Diagnosis**

1. **Clinical signs**
   a. **Dogs**
      (1) **Early signs** include anorexia and vomiting.
      (2) **Intermediate signs.** Lethargy and diarrhea develop within several days.
      (3) **Advanced signs** include moderate anemia, hemoglobinuria, and icterus. If not treated, some dogs may die.
   b. **Livestock**
      (1) **Early signs** include anorexia, diarrhea, and lethargy.
      (2) **Intermediate signs** include a decreased rate of gain or decreased milk production. In foals, lameness, epiphyseal swelling, and stiffness are prominent signs.
      (3) **Advanced signs** include moderate anemia and icterus. Polydipsia, polyphagia, exophthalmia, and seizures have also been reported.

2. **Lesions**
   a. Most species show some degree of hemolytic anemia with regenerative response in the erythrocytes.
   b. Hematuria, proteinuria, urinary casts, and uremia indicate renal damage.
   c. Postmortem lesions include gastroenteritis, renal tubular necrosis, and hepatocyte necrosis.
   d. The presence of radiodense materials in the stomach suggests the possibility of zinc toxicosis in small animals.

3. **Laboratory diagnosis**
   a. **Serum bilirubin and AP levels** are elevated.
   b. **Serum zinc levels.** Elevated serum zinc levels indicate recent high exposure or long-term elevated zinc intake. Trace element–free tubes and syringes should be used for sampling, because some rubber stoppers on blood collection tubes and rubber grommets in plastic syringes may contain zinc stearate as a component of the lubricant.
   c. **Zinc concentrations in the liver, kidney,** and **urine** are elevated.
   d. **Copper concentrations in the liver** may be depressed in chronic zinc toxicosis.

H. **Treatment**

1. **Detection and removal of zinc objects** from the gastrointestinal tract is the first step.

2. **Symptomatic and supportive therapy** addresses the gastroenteritis and anemia.

3. **Chelation therapy.** Calcium disodium EDTA or D-penicillamine may be given orally (see Table 6-1 for standard dosages).

X. **SELECTED METALS OF LIMITED IMPORTANCE IN VETERINARY MEDICINE**

A. **Cadmium**

1. **Sources**
   a. Cadmium is a by-product of zinc or lead production.
   b. It is used in metal plating, alloys, small cadmium–nickel batteries, and antiseborrheic shampoos (cadmium sulfide).
   c. Cadmium accumulates moderately in plants fertilized with cadmium-contaminated sewage sludge or fertilizers.

2. **Exposure.** Cadmium toxicosis is of limited significance in veterinary medicine; most exposure takes place when pets ingest cadmium–nickel batteries.

3. Toxicokinetics

   a. Transport. Most cadmium is transported in plasma bound to albumin or gamma globulin. A limited amount is carried by erythrocytes.

   b. Absorption. Cadmium is poorly absorbed (less than 10%), primarily by the gastrointestinal tract.

   c. Deposition

   (1) Cadmium is concentrated in the kidney tubules and, to a lesser degree, in the liver.

   (2) It also accumulates in the placenta.

   d. Excretion. Most cadmium is excreted in the feces; excess is excreted in the urine.

4. Mechanism of toxicologic damage. Cadmium induces the formation of metallothionein and binds to it in the tissues. The cadmium–metallothionein complex promotes renal accumulation. Metabolism releases free cadmium, which is nephrotoxic.

5. Toxicity

   a. Dietary zinc reduces the toxicity of cadmium.

   b. Milk production in cows is reduced by dietary cadmium levels exceeding 300 ppm.

   c. Turkeys and calves can tolerate 20 ppm and 40 ppm dietary cadmium, respectively.

6. Diagnosis. In most cases, cadmium toxicosis is chronic and degenerative.

   a. Clinical signs include anemia, retarded growth, testicular degeneration and necrosis, arthropathy and osteoporosis, proteinuria, glycosuria, and hyperphosphatemia. High dosages can cause vomiting and diarrhea, but acute poisoning is rare.

   b. Lesions include hepatic damage and nephrosis.

   c. Laboratory diagnosis. Urinary threonine and serine excretion is increased. Urinary cadmium levels are elevated.

7. Treatment. There are no effective antidotes for cadmium poisoning; treatment is supportive.

   a. Selenium forms a selenium–cadmium–protein complex that protects against testicular necrosis.

   b. Vitamin D may be used to reduce the effects of osteoporosis.

B. **Antimony** resembles arsenic both chemically and biologically.

1. Sources. Antimony is used in batteries, alloys, rubber, ceramics, paints, and an older medication known as tartar emetic.

2. Toxicokinetics. Antimony is absorbed slowly from the gastrointestinal tract and excreted slowly by the kidneys.

3. Mechanism of toxicologic damage. Antimony inhibits sulfhydryl-containing enzymes, causing signs and lesions similar to those of arsenic toxicosis.

C. **Barium**

1. Sources. Barium is present in alloys, paints, soap, paper, ceramics, and certain obsolete insecticides and rodenticides (e.g., barium fluosilicate, barium carbonate).

2. Toxicity is related to solubility, which varies widely among barium salts.

   a. Barium sulfate, which is used as a contrast medium for gastrointestinal radiology, is very insoluble and nearly nontoxic.

   b. Barium carbonates, chlorides, nitrates, and acetates are very acid-soluble and highly cardiotoxic.

3. Diagnosis. Signs of acute barium toxicosis include gastroenteritis and hyperperistalsis, followed by ventricular fibrillation and extrasystoles associated with hypokalemia.

4. Treatment of acute toxicosis involves gastrointestinal detoxification followed by the administration of potassium to counteract the hypokalemia.

D. **Chromium.** Trivalent chromium is an essential nutrient, but hexavalent chromium (chromate) is toxic.

    1. Sources. Chromium is used in paints, pigments, leather tanning, and wood preservatives.

    2. Diagnosis. Clinical signs of chromium toxicosis include contact dermatitis, irritation of the nasal passages, and acute gastroenteritis.

E. **Thallium** is very toxic and highly cumulative.

    1. Sources. Thallium has been used most recently as a rodenticide and an insecticide; however, all uses are currently banned in the United States.

    2. Exposure. Ingestion of baits by pets has led to thallium toxicosis in the past.

    3. Diagnosis
        a. Clinical signs. At sufficient dosages, thallium is necrotizing to many different epithelial and endothelial cells.
            (1) Acute toxicosis is characterized by severe hemorrhagic gastroenteritis, dermal erythema, congested oral mucosae, dilated scleral blood vessels, and necrotizing pneumonia.
            (2) Subacute or chronic toxicosis is characterized by chronic dermatitis, dermal necrosis, and peeling of the epidermis. Subacute or chronic exposure can cause liver and kidney damage.
        b. Laboratory diagnosis. Elevated thallium concentrations in the urine, feces, or tissues confirm the diagnosis.

    4. Treatment. In the past, dithizone and potassium ferricyanide (Prussian blue) have been used to treat thallium toxicosis, but these treatments are relatively ineffective when clinical signs are already present.

DIRECTIONS: Each of the numbered items or incomplete statements in this section is followed by answers or by completions of the statement. Select the **one** numbered answer or completion that is **best** in each case.

1. Which type of toxicosis is associated with red cell fragility and hemolysis?

(1) Arsenic toxicosis
(2) Copper toxicosis
(3) Cadmium toxicosis
(4) Lead toxicosis
(5) Mercury toxicosis

2. Which of these compounds contains a trivalent toxicant?

(1) Mercuric chloride
(2) Ferrous sulfate
(3) Sodium arsenite
(4) Lead arsenate
(5) Copper oxide

3. On average, what percentage of most inorganic metal salts is absorbed from the gastrointestinal tract?

(1) > 90%
(2) 60%–80%
(3) 40%–60%
(4) 20%–40%
(5) 0%–20%

4. Lead absorption is most affected by which of the following?

(1) Calcium
(2) Potassium
(3) Sodium
(4) Arsenic
(5) Selenium

5. In a group of swine with anterior hemiparesis, ataxia, and sternal recumbency, but no central nervous system (CNS) depression or visual disturbances, the two agents most important to consider are:

(1) arsanilic acid and cadmium.
(2) cadmium and lead.
(3) lead and mercury.
(4) mercury and selenium.
(5) selenium and arsanilic acid.

6. Deferoxamine is recommended to treat which of the following poisonings?

(1) Selenium
(2) Zinc
(3) Iron
(4) Copper
(5) Cadmium

7. Which metal is least likely to accumulate in edible tissues of domestic animals as the result of prolonged exposure?

(1) Arsenic
(2) Cadmium
(3) Copper
(4) Lead
(5) Zinc

8. In which of these toxicoses is a blood sample least useful for diagnosis?

(1) Chronic copper toxicosis
(2) Acute iron toxicosis
(3) Acute arsenic toxicosis
(4) Acute selenium toxicosis
(5) Lead toxicosis

DIRECTIONS: The group of items in this section consists of numbered options followed by a set of numbered items. For each item, select the **one** numbered option that is **most** closely associated with it. Each numbered option may be selected once, more than once, or not at all.

Questions 9–14

Match each description of clinical signs and lesions with the appropriate metal or metal compound.

(1) Lead
(2) Methyl mercury
(3) Selenium
(4) Arsanilic acid
(5) Copper
(6) Molybdenum

9. Rhythmic facial and ear tics in cattle with ruminal stasis and complete anorexia are characteristic. Some animals may have acute, violent tonic–clonic seizures.

10. Chronic poisoning produces abnormal hoof growth, loss of hair from mane and tail, and chronic weight loss in horses.

11. Bluish-black kidneys, generalized icterus, and anemia are characteristic gross lesions. Urine in the bladder is a dark port-wine color.

12. Poisoned swine are blind, comatose, recumbent, and may assume abnormal postures. Some affected animals may have mild dermatitis and conjunctivitis.

13. A nine-month-old puppy has had periodic vomiting, abdominal pain, and loss of appetite, along with intermittent tonic–clonic seizures and a distinct personality change.

14. A group of beef cows exhibits gradual loss of hair coat color and chronic greenish diarrhea that is unresponsive to antibiotics.

1. The answer is 2 *[III B 2 b (1)]*. Excessive amounts of copper, a strong oxidant of erythrocyte membranes and hemoglobin, induce the formation of Heinz bodies and compromise the flexibility of the erythrocyte membrane. When large amounts of copper are released from liver storage, as in acute ovine copper toxicosis or chronic canine copper toxicosis, damage and hemolysis result in a hemolytic crisis and the animal dies of anemia and hemoglobinuric nephrosis. Arsenicals affect the vascular system and cause congestion, but little erythrocyte damage. Cadmium and mercury primarily affect epithelial cells. Lead interferes with key enzymes in heme synthesis, causing release of immature nucleated erythrocytes from the bone marrow; however, lead has little effect on the red blood cell membrane.

2. The answer is 3 *[II A 2 a (2)]*. The arsenites are water-soluble, trivalent salts that interfere with the utilization of lipoic acid in the conversion of pyruvate to acetyl coenzyme A (acetyl CoA) for entry into the tricarboxylic acid cycle (TCA). The rest of the metals in the compounds listed are divalent, except for sodium, which is monovalent, and arsenate, which is pentavalent. The valence state of a metal is an important determinant of toxicity, and the expression of toxicity is not accurate without definition of the valence state of the metal.

3. The answer is 5 *[I A 3 d (1) (a)]*. In general, most inorganic metallic compounds are poorly absorbed (i.e., less than 10%) from the gastrointestinal tract. They are relatively insoluble in the alkaline medium of the intestine, although prolonged time in the acidic environment of the stomach may favor solubility and absorption. Organic forms of metals, however, are usually less polar and more lipophilic, allowing for greater absorption of the organic metallic toxins (e.g., methyl mercury, arsanilic acid).

4. The answer is 1 *[V D 1 a (2)]*. Calcium, like lead, is a divalent cation and utilizes the same transport system for enteric absorption as does lead. Experimental work has confirmed that dietary calcium deficiency enhances the absorption and toxicity of lead, while elevated calcium concentrations can reduce the apparent toxicity of lead by competing for the transport mechanism. Potassium, sodium, arsenic, and selenium are of different valences than

calcium or lead and generally are absorbed by different mechanisms.

5. The answer is 5 *[II C 3, F 1 b; VIII G 2 b]*. Selenium and arsanilic acid should be considered first. The affected swine appear to have a spinal cord or peripheral nerve problem, which in this case is more severe in the thoracic region as evidenced by the anterior hemiparesis. Because there is no apparent blindness or central nervous system (CNS) depression, there is likely little or no involvement of the brain. Both arsanilic acid and selenium are available as feed additives for swine, and mixing errors can occur. Both cause spinal or peripheral nerve dysfunction and degeneration. Selenium causes bilateral symmetrical focal poliomyelomalacia, whereas arsanilic acid causes peripheral nerve demyelination. In both cases, there is little or no CNS depression, but arsanilic acid-poisoned pigs are often blind. The best clinical choice would be selenium toxicosis, but both selenium and arsanilic acid are valid differentials. Cadmium is primarily a nephrotoxin and swine are relatively unlikely to be exposed to it. Lead is of very low toxicity to swine and, if toxic, would cause mainly visual and CNS effects. Inorganic mercury is classically a gastrointestinal or renal toxicant, and organic mercurials cause blindness, coma, and death. Mercury exposure is unlikely in most circumstances of modern farming, because mercurial fungicides have been banned for over 20 years.

6. The answer is 3 *[IV F 3]*. Deferoxamine is used almost exclusively for removal of excessive iron. It has a very high affinity for ferric iron, which is the more toxic valence and the form that predominates when iron toxicosis occurs.

7. The answer is 1 *[II C 3, F 3 d (2)]*. Arsenic has a very short half-life in blood and tissues of domestic animals. Significant residues occur in the kidney and liver during acute poisoning, and accumulation can occur in inedible tissues (e.g., hair, hooves, nails) of animals. Cadmium, which has a long half-life, accumulates in the kidney. Copper accumulates to high levels in the liver and remains for weeks after toxic exposure has stopped. Lead accumulates in soft tissues initially, and is then deposited in bone where it causes relatively little public health risk, but could be released to soft tissues during periods of stress, calcium deficiency, or metabolic acidosis. Zinc accumulates in certain soft tissues such as the kidney, pancreas, prostate, and others; in those tissues, it could be passed to animal by-products or human specialty foods, although the risk from zinc residue is minimal because of the relatively low toxicity of zinc.

8. The answer is 3 [III B 4 c; IV E 3 a; V F 3; VIII G 3]. Of the choices presented, only arsenic toxicosis is not readily confirmed by detection of high concentrations in the blood. Arsenic in domestic animals has a high affinity for many epithelial tissues and is excreted rapidly in the urine. Copper accumulates in erythrocytes just prior to and during the acute hemolytic crisis. Iron is transported in the blood bound to transferrin, and both bound iron and total iron increase as dosage increases. Selenium is present in both erythrocytes and serum or plasma and responds quickly to dietary or parenteral dosing. Lead is primarily associated with erythrocytes and is consistently elevated in lead poisoning.

9–14. The answers are: 9-1 [V F 2; Table 17-2], **10-3** [VIII G; Table 17-5], **11-5** [III B 4], **12-2** [VI G], **13-1** [V F; Table 17-2], **14-6** [VII E]. In cattle and dogs, lead is a neurotoxicant and gas-trointestinal toxicant. Characteristic signs include anorexia, colic, and a variety of neurologic signs that usually include intermittent seizures, facial tics, and blindness. Signs in dogs often occur most frequently in puppies.

In horses and cattle, selenium has a strong predilection for epithelial and dermal tissues (e.g., hooves, skin, and hair). Both selenium and arsanilic acid can cause ataxia and paralysis, but arsanilic acid can be differentiated from selenium because it produces blindness but does not cause hoof or hair lesions.

Icterus, dark urine and kidneys (from either hemoglobinuria or myoglobinuria), and anemia are signs of an acute hemolytic crisis, which is characteristic of ovine copper toxicosis.

Blindness, coma, evidence of severe brain damage, and a high mortality rate are typical of organic mercury toxicosis. Mercury accumulates to dangerous concentrations in the kidneys and muscle and is retained indefinitely, making residues in poisoned animals a serious public health threat.

Beef cows exhibiting loss of hair coat color (achromotrichia) and chronic, greenish diarrhea are most likely victims of chronic molybdenum toxicosis, which induces a copper deficiency.

Chapter 18

Industrial and Commercial Toxicants

I. INTRODUCTION

A. Pets and livestock have limited access to chemicals used in business and industry. Current restrictions governing the use of these chemicals, along with better safety testing and risk analysis, have further reduced the threat of industrial chemical exposure.

B. The chemicals discussed in this chapter are, or have been, of significant veterinary importance. Knowledge of their characteristics and impact on animal health is important for veterinarians, especially because of the related human health and environmental issues that exist.

II. PETROLEUM PRODUCTS

A. Sources

1. **Crude (raw) oil**
   a. **Sweet crude oil** is crude oil that contains relatively high levels of gasoline, naphtha, and kerosene.
   b. **Sour crude oil** is crude oil that contains relatively low levels of gasoline, naphtha, and kerosene. Sour crude oil has high levels of gas oil, lubricating distillates, residue, and sulfur.

2. **Refined petroleum products**
   a. **Aliphatic hydrocarbons**
      (1) **Short-chain aliphatics** (1–4 carbons) include **methane, ethane, propane,** and **butane**.
      (2) **Long-chain aliphatics** (greater than 5 carbons) include **gasoline, kerosene, petroleum distillates, mineral seal oil,** and **Stoddard solvent**. Petroleum distillates are used as carriers for **insecticides**.
      (3) **Chlorinated aliphatic hydrocarbons** [e.g., **carbon tetrachloride, chloroform, trichloroethane, trichloroethylene (TCE), tetrachloroethylene**] are found in **dry cleaning** and **degreasing solvents**.
   b. **Aromatic hydrocarbons** (e.g., **benzene, toluene, xylene**) contain one or more benzene rings and are used in **quick-drying paints, resins, lacquers, glues,** and **plastics**.

B. Exposure

1. **Crude oil.** Exposure to crude oil is often associated with oil exploration and production activities.
   a. **Cattle and horses.** Access to industrial sites or oil fields, or contamination of feeds, may lead to toxicosis.
   b. **Aquatic wildlife and birds** are often the victims of environmental contamination (e.g., oil spills).

2. **Refined petroleum products.** Small and large animals gain access to refined petroleum products through home or commercial use. Kerosene and other petroleum distillates

TABLE 18-1. Toxicity and Effects of Common Refined Petroleum Products

Name	Sources	Toxicity	Clinical Effects	Characteristics
Acetone	Paint products and solvents	Oral LD_{50}: 5–10 mg/kg Dermal LD_{50}: 20 g/kg	CNS depression, narcosis, dermatitis	Highly flammable; excreted unchanged in expired air and urine; odor threshold: 20 ppm
Carbon disulfide	Solvents for pesticides, waxes, resins; degreasers; fumigants	LC_{50}: 15 mg/L air	Tremor, prostration, dyspnea, cyanosis, vascular collapse, convulsions, coma	Metabolized rapidly; may chelate copper
Ethyl alcohol (ethanol, methyl carbinol, ethyl hydrate, grain alcohol)	Drug formulations, cosmetics, feed additives	Oral LD_{50}: 5–15 g/kg	CNS depression, hepatic lipidosis, hepatic and myocardial fatty change	Metabolized to acetaldehyde, which is also toxic; crosses the placenta and is toxic to the fetus
Isopropyl alcohol (isopropanol), 2-propanol, dimethyl carbinol)	Rubbing alcohol, skin lotions, deicing solutions, window cleaners	Oral LD_{50}: 5–8 g/kg	Similar to ethanol	Metabolized to acetone; odor threshold: 50 ppm
Methyl alcohol (methanol, wood alcohol, carbinol)	Solvents, cleaning agents, paints, varnishes, deicers	Oral LD_{50}: 6–13 g/kg LC_{50}: 30,000 ppm	Respiratory stimulation, ataxia, CNS depression, weakness, coma, death; acidosis possible in neonates	Metabolized to formic acid in primates, which causes severe acidosis and ocular injury
Turpentine (gum turpentine, spirits of turpentine)	Paints, waxes, polishes	Strong irritant at all dosages; readily absorbed through skin and respiratory tract	Irritation of skin, mucous membranes, and GI tract; respiratory irritation, dyspnea, CNS depression, narcosis	Contains isomers of pinene and terpene

Toluene (methylbenzene, phenylmethane)	Anthelmintics, industrial solvents, inks, dyes, varnishes, paints, adhesives	Oral LD_{50}: 6–8 ml/kg LC_{50}: 8000 ppm	Ataxia, depression; cerebellar, liver, and kidney damage	Odor threshold: 2.5 ppm
Xylene (xylol)	Thinners, solvents for rubber and resins, adhesives, lacquers	Oral LD_{50}: 4 ml/kg LC_{50}: 6500 ppm	Ocular and skin irritation, dermal vasodilation, impaired vision, tremors, salivation, CNS depression, coma	Odor threshold: 1 ppm
Varnish maker's and painter's (VM & P) naptha (dry cleaner's naphtha)	Solvent for lacquers and quick-drying paints	No data	CNS signs, ataxia, depression	Odor threshold < 1 ppm
Petroleum spirits (mineral spirits)	Common painting and refinishing solvent	Air concentrations of 360 ppm cause no ill effect	Dermal and GI irritation	
Stoddard solvent (white spirits)	Dry cleaning and general cleaning solvent	No data	Dermal hyperemia (acute exposure), dry, scaling skin (chronic exposure)	Odor threshold: 9 ppm

CNS = central nervous system; GI = gastrointestinal; LC_{50} = median lethal concentration; LD_{50} = median lethal dose.

2. **Refined petroleum products.** Small and large animals gain access to refined petroleum products through home or commercial use. Kerosene and other petroleum distillates have been used as a home remedy for digestive disturbances in ruminants.

C. **Toxicokinetics**

1. **Absorption**
   a. Petroleum products are highly **lipophilic,** and many are readily absorbed through intact skin and the gastric and intestinal mucosae.
   b. Aliphatic and aromatic hydrocarbons, which are highly **volatile,** are readily absorbed through the lungs.

2. **Excretion**
   a. **Excretion of aromatic hydrocarbons** is by metabolism to phenols or carboxylic acids and conjugation with sulfates, glucuronides, or glycine.
   b. **Excretion of volatile aliphatic hydrocarbons** may take place, in part, through the lungs.

D. **Mechanism of toxicologic damage**

1. **Direct irritation.** Both crude and refined petroleum are highly irritating to mucous membranes and skin.
   a. Because of their irritant and volatile nature, crude oils and refined products cause **upper respiratory irritation** and **aspiration pneumonia**.
   b. Low-viscosity refined petroleum products (e.g., gasoline, petroleum distillates) are more likely to cause pulmonary damage than highly viscous products (e.g., oils, greases) because small amounts spread over a large surface area in the lung.

2. **Transfer of microorganisms into the lungs.** Oil can carry microorganisms in the respiratory tract into the lungs, leading to infection.

3. **Stimulation of vomiting or bloat.** Oils or distillates may induce vomiting or cause bloat, contributing to the likelihood that the oil will be aspirated. Abnormal eructation may introduce petroleum products into an open glottis.

E. **Toxicity**

1. The toxicity of **crude oil** correlates with the relative content of kerosene, naphtha, and gasoline. Dosages of 48 ml/kg (sweet crude oil), 56 ml/kg (kerosene), or 74 ml/kg (sour crude oil) over the course of 1 week cause aspiration pneumonia and, eventually, death.

2. **Refined petroleum products** have variable toxicity (Table 18-1).
   a. **Short-chain aliphatics** have low toxicity, but they are very volatile and may contribute to asphyxia.
   b. **Long-chain aliphatics.** Less than 1 ml of the volatile, low-viscosity aliphatic hydrocarbons can cause aspiration pneumonia if aspirated directly into the trachea.
   c. **Chlorinated aliphatics.** Highly saturated compounds (i.e., those with more chlorines) are the most toxic. From most to least toxic, these compounds are carbon tetrachloride, chloroform, tetrachloroethane, trichloroethane, trichloroethylene, and tetrachloroethylene.
   d. **Aromatic hydrocarbons.** Prolonged exposure to more than 60 ppm in the air can cause bone marrow depression, anemia, leukopenia, and thrombocytopenia.

F. **Diagnosis**

1. **Clinical signs**
   a. **Crude oil**
      (1) **Gastrointestinal signs**
         (a) **Bloat.** Cattle consuming sweet crude oil develop bloat, and death may occur in a few hours. Bloat relieved by intubation does not recur.

    (b) Vomiting. Sweet crude oil causes vomiting in monogastrics or attempts to vomit in ruminants.

    (c) Anorexia and weight loss occur over a period of several days to weeks.

    (d) Oil, kerosene, or other distillates may appear in the feces after 1–2 weeks; animals may have dry but formed feces if more refined products are consumed.

  (2) Central nervous system (CNS) signs include incoordination, muscle tremors, head shaking, and confusion.

  (3) Respiratory signs. Pneumonia develops and becomes increasingly intense, leading to death.

b. Refined petroleum products

  (1) CNS signs. Low molecular weight hydrocarbons are more likely to cause CNS effects.

    (a) Chlorinated aliphatic hydrocarbons. Early prominent CNS effects include **anesthesia, depression, disorientation,** and **narcosis.**

    (b) Aromatic hydrocarbons. Early effects are **incoordination, ataxia, depression,** and **coma.**

  (2) Cardiovascular signs. Cardiac arrhythmias and myocardial degeneration are associated with chlorinated aliphatic hydrocarbon toxicosis.

  (3) Respiratory signs. The irritant and lipophilic properties of refined petroleum products cause **chemical pneumonitis.**

2. Laboratory diagnosis

a. Blood glucose levels are decreased because of anorexia associated with crude oil toxicosis.

b. Hematologic changes

  (1) Hemoconcentration accompanied by increased blood urea nitrogen (BUN) levels and increased levels of serum hepatic transaminase enzymes are changes associated with pneumonia.

  (2) Initial leukopenia is followed within 2–3 days by a relative increase in neutrophils, but the total white blood cell count is depressed.

  (3) Aromatic hydrocarbons cause bone marrow depression, anemia, leukopenia, and thrombocytopenia (i.e., pancytopenia); signs are similar to excessive exposure to ionizing radiation.

3. Necropsy findings

a. Gastrointestinal lesions

  (1) Both kerosene and sweet crude oil may cause ulcerations and raised yellow-green plaques in the ventral tracheal mucosa.

  (2) Oil or kerosene may be visible in the gastrointestinal tract, and evidence of rumen atony or bloat may be present.

  (3) The contents of the stomach or rumen may be vigorously mixed with warm water.

    (a) If oil, kerosene, or petroleum distillates are present, they will rise to the surface.

    (b) Gas–liquid chromatography, infrared spectrophotometry, or mass spectrometry may be used to identify the oil or petroleum distillate.

b. Pulmonary lesions are bilateral and include the caudoventral apical, cardiac, cranioventral diaphragmatic, and intermediate lobes.

  (1) The lungs are congested and consolidated. In animals that survive for several days, the lungs contain multiple abscesses that may eventually become heavily encapsulated.

  (2) Oil may be grossly visible in pulmonary tissue.

  (3) Foreign-body pneumonia lesions are the expected necropsy finding, and may be accompanied by localized fibrinous pleuritis, hydrothorax, or both.

c. Hepatic and renal cellular degeneration and necrosis are associated with exposure to aliphatic hydrocarbons. Hepatic fatty change and swollen pale kidneys are visible upon necropsy.

G. Treatment

1. **Domestic animals and livestock.** The best approach in petroleum toxicosis is to prevent absorption of ingested materials and to treat the symptoms.
   a. **Reduction of absorption**
      (1) If treatment is initiated within 2–4 hours following consumption of the oil, **activated charcoal or a nonabsorbable oil** (e.g., mineral oil) may be used to reduce absorption.
      (2) **Emesis or gastric lavage** usually **is not recommended,** because the volatile and irritating components of the petroleum or oil increase the risk of aspiration pneumonia.
      (3) In cases of dermal exposure, **bathing the animal in warm water and a mild detergent may reduce absorption** (see II G 2 d).
   b. **Supportive treatment** involves the administration of:
      (1) Antibiotics to prevent secondary pneumonia
      (2) Intravenous fluid and electrolytes
      (3) CNS and cardiac stimulants if necessary
      (4) Blood transfusions, as appropriate

2. **Birds and wildlife exposed to crude oil spills**
   a. The animal must be examined to determine the extent of contamination and whether or not oil has been ingested or inhaled.
   b. The eyes and mouth should be flushed, and the nares cleaned. The animal may be tube-fed a warm electrolyte solution.
   c. Demulcents or gastrointestinal protectants (e.g., bismuth subsalicylate, 2 ml/kg body weight) may be administered.
   d. The animal should be bathed in a solution of warm (103°F–104°F) water and 5%–10% liquid dishwashing detergent. The solution is squeezed through the feathers or hair, the contaminated water is removed, and the process is repeated until all the oil is removed.
   e. The animal should be maintained in a warm, quiet environment.

III. DIOXINS

A. Sources

1. **Commercial products.** Dioxin-containing products currently are banned from use or carefully restricted. These products include:
   a. **Chlorinated phenoxy herbicides** [especially **2,4,5-T (Agent Orange),** which is no longer available]
   b. Antibacterial **hexachlorophene soaps**
   c. **Wood preservatives** containing pentachlorophenol

2. **Industrial processes**
   a. The **manufacture of trichlorophenol,** which was used as a source for the manufacture of Agent Orange, led to the formation of **polychlorinated dibenzodioxins.** There are **75 possible isomers** of polychlorinated dibenzodioxins. These isomers differ only in the number and location of chlorine atoms on the dioxin nucleus.
      (1) **Tetrachlorodibenzodioxin (TCDD)** is a dioxin isomer chlorinated at the 2,3,7,8 positions (Figure 18-1). TCDD is generally considered the most toxic synthetic molecule known, and it is a highly stable contaminant in the environment.
      (2) **Hexachlorodibenzodioxin (HCDD), heptachlorodibenzodioxin (HpCDD),** and **octachlorodibenzodioxin (OCDD)** are present in pentachlorophenol wood preservatives.
   b. The **manufacture of chlorophenols** can release dioxins to the environment.
   c. **Combustion processes** can release TCDD and other dioxins to the environment.

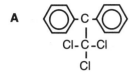

FIGURE 18-1. Comparative structures of common chlorinated industrial and commercial compounds. (*A*) Dichlorodiphenyltrichloro ethane (DDT). (*B*) Polychlorinated biphenyl (PCB). The number and position of the chlorines vary among commercial products. When bromine replaces chlorine, the compound is a polybrominated biphenyl (PBB). (*C*) Tetrachlorodibenzodioxin (TCDD) is chlorinated at positions 2, 3, 7, and 8. Additional chlorination (i.e., from five to eight chlorines) generally reduces toxicity.

B. | Exposure

1. Waste oils contaminated with dioxin were used to control dust in horse arenas in the St. Louis area.

2. 2,4,5-T was used for jungle defoliation during the Vietnam war and as an agricultural and forestry herbicide.

3. Both acute and severe chronic dioxin toxicosis are rare in livestock; but because of public health concerns, veterinarians should be aware of the danger dioxin poses to humans.

C. | Toxicokinetics

1. **Absorption.** TCDD is readily absorbed orally or dermally.
   a. Inhalation of TCDD is not as hazardous because TCDD has a low vapor pressure.
   b. Absorption is influenced by the formulation of the carrier.
   c. Soil and activated charcoal bind strongly to TCDD and inhibit its absorption.

2. **Fate.** TCDD accumulates primarily in the liver and adipose tissue.
   a. The half-lives of TCDD in rats and guinea pigs are 31 ± 6 days and 22–43 days, respectively.
   b. Small amounts of metabolites have been identified. The chemical structure of TCDD metabolites is unknown; however, these metabolites appear to be glucuronides of hydroxylated TCDD.

3. **Elimination**
   a. TCDD is eliminated primarily in the feces.
   b. Small amounts are detectable in urine. Urine and bile contain only unmetabolized TCDD.

D. | Mechanism of toxicity

1. **TCDD,** which may be bound in a cytosolic enzyme that is transferred to the nucleus, **affects many biologic activities**.
   a. TCDD induces microsomal mixed function oxidases (MFOs) and increases the amount of smooth endoplasmic reticulum (sER) in the liver and kidney.
   b. TCDD and other highly toxic chlorinated dibenzodioxins **induce hepatic δ-amino-levulinic acid synthetase (δ-ALAS)** and **aryl hydrocarbon hydroxylase,** which may affect metabolism of some xenobiotics.
   c. **Adrenocortical function, thyroid function,** and **immunocompetence** are affected.

    (1) Exposure to TCDD and other dioxins causes thymic and peripheral lymph node atrophy. A decrease in thymic weight in mice, rats, and guinea pigs is the most sensitive indicator of TCDD exposure.

    (2) Cell-mediated immunity is altered more than humoral immunity.

2. Teratogenesis. Dioxins are teratogenic in hamsters, mice, and rats.

    a. Dosages of 1–3 µg/kg induce hydronephrosis and cleft palate.

    b. Dosages ranging from 0.125–2 µg/kg/day induce fetal mortality and resorption in rats.

    c. Dosages of 0.2–5 µg/kg/day cause spontaneous abortions in monkeys without producing fetal abnormalities.

3. Carcinogenesis. TCDD appears to be carcinogenic in rodents. Evidence that TCDD is a promoter or cocarcinogen is equivocal.

    a. Carcinogenesis does not occur except when dosages are high enough to induce toxicity (see III E 3 a).

    b. The liver is the target organ in rats and mice.

E. Toxicity

1. Structure

    a. Dioxin isomers with at least three of the four lateral ring positions (i.e., 2,3,7,8) occupied are the most toxic.

    b. Toxicity is enhanced if one or more of the ring positions adjacent to the 2,3,7,8 positions is not halogenated.

    c. The higher the number of chlorine atoms, the less toxic the isomer.

2. Acute toxicity. Dosages necessary to produce acute dioxin toxicity vary widely among the isomers and among species.

3. Chronic toxicity is of greater concern than acute toxicity. Chlorinated dioxins are cumulative toxins. A long lag phase or exposure period is typical of dioxin toxicosis.

    a. TCDD

        (1) Dosages of 1 µg/kg/day of TCDD for 90 days cause death in rats.

        (2) Toxicity of TCDD in domestic food animals is not known.

    b. HCDD, HpCDD, OCDD. Highly chlorinated dioxins are contaminants in pentachlorophenol (PCP).

        (1) PCP typically contains 5–200 ppm HCDD, 100–400 ppm HpCDD, and 1000–2000 ppm OCDD.

        (2) Calves given 80 µg/kg HCDD and 8000 µg/kg OCDD extracted from PCP develop chronic toxicosis. These dosages are equivalent to the dioxins in a dosage of 80 mg/kg PCP.

F. Diagnosis

1. Clinical signs and lesions are similar for all isomers, although the toxic dose for each isomer varies widely.

    a. Chloracne is typical in humans, rabbits, and monkeys.

        (1) Hyperkeratosis takes place and comedones form on skin lacking significant hair growth.

        (2) In monkeys and rabbits, the dermal lesions are manifested as edema of the eyelid and orbit.

    b. Wasting. The characteristic loss of body weight is not accounted for by decreased food intake.

    c. Porphyria and photosensitivity. Liver damage and depression of δ-ALAS increase plasma porphyrins. Porphyria can lead to photosensitivity; the most susceptible species include rats, mice, and humans.

    d. Liver necrosis occurs in rats. Mice, guinea pigs, and monkeys develop only minimal hepatic damage.

    e. Impaired biliary excretion

f. Kidney damage

g. Immunosuppression

h. Hematopoietic depression occurs in chronic toxicosis, leading to **anemia** and **thrombocytopenia**. **Pancytopenia** and **widespread hemorrhages** occur in monkeys.

i. Chick edema disease is characterized by **listlessness, anorexia, reduced growth rate, anemia, ventral edema,** and **decreased egg hatchability**. **Subcutaneous edema, hydropericardium,** and **ascites** occur in poultry because vascular integrity is lost.

2. **Laboratory diagnosis.** Clinical signs alone are insufficient to establish a diagnosis. Analysis of tissues is necessary to confirm exposure; unfortunately, few laboratories offer routine dioxin analysis.

   a. Gas–liquid chromatography and **mass spectroscopy** are used to identify dioxins in the tissues.

   b. Hepatic, renal, and **adipose tissues** are the specimens of choice.

IV. FLUORIDE

A. Sources

1. Fluorine is usually **found in nature** as fluoride.

2. **Industry.** Plants that produce aluminum, steel, mineral supplements, or fertilizers may contaminate nearby areas.

   a. Fluorine-containing materials are heated to high temperatures to expel fluorides.

   b. Fluoride combines with water and particulates in the air, settling on vegetation. Direct inhalation is not a significant problem.

   c. Rainfall or leaf loss reduces fluoride contamination of plants.

B. Exposure

1. **Chronic toxicosis** is seen most often in herbivores, especially dairy cattle.

   a. Livestock may consume forages subjected to airborne contamination.

   b. Drinking water may have high natural levels of fluoride.

   c. Some feed supplements and mineral mixtures are high in fluoride-containing rock phosphate. The American Association of Feed Control Officials (AAFCO) has set the minimum phosphorus:fluoride ratio at 100:1. These supplements can be added to feeds at normal levels (0.1%–0.3%) without risking fluoride toxicosis.

   d. Rarely, exposure may occur from vegetation grown on soil with a high fluoride content.

   (1) Plants accumulate fluorides poorly.

   (2) Natural fluoride concentrations range from 1–3 ppm in grains and 1–36 ppm in forages with a mean of less than 4 ppm.

2. **Acute toxicosis** is rare but may result from ingestion of:

   a. Sodium fluorosilicate, occasionally used as a rodenticide

   b. Sodium fluoride, used as an ascaricide in swine

   c. Water, vegetation, or **feeds** containing extremely high fluoride levels

C. Toxicokinetics

1. **Absorption.** Fluoride is absorbed from the gastrointestinal tract.

2. **Fate.** 96%–99% of the absorbed fluoride is incorporated into the hydroxyapatite crystalline structure of bone.

   a. Fluoride accumulation in calcified tissue varies directly with both the duration and rate of fluoride intake.

   b. Bone fluorides are depleted slowly over months or years after exposure ceases.

    c. The normal concentration of fluoride in adult bovine bones ranges from 1000–1500 ppm on a dry fat-free basis.

    d. Fluoride accumulation in the fetal skeleton is not toxicologically significant.

3. Excretion. Fluoride that is not stored is excreted rapidly by glomerular filtration.

D. **Mechanism of toxicity.** Excessive amounts of fluoride result in delayed and impaired mineralization of the teeth and skeleton.

1. Teeth

    a. Developing. Fluoride damages ameloblasts and odontoblasts during tooth development.

        (1) The degree of damage varies directly with the level of fluoride exposure.

        (2) Matrix laid down by damaged ameloblasts and odontoblasts fails to accept minerals normally.

    b. Mature. In fully formed teeth, enamel formation is not occurring and enamel lesions do not develop.

        (1) Malformed enamel and dentin produced during tooth eruption allow rapid and excessive wear of molars and incisors in the adult.

        (2) Oxidation of organic material in areas where the enamel is defective results in brown or black discoloration.

2. Bone. Skeletal fluorosis results in disrupted osteogenesis, acceleration of bone remodeling, production of abnormal bone (e.g., exostosis, sclerosis) and, occasionally, accelerated resorption (i.e., osteoporosis).

    a. High fluoride levels affect osteoblastic activity, leading to inadequate matrix formation and defective, irregular mineralization.

    b. Bone lesions may result from the replacement of hydroxyl radicals by fluoride ions in the hydroxyapatite crystal structure of bone substance.

E. **Toxicity**

1. The response to fluoride ingestion is influenced by the:

    a. Level or amount of fluoride in the diet

    b. Duration of exposure

    c. Solubility of the ingested fluoride

    d. Age of the animal

    e. Nutritional status of the animal

2. Toxic levels for most large animals range from 30–60 ppm. Intermittent exposures in excess of tolerances may increase the incidence of bone and tooth lesions, even if the average annual exposure is within tolerance limits.

F. **Diagnosis**

1. Clinical signs

    a. Acute fluoride toxicosis. Signs may develop within 30 minutes of ingestion and include excitement, clonic convulsions, bladder and bowel incontinence, stiffness and weakness, weight loss, decreased milk production, excessive salivation, nausea or vomiting, severe depression, cardiac failure, and death.

    b. Chronic fluoride toxicosis. Clinical signs may not be apparent until several months or years after the initial exposure.

        (1) Mottled or pitted enamel and **unevenly worn teeth** are characteristic of animals exposed during active dentition of permanent teeth. The concurrent formation and eruption of certain incisors and molars (i.e., first incisor–second molar; second incisor–third molar; third incisor–second premolar) permit evaluation of the severity of fluorosis based on the condition of the incisors.

        (2) Lapping of water is indicative of dental pain.

    (3) Appendicular lameness, an unnatural posture (i.e., **an arched back**), and **generalized stiffness** may all result from exostoses that cause spurring and bridging at joints. Affected animals typically show brief periods of remission.

    (4) Cachexia and poor performance (i.e., **decreased milk production, reproduction**)

        (a) Malnutrition resulting from dental wear and difficulty chewing is manifested as **weight loss** and **a dull haircoat**.

        (b) Severe lameness reduces mobility and causes pain.

2. Lesions

  a. Dental lesions. The teeth of affected animals have periodic radiolucent regions.

  b. Bone lesions initially appear bilaterally on the medial surfaces of the proximal third of the metatarsals. Later, the mandible, metacarpals, and ribs are affected.

    (1) Affected bones are enlarged and chalky with a roughened periosteal surface.

    (2) Lesions are diffuse.

    (3) Histopathologic changes include cortical thickening, periosteal hyperostosis, uneven mineralization, resorption of endosteal bone, and excessive osteoid tissue.

3. Laboratory diagnosis

  a. Skeletal and dental tissues can be analyzed for fluoride content.

    (1) Samples may be obtained by either biopsy or necropsy.

        (a) Recommended sampling sites include the metatarsals, metacarpals, ribs, pelvis, mandible, or coccygeal vertebrae.

        (b) Generally, cancellous bone contains higher levels of fluoride than cortical bone.

    (2) A positive diagnosis is one exceeding 1500 ppm/dry fat-free bone.

  b. Bony structures may be examined radiographically or microscopically.

  c. Urine fluoride analysis reflects recent exposure. Cows with fluorosis void urine containing 15–20 ppm of fluoride, as compared with 2–6 ppm for normal cattle.

  d. Feed and water consumed by the suspect animals should be analyzed for fluoride.

G. Treatment and prevention

1. Treatment. Aluminum sulfate, aluminum chloride, calcium aluminate, calcium carbonate, and defluoridated phosphate are recommended to reduce absorption of fluoride. Treatment is ineffective once dental and skeletal lesions have developed.

2. Prevention. If animals must ingest feeds or water with a high fluoride content, noncontaminated feeds or water should be added to decrease the fluoride concentration.

V. POLYBROMINATED BIPHENYLS (PBBs)

A. Sources. PBBs are man-made chemicals that have fire retardant properties. PBBs include many isomers.

B. Exposure. PBBs are no longer manufactured in the United States, but these compounds are persistent in the environment and in the adipose tissue of animals.

1. In 1973, a fire retardant known as "Firemaster" was accidentally mixed in animal feed intended primarily for dairy cattle and poultry.

2. Losses from illness and contamination were estimated between $25 million and $45 million.

C. Mechanism of toxicologic action. PBBs are believed to activate ribonucleic acid (RNA) synthesis in the cell nucleus and lead to the induction of mono-oxygenase enzymes. The relationship of enzyme induction to PBB effects is not clear.

D. **Toxicity.** Toxicosis in dairy cattle is likely at dosages exceeding 50 mg/kg body weight for 60 days. Biologic effects of toxic doses are similar to those for chlorinated dioxins and polychlorinated biphenyls (see III F 1; IV F).

E. Diagnosis

1. **Clinical signs**
   a. **Clinical signs in most species** include retarded growth, neuroendocrine disturbances, abnormal lipid metabolism, acneform eruption and pigmentation, reproductive failure, and immunosuppression. Because of poor nutrition and immunosuppression, there is an increased incidence of infectious disease.
   b. **Clinical signs in dairy cows** include anorexia, depressed milk production, frequent urination, lacrimation, lameness, excessive hoof growth, infertility, abortion, early embryonic resorption, prolonged gestation, subcutaneous hematomas and abscesses, alopecia, and wrinkling and thickening of the skin.

2. **Lesions**
   a. **Gross lesions** include emaciation, subcutaneous emphysema, thymic atrophy, placental and caruncular necrosis, hepatic fatty change, and pale, enlarged kidneys.
   b. **Microscopic lesions** include renal tubular degeneration, hepatocyte vacuolation and fatty change, amyloidosis, hyperkeratosis, and dermal squamous metaplasia.

3. **Laboratory diagnosis**
   a. **Blood work.** There are no consistent changes in complete blood count, but serum clinical chemistries show increased blood urea nitrogen (BUN) levels, increased levels of hepatic enzymes [e.g., aspartate transaminase (AST)], and hypercholesterolemia.
   b. **Gas–liquid chromatography** can be used to detect PBB residues in body fat, milk fat, and eggs. The half-life of PBB in milk fat is approximately 12 weeks.

G. Treatment and prevention

1. **Treatment.** No useful treatment has been identified. Disposal of the contaminated animals and decontamination of the premises are the only available course of action.
   a. Adsorbents are ineffective for the removal of residues.
   b. Enzyme induction by phenobarbital does not enhance residue excretion.
   c. Reduced consumption of calories helps to deplete fat storage sites, but PBB levels in the milk of lactating dairy cows may increase.

2. **Prevention.** Good husbandry and nutritional management may reduce the adverse effects of PBB exposure.
   a. Stress resulting from crowding and weather conditions should be minimized.
   b. The diet may be supplemented with fat-soluble vitamins, especially vitamin A.

VI. **POLYCHLORINATED BIPHENYLS (PCBs)**

A. Structure and characteristics

1. PCBs are **similar in structure to DDT** (see Figure 18-1).

2. PCBs are **chemically inert** (i.e., they are not hydrolyzed by water and they resist alkalis, acids, and corrosive chemicals). Therefore, they are persistent in the environment and they accumulate in the environmental food chain, where they concentrate in fish-eating birds.

B. Sources. PCBs were first described in 1881 and commercial production began in 1929. Commercial PCB products comprise several compounds and include:

1. Nonflammable oils in transformers, condensers, and electrical insulators

2. Closed heat transfer systems

3. Plasticizers, flame retardants, pressure-sensitive adhesives, paints, and silo sealants

4. Chemical oxidation inhibitors

C. **Exposure.** Production of PCB-containing products was discontinued in the United States in 1979, but the environmental stability of PCBs has made them an ongoing problem.

1. Acute and subacute diseases and death of cattle have resulted from the use of contaminated oil in a cattle oiler.

2. The use of contaminated sealants inside silos has led to residues in milk.

3. Contaminated fish meal used in poultry feed has resulted in residues in poultry and eggs.

4. Contamination of rice oil in Japan in 1968 affected both chickens and humans. Known as **Yusho disease in humans,** PCB toxicosis produces clinical signs of dark pigmentation of the nails and skin, acne, swelling of the limbs, lacrimation, conjunctivitis, jaundice, peripheral neuropathy, fever, headache, vomiting, and diarrhea. Infants born to mothers exposed to excessive levels of PCBs during pregnancy are "cola-colored."

D. **Mechanism of toxicity.** PCBs are strong inducers of MFOs, although the relationship of this effect to toxicity is not clear.

E. **Toxicity**

1. Dosages of 2–10 g/kg body weight in mammals can produce acute toxicity.

2. Toxicity increases as the chlorine content of the PCB increases. In highly toxic compounds, the placement of the chlorines is similar to the placement of chlorines in the TCDD molecule.

F. **Diagnosis**

1. **Clinical signs** are very similar to those of chlorinated dioxin toxicosis.
   a. **Cattle** develop anorexia, polypnea, salivation, polydipsia, diarrhea, colic, recumbency, and depression.
   b. **Poultry** develop chick edema disease (see III F 1 i).

2. **Clinical effects** include:
   a. Reduced viability of piglets
   b. Embryotoxicity and teratogenicity
   c. Increased estrogenic activity in rats
   d. Immunosuppression
   e. Secondary bacterial pneumonia in mammals

3. **Lesions.** Microscopic changes include intestinal submucosal and muscular hemorrhage, hepatic fatty change, thymic hypoplasia, interstitial myocarditis, endocarditis, and colitis.

4. **Laboratory findings.** Gas–liquid chromatography can detect PCBs that have accumulated in body lipids.

G. **Treatment and prevention**

1. **Treatment.** There is no specific effective therapy for PCB toxicosis. Attempts to deplete animal residues using charcoal, phenobarbital, or dietary restriction are not economically feasible or particularly effective.

2. **Prevention.** Efforts should concentrate on identification of contaminated animals and environments for prevention of further contamination. Because PCBs have been associated with human poisoning, contaminated animals should never be recommended for human consumption.

VII. TRIARYL PHOSPHATE AND OTHER NEUROTOXIC PHOSPHATE ESTERS

A. **Source.** Esters of organic phosphorus compounds are used as fire retardants; solvents; stabilizers; antioxidants in lubricants, rubber, or plastics; gasoline additives; plasticizers; and pressure additives in lubricants.

B. **Exposure**

1. **Humans.** In 1930, an extract of Jamaica ginger was contaminated with tri-ortho-cresyl phosphate esters. Consumption of the ginger extract or contaminated cooking oil poisoned more than 40,000 people. Tri-ortho-cresyl phosphate toxicosis in humans is also known as **Jamaica ginger paralysis**.

2. **Cattle and swine** are poisoned occasionally by exposure to lubricants containing tri-ortho-cresyl phosphates.

C. **Mechanism of toxicity**

1. Most organophosphorus esters **inhibit acetylcholinesterase (AChE),** although inhibition of AChE is not directly related to development of neurotoxicity.

2. Hydrophobic phosphate esters enter the nervous system and phosphorylate or alkylate macromolecules. Large peripheral nerves develop **axonal degeneration followed by demyelination**. Lesions are usually irreversible.
   a. **Initial injury** occurs at the distal ends of both sensory and motor nerves, causing "dying back" neuropathy (see Chapter 7 II C 2).
   b. **Advanced injury.** Lesions extend into the spinal cord, affecting axons in the spinocerebellar and corticospinal tracts, and into the medulla, affecting fiber tracts in the lateral portion. Motor end-plates and muscle fibers are not involved in the primary lesion.

3. Organophosphorus esters that **inhibit neurotoxic esterase,** an enzyme present in the brain and peripheral nerves, are associated with delayed neurotoxicity (i.e., peripheral axonopathy). Although inhibition of neurotoxic esterase may not play a primary role in the development of the nerve lesions, it serves as a marker for potential damage. Chickens are often used as test animals for this effect.

D. **Toxicity**

1. Toxicity depends on **compound structure** (Figure 18-2).
   a. **Aliphatic phosphorus esters**
      (1) In order of greatest to least effect, the following compounds **cause delayed neurotoxicity:** Phosphonates, phosphorofluoridates, phosphonofluoridates, phosphorodiamidofluoridates, phosphoroamidofluoridates, phosphates, phosphorotrithioates, phosphorotrithioites, and phosphites.
      (2) Aliphatic phosphorus esters that **do not cause delayed neurotoxicity** include phosphorothioates, phosphonothioates, phosphinates, phosphinofluoridates, and phosphorochloridates.
   b. **Triaryl phosphate esters.** The length, position, and number of substitutions determine neurotoxicity. Unsubstituted triphenyl phosphates are not active.
      (1) Generally, the shorter the alkyl side chain, the more potent the delayed neurotoxicity activity.
      (2) Substitution in the ortho position on one or more rings increases activity.
      (3) Compounds substituted in the meta position, but not in the ortho position, are inactive.
   c. **Saligenin cyclic phosphate esters** are neurotoxic.

2. **Dosage.** Single doses or repeated small exposures can induce toxicosis.

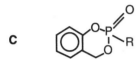

A

B

C

FIGURE 18-2. Structures of phosphate esters that produce delayed neurotoxicity. (*A*) Aliphatic phosphorus ester. (*B*) Triaryl phosphate ester. (*C*) Saligenin cyclic phosphate ester.

3. **Susceptibility**
   a. **Birds,** including chickens, pheasants, and mallard ducklings, **are highly susceptible**.
      (1) Young chickens (i.e., less than 10 months of age) are resistant.
      (2) Adult chickens are a model for the syndrome in humans. Lesions are similar in both.
   b. **Mammals**
      (1) Cats, cows, lambs, adult sheep, and water buffalo are susceptible.
      (2) Rats, mice, rabbits, guinea pigs, hamsters, dogs, and gerbils are resistant.

E. **Diagnosis**

1. **Clinical signs.** There is usually a latent period of 1–2 weeks before the onset of clinical signs.
   a. **Early signs** include numbness and loss of sensation in the distal part of limbs.
   b. Posterior paresis, knuckling of fetlocks, and ataxia follow.
   c. **Advanced signs** include ascending bilateral paresis leading to hemiplegia and, eventually, quadriplegia.

2. **Lesions** occur mainly in axons that are long and have a large diameter.
   a. The pattern of degeneration is distal to proximal.
   b. Microtubules and microfilaments are replaced by granular masses.
   c. Myelin is degenerated.

3. **Laboratory diagnosis**
   a. Detection of the initiating organophosphate is difficult or impossible because residues may be minimal or absent by the time signs develop.
   b. Determination of neurotoxic esterase levels is possible, but such analysis is expensive and available in only a few laboratories.

F. **Treatment and prevention**

1. **Treatment.** No antidote or effective treatment is available; therefore, the prognosis for animals with advanced signs is poor. Early removal of the animal from the source of the toxicant may slow degeneration and allow partial recovery.

2. **Prevention.** Educating clients about how to avoid potential sources is the best preventive measure.

STUDY QUESTIONS

DIRECTIONS: Each of the numbered items or incomplete statements in this section is followed by answers or by completions of the statement. Select the **one** numbered answer or completion that is **best** in each case.

1. What single diagnostic specimen would best confirm a clinical diagnosis of chronic fluorosis?

(1) Blood
(2) Urine
(3) Bone
(4) Hay
(5) Soil

2. Which of the following potential toxicants is most likely more toxic to cats than to other domestic animals?

(1) Benzene
(2) Chloroform
(3) Kerosene
(4) Trichloroethylene
(5) Mineral oil

3. Which of the following could be a source of fluorosis?

(1) Soil
(2) Hay
(3) Grains
(4) A salt–trace mineral mixture fed *ad libitum*
(5) A vitamin premix added to the grain ration

Questions 4–5

The owner of the local automotive repair and body shop keeps several cats on the premises to control mice. Recently, two of the cats have been somewhat ataxic and incoordinated, with poor appetites and little energy. In the last few days, they have vomited occasionally and the stools have been dark and soft.

4. Which one of the following courses of action would not be useful?

(1) A complete blood count on both normal and affected cats
(2) A neurologic examination
(3) Evaluation of liver and kidney function with a clinical chemistry panel
(4) Evaluation of electrolyte levels, acid–base balance, and serum cations
(5) Testing for feline leukemia

5. What therapeutic measure would be most useful prior to reaching a definitive diagnosis?

(1) Administration of activated charcoal
(2) Bathing all the cats in a mild detergent
(3) Blood transfusions
(4) Gastric lavage
(5) Maintaining the affected cats in a warm, quiet environment

DIRECTIONS: Each group of items in this section consists of numbered options followed by a set of numbered items. For each item, select the **one** numbered option that is most closely associated with it. Each numbered option may be selected once, more than once, or not at all.

Questions 6–10

Match each description with the toxicant it describes.

(1) Polychlorinated biphenyls (PCBs)
(2) Tetrachlorodibenzodioxin (TCDD)
(3) Tri-ortho-cresyl phosphate
(4) Kerosene
(5) Fluoride

6. Produces permanent ascending paresis and paralysis

7. Produces chronic degenerative and proliferative disease resulting in exostoses, lameness, and excessive dental wear

8. Highly lipophilic contaminant that is poorly metabolized and excreted and accumulates to high levels in fat

9. Ingestion of this toxicant is likely to cause severe aspiration pneumonia

10. Associated with chloracne (in primates), porphyria, and liver necrosis

ANSWERS AND EXPLANATIONS

1. The answer is 3 *[IV F 3 a]*. Bone would be the specimen of choice to confirm a clinical diagnosis of fluoride toxicosis. Chronic fluorosis requires months or years to develop. Bony changes are the consequence of long-term fluoride accumulation; therefore, bone reflects specific histologic changes that can be used, in part, to corroborate toxicosis. Blood fluoride levels and urinalysis reflect only recent exposure. Analysis of hay and soil samples is useful for establishing liability and determining the source of the fluoride.

2. The answer is 1 *[II A 2 b, C 2]*. Benzene is an aromatic hydrocarbon. Aromatic hydrocarbons are metabolized by hydroxylation and glucuronidation, which facilitates excretion. Because cats lack glucuronide conjugating ability, the aromatic compounds would most likely be more toxic to cats than to other domestic animals at comparable body weight dosages.

3. The answer is 2 *[IV A–B]*. Of the choices given, the only logical choice is the hay. Soil may be contaminated with airborne fluorides, but uptake by plants or grains is minimal. Hay and other forages with a large leaf surface area serve as receptacles for airborne fluorides that are released from industrial processes. The fluorides combine with water and particulates in the air, and then settle out to contaminate the forages. Grain has limited surface area and is usually not contaminated by airborne fluorides. Neither salt–trace mineral mixtures nor vitamin premixes contain the macromineral phosphates that are most likely to have fluoride residues. Furthermore, most mineral products are regulated and contain fluoride in a phosphorus:fluoride ratio of 100:1.

4–5. The answers are: 1-4 *[II A 2, F]*, **2-2** *[II G]*. The history and clinical signs indicate neurologic involvement (and, possibly, systemic disease) compatible with exposure to cleaning solvents, vapors, or petroleum products. Although the animals' environment could suggest antifreeze toxicosis, the presentation is more prolonged than that associated with antifreeze toxicosis, and there is little evidence of acidosis, which is typical of antifreeze toxicosis. Because the gastrointestinal signs are minimal at this time, electrolyte and acid–base disturbances would not be expected. However, petroleum products include aromatic and chlorinated compounds, which are likely to cause neurologic signs (e.g., ataxia), hematopoietic suppression, and hepatic and renal cellular degeneration and necrosis. Therefore, a complete blood count and evaluation of liver and kidney function would be logical steps in arriving at a diagnosis. In addition, the possibility of infectious diseases such as feline leukemia should always be considered.

The most probable route of exposure in this case is inhalation or dermal absorption. Therefore, bathing all of the cats in a solution of warm water and liquid dishwashing detergent may eliminate residual contaminants that might continue to be absorbed through the skin. Because of the demonstrated extended course of the disease and the existing damage and clinical signs, administration of activated charcoal would likely be ineffective. Gastric lavage is not recommended because of the risk of aspiration pneumonia. Temporarily removing all of the cats from the premises until the source of the toxicosis is identified would be wise; the affected cats should be maintained in a warm, quiet environment after they have been bathed and supportive treatment is underway.

6–10. The answers are: 6-3 *[VII E 1]*, **7-5** *[IV F 1 b]*, **8-1** *[VI A 2, F 4]*, **9-4** *[II D 1 a]*, **10-2** *[III F]*. Tri-ortho-cresyl phosphate is a triphenyl phosphate ester. Prolonged exposure to aliphatic, triphenyl, or cyclic phosphate esters, which are found most commonly in hydraulic fluids and other lubricant products, causes a syndrome of peripheral axonopathy known as organophosphate-induced delayed neurotoxicity. The lesion begins peripherally and moves in a retrograde manner up the peripheral nerves to the spinal tracts. The lesion is permanent; recovery is unlikely.

The classic lesion of fluoride toxicosis is caused by damage to ameloblasts, osteoblasts, odontoblasts, and osteoclasts, resulting in poorly formed tooth enamel and dentin as well as impaired bone remodelling and periosteal new bone growth (i.e., exostosis). These changes lead to the clinical signs of lameness, thickened long bones, and excessive wear of both incisor and molar teeth that were formed during fluoride exposure.

Polychlorinated biphenyls (PCBs) have a high chlorine content and are highly lipophilic; therefore, they accumulate in body fat and milk fat. Food-producing animals may experience toxicosis without any overt clinical signs, leading to residues in products such as eggs and milk.

Kerosene is a volatile, highly lipophilic, refined aliphatic hydrocarbon of very low viscosity. Small amounts enter the lung by inhalation, or by partitioning from the blood after absorption. Because of its low viscosity, small amounts of kerosene can spread widely over the alveolar membranes. In addition, foreign materials and bacteria may be carried into the lung from the pharynx or from rumen contents following eructation.

Tetrachlorodibenzodioxin (TCDD) is one of the most toxic synthetic molecules known. It causes a wide range of clinical and pathologic effects, depending on the species of animal. Chloracne is typical in primates. Other effects include porphyria, wasting, immunosuppression, hematopoietic depression, and chick edema disease. Some products such as PCBs, chlorophenols, waste oils, and phenoxyherbicides manufactured before 1970 may contain TCDD. Inadvertent exposure to these obsolete compounds, or exposure to contaminated environments (TCDD biodegrades very slowly) can cause toxicosis.

Chapter 19
Insecticides and Molluscacides

A. Chemical structure

    1. **Organophosphorus insecticides** are either aliphatic carbon, cyclic, or heterocyclic phosphate esters (Figure 19-1). In **organothiophosphates,** the double-bonded oxygen is replaced with a sulfur molecule.

        a. Esters with the P=S functional group are usually less toxic than those with a P=O group.

        b. Oxidative desulfuration (i.e., conversion from a P=S to a P=O functional group) increases the anticholinesterase activity of the insecticide.

        c. Organothiophosphates are usually more resistant to nonenzymatic hydrolysis, such as might occur in the environment.

    2. **Carbamates** are cyclic or aliphatic derivatives of carbamic acid. Usually, they are not sulfurated (see Figure 19-1).

B. Sources

    1. Organophosphorus and carbamate insecticides are commonly used on **crops, stored grain, soils, structures,** and **animals** to prevent or treat insect or nematode infestation.

    2. They are the active ingredient of **flea collars** for pets. Higher concentrations are approved for dogs as compared with cats.

    3. They are active ingredients in **fly, ant,** and **roach baits.**

C. Exposure

    1. **Sources of exposure**

        a. Contamination of feedstuffs with concentrated granular insecticides is a major source of livestock poisoning.

            (1) Granular insecticides may be **mistaken for feed additives** or **vitamin and mineral supplements**.

            (2) Insecticides may be **added to feeds maliciously;** the highly toxic nature of these products is well-known.

        b. Excessive application to crops, or **failure to observe the posttreatment withdrawal period before using treated grain as feed for animals,** can lead to toxicosis.

        c. Improper use

            (1) Poisoning may occur when **insecticides** are **used as rodenticides** and pets have access to the rodents.

            (2) Use of products on species for which the product is not cleared (e.g., using plant insecticides on animals or canine insecticides on cats) often leads to toxicosis.

        d. Residues in the environment. Toxic residues from label-approved uses are unlikely. Because they are degraded by sunlight and soil microbes, organophosphorus and carbamate insecticides generally have a short residue life in the environment; however:

            (1) They **may bind strongly to organic matter and minerals in certain soils,** increasing their environmental persistence.

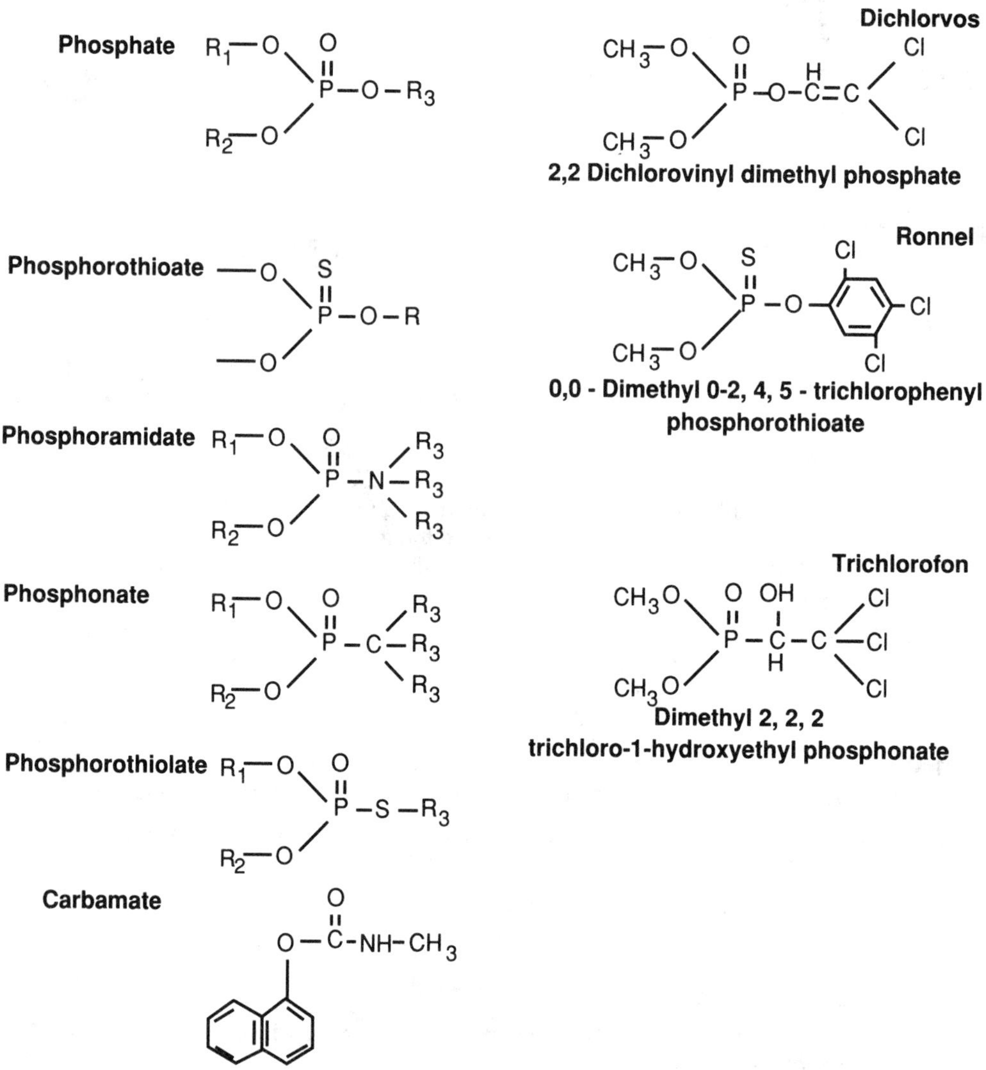

FIGURE 19-1. Basic structural features of the organophosphorus and carbamate insecticides. R groups are commonly methyl or ethyl groups, but they may also include aryls or chlorine. The basic structure of an organophosphorus insecticide can be determined by finding the root word (e.g., phosphorothioate) in the chemical name.

(2) **Acidic soils favor stability of organophosphorus insecticides** (whereas alkaline soils promote hydrolysis of the ester linkage, contributing to detoxification).

(3) **Concentrated spills** from grain planters or trucks **can persist in the environment** for months beyond the normal degradation time.

e. **Secondary (relay) toxicosis.** The stomach contents of deceased, poisoned animals may contain sufficient insecticide to poison scavengers. Tissue residues are low, and toxicosis from consumption of muscle or organs is unlikely.

2. **Product formulation**

a. **Topical products** remain on the surface and are not absorbed.

b. **Systemic products** are absorbed and distributed widely in an active form.

c. **"Pour-on" formulations** are systemically active after application to limited areas of the skin.

3. **Routes of exposure**
   a. **Oral.** Most serious acute poisonings result from ingestion of the poison, or from a combination of oral and dermal exposure.
   b. **Dermal.** Excessive dosages of spray or pour-on products can cause toxicosis.
   c. **Inhalation.** Spraying animals in inadequately ventilated areas can lead to the inhalation of mist.

D. Toxicokinetics

1. **Absorption** can occur from all body surfaces, especially the gastrointestinal tract, skin, lungs, and eyes.

2. **Distribution** is rapid, but organophosphorus and carbamate products do not accumulate in fat depots.

3. **Metabolism**
   a. **Conditions that promote phase I or mixed function oxidase (MFO) activity** are likely to **increase the toxicity of organothiophosphates** by converting them to the corresponding oxygen analog.
   b. **Hydrolysis of the ester linkage** in organophosphates or carbamates **markedly decreases toxicity**.

4. **Excretion.** Most organophosphates and carbamates are **rapidly and nearly completely eliminated**.
   a. Tissue or blood residues are minimal within a few hours of exposure.
   b. Chlorinated organophosphates (e.g., chlorpyrifos) are more lipid-soluble; therefore, residues persist longer than for other organophosphorus insecticides.
   c. Acidic conditions (e.g., in the stomach or rumen) enhance the stability of organophosphates and promote their persistence.

E. Mechanism of toxicologic damage.
Organophosphorus and carbamate insecticides **competitively inhibit acetylcholinesterase (AChE)** and **other cholinesterases**.

1. **Normal AChE function**
   a. **Acetylcholine (ACh)**, a neurotransmitter released at synapses or neuromuscular junctions, mediates the physiologic transmission of nerve impulses from:
      (1) Preganglionic to postganglionic neurons of the parasympathetic and sympathetic nervous systems
      (2) Postganglionic parasympathetic and sympathetic fibers to effector organs and sweat glands, respectively
      (3) Motor nerves to skeletal muscle
   b. **AChE** at cholinergic nerve endings and neuromuscular junctions rapidly hydrolyzes ACh to control the level and duration of synaptic transmission (Figure 19-2A).

2. **Toxic action of AChE inhibitors.** Without AChE, ACh accumulates and causes excessive synaptic neurotransmitter activity in the parasympathetic (cholinergic) nervous system and at neuromuscular (nicotinic) sites.
   a. Organophosphates and carbamates phosphorylate the enzyme by binding to the esteratic site (Figure 19-2B). Some organophosphorus compounds engage in a reaction known as **"aging."**
      (1) Aging causes the organophosphate to lose an esterified moiety, rendering the phosphorylated enzyme very stable.
      (2) When aging occurs, recovery of cholinesterase activity occurs only through the synthesis of new enzyme.
   b. **Reversal.** In general, inhibition by the organophosphates tends to be irreversible, whereas inhibition by the carbamates is reversible. **Spontaneous hydrolysis** of the phosphorylated or carbamylated cholinesterase reverses the inhibition and allows return to normal function.

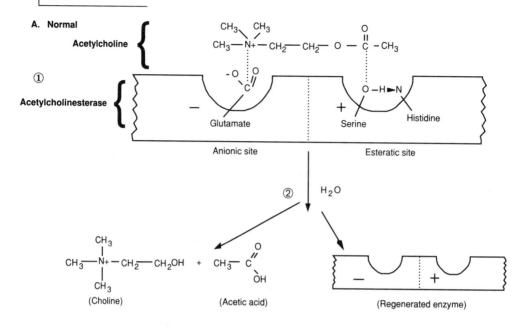

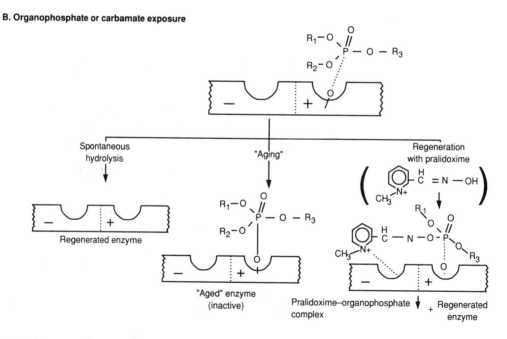

FIGURE 19-2. (*A*) The inactivation of acetylcholine (ACh) by acetylcholinesterase (AChE). (*1*) Formation of the enzyme–substrate complex. A positively charged quaternary nitrogen on the choline moiety of ACh forms an electrostatic linkage with the anionic site of AChE. A covalent bond forms between the carbonyl atom of the acetate group and the esteratic site of the enzyme to fully acetylate the enzyme. (*2*) Hydrolysis of the ester linkage. The acetylated enzyme reacts with water to regenerate the enzyme and release acetic acid. (*B*) Phosphorylation of AChE by an organophosphate or carbamate. Spontaneous hydrolysis or the administration of pralidoxime (2-PAM) leads to regeneration of the enzyme and reversal of toxicity. When "aging" occurs, recovery of cholinesterase activity occurs only through the synthesis of new enzyme.

F. **Toxicity**

1. **Acute toxicity** of organophosphates and carbamates varies widely among compounds and species of animals.
   a. **Exposure to small amounts of commercial insecticides is highly hazardous.** The most toxic commercial products are those for soil nematodes, such as the corn rootworm insecticides (e.g., phorate, fonofos, carbofuran).
      (1) Acute toxicity in most species ranges from 1–20 mg/kg.
      (2) The concentration of active ingredients in these products is 5%–50%.
   b. Acute toxicosis is the **most likely clinical problem in animals**.

2. **Subacute toxicity**
   a. Constant subclinical exposure may reduce cholinesterase activity over a period of days, with eventual manifestation of mild toxicosis.
   b. More persistent organophosphates (e.g., chlorpyrifos) are more likely to cause subacute toxicosis.

3. **Chronic toxicity** (see Chapter 18 VII C) occurs occasionally with modern organophosphorus insecticides (e.g., leptophos, mipafox) and rarely with carbamate insecticides. The most probable cause of chronic toxicity is continuous, excessive use of the agent over an extended period of time.

4. **Potentiators of toxicity**
   a. **Phenothiazine tranquilizers** enhance the toxicity of organophosphates.
   b. **Haloxon,** an organophosphate anthelmintic used in other countries, is a cholinesterase inhibitor that would potentiate the effects of other organophosphate insecticides.
   c. **Neuromuscular blocking agents**
      (1) **Succinylcholine** or other neuromuscular blocking agents may potentiate the nicotinic effects of organophosphates.
      (2) **Levamisol,** a nicotine-like neuromuscular blocking anthelmintic, may enhance the nicotinic effects of organophosphates.
      (3) **Nicotine** and **curare** enhance the nicotinic effect of organophosphates.
   d. **Aminoglycoside antibiotics** block synaptic transmission either by inhibition of ACh release or by postsynaptic neuromuscular blockade.
   e. **Enzyme inducers of the microsomal MFOs** enhance the oxidative desulfuration of organothiophosphates.

5. **Susceptibility**
   a. Cats are generally more susceptible than dogs.
   b. Brahman cattle are more susceptible than English breeds. Bulls are more sensitive to some organophosphates (e.g., chlorpyrifos) than females.
   c. Poultry may have lower tolerance than mammals to some organophosphates (e.g., dichlorvos).

G. **Diagnosis**

1. **Clinical signs**
   a. **Muscarinic signs** (e.g., **vomiting, diarrhea, salivation, lacrimation, miosis, dyspnea, micturition, bradycardia**) result from stimulation of the parasympathetic nervous system.
   b. **Nicotinic (neuromuscular) signs** include **muscle tremors and twitching** and **paresis progressing to paralysis**.
   c. **Central nervous system (CNS) signs** (e.g., **depression, behavioral or personality changes, hyperactivity, seizures**) are relatively rare.

2. **Laboratory diagnosis**
   a. **Evaluation of cholinesterase activity.** Cholinesterase depression resulting from organophosphate poisoning is relatively stable; however, that resulting from carbamate poisoning is labile—cholinesterase activity often spontaneously returns to normal before or during laboratory determination.

        (1) Blood. Depression of cholinesterase activity in blood indicates exposure, but correlates only moderately with the severity of clinical signs.
          (a) In most domestic animals, blood AChE activity is greatest in erythrocytes; therefore, whole blood is used for diagnosis.
          (b) Cats exhibit pseudocholinesterase activity in the plasma.
        (2) Brain. Cholinesterase activity of the whole brain or caudate nucleus is commonly used for **postmortem diagnosis**.
    b. Analysis for insecticides or their metabolites
        (1) Tissue residues are low and often analysis is negative.
        (2) Stomach or rumen contents can be used to confirm exposure if the insecticide was ingested.
        (3) Hair and skin samples are useful when dermal exposure has taken place.
        (4) Urine may contain organophosphorus metabolites.

3. Lesions resulting from organophosphate or carbamate toxicosis are **limited** and they are **not diagnostic**.
    a. Pulmonary edema may be present.
    b. The **intestinal tract** may be dilated and filled with fluid.

H.   **Treatment, prognosis, and prevention**

1. Treatment
    a. Detoxification
        (1) Dermal exposure
          (a) The animal should be washed with soap (or mild detergent) and water and rinsed thoroughly, taking care to protect owners and health care personnel from exposure.
          (b) For long-haired animals, clipping may be advisable.
        (2) Ingestion
          (a) Emesis or **gastric lavage** is indicated if exposure has been less than 4 hours.
          (b) Activated charcoal is a highly effective adsorbent for pesticides.
    b. Emergency therapy. Death is usually the result of cardiac arrhythmias and hypoxia (caused by bronchoconstriction and excessive pulmonary secretions).
        (1) Atropine is effective for counteracting muscarinic signs (e.g., bronchoconstriction, bronchosecretion, bradycardia), but does not correct muscarinic signs (e.g., muscle tremors).
          (a) The **dosage (0.1–0.5 mg/kg)** may be repeated in 6 hours if muscarinic signs return. **Overtreatment with atropine should be avoided because atropine toxicosis can occur.**
          (b) Administration. It is safest to administer one quarter of the dosage intravenously, wait 15 minutes to observe effects, and administer the remainder of the dosage intramuscularly or subcutaneously.
          (c) Contraindications. Atropine is contraindicated for **cyanotic cats**.
        (2) Diphenhydramine (4 mg/kg orally, 3 times daily) may help to control refractory nicotinic signs. It **should not be used in combination with atropine**.
    c. Specific antidotes. Pralidoxime chloride (2-PAM) accelerates the hydrolysis of phosphorylated AChE and aids in the regeneration of active cholinesterase (see Figure 19-2); however, this product is not approved by the Food and Drug administration (FDA) for use in animals. 2-PAM is not recommended for use with carbamate poisoning, because reversal is often spontaneous.
        (1) Oximes will not reverse phosphorylated enzymes that have "aged."
        (2) Early treatment is essential for positive results.
        (3) For small animals, the recommended dosage of 2-PAM is 20 mg/kg intramuscularly twice daily.
        (4) Anecdotal reports indicate that bulls with chronic toxicosis from chlorpyrifos appear to benefit from 2-PAM administration.
    d. Supportive therapy. Cats may have prolonged anorexia and require extensive nutritional and fluid therapy.

2. Prognosis. The mortality rate is high with many types of organophosphate and carbamate insecticide poisoning. The prognosis improves with good supportive and detoxification therapy. Early treatment also improves the prognosis.

3. Prevention
    a. To prevent toxicosis, client education is crucial.
        (1) Owners should be advised against using several cholinesterase inhibitor products simultaneously.
        (2) They should be aware of safe procedures for handling and storing pesticides.
    b. To prevent recurrence, all potential sources of insecticides should be removed from the animal's environment.
        (1) Feeds should be changed if the diet is suspect.
        (2) The premises should be washed.
        (3) Contaminated soil should be removed.
        (4) Retreatment with organophosphate or carbamate products should be avoided for 4–6 weeks.

I. Public health concerns

1. Humans may be exposed to dips, spray mists, or dusts.

2. Caution should be used when washing poisoned animals.

3. Milk from poisoned animals should not be used until analysis indicates no evidence of residue. Residues in foods of animal origin are usually not a problem because organophosphate and carbamate insecticides are rapidly metabolized and excreted.

J. Environmental concerns

1. The careless use of granular insecticides on lawns or crops may by harmful to wild birds.

2. Pesticide spills and runoff can poison fish and aquatic animals.

II. ORGANOCHLORINE (CHLORINATED HYDROCARBON) INSECTICIDES

A. Chemical structure (Figure 19-3)

1. Diphenyl aliphatic compounds include DDT, methoxychlor, perthane, and dicofol.

2. Aryl hydrocarbons include lindane, mirex, kepone, and paradichlorobenzene.

3. Cyclodiene insecticides include aldrin, dieldrin, endrin, chlordane, heptachlor, and toxaphene.

B. Sources

1. Environmental residues. These agents were heavily used in pest control and agriculture from the 1950s through the early 1970s. Contaminated soils or leakage from old dump sites occasionally leads to residues.
    a. Toxic contamination of food and water is no longer likely, but the organochlorine insecticides already in the environment are slowly degraded, and low-level residues may persist in selected areas (e.g., lake sediments).
    b. The highly lipid-soluble nature of these agents, combined with their environmental persistence, favors bioaccumulation upward in food chains from environmental to animal or human hosts.

2. Lindane and **methoxychlor** are currently approved for limited uses.

C. Exposure

1. Availability in food or the environment is decreasing slowly as contaminated areas are biodegraded and continuing sources are not generally available.

Diphenyl aliphatic type

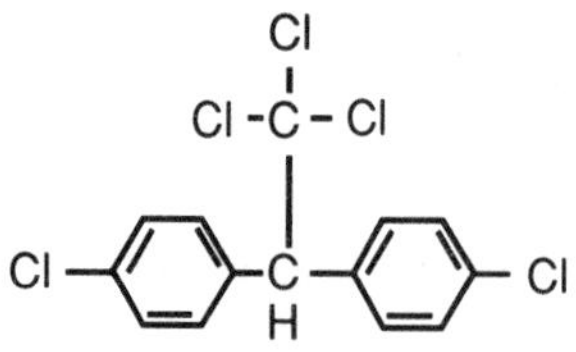

DDT

Cyclodiene type

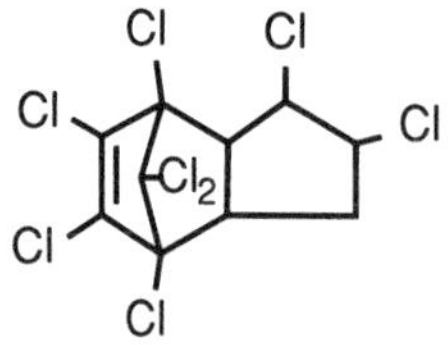

Chlordane

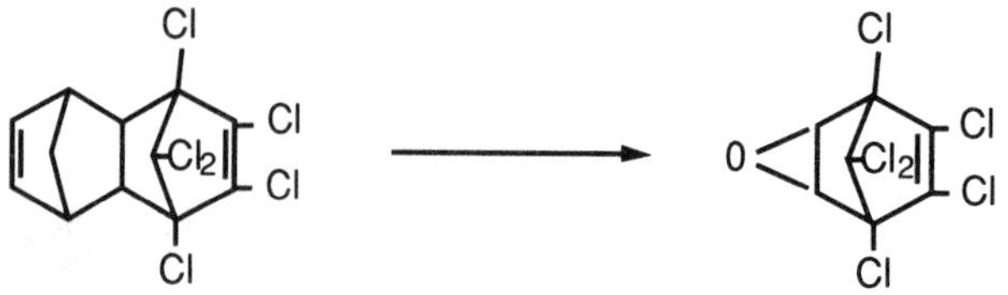

Aldrin

Dieldrin
(epoxide of aldrin)

FIGURE 19-3. Organochlorine insecticides.

2. Accidental toxic exposures occur occasionally when old products stored carelessly gain access to animal foods or leak into the environment.

3. Owners may fail to properly dilute currently approved sprays and dips.

4. Some organochlorines (e.g., endrin) have been used intentionally as avicides.

D. **Toxicokinetics**

1. **Absorption.** Because they are lipid-soluble, the organochlorines are readily absorbed by the **skin and mucous membranes**. Inhalation does not pose a significant problem because the organochlorines are not highly volatile.

2. **Distribution.** Organochlorines are found in the liver, kidney, and brain; they rapidly accumulate in lipid depots (e.g., adipose tissue).

3. **Metabolism**
   a. Cyclodiene insecticides are converted to epoxides by MFOs. Diphenyl aliphatics are dechlorinated by MFOs.
   b. Metabolites may be more toxic than the parent compound.

4. **Excretion**
   a. Metabolites are slowly released from lipid storage depots until equilibrium with the blood is achieved.
   b. The major excretory route is from bile to the digestive tract. Some enterohepatic recycling takes place.

    c. Lactating animals excrete organochlorine insecticides in milk fat.

    d. The half-life of some diphenyl aliphatics (e.g., DDT) and the cyclodienes may range from days to weeks. Residue elimination may be described by a two-compartment model, where the first phase is relatively rapid and the second is prolonged.

E. Mechanism of toxicologic damage

    1. Diphenyl aliphatics

       a. Diphenyl aliphatics **interfere with sodium channel kinetics in nerve membranes.** Sodium inflow is enhanced and potassium outflow is inhibited, leading to enhanced initiation of action potentials and an increased tendency for seizures.

       b. DDT metabolites (e.g., **o,p' DDD**) **inhibit the output of the adrenal gland** by selective necrosis of the zona fasciculata and zona reticularis. In patients with Cushing's disease, these agents may be used therapeutically.

    2. Heptachlor and **lindane** may **inhibit the binding of** the inhibitory neurotransmitter **γ-aminobutyric acid (GABA).**

    3. Cyclodiene insecticides. The mechanism of action of these agents is unknown, but they cause intense stimulation of the nervous system.

F. Toxicity

    1. Acute toxicity of organochlorines

       a. Agents in the **cyclodiene group** are **generally the most toxic;** the LD_{50} in dogs ranges from 15–65 mg/kg. The toxic dosage for cattle and swine ranges from 20–100 mg/kg.

       b. Cats are more susceptible than other common domestic animals to organochlorine insecticides. For example, the oral LD_{50} for endrin in the cat is 3–6 mg/kg.

    2. Subacute toxicity occurs when a sublethal dosage is encountered over a period of several days. Enzyme induction can enhance the toxicity of insecticides acquired during that time period.

    3. Chronic toxicity has been difficult to confirm. Most chronic low-level exposure has been associated with reproductive dysfunction in wild birds (i.e., eggshell thinning, reduced fertility) or with potential carcinogenic effects in animals.

    4. Potentiators of toxicity. Agents that cause MFO enzyme induction could potentiate organochlorine toxicosis.

G. Diagnosis

    1. Clinical signs of acute toxicosis are mainly referable to the nervous system. The severity of clinical signs is not well-correlated with prognosis.

       a. Early signs include **salivation, nausea,** and **vomiting,** but these are inconsistent. Early neurologic signs include **nervousness, agitation, apprehension, tremors, hyperexcitability, incoordination,** and **tremors.**

       b. Advanced signs

          (1) Intermittent clonic-tonic seizures are seen in advanced acute toxicosis. **Cranial to caudal epileptiform seizures** with **opisthotonus, paddling,** and **champing of the jaws** are common.

            (a) Acute seizures **may persist for 48–72 hours.**

            (b) Hyperthermia (106°F–108°F) may be present during or after seizures.

          (2) Affected animals may have **intermittent periods of depression** or appear almost normal between seizures.

          (3) Cattle may assume **abnormal postures, walk backwards,** or **chew or lick excessively.**

          (4) Intoxicated birds may show **sudden death, depression, disorientation, abnormal postures,** and **apparent blindness.**

2. Laboratory diagnosis

　a. Hematology values and **clinical chemistry** are usually not helpful, although dogs may have liver damage.

　b. Gas chromatography will confirm acute cases if the insecticide is in the blood, liver, or brain.

　c. Tissue concentrations of insecticide confirm exposure, but are poorly correlated with the severity of signs or survival.

　　(1) Chronic accumulation of residues can be detected in **milk fat** or **adipose tissue,** including fat obtained during biopsy.

　　(2) Tissues submitted for analysis should be packaged in clean glass containers or wrapped in aluminum foil to avoid contamination from plastic containers.

3. Lesions of organochlorine insecticide toxicosis are unreliable for diagnosis.

　a. Animals may show signs of trauma resulting from seizures.

　b. Pale musculature may result after seizures or hyperthermia.

　c. Dogs may have liver necrosis or hemorrhage of the adrenal gland.

H. | **Treatment, prognosis, and prevention**

1. Treatment

　a. Detoxification is essential to shorten the clinical course of intoxication.

　　(1) Dermal exposure

　　　(a) The animal should be washed with water and soap or detergent.

　　　(b) The hair of heavily contaminated, long-haired animals should be clipped.

　　　(c) Animal care personnel should wear gloves and aprons or raincoats, because these products readily absorb through the skin.

　　(2) Ingestion. Activated charcoal (1–2 g/kg) should be administered orally to adsorb the insecticide.

　　　(a) Mineral oil, which solubilizes the insecticide but is not absorbed, is a less preferable **alternative to charcoal**.

　　　(b) Adsorbents or nonabsorbable oils are **most effective when given within 4 hours of ingestion** of the pesticide.

　b. Supportive therapy. Diazepam, phenobarbital, or **pentobarbital** is used as needed to control seizures (see Chapter 5 III B 4). Animals should be placed in a **comfortable, warm area to minimize trauma** from seizures.

　c. Specific antidotes are not available for organochlorine insecticides.

　d. Management of recovered contaminated animals. Residues can persist for months or years.

　　(1) Loss of body fat accelerates reduction of residues in adipose tissue.

　　(2) Feeding activated charcoal (500–1000 g/day) to large animals may reduce enterohepatic recycling, but benefits often are limited.

　　(3) Administration of phenobarbital may enhance biotransformation in some animals, but phenobarbital's effectiveness for removing residues is minimal.

2. Prognosis is guarded to good, depending on the dosage received and how quickly detoxication is accomplished.

3. Prevention

　a. Clients should be instructed regarding how to properly contain, store, and dispose of organochlorine insecticides.

　b. Local or state environmental authorities should be contacted for assistance in disposing of contaminated animals, soil, or materials.

I. | **Public health concerns**

1. Potential human exposure to these products is regulated by the Environmental Protection Agency (EPA) and state public health authorities.

2. The high lipid solubility and slow elimination of the organochlorines favor the accumulation of unacceptable residues in the edible tissues of food animals.

a. Immediate sale or consumption of products from animals that have recovered from toxicosis is not recommended.

b. Other potentially exposed food animals should be evaluated to determine if residues exist.

J. Environmental concerns

1. Organochlorine insecticides cause eggshell thinning in raptors (e.g., eagles, hawks) and estrogenic effects in birds, leading to infertility.

2. Their persistence in soils and sediments leads to accumulation by organisms of the food chain and upward biomagnification of residues:
   a. 1× concentration in lake sediment
   b. 500× concentration in plankton
   c. 50,000× concentration in small fish
   d. 100,000× concentration in large fish and predators

III. PYRETHRINS AND PYRETHROIDS

A. Sources

1. Pyrethrins are natural insecticides produced from extracts of pyrethrum flowers (of the genus *Chrysanthemum*).

2. Pyrethroids are synthetic insecticides that resemble pyrethrins in structure and action.
   a. Type 1 pyrethroids do not contain an alpha-cyano moiety.
   b. Type 2 pyrethroids contain an alpha-cyano moiety.

B. Exposure

1. Environment
   a. Pyrethrum flowers are cultivated in the United States, but under North American conditions, the pyrethrin content is low.
   b. Agricultural use rarely results in residues or toxicosis. Low environmental persistence limits probability of toxic residues in plants or foods.

2. Products for commercial and home pest control
   a. Applications
      (1) Pyrethrins and pyrethroids are used for flea control and as insecticidal premise sprays when small animals are present.
      (2) They are used for sprays and other products where persistent pesticides are not desirable (e.g., dairies).
   b. Circumstances of poisoning
      (1) Excessive use of flea control sprays or dips can lead to dermal exposure.
      (2) Spraying in enclosed spaces can lead to inhalation of mists or vapors. Contamination of open aquariums by sprays or mists could lead to intoxication of fish.
      (3) Concentrated pesticides may be accidentally consumed by pets or livestock.

3. Secondary (relay) toxicosis. The potential for secondary toxicosis is very limited because of the low acute toxicity and rapid detoxification of pyrethroids.

C. Toxicokinetics

1. Absorption. Pyrethrins are lipophilic and readily absorbed orally, dermally, or via the lungs.

2. Distribution. Because of their rapid metabolism, the distribution of pyrethrins and pyrethroids is relatively unimportant.

3. **Metabolism.** Plasma and liver esterases rapidly hydrolyze the ester linkages of the insecticide.
   a. Hydrolyzed insecticide is **less toxic.**
   b. Metabolism **occurs readily in the intestinal tract,** so **oral toxicity** is **very low.**

4. **Excretion.** Metabolites are conjugated with glycine, glucuronic acid, or sulfates and excreted in the urine.

D. Mechanism of toxicologic damage

1. The **pyrethrins act on sodium channels in the axonal membrane,** decreasing and slowing inward sodium conductance and suppressing potassium outflow. They **may also inhibit adenosine triphosphatases (ATPases),** which may affect cation conduction at axonal membranes. The net result is decreased action potential amplitude and the generation of repetitive nerve impulses.

2. In addition, **type 2 pyrethroids interfere with binding of GABA and glutamic acid** at receptor sites.

E. Toxicity

1. **Acute toxicity**
   a. **Type 2 pyrethroids** (i.e., those with the alpha-cyano moiety) **are generally more toxic** than type 1 pyrethroids.
   b. **Acute oral toxicity** of common pyrethrins ranges generally from 100–2000 mg/kg body weight.

2. **Subacute** and **chronic toxicity** are not described.

3. **Potentiators of toxicity.** Drugs, chemicals, and nutritional changes that alter the effectiveness of the MFO system can change toxicity of the pyrethrins and pyrethroids.
   a. MFO inhibitors [e.g., piperonyl butoxide, N-octyl-bicycloheptene dicarboximide (MGK-264)] suppress the hydrolysis of pyrethrins and pyrethroids, increasing their toxicity.
   b. Commercial pyrethrin insecticides contain synergists.

F. **Diagnosis** of pyrethrin or pyrethroid toxicosis is difficult and usually depends on a compatible history, clinical signs, and elimination of differential diagnoses.

1. **Clinical signs** are apparent mainly in the nervous system.
   a. **In experimental animals** (e.g., rats), the clinical signs vary slightly with the type of pyrethroid.
      (1) **Type 1 pyrethroids** cause increased response to stimulation, muscle tremors, excitement, and paralysis.
      (2) **Type 2 pyrethroids** induce salivation, weakness, and a distinctive "writhing" (burrowing) syndrome.
   b. **In dogs, cats, and large animals,** the clinical signs are usually similar for both types of pyrethroids. Signs include:
      (1) Salivation, vomiting
      (2) Hyperexcitability, tremors, and seizures
      (3) Dyspnea
      (4) Weakness, prostration, death
   c. **Onset of signs** occurs in all species within minutes to hours of exposure, depending on the route of exposure.
   d. **Clinical signs resolve, in either death or recovery, within 24–72 hours.**

2. **Laboratory diagnosis**
   a. **Hematology values** and **clinical chemistry** are normal, except for possible stress-related responses (e.g. neutrophilia, hyperglycemia).
   b. **Tissue analysis.** Pyrethrins are difficult to detect and confirm in blood or tissue.

(1) The presence of pyrethrins, pyrethroids, or their metabolites confirms exposure, but tissue levels are not well-correlated with the severity of signs or death.

(2) Brain and liver tissue have been used for analysis.

3. Lesions are not usually associated with clinical toxicosis.

4. Differential diagnoses include chlorinated hydrocarbon and organophosphate toxicosis, metaldehyde poisoning, strychnine, nicotine, and aminopyridine poisoning, pseudorabies, and meningitis.

G. **Treatment, prognosis, and prevention**

1. Treatment

a. Detoxification

(1) Dermal exposure. The animal should be bathed with soap or detergent and water if exposure is dermal.

(2) Ingestion

(a) Emetics or gastric lavage can be used to empty the stomach if exposure is recent (i.e., within the previous 4 hours) and the animal is not having seizures.

(b) Activated charcoal and a saline or sorbitol cathartic reduce oral absorption and aid elimination.

b. Supportive therapy

(1) Diazepam or **barbiturates** can be used to control seizures and hyperexcitability. **Phenothiazine tranquilizers should be avoided because they may lower the seizure threshold.**

(2) Atropine can be used sparingly to alleviate excessive salivation or gastrointestinal hypermotility.

c. Specific antidotes are not available for pyrethrins. Generally, they are not needed because toxicosis is mild or moderate.

2. Prognosis is excellent unless exposure is massive or the animal is otherwise compromised.

3. Prevention

a. Clients should be educated regarding the accurate dilution and application of pesticides.

b. They should be cautioned against using several pesticides concurrently to address the same problem.

H. **Public health concerns**

1. Human exposure to these products can occur through careless use. Because pyrethrins have a reputation for being "safe," carelessness may result.

2. Residues in foods of animal origin are not likely because of the rapid metabolism and excretion of pyrethrins and pyrethroids.

I. **Environmental concerns**

1. Improper disposal can contaminate aquatic environments; fish (and some birds) are very sensitive to pyrethroids.

2. Excessive reliance on a relatively "safe" pesticide can result in ignoring principles of pest management and environmental protection.

IV. **ROTENONE** is prepared from extracts of the root of the *Derris* plant. Historically, rotenone was used to treat arrowheads used for fishing.

A. **Chemical structure.** Rotenone is unstable in light and air.

B. **Sources.** Rotenone is used in flea control products and premise insecticides, and as a topical product for the eradication of bovine *Hypoderma* larvae.

C. **Exposure**

1. **Excessive use of topical powders or dips** can cause toxicosis. Cats are most commonly affected.

2. Rotenone **may be intentionally added to bodies of water** to kill unwanted fish.

3. **Accidental exposures** from ingestion **are rare.**

4. **Secondary (relay) toxicosis** is **not likely.**

D. **Toxicokinetics**

1. **Absorption.** Oral absorption is limited but may be increased by oily or fatty foods.

2. **Metabolism.** Rotenone is metabolized in the liver by hydroxylation and demethylation to toxic or nontoxic products, respectively.

3. **Elimination.** Rotenone is eliminated primarily in the feces.

E. **Mechanism of toxicologic damage**

1. Rotenone **forms a complex with reduced nicotinamide adenine dinucleotide (NADH) dehydrogenase** and inhibits electron transfer between flavoprotein and ubiquinone.

2. It **inhibits mitosis,** probably by binding to the mitotic spindle apparatus.

F. **Toxicity**

1. **Acute toxicity** is most common. The **acute oral LD$_{50}$** is 100 mg/kg in guinea pigs, 300 mg/kg in dogs, and 1600 mg/kg in rabbits.
   a. Birds, fish, and cats are considered the most sensitive species. The LD$_{50}$ for fish is 12–75 µg/L.
   b. Chickens are resistant, with lethal doses ranging from 1000–3000 mg/kg.

2. **Potentiators of toxicity**
   a. Toxicity may be enhanced by combination with **pyrethrins.**
   b. **Intravenous administration** renders rotenone much more toxic to mammals.

G. **Diagnosis**

1. **Clinical signs** include vomiting and gastric irritation, lethargy and stupor, dyspnea and respiratory depression, and, possibly, tremors and seizures.

2. **Laboratory diagnosis**
   a. **Hematologic workup** may reveal hypoglycemia.
   b. **Chemical analysis** may confirm exposure, but exposure is not well-correlated with the severity of clinical signs. **Vomitus, blood, urine,** or **feces** may be analyzed.

3. **Lesions** include the following:
   a. Mild to moderate nonspecific gastroenteritis
   b. Pulmonary congestion
   c. Microscopic passive congestion of the liver with midzonal hepatic necrosis (chronic exposure)

H. **Treatment and prognosis**

1. **Treatment**
   a. **Detoxification** should be carried out as for other acute insecticide exposures (see III G 1 a).
   b. **Supportive therapy**
      (1) **Diazepam** can be used to control seizures. **Phenothiazine tranquilizers should be avoided.**
      (2) **Dextrose** can be administered intravenously if blood glucose levels warrant it.

c. **Specific antidotes** are not available. Usually supportive and detoxification therapy are sufficient to aid recovery.

2. **Prognosis** is excellent in most cases.

I. **Public health concerns.** Premise sprays or lawn and garden products are the most likely sources of human exposure. Residues in foods of animal origin are unlikely.

J. **Environmental concerns**

1. Rotenone is toxic to fish, and use near water may be hazardous to aquatic life.

2. Secondary effects (e.g., botulism) can occur when animals consume fish killed by rotenone.

V. **AMITRAZ** is a newer formamidine insecticide cleared for use on cattle, dogs, and pigs.

A. **Chemical structure.** The chemical formula is N'-(2,4-dimethyl)-N-(2,4-dimethylphenyl) [imino] methyl-N-methyl methanimidamide.

B. **Sources.** Amitraz, a topical miticide, is used in flea collars and for ectoparasite control in swine.

C. **Exposure**

1. Careless use as a spray or dip can lead to toxicosis.

2. Dogs may eat treated flea collars.

3. Contamination of food or the environment is unlikely.

4. Secondary (relay) toxicosis is unlikely.

D. **Toxicokinetics**

1. **Absorption.** Amitraz is readily absorbed both orally and parenterally. Blood levels peak within 2–6 hours following exposure.

2. **Distribution.** Amitraz appears to concentrate in the skin, liver, eyes, bile, kidney, cerebellum, lungs, spleen, and gonads.

3. **Metabolism and excretion.** Amitraz is metabolized to 4-amino-3-methylbenzoic acid, which is excreted in the urine.

E. **Mechanism of toxicity.** Amitraz is believed to act as an α_2-**adrenergic agonist** and a **weak monoamine oxidase (MAO) inhibitor**. The central nervous and cardiovascular systems are the main target tissues, resulting in **cardiovascular collapse** and **respiratory depression**.

F. **Toxicity**

1. **Acute toxicity.** The acute oral LD_{50} is 100 mg/kg for dogs, 400–800 mg/kg for guinea pigs, 515–938 mg/kg for rats, and greater than 1600 mg/kg for mice.

2. **Subacute toxicity**
   a. Dogs may experience transient clinical signs at dosages of 20 mg/kg.
   b. Some dogs (less than 10%) with demodicidosis experience transient sedation when treated with the recommended concentration of dip. Sedation usually occurs 2–6 hours following treatment and is generally resolved within 24–72 hours.

3. **Chronic toxicity** is not described.

4. **Potentiators of toxicity.** Interactions with meperidine or sympathomimetic amines (e.g., isoproterenol) have been reported.

G. Diagnosis

1. **Clinical signs** are similar to those caused by cholinesterase inhibitors or pyrethrins and include bradycardia, ataxia, depression, disorientation, vomiting, anorexia, polyuria, diarrhea, vocalization, and seizures.

2. **Laboratory diagnosis**
   a. **Hematologic workup.** Insulin release may cause hyperglycemia.
   b. **Gas chromatography** can detect and quantitate amitraz.
   c. **Tissue analysis.** Samples may be taken from the liver, kidney, skin, brain, lungs, adipose tissue, or spleen.

3. **Lesions**
   a. The size or weight of the liver may be increased.
   b. Chronic exposure to low dosages (1–4 mg/kg) may produce hepatic periportal hyperplasia and thinning of the adrenal zonae fasciculata and reticularis.

H. Treatment, prognosis, and prevention

1. **Treatment**
   a. **Detoxification**
      (1) **Dermal exposure.** The animal should be bathed in soap and water.
      (2) **Ingestion.** Emetics or activated charcoal and saline cathartics may be administered.
   b. **Supportive therapy** is similar to that recommended for pyrethrins and rotenone (see III G 1 b, IV H 1 b). The animal's temperature should be monitored to detect hypothermia.
   c. **Specific antidotes** are not available.

2. **Prognosis** is good; mildly affected animals may recover spontaneously.

3. **Prevention.** Clients should be reminded to follow label directions; **amitraz should never be used on cats**.

I. Public health concerns

1. Toxicosis in humans has occurred from intentional or accidental ingestion or accidental immersion in cattle dip.

2. Residues in foods of animal origin are unlikely because of amitraz's rapid metabolism. Label indications should be followed to avoid potential residue problems.

VI. CITRUS OIL EXTRACTS are derived from citrus fruit and peels.

A. Sources

1. **Crude citrus oils**

2. **Refined products** are marketed as aids for the control of lice, ticks, and fleas, as well as food additives.
   a. **Limonene** is a colorless liquid with a lemon-like odor.
   b. **Linalool** (3,7-dimethyl-16-octadiene-3-ol) is a tertiary alcohol used as a fragrance and food additive.

B. Exposure. Poisoning is uncommon under most circumstances.

1. **Misuse**
   a. Toxicosis occurs primarily in cats treated with citrus oil extracts at dosages recommended for dogs.

   b. Excessive exposure to products containing limonene or linalool can lead to toxicosis, especially when the synergist piperonyl butoxide is included in the spray or dip.

   2. Environmental residues are unlikely because the refined products are food additives with a GRAS ("generally recognized as safe") classification.

   3. Secondary (relay) toxicosis. There is no indication of secondary toxicosis.

C. **Toxicokinetics**

   1. Absorption. Citrus oil extracts are rapidly absorbed orally and dermally.

   2. Distribution. The distribution of citrus oil extracts is similar to that of other lipid-soluble compounds.

   3. Metabolism
   a. Phase I metabolism is by hydroxylation, acetylation, or reduction.
   b. Phase II metabolism. Citrus oil extracts are conjugated with glucuronides or sulfates. Linalool is partially metabolized to carbon dioxide.

   4. Excretion. Most of the dose is excreted in the urine; less than 10% of the dose is excreted in the feces. Enterohepatic recycling may occur.

D. **Mechanism of toxicologic damage** is unknown for citrus oil extracts. Central and peripheral vasodilatation may occur secondary to a neurologic mechanism.

E. **Toxicity**

   1. Acute toxicity
   a. Limonene. The oral toxic dosage in dogs is 680 g/kg.
   b. Crude citrus oils are toxic to cats at 5 times the recommended concentration. The suggested canine dosage of some products is lethal to cats.

   2. Subacute toxicity. Multiple exposures at high dosages (greater than 2000 mg/kg) may be **teratogenic**.

   3. Potentiators of toxicity. Citrus oil products appear to be potentiated by **piperonyl butoxide,** and presumably by **other MFO inhibitors**.

F. **Diagnosis**

   1. Clinical signs include ataxia, weakness, recumbency, generalized paralysis, vasodilation and hypotension, CNS depression, and hypothermia. Self-induced trauma or perineal dermatitis may occur in male cats.

   2. Laboratory diagnosis. Gas chromatography or **mass spectrometry** may detect metabolites of linalool or limonene; however, good correlation between quantitation of metabolites and clinical signs has not been established.

   3. Lesions. Renal tubular degeneration may occur in rats, but diagnostic lesions are usually not found in cats or dogs.

G. **Treatment, prognosis, and prevention.** Sublethal toxicosis usually resolves within 6–12 hours.

   1. Supportive therapy. The animal should be bathed in warm, soapy water and kept warm and well-ventilated.

   2. Prognosis is excellent.

VII. **OTHER INSECTICIDES.** Table 19-1 lists uncommon insecticides and those that pose less of a hazard.

TABLE 19-1. Characteristics of Four Minor Insecticides

	Boric Acid	Deet	Naphthalene	Nicotine
Chemical characteristics	Trihydroxy compound containing boron	N, N-diethyltoluamide	Highly volatile coal tar or petroleum hydrocarbon with two benzene rings	Alkaloid derived from tobacco plant (*Nicotiana tabacum*)
Sources	Ant and roach baits, cleaning compounds, denture cleaners	Common synthetic insect repellent, often combined with fenvalerate in flea control products for dogs and cats	Commercial mothproofing products	Tobacco leaves or plugs, nicotine sulfate ("Black leaf 40"), an older insecticide
Toxicokinetics	Concentrated in kidneys and slowly excreted in urine	Metabolized in liver and excreted in urine	Skin absorption enhanced by oils	Readily absorbed through skin and mucous membranes
Toxicity	Rat oral LD_{50}: 2.7–4.0 g/kg	Rat oral LD_{50}: 1–2 g/kg Rabbit dermal LD_{50}: 3 g/kg Dogs and cats show signs after exposure to 0.05 oz of a 0.09% fenvalerate/9% DEET solution; cats may be more sensitive than dogs	> 400 mg/kg to dogs; cats are more susceptible	1–2 mg/kg
Mechanism of toxicologic action	Unknown, but acts as an irritant in concentrated solutions (e.g., urine)	Increases dermal absorption of some chemicals (e.g., fenvalerate) Causes neurotoxicity, hypotension, bradycardia	Oxidation products of naphthalene cause hemolytic anemia and methemoglobinemia	Stimulates sympathetic and parasympathetic ganglia
Clinical signs	Vomiting, diarrhea, muscle weakness, ataxia, seizures, tremors, oliguria, anuria, hematuria, acidosis, depression, erythematous dermatosis (in primates)	Vomiting, anorexia, tremors, excitation, seizures, hypersalivation; signs develop within hours	Vomiting, malodorous breath, methemoglobinemia, acute hemolytic Heinz body anemia, hemoglobinuria, hepatic damage, nephrosis secondary to hemoglobinuria, cataracts (in neonates)	Rapid onset of hyperactivity, vomiting, and salivation, progressing to tremors, dyspnea, tachycardia, weakness, paralysis, and death

Diagnosis	Lesions of gastroenteritis and hepatic and renal lipidosis; urinalysis results typical of tubular damage; boric acid in urine confirms exposure	Protein and glucose levels may be increased in cerebrospinal fluid; urine, skin, blood, stomach contents, and vitreous humor may be analyzed; 20 ppm in serum is considered diagnostic	Hematologic workup reveals Heinz bodies, hemolysis, methemoglobinemia; odor of mothballs on skin or breath	No characteristic lesions; nicotine may be detectable in stomach contents, skin, or urine
Treatment and prognosis	Emesis and administration of activated charcoal; fluids for diuresis; symptomatic treatment for renal failure; peritoneal dialysis	Decontamination and supportive therapy similar to that used for pyrethrins; sublethally exposed animals recover in 24–72 hours	Emesis; administration of activated charcoal and a saline cathartic; ascorbic acid (20 mg/kg) to treat methemoglobinemia; fluids and bicarbonate to reduce precipitation of hemoglobin in kidney; blood transfusion	Emesis early if not contraindicated by the animal's clinical condition; gastric lavage and administration of activated charcoal; soap and water to cleanse skin if dermal exposure; atropine if parasympathetic effects are present; artificial oxygen therapy

VIII. METALDEHYDE

A. **Sources.** Metaldehyde is an active component of **slug** and **snail baits**.

   1. The pelleted or meal-style baits contain 3.5% metaldehyde.

   2. Baits of this type are used most frequently in temperate coastal areas and the southern lowlands of the United States.

B. **Exposure.** Careless placement of baits by homeowners can lead to toxicosis, because dogs find the meal and pellets attractive and readily consume them. Poisoning is most common in dogs; it is also reported in cats and sheep.

C. **Toxicokinetics.** Metaldehyde is **readily absorbed from the intestines** and **metabolized to acetaldehyde** (a metabolite similar to that of ethanol). The acetaldehyde metabolite is **excreted in urine**.

D. **Mechanisms of toxicologic damage**

   1. Metaldehyde **decreases concentrations of 5-hydroxytryptamine (5-HT, serotonin)** in the brain.

   2. It also **decreases GABA levels**.
      a. Loss of GABA allows excitatory signs to predominate in the CNS.
      b. As GABA levels decrease, the chance of survival is reduced.

E. **Toxicity. Acute toxicity** for most species ranges from 100–500 mg/kg. For example, the minimum lethal dosage is 100 mg/kg for dogs, 200 mg/kg for cattle, 60–360 mg/kg for horses, and 300 mg/kg for ducks.

F. **Diagnosis**

   1. Clinical signs
      a. Dogs. Signs may appear similar to those of organophosphate toxicosis, except vomiting and diarrhea are not likely.
         (1) Early signs include **anxiety** and **restlessness**.
         (2) Intermediate signs include **salivation, mydriasis, tremors, ataxia,** and **incoordination**.
         (3) Advanced signs include **polypnea, tachycardia, muscle tremors** leading to **opisthotonos** and **continuous convulsions, cyanosis, nystagmus,** and **hyperthermia**. Dogs are not as hyperesthetic as with strychnine toxicosis (see Chapter 22 V G).
      b. Cats exhibit signs similar to those exhibited by dogs; nystagmus is prominent.
      c. Cattle and sheep
         (1) Ataxia and **tremors** predominate.
         (2) Cattle may display **salivation, diarrhea,** and, possibly, **blindness**.
      d. Horses exhibit **colic, diarrhea, sweating, tremors,** and **hyperesthesia**.

   2. Laboratory diagnosis
      a. Acidosis may result from the metabolism of metaldehyde to acetaldehyde.
      b. Blood cholinesterase levels should be evaluated to rule out organophosphate toxicosis.
      c. Chemical analysis. Acetaldehyde may be evident in the stomach contents or lavage fluid. Residues are difficult to detect in tissues and may not be reliable for diagnosis.

   3. Lesions
      a. Gross lesions include **hepatic, renal,** and **pulmonary congestion, pulmonary** and **nonspecific hemorrhages,** and **gastrointestinal petechiae** and **ecchymoses**. The stomach contents may have an **odor of acetaldehyde**.
      b. Microscopic lesions are nonspecific, but include **hepatic swelling** and **degeneration,** and **neuronal degeneration in the brain**.

G. | **Treatment and prognosis**

1. **Detoxification therapy** involves **emesis** or **gastric lavage** and **activated charcoal** followed by a **saline** or **sorbitol cathartic**.

2. **Supportive therapy**
   a. **Sedation and seizure control. Diazepam** (2–5 mg/kg) should be administered first; if diazepam is ineffective, **barbiturates** may be used. Muscle relaxants (e.g., **methocarbamol**) may be useful to control severe tremors.
   b. **Artificial respiration**
   c. **Fluid therapy** should be initiated to maintain hydration and correct acidosis. **Magnesium-sodium lactate (1.6%)** should be administered intravenously (22 ml/kg given slowly over a 12-hour period).

3. **Antidotal therapy.** No specific antidotes are available.

4. **Prognosis** depends on the dosage received, the elapsed time since ingestion, and the timeliness of detoxification and supportive therapy.

DIRECTIONS: Each of the numbered items or incomplete statements in this section is followed by answers or by completions of the statement. Select the **one** numbered answer or completion that is **best** in each case.

1. After binding to cholinesterase, an organophosphate may lose an esterified moiety. What is the term for this process and why is it clinically significant?

(1) Known as "phase I metabolism" or induction, it increases the toxicity of organophosphates

(2) Known as "phase I metabolism" or induction, it decreases the toxicity of organothiophosphates

(3) Known as "aging," it enhances the spontaneous release of the organophosphate from cholinesterase

(4) Known as "aging," it increases the binding affinity and stability of the organophosphate–cholinesterase complex

(5) Known as "free radical synthesis," it enables the organophosphate to bind to postsynaptic neuronal membranes

2. Which one of the following is a well-known biological effect of organochlorine insecticides?

(1) Delayed peripheral neuropathies in wild mammals

(2) Overkill of desirable insect predators

(3) Development of birth defects in waterfowl

(4) Behavioral changes in wild birds

(5) Bioaccumulation and reproductive failure in wild birds

3. Which one of the following is the treatment of choice for carbamate toxicosis?

(1) Atropine

(2) Diazepam

(3) Pentobarbital

(4) Pralidoxime chloride (2-PAM)

(5) Diphenhydramine plus atropine

4. Which one of these products is formulated with a metabolic inhibitor to enhance its insecticidal activity?

(1) Amitraz

(2) DDT

(3) Nicotine

(4) Chlorpyrifos

(5) Pyrethrin

5. Which one of the following would not be improved by treatment with atropine?

(1) Excessive salivation

(2) Miosis

(3) Bradycardia

(4) Dyspnea

(5) Paresis

6. Which of the following natural compounds is sometimes intentionally added to water as a fish toxicant?

(1) Amitraz

(2) Limonene

(3) Nicotine

(4) Pyrethrin

(5) Rotenone

7. The most likely cause of the excitatory clinical signs seen in metaldehyde toxicosis of dogs is:

(1) acidosis resulting from the metabolism of metaldehyde to acetaldehyde.

(2) enhancement of sodium transport at the neuronal membrane.

(3) decreased brain serotonin levels.

(4) decreased γ-aminobutyric acid (GABA) levels.

(5) inhibition of glycine in the brain.

DIRECTIONS: The numbered item or incomplete statement in this section is negatively phrased, as indicated by an italicized word such as *not, least,* or *except.* Select the **one** numbered answer or completion that is **best**.

8. Which of the following statements is *not* true about organophosphate insecticides?

(1) Brahman cattle are more susceptible than the English breeds.
(2) Dogs are usually more susceptible than cats.
(3) Bulls are more susceptible than heifers to some organophosphates.
(4) Phenothiazine tranquilizers enhance the toxicity of organophosphates.
(5) Inducers of microsomal mixed function oxidases (MFOs) increase the toxicity of organothiophosphates.

1. The answer is 4 *[I E 2 a]*. Loss of one or more of the esterified moieties from the cholinesterase-bound organophosphate increases the stability of the phosphate–ester bond and inhibits or slows the release of the organophosphate from the bound enzyme. While bound, the cholinesterase enzyme is unable to hydrolyze acetylcholine (ACh), and the signs of organophosphate poisoning persist. Furthermore, oximes [e.g., pralidoxime (2-PAM)] are not effective at regenerating cholinesterase once the aging process has occurred. Thus, if treatment with 2-PAM is not prompt, the ability to regenerate cholinesterase is lost. Phase I metabolism is the term applied to microsomal oxidations, which, for organothiophosphates, result in oxidative desulfuration of the organophosphate and increased cholinesterase inhibiting activity. Free radical synthesis is not a feature of organophosphate toxicosis.

2. The answer is 5 *[II I 1–2]*. The tendency toward bioaccumulation of organochlorine insecticides in birds, combined with the estrogenic effects of organochlorines (i.e., infertility, eggshell thinning, and the loss of incubating eggs) leads to serious reproductive losses and reduction in the bird population (especially raptors). Organochlorines do not cause peripheral neuropathies such as those associated with some of the organophosphates. Birth defects in waterfowl have been associated with excess selenium uptake from contaminated marshes. Interference with protein synthesis in the brain is associated with organomercurials, which were a component of some fungicides prior to the 1970s.

3. The answer is 1 *[I H 1 b]*. Atropine is useful to counteract the muscarinic signs of carbamate toxicosis, especially the life-threatening effects of bronchoconstriction, bronchosecretion, severe vomiting, and diarrhea. Diazepam and pentobarbital are recommended to control seizures resulting from organochlorine or pyrethrin toxicosis. The oximes [e.g., pralidoxime chloride (2-PAM)] are not recommended for carbamates because the carbamate–cholinesterase bond is readily and spontaneously reversed, so the oximes are largely unnecessary. In addition, some early reports indicated specifically that treatment with oximes worsened toxicosis caused by carbaryl (Sevin), a common carbamate insecticide. Thus, most authorities have continued to stress the lack of efficacy or need for oximes against carbamates and the potential, although largely undocumented, adverse effects they may cause when used with specific carbamates. Diphenhydramine may help control refractory nicotinic signs, but it is not the agent of first choice for the treatment of carbamate toxicosis and it should never be administered with atropine.

4. The answer is 5 *[III E 3 a–b]*. Pyrethrins are metabolized and detoxified by mixed function oxidases (MFOs). Piperonyl butoxide and MGK-264, inhibitors of microsomal MFOs in insects as well as mammals, are often added to commercial pyrethrin insecticides. Thus, preventing the detoxifying effects of the MFO enzymes increases the insecticidal activity of the pyrethrins, but it also increases their mammalian toxicity.

5. The answer is 5 *[I G 1 a–b, H 1 b (1)]*. Salivation, miosis, bradycardia, and dyspnea are muscarinic signs of organophosphate cholinesterase inhibition that are counteracted by atropine. Paresis is a nicotinic (neuromuscular) effect and is not altered by atropine. As a result, even though the parasympathetic signs of organophosphate toxicosis are controlled by atropine, animals may still have muscle tremors, weakness, and even dyspnea (as a result of weakness or paralysis of the striated muscles of respiration).

6. The answer is 5 *[IV C 2]*. Both pyrethrins and rotenone are very toxic to fish, but rotenone has traditionally been used to control unwanted fish and to clear ponds and lakes for restocking. Amitraz is a synthetic pesticide approved for use on dogs and pigs. Limonene, one of several extracts from citrus rinds, is used in a number of food additives and natural aids to control ticks and fleas. Nicotine is a potent ganglionic blocker; its use is limited to direct application to animals to treat ectoparasite infestation. Nicotine is rarely used because it has a narrow margin of safety.

7. The answer is 4 *[VIII D 2]*. Metaldehyde decreases levels of the inhibitory neurotransmitter γ-aminobutyric acid (GABA), allowing excitatory influences to predominate in the central nervous system (CNS). Methaldehyde does cause acidosis as a result of metabolism to acetaldehyde, but acidosis is a depressive influence, and there is little evidence to link it to the known neurologic effects of metaldehyde. Brain serotonin levels are reduced, but a causative relationship has not been established. Glycine is an inhibitory neurotransmitter that is affected in strychnine toxicosis. Inhibition in the reflex arc is released resulting in uncontrolled response to stimuli.

8. The answer is 2 *[I D 3 a, F 4 a, 5]*. Cats are usually more susceptible than dogs to organophosphates. Brahman cattle appear to have greater cholinesterase binding by organophosphate compounds, thus increasing their susceptibility. Bulls are more susceptible than heifers to organophosphates that are metabolized by the mixed function oxidases (MFOs) to more toxic intermediates, because testosterone increases the activity of the microsomal enzymes. Phenothiazine tranquilizers have historically been thought to increase susceptibility to organophosphates, although clearly documented experimental evidence of such an effect is generally lacking. Microsomal MFOs increase the toxicity of organothiophosphates by replacing sulfur with oxygen.

Chapter 20

Herbicides

I. **INTRODUCTION.** Certain herbicides are of interest in veterinary medicine because of their toxicity, widespread use, or historical significance; these agents are discussed in II–III. Other herbicides are summarized in Tables 20-1 and 20-2.

A. **Types of herbicides.** Representative chemical groupings of common herbicides tested for toxicity in cattle and sheep are presented in Table 20-1. **Inorganic** and **organic synthetic herbicides** are recognized.

1. **Inorganic herbicides** include arsenicals and chlorates. Most of these agents are banned from use; those not banned from use are used infrequently.

2. **Organic synthetic herbicides** are most commonly used in modern agriculture.

B. **Applications.** Herbicides are the most commonly used pesticide chemicals in agriculture. **Post-emergent herbicides** are applied directly to growing plants, whereas **pre-emergent herbicides** are incorporated in soil to prevent germination.

1. **Agriculture.** Herbicides are commonly applied to **row crops** (e.g., corn, soybeans, cotton, sorghum) and used for selective weed control in **small grain crops** (e.g., wheat, barley, rye) and **forages**.

2. **Commercial use** has been increasing steadily.
   a. Herbicides are used for **weed control in residential lawns** and **at industrial sites**.
   b. **Road crews** use herbicides to maintain visibility at intersections.

C. **Exposure.** Relatively few herbicides are considered hazardous to livestock at recommended conditions of use.

1. **Environmental residues.** Herbicides are degraded by photolytic activity and soil microbes. Therefore, they generally do not persist in soil beyond the normal growing season.
   a. **Excessive application rates** or **use outside of label restrictions** can result in residues in soil or ground water.
   b. **Urban runoff** into storm sewers is an occasional problem.

2. **Inadvertent consumption of concentrated or mixed herbicide is rare,** but when it does occur, cattle and, occasionally, dogs, are most often affected.

3. **Grazing freshly sprayed pastures or eating treated hay** that was cut before the post-application harvest interval is completed can lead to toxicosis.
   a. Herbicides may drift from an adjoining field.
   b. Pets may have access to treated lawns. Table 20-2 compares the toxicity of selected lawn and turf herbicides.

D. **Diagnosis.** Clinical signs and lesions are nonspecific and remarkably similar among herbicides.

1. Toxicosis by most herbicides cannot be diagnosed based on circumstantial evidence alone; evidence of substantial and repeated exposure is necessary.

TABLE 20-1. Selected Herbicides Toxic to Ruminants at Dosages Less Than 100 mg/kg

Category	Exposure (days)	Characteristics of Intoxication
Acetamides Propachlor	3–9	Relatively toxic, producing anorexia, depression, salivation, muscle tremors, prostration. Lesions include an enlarged, pale liver, renal congestion, enlarged adrenals, green undigested rumen contents, and petechial hemorrhages in the urinary bladder.
Benzoic acids Chloramben	1–2	Low dosages cause weight loss and anorexia. Higher dosages cause bloat, diarrhea, lameness, prostration, and death. Lesions include hepatic adrenal congestion, intestinal hyperemia, an enlarged spleen, subepicardial hemorrhages, and, occasionally, hydropericardium and ascites.
Bipyridyls Paraquat	10	Depression, ataxia, and diarrhea are acute signs. Progressive dyspnea and labored breathing, weakness, cyanosis, and death may occur over 7–21 days.
Carbamates Chloropropham	2–10	Anorexia and salivation are prominent; unexpected deaths may occur. Lesions are pulmonary, hepatic, renal, and intestinal congestion.
Dinitroanilines Benefin	2–6	Anorexia, weight loss, diarrhea, bloat, depression, ataxia, and tachypnea are major clinical signs. The lymph nodes and liver are congested and enlarged.
Diphenyl esters Nitrofen	3	Anorexia, depression, ataxia, diarrhea, and hematuria are seen in toxicosis. Necropsy findings include pulmonary congestion and edema, hydropericardium, and epicardial hemorrhages.

Class / Compound	Structure	Dosage	Clinical signs and lesions
Nitriles Dichlobenil		1–4	Anorexia, weight loss, salivation, and depression are major clinical signs. Lymphatic, intramuscular, and epicardial hemorrhages occur along with congestion of the liver, kidney, and intestinal tract.
Organoarsenicals MSMA (methyl-arsonic acid)		2–3	Acute, severe gastroenteritis with watery to hemorrhagic diarrhea is typical. Lesions of mucoid to hemorrhagic and necrotic gastritis and enteritis are followed in subacute stages by pale, swollen kidneys with tubular degeneration and necrosis.
Phenoxys 2,4-D		2–10	Gradual onset of anorexia, weight loss, rumen stasis, and weakness; signs may appear similar to those of malnutrition or starvation. Rumen at necropsy is atonic and filled with fresh-appearing undigested forages. The kidneys may be pale and the liver and intestines are congested.
Phthalamic acids Naptalam		3–6	Anorexia, diarrhea, and weight loss are common. Lesions are primarily congestion of the liver, kidneys, and intestines.
Thiocarbamates EPTC Triallate		1–2 2–5	Some members of this group (e.g., EPTC) have anticholinesterase activity. Signs are anorexia, weight loss, diarrhea, ataxia, muscle tremors, salivation, and bloating. Atropine may be used cautiously as an antidote. Lesions are nonspecific congestion of the intestinal tract and other organs.
Triazines Atrazine Simazine		2–10 3–10	Relatively toxic to ruminants. Central nervous stimulation may be prominent, with muscle tremors, seizures, ataxia, weakness, and recumbency. Diarrhea and salivation sometimes occur. Necropsy reveals an enlarged and friable liver; pulmonary edema and hydrothorax are possible.

TABLE 20-2. Comparative Toxicities of Selected Lawn and Turf Herbicides in Dogs

Generic Name	Expected Concentration (ppm) in Grass from Recommended Application Rates*	No-effect Dietary Concentration (ppm)†	Toxic Dietary Concentration (ppm)	Toxic Effects
Alachlor	225–600	200	No information	Not reported in dogs
Atrazine	150	150	No information	Not reported in dogs Mucosal irritation, vomiting, diarrhea, weakness, ataxia in rodents
Benefin	150	5000	80,000 (lethal)	Not reported in dogs Wide margin of safety
Bensulide	1000	12	8000 (lethal)	Dose-related decrease in cholinesterase
Chloroflurenol	5–7	3000	No information	Not reported in dogs Wide margin of safety
2,4-D	150	500	No information	Adequate margin of safety
Dicamba	15–40	50	250	Mild hepatic jaundice, no other health effects
Glyphosate	150	2000	No information	Not reported in dogs Wide margin of safety
MCPA, MCPP	300–450	160	640 (chronic) 2560 (acute)	Decreased weight gains Anemia and decreased weight gains
Paraquat	75–150	34	300 (chronic)	Long-term exposure leads to chronic pulmonary fibrosis Narrow margin of safety for chronic effects
Pendimethalin	80–120	500	2000–8000	Dose-related increase in serum alkaline phosphatase, no other health effects
Propachlor	450–900	1000	No information	Not reported
Triclopyr	5–7	400	No information	Wide margin of safety Anorexia and reduced weight gain, enlarged liver and kidneys, mild nephrosis reported at high dosages

*Based on actual analysis, or estimated at 150 ppm for each pound applied per acre.
†Based on prolonged feeding trial.

2. Veterinarians should make rigorous efforts to rule out other diagnoses before making a diagnosis of herbicide toxicosis.

3. Chemical analysis helps to establish exposure, but in many cases will not confirm the diagnosis.

E. | Public health considerations

1. Currently there is no evidence that herbicides pose a residue problem in meat, milk, or eggs.

2. Surveys in some agricultural areas demonstrate very low levels of common herbicides in ground waters.

II. | PHENOXY HERBICIDES (e.g., **2,4-D, MCPA, silvex**) are chlorinated phenoxy derivatives of fatty acids.

A. | Chemical structure

1. The phenoxy herbicides contain from one to three chlorine atoms and, sometimes, a methyl group.

2. The chlorophenoxy ring is esterified to simple acids (e.g., acetic, propionic, butyric).

3. Some early formulations (e.g., 2,4,5-T) contained dioxin contaminants that increased the toxicity of the technical material.

B. | Exposure

1. Anecdotal reports of toxicosis in **dogs with access to freshly sprayed lawns** have been made, although verification of toxicosis is usually lacking.

2. **Cattle** may **drink concentrates or tank mixes**.

3. In addition to their own toxic properties, phenoxy herbicides can **potentiate the toxic effects of some plants:**
   a. They may **increase the nitrate content of certain plants** (e.g., red root pigweed).
   b. Phenoxy derivatives can **increase the palatability of certain toxic plants** (e.g., Sudan grass, larkspur), thus increasing poisoning risk from those plants.

C. | Toxicokinetics

1. **Absorption** occurs readily from the stomach and intestines. Dermal absorption is slower and less complete.

2. **Distribution.** Phenoxy herbicides are protein-bound in vivo and rapidly distributed to the liver, kidney, and brain.

3. **Metabolism**
   a. Esters may be metabolized by hydrolysis.
   b. Small amounts of herbicide may be conjugated to glycine or taurine.

4. **Excretion** is by tubular secretion using the organic anion transport system. A major portion of the dose is excreted unchanged in the urine.
   a. Canines excrete phenoxy herbicides relatively slowly.
   b. Excretion is markedly enhanced by ion-trapping using alkaline diuresis, because phenoxy herbicides are organic acids.
   c. The half-life of 2,4-D is brief, approximately 18 hours.

D. Mechanism of toxicologic damage

1. The phenoxy herbicides **depress ribonuclease synthesis, uncouple oxidative phosphorylation,** and **increase the number of hepatic peroxisomes.** The relationship of these biochemical changes to clinical effects is unknown.

2. In **dogs,** the phenoxy herbicides **may directly affect muscle membranes,** causing changes visible on the electromyogram.

E. Toxicity

1. **Acute toxicity**
   a. The acute toxic dose is 200 mg/kg in cattle and 100 mg/kg in pigs.
   b. The oral LD_{50} is 500 mg/kg in rats and approximately 100 mg/kg in dogs.
   c. The multiple lethal dosage in dogs is 25 mg/kg for 6 days.

2. **Chronic toxicity**
   a. Dogs can tolerate dietary dosages of 500 ppm for 2 years with no adverse effects.
   b. Long-term feeding of diets containing 2000 ppm has been tolerated by cattle. The toxic dosage in cattle is 100 mg/kg for 10–30 days.

F. Diagnosis

1. **Clinical signs** for various species are summarized in Table 20-3.

2. **Laboratory diagnosis**
   a. **Hematologic workup** does not reveal any characteristic changes.
   b. **Alkaline phosphatase (AP), lactate dehydrogenase (LDH),** and **creatine phosphokinase levels** are consistent with liver, kidney, and muscle damage.
   c. **Chemical analysis of forages, urine,** or **renal tissue** confirms exposure to phenoxy herbicides; however, the concentration of phenoxy herbicide in tissue or urine that confirms toxicosis is not well-established.

3. **Lesions**
   a. Oral ulcers are occasionally present.
   b. There is evidence of rumen stasis; bright green, undigested feed may be present in the rumen.
   c. The liver is swollen and friable.
   d. The kidneys are enlarged and show renal congestion and tubular degeneration.
   e. The mesenteric lymph nodes and vessels are hyperemic and enlarged.
   f. There may be evidence of epicardial hemorrhage.
   g. Hydropericardium may be present.

TABLE 20-3. Clinical Signs of Phenoxy Herbicide Toxicosis

Species	Signs	
	Gastrointestinal	**Neuromuscular**
Cattle	Anorexia, rumen atony, diarrhea, ulceration of oral mucosa, bloat, rumen stasis	Depression, muscle weakness
Swine	Vomiting, diarrhea, salivation	Tremors, ataxia, weakness
Dogs	Vomiting, diarrhea, bloody feces	Myotonia, ataxia, posterior weakness, periodic clonic spasms (only at high dosages), altered electromyogram with increased insertional activity

G. **Treatment and prognosis**

1. **Treatment**
   a. **Detoxification**
      (1) **Dermal exposure.** Skin and hair should be washed with soap and water.
      (2) **Ingestion.** Activated charcoal is effective, especially in ruminants, if exposure is recent (i.e., less than 2 days).
   b. **Supportive therapy**
      (1) Symptoms of diarrhea and rumen atony should be treated.
      (2) Renal function should be monitored, and intravenous fluids should be administered to promote diuresis.
      (3) Convalescing animals require a bland, high-quality diet. Rumen activity should be monitored; treatment with rumen inoculants may be necessary.
   c. **Specific antidotes** are not available.

2. **Prognosis** is good if exposure is moderate and decontamination therapy is instituted promptly.

H. **Public health concerns**

1. Pesticide applicators and farm workers are at greatest risk for exposure. Some epidemiological reports have linked phenoxy herbicide use to increased incidence of non-Hodgkin's lymphoma in humans.

2. Residues in foods of animal origin are infrequent because of the rapid excretion and short tissue half-life of the phenoxy herbicides. In addition, the incidence of animal exposure to these agents is low.

III. DIPYRIDYL HERBICIDES (e.g., PARAQUAT, DIQUAT)

A. **Chemical structure and characteristics**

1. **Structure.** The dipyridyl structure is unique among the herbicides (see Table 20-1).

2. **Characteristics.** Dipyridyl herbicides are:
   a. Nonvolatile, water-soluble, and stable at temperatures up to 300°C
   b. Degradable in sunlight within 3 weeks
   c. Rapidly and completely inactivated in soil by bacterial activity
   d. Strongly bound to clays in soil

B. **Sources**

1. The dipyridyl herbicides are available in **concentrated forms (5%–20% solutions) for agricultural use** and **dilute forms for home lawns and gardens**.

2. They are applied to foliage as a **contact (desiccant) herbicide** to kill vegetation prior to planting and to defoliate cotton prior to harvest.

C. **Exposure.** The agricultural application rate is low (0.5 lb/acre), which limits risk and makes poisoning from sprayed forage unlikely.

1. Poisoning of livestock occurs when animals consume concentrates or tank mixes.

2. The dipyridyl herbicides are frequently implicated in cases of malicious poisoning of dogs.

D. **Toxicokinetics**

1. **Absorption** is limited.
   a. Less than 20% of an ingested dose is absorbed.
   b. In cases of dermal exposure, less than 10% of the dose is absorbed through the skin.

2. **Distribution.** Paraquat concentrates in the lung; the concentration in lung tissue is up to 10 times that of other tissues.

3. **Metabolism** is minimal, except for oxidation–reduction reactions (see III E).

4. **Excretion.** Dipyridyl herbicides are excreted primarily in the urine as unmetabolized compounds.

E. **Mechanism of toxicologic action.** The dipyridyl herbicides are reduced by reduced nicotinamide–adenine dinucleotide phosphate (NADPH). Electron transfer occurs from paraquat to oxygen.

1. Singlet oxygen reacts with lipids in cell and organelle membranes to form lipid hydroperoxides.

2. Lipid free radicals are generated, which lead to additional free radical production, membrane damage, cellular degeneration, and necrosis.

3. The lungs are most affected.

F. **Toxicity**

1. **Acute toxicity**
   a. The **oral LD$_{50}$** ranges from 25–75 mg/kg in cats, dogs, pigs, sheep, and humans. It is 100 mg/kg in rats and 290 mg/kg in turkeys.
   b. The **dermal LD$_{50}$** for turkeys and rabbits is approximately twice the oral LD$_{50}$; in rats, the dermal LD$_{50}$ is similar to the oral LD$_{50}$.
   c. The **minimum lethal dose for humans** is approximately 30 mg/kg.

2. **Chronic toxicity** poses a hazard. Dogs consuming 170 ppm dietary paraquat for 2 months developed anorexia, respiratory distress, and pulmonary lesions, leading to death.

3. **Factors affecting toxicity.** Clay soils limit paraquat's toxicity because paraquat binds strongly to clay, which limits its availability and toxicity.

G. **Diagnosis**

1. **Clinical signs**
   a. **Acute toxicosis**
      (1) **Early signs** after ingestion may include vomiting and depression. High dosages cause early signs of ataxia, dyspnea, and seizures.
      (2) **Respiratory signs** are usually **delayed for 2–7 days**.
         (a) Early respiratory signs are tachypnea, dyspnea, moist rales, and cyanosis.
         (b) Hypoxia, cyanosis, pneumomediastinum, reduced pulmonary compliance, and death may occur within 8 days of ingestion.
   b. **Subacute or chronic toxicosis.** Signs may develop after 7 days and gradually worsen for up to 3 weeks. In the chronic phase, there is progressive pulmonary fibrosis and increasing respiratory distress.

2. **Laboratory diagnosis**
   a. **Radiographic changes in the lungs** are mild relative to the degree of respiratory distress shown.
   b. **Analysis of urine, herbicide solutions,** or **suspect baits** will help to establish exposure, but may not be well-correlated with severity of signs. Paraquat is only detectable in the urine for 2–3 days following the onset of clinical signs.

3. **Lesions** are primarily in the respiratory tract.
   a. **Gross lesions** include pulmonary congestion, hemorrhage, atelectasis, broncho-dilatation, and bullous emphysema.
   b. **Microscopic lesions** include necrosis of the alveolar type I epithelium, followed by progressive alveolar and interstitial fibrosis and alveolar emphysema. Renal proximal tubular degeneration and moderate centrilobular hepatic degeneration may be seen.

H. **Treatment and prognosis**

1. **Treatment**
   a. **Detoxification**
      (1) **Emetics** should be used soon after ingestion.
      (2) **Bentonite** or **Fuller's earth** is the preferred adsorbent because of the high absorptive capacity of clays for paraquat.
         (a) **Activated charcoal** should be used if a clay adsorbent is not available.
         (b) **Ground clay-based kitty litter** has been suggested as an emergency detoxicant, but its efficacy is uncertain.
      (3) **Saline cathartics** should follow the adsorbents to remove as much paraquat as possible from the gastrointestinal tract.
   b. **Supportive therapy**
      (1) **Assisted ventilation** may be of some benefit because pulmonary compliance is usually compromised. **Oxygen is contraindicated** because it may exacerbate oxidative damage to the lung.
      (2) **Renal function should be monitored.** Fluids should be provided as needed and used to force diuresis.
   c. **Specific antidotes** are not available, but **biochemical antagonists** have been recommended.
      (1) **Superoxide dismutase (orgotein)** scavenges superoxide free radicals.
      (2) **Acetylcysteine** may serve as a substitute for glutathione in the reduction of free radicals.
      (3) **Niacin** and **riboflavin** may be helpful, but their specific benefits are not documented.
      (4) **Ascorbic acid** may be useful as a general antioxidant to combat free radical damage.

2. **Prognosis** is **guarded or grave** in spite of therapy. Early detoxification may be the most beneficial approach.

I. **Public health concerns.** Residues in foods of animal origin are not likely because of paraquat's low concentration in edible tissues and its relatively short half-life.

STUDY QUESTIONS

DIRECTIONS: Each of the numbered items or incomplete statements in this section is followed by answers or by completions of the statement. Select the **one** numbered answer or completion that is **best** in each case.

1. Which one of the following procedures could be used to detect early or mild effects of 2,4-D in dogs?

(1) Electrocardiography
(2) Electroencephalography
(3) Electromyography
(4) Radiography
(5) Ultrasound

2. Which herbicide is associated with lesions of oral ulcers, rumen stasis with bright green undigested forages, and liver and kidney congestion?

(1) Arsenic
(2) 2,4-D
(3) Paraquat
(4) Chloropropham
(5) Atrazine

3. Which herbicide is known to increase the nitrate content of some plants?

(1) Arsenic
(2) 2,4-D
(3) Glyphosate
(4) Paraquat
(5) Benefin

DIRECTIONS: The numbered item or incomplete statement in this section is negatively phrased, as indicated by an italicized word such as *not, least,* or *except.* Select the **one** numbered answer or completion that is **best**.

4. Which one of the following statements is *not* true about paraquat herbicide?

(1) It initiates the formation of singlet oxygen.
(2) Paraquat is often mixed with hamburger to maliciously poison dogs.
(3) Paraquat is preferentially concentrated in the liver and kidney.
(4) The prognosis for recovery is often very poor.
(5) Paraquat is strongly adsorbed to clays and bentonite.

ANSWERS AND EXPLANATIONS

1. The answer is 3 *[II D 2]*. 2,4-D affects the muscle membranes of dogs by an unknown mechanism, leading to myotonia or stiffness and changes detected by electromyography. To date, these muscular changes are a sensitive and early effect of 2,4-D that is unique to dogs.

2. The answer is 2 *[II F; Table 20-3]*. The phenoxy herbicides (e.g., 2,4-D) have been observed experimentally and clinically to inhibit ruminal digestion of forages, leading to rumen hypoactivity (atony) and persistence of bright green undigested forages in the rumen. Arsenic is absorbed readily and causes acute abomasitis and enteritis with fluid to hemorrhagic diarrhea. Death is often acute, before any rumen consequences can occur. Paraquat concentrates preferentially in lung tissue, rather than remaining in and affecting the rumen. The lesions associated with chloropropham are primarily pulmonary, hepatic, renal, and intestinal. Atrazine is associated with central nervous system (CNS) stimulation. Lesions include an enlarged and friable liver and, possibly, pulmonary edema and hydrothorax.

3. The answer is 2 *[II B 3 a]*. Phenoxy herbicides (e.g., 2,4-D) are plant growth regulators, and at low to moderate rates or early in the plant damage cycle, they may increase nitrate accumulation in some plants. This is not true for all plants, but the possibility should always be kept in mind when investigating potential herbicide overspraying of pastures or crops.

4. The answer is 3 *[III C 2, D 2, E, H 2]*. Paraquat is unique among the common herbicides because it preferentially accumulates in lung tissue. In the lung, it stimulates the formation of free radicals and lipid peroxides, leading to lung damage and progressive pulmonary fibrosis. Dogs are particularly susceptible to toxicosis, and paraquat has been used in baits such as fresh hamburger by malicious poisoners. Treatment of poisoned dogs is ineffective and the prognosis for recovery is very guarded.

Chapter 21
Fungicides

I. **GENERAL CONSIDERATIONS.** The specific chemical characteristics, uses, toxicity, and effects of common fungicides are summarized in Table 21-1.

A. **Applications.** Fungicides are used to prevent or treat fungal infections in plants or plant products.

   1. They are used to protect tubers, fruits, and vegetables during storage.

   2. Soil fungicides are used at the time of planting.

   3. They are applied directly to ornamentals, trees, field crops, cereals, and turf grasses.

B. **Potential for toxicosis.** Use restrictions and the low toxicity of modern fungicides generally prevent poisoning in animals. **Flagrant misuse, accidents,** and **carelessness** are the principal causes of toxicosis in pets and livestock.

C. **Toxicity.** Fungicides vary in toxicity from barely toxic to highly lethal.

   1. Most available toxicity data are for laboratory animals; little information is available for farm animals and pets.

   2. Fungicides are commonly marketed and used in combination with other fungicides and with insecticides.

   3. The carriers or solvents, also known as "inert ingredients," may be toxic.

D. **Diagnosis of fungicide toxicosis**

   1. **Clinical signs** are often **nonspecific.** They may include **anorexia, depression, weakness,** and **diarrhea.**

   2. **Laboratory diagnosis. Chemical analysis** of **treated or contaminated feeds and forages** is usually more effective than analysis of animal tissues.

   3. **Lesions,** which are commonly **mild or generalized,** include **gastroenteritis** (from acute exposure), **rumen stasis,** and **hepatic, renal,** and **pulmonary congestion.**

E. **Treatment and prevention of fungicide toxicosis**

   1. Treatment
      a. Detoxification and supportive therapy should be carried out for known or suspected exposures.
      b. Specific antidotes are generally not available.

   2. Prevention. Adverse effects are not likely if these products are used according to label restrictions. Alternatively, the suppliers or manufacturers of the chemical can supply details regarding the proper application, storage, and disposal of the fungicide.

TABLE 21-1. Selected Common Fungicides

Name	Chemistry	Uses	NOAEL	Acute (Oral LD_{50})	Chronic	Effects
Benzimidazoles						
Benomyl	(1-[(butylamino) carbonyl] - 1H-benzimida-zol-2-yl)-carbamic acid	Systemic fungicide for fruits, nuts, vegetables, field crops, turf, ornamentals	Rats: 2500 ppm Dogs: 500 ppm	Rats: > 10,000 mg/kg		
Thiophanate-methyl	Dimethyl [(1,2-phenylene) bis-(imino-car-bonothioyl)] biscarbamate Dimethyl 4,4'o-phenylenebis [3-thioallo-phanate]	Systemic fungicide used for fruits, vegetables, field crops, nuts		Rats: 7500 mg/kg Dogs: 4000 mg/kg	Dogs: 2500 ppm	Liver damage, cirrhosis
Binapacryl	[1,2-phenylenebis (imino-carbonothioyl)] b as the carbamic acid or dimethyl ester 2-sec-butyl-4,6-dinotrophenyl-3-methyl-2-butenoate			Rats: 421 mg/kg		
Bordeaux mixture*	Mixture of hydrated lime and copper sulfate (1%); old formulations may contain lead arsenate	Historically used in orchards and vineyards where soils may be contaminated with copper and lead				Gastroenteritis and hepatic damage
Cadmium-containing fungicides	Cadmium chloride or succinate; formulations may contain up to 12.3% elemental cadmium					
Chloroneb	1,4-dichloro-2,5-dimethoxybenzene	Seed treatment and turf fungicide	Rats: 2500 ppm	Rats: 660 mg/kg		Nephrosis, anuria, and depression
Chlorothalonil	Tetrachloroisophthalonitrile	Broad-spectrum fungicide for fruits and vegetables	Dogs: 120 ppm	Rats: > 5000 mg/kg Rats: > 10,000 mg/kg		
Copper-containing fungicides†				Rats: 400–1200 mg/kg	Dogs: 15,000–30,000 ppm for 2 years	Anorexia, weight loss, increased liver, kidney, and thyroid weights
Cyclohexamide	3-[2-(3,5-dimethyl-2 oxocyclohexyl) 2-hydroxyethyl-] glutarimide	Ornamentals and grass, antibiotic action as well as fungicidal activity		Rats: 2 mg/kg		
DCNA	2,6-dichloro-4-nitroaniline	Fruits and vegetables		Rats: > 5000 mg/kg		
Diclobutrazol	1-(2,4-dichlorophenyl) 4,4-dimethyl-2-(1,2,4-triazol-1-yl) pentan-3 ol	Systemic fungicide for cereal crops		Rats: 4000 mg/kg	Dogs: 25–50 mg/kg for 6 weeks	Sunlight-activated corneal and lens opacities
Dinocap	Mixture of 2,4-dinitro-6-octyl-phenyl croto-nate; 2,6-dinitro-4-octyl-phenyl crotonate; and nitrooctyo phenols	Fruit and vegetable fungicide; also active against mites		Rats: 980 mg/kg		

Compound	Chemical name	Use	Dose	LD50	Chronic	Effects
Dithiocarbamates	Metal salts of dithiocarbamic acid					
Ferbam	Ferric dimethyldithiocarbamate		Rats: 250 ppm	Rats: 4000–17,000 mg/kg		Mild brain lesions
Maneb	Manganese ethylenebisdithiocarbamate			Rats: 6750 mg/kg	Rats: 2500 ppm for 2 years	Suspected carcinogen at high dosages; Growth inhibitor; Irritant to skin, eyes, mucous membranes
Nabam	Disodium ethylene-1,2 bisdithiocarbamate			Rats: 395 mg/kg	Rats: 2500 ppm for 2 years	Skin irritation, peripheral neurologic damage possible
Thiram	Bis (dimethylthio-carbamoyl) disulfide Tetramethylthiuram disulfide	Fungicide, seed protectant, animal repellant, bacteriostat in soap	Rats: 125 mg/kg	Rats: 780 mg/kg		Hepatotoxic; may produce alopecia, skin irritant and sensitizer
Zineb	Zinc ethylenebisdithiocarbamate			Rats: > 5200 mg/kg		Carcinogenic only at very large doses
Ziram	Zinc dimethyldithiocarbamate		Rats: 250 ppm	Rats: 1400 mg/kg	Rats: 2500 ppm for 2 years	Irritant to skin and mucous membranes; Reduced weight gain
Feraminosulf	Sodium [4-(dimethylamino) phenyl] diazene sulfonate or para-(dimethylamino)-benzenediazosulfonic acid	Turf and soil fungicide		Rats: 75 mg/kg		
Hexachlorobenzene	Perchlorobenzene	Historically used for seed treatment on wheat		Cats: 1700 mg/kg Rats: 3500 mg/kg Mice: 4000 mg/kg	Dogs: 1000 ppm for 1 year > 100 ppm for 1 year Pigs: 50 mg/kg per day	Dermal irritation, hepatotoxic, nephrotoxic; Death, anorexia, weight loss; Anemia, hypoglycemia, hypocalcemia; Porphyria, increased liver weight, death within 90 days
Hexachlorophene	2,2'methylene bis (3,4,6-trichlorophenol)	Foliar and soil fungicide		Rats: 56 mg/kg		Vacuolization, demyelination, and peripheral neuropathy (neonates)

Name	Chemistry	Uses	NOAEL	Acute (Oral LD$_{50}$)	Chronic	Effects
Metalaxyl	N-(2,6-dimethylphenyl)-N (methoxyacetyl)-alanine methyl ester	Soil fungicide, occasionally used on crops and ornamentals		Rats: 669 mg/kg		
PCNB	Pentachloronitrobenzene	Soil fungicide, seed dressing		Rats: 15,000 mg/kg	Dogs: > 180 ppm	Cholestatic hepatosis, secondary biliary nephrosis
Phthalimides						
Captan	N-sulfenyl phthalimide 3a,4,7,7a-tetrahydro-2 ((trichloromethyl) thio]-1 H-isoindole-1,3 (2H)-dione or cis N-trichloromethylmercapto-4-cyclohexene 1,2 dicarboxamide	Widely used in agriculture‡ and home gardening		Rats: 9000–12,500 mg/kg Ruminants: 250–500 mg/kg		Labored respiration, anorexia, depression, hydrothorax, ascites, hemorrhage of the gallbladder, gastroenteritis
Folpet	N-(trichloromethylthio) phthalimide or 2-[(trichloromethyl) thio]-I H-isoindole-1,3 (2H)-dione	Fruits, vegetables, ornamentals		Rats: > 10,000 mg/kg	Rats: > 10,000 ppm for 17 months	Reduced weight gain
Captafol	Cis-N-((1,1,2,2-tetrachloroethyl) thio) 4 cyclohexene-1,2 dicarboximide			Rats: 5000–6200 mg/kg	Rats: > 1500 ppm/day	Dermatitis Reduced growth rate, mild hepatic and renal damage
Pyrazophos	0,0 Diethyl-0-(5-methyl-6-ethoxycarbonyl-pyrazolo-[1,5,-a]-pyrimid-2-yl)-thionophosphate	Systemic fungicide		Rats: 415–778 mg/kg		Signs of cholinesterase inhibition, antidote is atropine plus Toxogonin
Sulfur (flowers of sulfur, sulfur flour)		Fungicide		Horses, cattle: 250 mg/kg		Gastroenteritis, superpurgation, colic, depression, renal and hepatic congestion
Terrazole	5-ethoxy-3-trichloromethyl 1,2,4-thiadiazole	Turf grass, seeds, vegetables		Rats: 1077 mg/kg	Dogs: 1000 ppm for 2 years	Decreased weight gain; increased serum cholinesterase, bromsulphalein retention, and liver weight; hepatosis, secondary biliary nephrosis
Triphenyltin	Formulated as acetate, chloride, or hydroxide	Algicide, molluscacide		Rats: 108–298 mg/kg depending on the chemical salt		Does **not** cause central nervous system effects like the lower trialkyl derivatives

NOAEL = no observed adverse effect level.

*See discussion of copper, arsenic, and lead toxicoses in Chapter 17 for more information.

†Agents include copper salts of fatty acids (e.g., copper lineolate), rosin acids (e.g., copper abietate), copper carbonate (malachite), copper hydroxide (cupric hydroxide), copper naphthenate, copper arsenite, copperized chromated zinc arsenate, and copper sulfate. Toxicosis is unlikely if label restrictions are observed, but continued use of copper salts can cause copper accumulation on soil, which may place sheep at risk when grazing.

‡Environmental Protection Agency restrictions prohibit feeding of captan-treated seed grains.

PENTACHLOROPHENOL

A. **Applications.** Pentachlorophenol was available on a limited basis as a **fungicide, herbicide, bacteriocide,** and **wood preservative** until the 1980s, when concerns regarding its toxicity and effects on the environment led the Environmental Protection Agency (EPA) to severely restrict its use.

    1. Structural wood preservation was the principal use of pentachlorophenol until the 1980s.
        a. Both oil-soluble pentachlorophenol and the water-soluble sodium salt are used in wood treatment.
        b. Treated wood contains from 0.4–0.6 pound of pentachlorophenol per cubic foot of wood.

    2. Pentachlorophenol was used most frequently to treat poles, decay-resistant lumber, and posts.

B. **Exposure**

    1. Under current conditions and restrictions, **some treated wood is available.** Livestock could be exposed to freshly treated wood, especially if used to build **fences** or **feedbunks.**

    2. Because public access to pentachlorophenol is restricted, the probability of acute poisoning is low.

C. **Source.** Pentachlorophenol is synthesized by the **successive chlorination of phenol.** The toxicity of pentachlorophenol is closely associated with the potential or actual dioxin content of penta.

    1. During the chlorination of phenol, a small amount of pentachlorophenol forms a dimer by means of an oxygen bridge, resulting in dioxin isomers containing from five to eight chlorines (see Figure 18-1).

    2. Photolysis and combustion of pentachlorophenol have also been implicated as generators of higher chlorinated dioxins.

D. **Toxicokinetics**

    1. Absorption is rapid; pentachlorophenol is readily taken up by the intestinal tract, skin, and lungs.
        a. The vapor pressure of pentachlorophenol is 1.1×10^{-4} mm Hg at 20°C, making pentachlorophenol a relatively volatile toxicant; however, inhalation of pentachlorophenol by cattle in barns built of treated wood contributes less than 10% to the body burden of pentachlorophenol.
        b. Pentachlorophenol in oils or hydrocarbon solvents is more readily absorbed than the water-soluble salts.

    2. Metabolism. Pentachlorophenol is conjugated with glucuronic acid to form glucuronides. Newborn animals, which lack the ability to conjugate glucuronides, are more susceptible to pentachlorophenol than adult animals.

    3. Excretion
        a. Glucuronides are readily excreted in the urine.
        b. Residues are rapidly depleted from the body.
            (1) The half-life of pentachlorophenol in cattle is approximately 2 days.
            (2) Pentachlorophenol in lipids is generally lost within 1 week of exposure.

E. **Mechanism of toxicologic damage**

    1. Pentachlorophenol **uncouples oxidative phosphorylation.**
        a. Oxygen consumption is increased, while adenosine triphosphate (ATP) formation is decreased.

b. Fever is a reflection of energy lost as heat instead of stored as high-energy phosphate bonds.

2. Like other phenols, pentachlorophenol is a **direct irritant,** especially to the skin and upper respiratory tract.

3. Neurotoxic effects (e.g., tremors) may result from cellular energy deficit and hyperglycemia.

F. Toxicity

1. Acute toxicity. The acute LD_{50} for most mammalian species is 100–200 mg/kg.

2. Subacute toxicity. Moderate toxicosis occurs in cattle at dosages of 15–20 mg/kg, and may be partially the result of the dioxin contaminants.

3. Chronic toxicity ranges from 40–70 mg/kg, indicating that pentachlorophenol has a very low chronicity factor. The chronic no observed adverse effect level (NOAEL) dosage in both rats and cattle ranges from 1–2 mg/kg body weight.

G. Diagnosis

1. Clinical signs
  a. Acute toxicity. Restlessness, fever, elevated blood pressure, and hyperperistalsis progress to weakness, seizures, and collapse. Newborn pigs in contact with treated wood floors develop hyperthermia, dermal irritation, and weakness, and usually die within a few hours of birth.
  b. Chronic toxicity. Signs include weight loss, reduced feed efficiency, progressive anemia, low thyroxine levels, and decreased milk production.
    (1) Chronic signs may result, in part, from higher chlorinated dioxins (e.g., hexa-, hepta- and octachlorodibenzodioxins).
    (2) High chronic exposure (e.g., 15 mg/kg for 160 days) causes villous hyperplasia of the urinary bladder in dairy cattle, probably as a result of the dioxin contaminants.

2. Laboratory diagnosis
  a. Analysis of **blood** or **urine** confirms recent or continuing exposure to pentachlorophenol. Background values in the blood of dairy cattle may be as high as 100 ppb, but as much as 2 ppm may be in the blood of clinically normal cattle.
  b. Postmortem analysis of **renal tissue, skin,** or both confirms antemortem exposure.

H. Treatment

1. Detoxification therapy for acute exposures should include emesis or lavage in the appropriate species, followed by the oral administration of activated charcoal or a non-absorbable oil.

2. Supportive therapy
  a. Hyperthermia is a threat to survival and must be controlled by applying cold water or alcohol to the skin.
  b. Balanced electrolyte solutions without glucose should be administered to prevent dehydration.

3. Specific antidotes are not available for pentachlorophenol toxicosis.

Chapter 22
Rodenticides

I. INTRODUCTION

A. **Sources.** Rodenticides are available commercially in several formulations.

1. **Pastes (paraffined blocks)** and **pellets** are consumed by rodents. **Concentrates for mixing with water** are also available, but are not used frequently.

2. **Tracking powders** are placed in areas of frequent rodent activity; the rodents consume the toxicant when they groom and clean their feet.

B. **Exposure.** Anticoagulant rodenticides with anti–vitamin K activity, **cholecalciferol (vitamin D$_3$)-based rodenticides**, and **zinc or aluminum phosphide preparations** are widely sold through lay outlets. These agents, along with **strychnine-based rodenticides** (sold mainly to control pocket gophers and ground squirrels), are responsible for most poisoning of domestic animals.

1. **Recommended safety precautions are often ignored.**
   a. Animals and small children should be excluded from baited areas.
   b. Protective bait stations should be used wherever exclusion of nontarget species is not feasible.
   c. Care must be taken to avoid spilling baits or powders on feeds for livestock.

2. **Homes and businesses may rely on heavy use of rodenticides rather than following good rodent control practices** (e.g., cleanup and removal of hiding and nesting areas, removal of available food and water sources, physical exclusion by plugging holes).

3. Rodenticides are commonly used for **malicious poisoning**.
   a. Many people are aware that rodenticides are very toxic.
   b. Rodenticides are readily available and can be obtained without raising suspicion.

C. **Risk of toxicosis.** Rodenticides are the **third most common source of toxicant exposure in dogs,** with approximately 20% of suspected exposures resulting in toxicosis. Toxicosis is very rarely reported in cats, and farm animals are rarely exposed to or poisoned by rodenticides. Several factors increase the likelihood of rodenticide toxicosis.

1. **Accessibility of toxicant.** Baiting for rodents **often occurs where pets, livestock, or desirable wildlife have access**.
   a. Homes (kitchen, basement, garage, gardens)
   b. Warehouses and food preparation businesses
   c. Docks, wharves, and grain elevators
   d. Livestock buildings and grain storage areas
   e. Public parks, recreation areas

2. **Intent of toxicant**
   a. Rodenticides are **designed to be toxic to mammals**.
   (1) Susceptible biochemical pathways are similar among all mammals, not just rodents.
   (2) There is often a narrow margin between the toxic dose and the lethal dose.
   b. Baits are **formulated to be attractive and palatable**.
   (1) **Aromas** (e.g., fish, peanut butter) are attractive to many animals.
   (2) **Grain baits** are readily consumed by birds and dogs.

D. **Prognosis.** Clinical signs of rodenticide toxicosis may be advanced when recognized by the owner, and at that point are not effectively treated.

II. ANTICOAGULANTS

A. Chemical structure

1. The anticoagulant rodenticides are **derivatives of 4-hydroxycoumarin** or **indane 1,3-dione** (Figure 22-1).
   a. The **coumarin derivatives** are **warfarin, brodifacoum, bromadiolone,** and **difenacoum**.
   b. Important **indanedione derivatives** are **pindone, chlorphacinone,** and **diphacinone**.

2. The addition of side chains or reactive groups affects the **potency and kinetics** of the anticoagulants.

3. Table 22-1 compares **first generation** and **second generation** anticoagulant rodenticides. Most anticoagulant rodenticides in current use are second generation rodenticides.
   a. Brodifacoum is used most frequently.
   b. Because of the emergence of warfarin-resistant rodents, warfarin, once used commonly, is now used very little.

B. **Sources. The concentration of toxicant in baits** ranges from 0.02%–1.0%; **0.05%** is the most common percentage.

C. Exposure

1. **Toxicosis occurs most frequently when pets, livestock, and wildlife have access to baits.**
   a. Cats occasionally ingest tracking powders during grooming.
   b. Unprotected bait stations permit access to bait blocks or grain mixes.
      (1) Animals may return to the same bait source several times.
      (2) Commercial formulations are designed to survive for weeks to months under adverse environmental conditions.

2. **Secondary (relay) toxicosis** is rare.
   a. Poisoned rodents may contain low residues.
   b. Animals or birds that consume large amounts of rodents (e.g., raptors, dogs, mink, cats) have been poisoned by diphacinone-poisoned rodents.

D. Toxicokinetics

1. **Absorption.** The rate of absorption is high (i.e., greater than 90%), and peak plasma levels may occur within 12 hours of ingestion.

A    **B**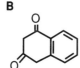

FIGURE 22-1. Chemical structure of (*A*) 4-hydroxycoumarin and (*B*) indane 1,3-dione.

TABLE 22-1. First Generation Versus Second Generation Anticoagulant Rodenticides

Characteristic	First Generation	Second Generation
Decade of development	Before 1970	1970s, 1980s
Potency as vitamin K antagonists	Relatively low	High
Excretion rate	Rapidly excreted	Retained in the body for a longer time
Number of doses required to produce toxicosis	Multiple dosages usually required	Effective after one feeding
Common products	Dicoumarol, warfarin, pindone, chlorphacinone, valone	Brodifacoum, bromadiolone, diphacinone

2. **Distribution** in the plasma is prolonged by strong binding to plasma proteins (90%–95% for warfarin).

3. **Metabolism and excretion.** Microsomal mixed function oxidases (MFOs) form inactive hydroxylated metabolites, which are excreted in the urine.

E. **Mechanism of toxicologic damage.** Anticoagulant rodenticides **competitively inhibit vitamin K epoxide reductase,** which is necessary to convert vitamin K epoxide to the reduced form.

1. The final carboxylation and activation of clotting factors II, VII, IX, and X are dependent on reduced vitamin K.

2. The activity of the coagulation system is maintained until natural decay of the clotting factors takes place (usually 24–36 hours postingestion).

F. **Toxicity** (Table 22-2)

1. **Susceptibility.** Ruminants are less susceptible to anticoagulants than simple-stomached animals.

2. **Potentiators of toxicity**
   a. **Drugs that reduce vitamin K synthesis** in the intestinal tract (e.g., sulfonamides, broad-spectrum antibiotics) are believed to exacerbate anticoagulant toxicosis.
   b. **Drugs that displace anticoagulants from plasma binding sites** may make more free toxicant available for toxicosis.
      (1) Drugs known to displace warfarin from plasma binding sites include phenylbutazone, diphenylhydantoin, sulfonamides, and adrenocorticosteroids.
      (2) Rapid displacement of warfarin by sulfamethazine actually protects against toxicosis by enhancing excretion of the unbound toxicant.
   c. Some products include **sulfaquinoxaline,** which enhances toxicity by inhibiting vitamin K synthesis in the intestine and colon.

G. **Diagnosis**

1. **Clinical signs,** which are always caused by some form of coagulopathy, become apparent 1–3 days after ingestion of the toxicant.
   a. Early signs include **subcutaneous hematoma, epistaxis, gingival hemorrhage, dark tarry stools,** and **hematemesis**.
      (1) Capillary hemorrhage may occur in the absence of trauma.
      (2) Hematomas often occur at points of trauma (e.g., submandibularly, periarticularly, laterally on the thorax). The blood may be clotted or unclotted.
      (3) Prolonged bleeding leads to **anemia, pale mucous membranes, weakness, ataxia,** and **dyspnea**.
      (4) The **heart rate is irregular** and the **pulse is weak**.

TABLE 22-2. Toxicity of Common Anticoagulant Rodenticides

Species and Agent	Single Dose	Multiple Doses
Cats		
Warfarin	5–50 mg/kg	5 days @ 1 mg/kg
Diphacinone	15 mg/kg*	
Brodifacoum	25 mg/kg*	
Dogs		
Warfarin	5–50 mg/kg	5–15 days @ 5 mg/kg
Diphacinone	3 mg/kg*	
Brodifacoum	0.25–3.6 mg/kg*	
Pigs		
Warfarin	3 mg/kg	7 days @ 0.05 mg/kg
Diphacinone	150 mg/kg*	
Brodifacoum	0.5–2.0 mg/kg*	
Ruminants		
Warfarin		12 days @ 200 mg/kg
Diphacinone		
Brodifacoum	25–33 mg/kg*	

Note that for warfarin, multiple dosing lowers the toxic dosage, especially in pigs.
*LD_{50} dosage.

    b. Hemorrhages may be slow and sustained or massive. They may be external or internal.

      (1) Sudden internal hemorrhaging can lead to **acute anemia, shock,** and **cyanosis.** Animals may be found dead with no premonitory signs.

      (2) Hemorrhage in the brain, spinal cord, or **subdural spaces** is reflected as **ataxia, paresis, depression, convulsions,** or **sudden death.** Manifestations depend on the location of the hemorrhage.

      (3) Placental hemorrhage may cause abortion.

      (4) Periarticular or **intraarticular hemorrhages** may cause **lameness, joint swelling,** and **pain.**

    c. Hematuria occurs in some cases.

  2. Laboratory diagnosis

    a. Hematology

      (1) The **activated coagulation time** is two to ten times longer than normal.

      (2) The **activated prothrombin time (PT)** is two to six times longer than normal. Activated PT is the earliest indicator of change.

      (3) The **activated partial thromboplastin time (APTT)** is two to four times longer than normal.

        (a) Elevation of the APTT occurs several hours after elevation of the activated PT.

        (b) Factor VII is measured by APTT and has a half-life of approximately 6 hours.

      (4) The **platelet count** is normal or marginally low.

      (5) Fibrin degradation products are not increased.

    b. Radiography may reveal massive hemorrhage in the abdomen or thorax.

    c. Thoracentesis (with a very small bore needle) confirms hemothorax.

    d. Chemical analysis may reveal anticoagulants or their metabolites in the **blood, renal or hepatic tissue,** or **urine.** Analysis of stomach or intestinal contents is not reliable because ingestion of the toxicant may have occurred 2–3 days earlier.

  3. Lesions

    a. Sudden deaths are often marked by massive hemothorax, hemomediastinum, hemopericardium, pulmonary edema, and pulmonary hemorrhage.

    b. Most hemorrhages are ecchymoses or suffusions, rather than petechiae.

    c. Centrilobular hepatic necrosis may result from anemia and hypoxia.

H. Treatment and prognosis

1. **Detoxification** should be carried out within 8 hours of ingestion of the toxicant. In symptomatic animals, detoxification is usually unnecessary, because of the delay between ingestion of the toxicant and the appearance of clinical signs. If continued consumption of the anticoagulant is suspected, activated charcoal and catharsis may be employed to detoxify the gastrointestinal tract.

2. **Supportive therapy**
   a. **Transfusion.** The animal should be transfused with whole blood (10–20 ml/kg body weight) if anemic. The first quarter of the dose should be administered rapidly; the rest is administered by slow intravenous drip.
      (1) Transfusion corrects anemia and hypovolemia and immediately provides clotting factors.
      (2) Either fresh blood or plasma will provide good clotting factor activity.
      (3) The animal should be kept warm; unnecessary manipulation or trauma should be avoided during treatment.
   b. **Thoracentesis** should be performed to prevent death from pulmonary or cardiac compression.

3. **Antidotal therapy. Phytonadione (vitamin K₁)** is the specific antidote (see Chapter 6 III L; Table 6-1).
   a. **Dogs and cats.** Phytonadione should be administered orally (2–5 mg/kg), followed by a fatty meal (e.g., moist dog food) to promote absorption.
      (1) Oral administration is more effective and rapid than parenteral administration and avoids potential hemorrhage from the injection.
         (a) If phytonadione must be administered parenterally (3–5 mg/kg intramuscularly or subcutaneously), the smallest bore needle available should be used.
         (b) Intravenous administration may cause anaphylaxis. If it is necessary to administer phytonadione intravenously, only approved products should be used and the antidote should be administered slowly over at least 15 minutes.
      (2) Convalescing animals should be administered phytonadione daily for at least 21–30 days, because some rodenticides (e.g., brodifacoum, diphacinone) may cause prolonged anticoagulation (e.g., 30 days). In addition, prolonged therapy provides a margin of safety when the toxic principle is not known.
   b. **Pigs** should be administered 2–5 mg/kg of phytonadione subcutaneously or intramuscularly. Swine diets are normally supplemented with menadione (vitamin K₃; 10–20 g/ton of feed) to prevent porcine hemorrhagic disease.
   c. **Horses.** The dosage of phytonadione for horses should not exceed 2 mg/kg. **Menadione may cause fatal renal failure in horses.**
   d. **Ruminants** should be administered 0.5–1.5 mg/kg of phytonadione subcutaneously or intramuscularly (not to exceed 10 ml per injection site). Menadione is ineffective.

4. **Prognosis** is good if hemorrhage is not massive and a full therapeutic and convalescent regimen is maintained.

I. Public health concerns.
Residues in foods of animal origin are not likely because these anticoagulants have a short half-life and low lipid solubility.

III. CHOLECALCIFEROL (VITAMIN D₃)

A. Chemical structure.
The sterol structure is activated by irradiation of 7-dehydrocholesterol.

B. **Sources**

1. **Baits for mice and rats** are available as "place packs" (i.e., packs designed to be dropped or thrown into areas frequented by rodents) and in 10- or 30-g packages to be mixed with seeds or grain.
   a. The usual **concentration of toxicant** is **0.075%**.
   b. Cholecalciferol-containing rodenticides produce delayed toxicosis and death in rodents 1–3 days after a single ingestion.

2. **Vitamin supplements**

3. **Feed additives**

C. **Exposure**

1. **Careless use of rodent place packs** is the most common cause of toxicosis in pets.

2. **Excessive cholecalciferol or ergocalciferol (vitamin D$_2$) in feed** is the most common cause of toxicosis in food animals. Increased feed levels may be accidental (e.g., because of miscalculation or equipment failure) or intentional (e.g., because of perceived benefits of increased vitamin D in dairy cattle).

3. **Excessive use as a growth promoter in large-breed dogs** has led to toxicosis.

D. **Toxicokinetics**

1. **Absorption** is rapid and complete in the small intestine, especially if the animal's diet is high in lipids.

2. **Distribution.** Cholecalciferol is carried by the plasma to the liver and kidney.

3. **Metabolism.** Cholecalciferol is metabolized to 25-hydroxyvitamin D in the liver; the liver metabolite is then converted to physiologically active 1,25-dihydroxyvitamin D in the kidney.

4. **Excretion.** Vitamin D$_3$ metabolites are excreted primarily via bile and in the feces, with less than one-third excreted in urine.

E. **Mechanism of toxicologic damage**

1. **Normal vitamin D$_3$ function.** Vitamin D$_3$ **promotes calcium retention** by:
   a. Increasing the absorption of calcium from the intestinal mucosa
   b. Stimulating the synthesis of a calcium-binding protein that participates in calcium absorption
   c. Interacting with parathyroid hormone (PTH) to promote the osteoclastic resorption of bone
   d. Increasing calcium reabsorption in the renal distal tubules

2. **Effects of vitamin D$_3$ overdosage**
   a. **Hypercalcemia** induces **conduction dysfunction** in the heart.
      (1) The Q-T segment is shortened and the P-R interval is prolonged on the electrocardiogram (EKG).
      (2) The cardiac rate is abnormally slowed; **hypercalcemic cardiac failure** may occur **when the serum calcium level exceeds 14 mg/dl**.
   b. Soft tissue receptors respond to 1,25-dihydroxyvitamin D, leading to **abnormal tissue mineralization**. Critical tissues that are affected include the renal tubules and small to medium arterioles.
   c. High concentrations of active vitamin D$_3$ may cause direct **cellular degeneration and necrosis** (e.g., in the renal tubules).

F. Toxicity

1. **Acute toxicity.** The oral LD_{50} for dogs is 85 mg/kg.
   a. Clinical reports indicate that toxicosis occurs at 0.5–3 mg/kg.
   b. Lethal intoxication can occur at dosages as low as 10–20 mg/kg.

2. **Chronic toxicity.** Accumulation of lower dosages can lead to toxicity. The dietary requirement for common domestic mammals ranges from 200–400 international units (IU)/kg diet (1 μg vitamin D = 40 IU).
   a. For long-term feeding of most species (i.e., longer than 60 days), the maximum safe level of vitamin D is only 4–10 times the dietary requirement.
   b. For short-term exposure, most species can tolerate up to 100 times the dietary requirement.

G. Diagnosis

1. **Clinical signs** often develop 12–36 hours after consumption of a toxic dose.
   a. Initial clinical signs (e.g., **depression, anorexia, vomiting, polydipsia, polyuria, diarrhea**) are often vague and mild or moderate. They worsen 24–36 hours after onset.
   b. As hypercalcemia increases, clinical signs worsen and **renal failure** may develop.
      (1) **Polyuria** and **hyposthenuria** are evident.
      (2) **Azotemia** with an elevated blood urea nitrogen (BUN) level may develop in acute, severe cases.
   c. **Heart sounds are slowed and prominent** as hypercalcemia increases.

2. **Laboratory diagnosis**
   a. A **serum calcium level higher than 2 mg/dl** is characteristic and highly suggestive of cholecalciferol toxicosis.
   b. An **elevated serum phosphorus level** may precede the hypercalcemia by as much as 12 hours and could serve as an early nonspecific indicator.
   c. The **urine specific gravity** is 1.002–1.006.
   d. **Increased BUN and creatinine levels** are common as toxicosis continues.
   e. **Excessive active 1,25-dihydroxyvitamin D metabolites** are present in renal tissue, but analysis is difficult and few laboratories offer it routinely.

3. **Lesions**
   a. **Gross lesions** include petechial hemorrhages in tissues, pale streaks in kidney tissue, and raised plaques in the intima of large vessels.
   b. **Microscopic lesions**
      (1) The kidney tubules, coronary arteries, gastric mucosa, parietal pleura, pulmonary bronchioles, pancreas, and urinary bladder are often mineralized.
      (2) The renal tubules may be degenerative or necrotic.

H. Treatment and prognosis. **Cholecalciferol overdose is a medical emergency.**

1. **Detoxification therapy,** which must be initiated as soon as possible (preferably within 3 hours of ingestion), should be carried out as follows:
   a. Emesis or gastric lavage
   b. Activated charcoal followed with an osmotic cathartic
   c. Continued administration of charcoal (0.5–1 g/kg three times daily) for 1–2 days to reduce enterohepatic recycling

2. **Supportive therapy**
   a. The animal's physiologic status and laboratory parameters (e.g., **serum calcium, BUN and creatinine levels, urine specific gravity, heart sounds, EKG) should be monitored.**
   b. **Hypercalcemia should be treated.**

(1) **Fluid therapy with normal saline and furosemide** (5 mg/kg intravenously followed by 3 mg/kg three times daily) should be initiated.
   (a) Saline diuresis promotes calcium excretion.
   (b) Furosemide is preferred over thiazide diuretics, which may promote hypercalcemia.
(2) **Corticosteroid administration (prednisone,** 2 mg/kg two or three times daily) inhibits the release of octeoclast-activating factors, reduces intestinal calcium absorption, and promotes hypercalciuria.
c. **Salmon calcitonin** may be administered to reduce excessive serum calcium levels (i.e., levels greater than 14 mg/dl), or when hypercalcemia is prolonged.
   (1) The initial dosage is 4–6 IU/kg subcutaneously every 3 hours until serum calcium is reduced.
   (2) The dosage may be increased to 10–20 IU/kg if the initial dosage is not effective.

3. **Prognosis** is guarded if the clinical signs are severe or advanced. Acutely poisoned animals usually die within 2–5 days of the onset of clinical signs.

IV. PHOSPHIDES OF ZINC, ALUMINUM, OR CALCIUM

A. Chemical structure and characteristics

1. **Synthesis.** Trivalent phosphorus binds to the metal salt to form the corresponding metal phosphide.

2. **Characteristics**
   a. Calcium, aluminum, and zinc phosphides are **brownish-red, gray to yellow,** or **dark gray crystals,** respectively.
   b. They are **unstable in acidic or moist environments**.
      (1) Environmental persistence is limited.
      (2) They decompose rapidly in stomach acids to form **phosphine** (PH_3), a flammable gas heavier than air (Figure 22-2). The odor imparted by phosphine is commonly described as similar to that of acetylene or decaying fish.

B. Sources

1. **Rodenticides.** Phosphide salts are often used as alternatives to anticoagulant rodenticides.
   a. They are used by professional exterminators and are available through lay markets.
   b. They are formulated in grain or sugar baits at concentrations of 2%–5%.

2. **Grain fumigants.** Phosphide salts are used in grain fumigants to control insects and rodents.

C. Exposure

1. Toxicosis is most often the result of accidental **ingestion of rodent baits** or **malicious baiting of dogs**.

2. Exposure to **phosphine gas** used as a fumigant may also cause toxicosis.

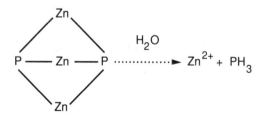

FIGURE 22-2. Production of phosphine (*PH₃*) from zinc phosphide. Phosphides of zinc, aluminum, and calcium are unstable in moist acidic environments. *Zn* = zinc; *P* = phosphorus; *H₂O* = water.

D. **Toxicokinetics**

1. **Absorption.** Stomach acid hydrolyzes intact phosphide salts to form phosphine, which is rapidly absorbed across mucous membranes.

2. **Metabolism and excretion.** Phosphine is labile and little is known of its metabolism and excretion.

E. **Mechanism of toxicologic damage.** Phosphide salts cause **respiratory and gastrointestinal irritation** and **inhibit cytochrome C oxidase,** but the relationship between cytochrome C oxidase inhibition and clinical effects is unclear.

F. **Toxicity**

1. **Acute toxicity**
   a. **Canine toxicity on an empty stomach** is 300 mg/kg (versus 40 mg/kg on a full stomach). Toxicity is increased in animals that consume phosphide with a meal or on a full stomach, because increased postprandial acid production enhances hydrolysis of phosphides to phosphine.
   b. The **lethal dosage to most animals** is between 20 and 50 mg/kg.

2. **Subacute** and **chronic toxicity** are not described.

G. **Diagnosis**

1. **Clinical signs** are usually acute in onset, occurring within 0.5–4 hours of ingestion.
   a. **Vomiting** occurs early.
   b. **Depression, tremors,** and **weakness progressing to recumbency** develop rapidly. **Hyperesthesia, seizures,** and **running** have been described. The exact mechanism of these effects is not known.
   c. **Salivation** may be present and, **with other signs, may give the impression of organophosphate toxicosis.**
   d. **Colic** is seen in **horses,** and **bloat** is seen in **cattle.**

2. **Laboratory diagnosis**
   a. **Hematology** and **clinical chemistry** values are not consistent.
      (1) Both **hyperphosphatemia** and **hypophosphatemia** are described.
      (2) **Hypoglycemia** may occur, and **hypocalcemia** has been observed inconsistently.
      (3) **Acidosis** occurs during intoxication.
   b. **Chemical analysis.** Analysis for zinc, aluminum, or phosphorus in stomach contents or tissues has been attempted, but is not consistent. Analysis for phosphine in tissues is not readily available.

3. **Lesions**
   a. The **stomach contents** may have a characteristic **acetylene** or **"dead fish" odor.**
   b. **Pulmonary congestion** and **edema** are mild to moderate and nonspecific.
   c. Other nonspecific and inconsistent lesions include **myocardial degeneration, a pale yellow liver,** and **fatty change and degeneration in the liver and kidneys.**

H. **Treatment and prognosis**

1. **Detoxification therapy.** General oral detoxification therapy and use of activated charcoal are recommended.

2. **Supportive therapy**
   a. **Fluids with bicarbonate** should be administered to combat acidosis.
   b. **Administration of oxygen** or **artificial respiration** may be necessary to overcome pulmonary irritation and edema.
   c. **Demulcents** and **protectants** may be administered to treat gastroenteritis.
   d. The **serum calcium level should be monitored.**
   e. Delayed hepatic or renal failure should be treated supportively and symptomatically.

3. **Specific antidotes** are not available.

4. **Prognosis** depends on the dosage received and the degree of supportive therapy. Outcome is difficult to predict.

V. STRYCHNINE

A. Chemical structure and characteristics

1. **Structure.** Strychnine is an **indole alkaloid** similar to brucine (Figure 22-3). The alkaloid is extracted from *Strychnos-nux vomica*, a tree found in southern Asia and northern Australia.

2. **Characteristics**
   a. It is **relatively stable** and **persists in food or the environment** when used as a bait.
      (1) Strychnine is **poorly soluble in water,** but **readily soluble in ethanol and other hydrocarbon solvents**.
      (2) Its salts (e.g., hydrochloride salts, sulfate salts) are more soluble in water.
   b. Strychnine tastes **bitter,** even in dilute solutions.

B. Sources. In the past, strychnine was used in medicine and veterinary medicine as an analeptic, circulatory stimulant, tonic, and ruminatoric. Its current use is as a **rodenticide**.

1. It is **approved to bait gophers** and **ground squirrels**.
   a. Strychnine is **restricted to below-ground use at concentrations less than or equal to 0.5%**.
   b. Strychnine is occasionally used illegally in rangelands to control predators.

2. It is **marketed as treated seeds** (e.g., peanuts, wheat) **or pellets** that look very much like alfalfa pellets. The seeds are often dyed green, pink, or yellow to signify their toxic nature and, in part, to deter consumption by birds.

C. Exposure

1. Strychnine is often added to hamburger or other baits and used as a **malicious poison for dogs**. Even though public access is heavily restricted, strychnine toxicosis is still one of the top five confirmed toxicologic diagnoses at the Iowa Veterinary Diagnostic Laboratory. The true incidence of toxicosis nationwide is unknown.

2. Toxicosis can result from the **careless use of baits** or when **pets gain access by burrowing below ground**.

3. Strychnine **may cause secondary (relay) toxicosis,** especially in raptors.

D. Toxicokinetics

1. **Absorption** is rapid from the gastrointestinal tract and upper respiratory tract mucous membranes.

2. **Distribution.** A small portion reaches the central nervous system (CNS), which is the site of action. Significant amounts can be found in the liver and kidney.

3. **Metabolism.** Strychnine is metabolized to **strychnine-N-oxide** by MFOs.

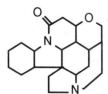

FIGURE 22-3. Chemical structure of strychnine.

4. Excretion is primarily in the urine.
    a. The half-life has been estimated at approximately 10 hours.
    b. Acidic urine enhances excretion by promoting ionization and ion trapping of the alkaloid.

E. | **Mechanism of toxicologic damage.** Strychnine **antagonizes** the inhibitory neurotransmitter glycine.

    1. The antagonism is **competitive** and **reversible**.

    2. The **major site of action** is the recurrent inhibitory interneurons (Renshaw cells) of the **reflex arc in the spinal cord and medulla**. Inhibitory effects in the reflex arc are lost, leading to uncontrolled excitation of the spinal reflex.
        a. Stimulation of the extensor muscles, which predominates, results in extensor rigidity and tonic seizures.
        b. Hypertonicity of the respiratory muscles causes asphyxia and death.

F. | **Toxicity** (Table 22-3). **Acute toxicity** is the only significant form of clinical poisoning.

    1. Dogs are more susceptible than cats.

    2. Large domestic animals are very sensitive.

    3. Poultry are relatively resistant.

G. | **Diagnosis**

    1. Clinical signs
        a. Premonitory signs may include nervousness, restlessness, muscle tremors, and muscle tics in response to noise or sudden, bright light.
        b. Early signs. Food in the stomach or consumed with the bait may delay the onset or minimize the severity of signs.
            (1) Acute, explosive onset of tonic to tetanic seizures may occur within 15 minutes to 2 hours of ingestion of a lethal dose.
            (2) Extreme sensitivity to external stimuli is characteristic.
            (3) Vomiting is rare, and dogs often retain stomach contents in fatal intoxications.
        c. Advanced signs include **spontaneous and nearly continuous tetanic seizures with marked rigidity,** sometimes known as a **"sawhorse stance."**
            (1) The **body temperature may be elevated**.
            (2) Poisoned animals are **conscious until near death**.
            (3) Myoglobinuria may result from muscle damage.

    2. Laboratory diagnosis
        a. Hematology and clinical chemistry values. Asphyxia and trauma may cause **acidosis,** an **elevated creatine phosphokinase level,** and **myoglobinuria**.
        b. Chemical analysis is readily available. Diagnosis is usually based on the presence of strychnine, but quantitation may not correlate well with the severity of clinical effects.
            (1) Urine from intoxicated animals may contain strychnine, unless death is so rapid that little excretion has occurred.

TABLE 22-3. Toxicity of Strychnine

Species	Toxic Dosage (mg/kg)
Cats	2.0
Dogs	0.75
Horses	0.5
Cows	0.5
Pigs	0.5
Poultry	5.0
Rats	3.0

(2) **Stomach contents or lavage fluids** contain strychnine.

(3) **Hepatic tissue** is usually positive for the presence of strychnine.

3. **Lesions.** Specific lesions are minimal or absent.

   a. Subcutaneous or intramuscular hemorrhages may result from trauma.

   b. Claws may be broken, indicating violent tetanic seizures.

   c. Strychnine-intoxicated dogs commonly have food or bait in the stomach.

   d. Cyanosis results from asphyxia.

   e. The onset of rigor mortis is rapid.

H. Treatment and prognosis

1. **Detoxification therapy**

   a. **Dogs in seizures must be relaxed and sedated before initiating detoxification therapy** (see V H 2 a).

      (1) Emetics may stimulate seizures.

      (2) Gastric lavage in an anesthetized animal with an endotracheal tube in place may be necessary.

   b. **Gastric lavage** should be followed by the administration of **activated charcoal** (2 g/kg) and a **saline cathartic.**

   c. **Fluid diuresis** should be initiated to stimulate urine flow and excretion of strychnine.

   d. If the animal is not acidotic (from hypoxia), the **urine should be acidified** with ammonium chloride to ionize the strychnine and promote excretion by ion trapping.

2. **Supportive therapy**

   a. **Animals must be relaxed as soon as possible to prevent asphyxia.**

      (1) **Pentobarbital** is usually given to effect for initial sedation.

      (2) **Muscle relaxants,** which reduce central respiratory depression, may be used to reduce reliance on barbiturates.

         (a) **Glyceryl guaiacolate** (110 mg/kg) may be administered as needed.

         (b) **Methocarbamol** (150 mg/kg initially, followed by 90 mg/kg as needed) is an alternative muscle relaxant.

      (3) **Ketamine and morphine are contraindicated in strychnine-intoxicated animals.**

   b. **Artificial respiration** may be necessary in cyanotic animals.

   c. Animals should be maintained in a **warm, quiet environment** away from external stimuli.

3. **Antidotal therapy.** Specific antidotes are not available.

4. **Prognosis** is good if the animal is treated promptly and supportive care is maintained for 24–48 hours.

VI. BROMETHALIN

A. Chemical structure and characteristics

1. The **chemical formula** is N-methyl-2,4-dinitro-N-[2,4,6-tribromophenyl]-6-[trifluoromethyl] benzeneamine (Figure 22-4).

2. **Characteristics**

   a. Bromethalin, a **pale yellow crystalline material,** is **insoluble in water,** but soluble in hydrocarbon solvents.

   b. It is **stable at room temperature.**

B. Sources. Bromethalin, which is available to the public, was developed in the 1980s as an **alternative rodenticide to use against warfarin-resistant rats and mice;** however, it is generally used less frequently than anticoagulant rodenticides or cholecalciferol.

1. It is usually **pelleted** and **dyed green.** The average pellet weight is approximately 140 mg, and a typical packet contains about 300 pellets.

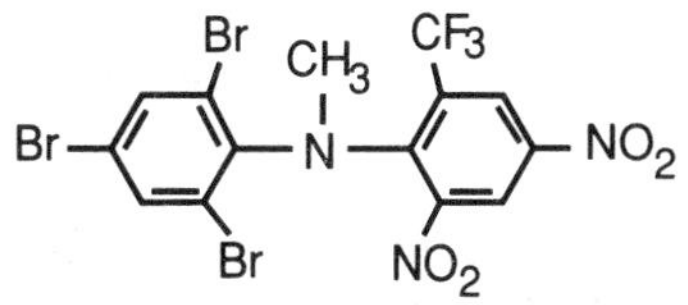

FIGURE 22-4. Chemical structure of bromethalin.

   2. It is often **packaged in place packs** that contain 16–42.5 g of bait with a bromethalin concentration of 0.01%.

C. **Exposure.** Toxicosis in dogs and cats usually results from the inadvertent consumption of carelessly placed rodenticide. The incidence of known malicious poisoning is very low.

D. **Toxicokinetics**

   1. **Absorption.** Bromethalin is **rapidly absorbed from the gastrointestinal tract.** Dermal exposure may lead to very low absorption.

   2. **Metabolism.** MFOs demethylate bromethalin to **desmethyl bromethalin,** which is at least as toxic as the parent compound, and possibly more toxic.

   3. **Excretion** is primarily via the bile. A small portion is eliminated in the urine. The approximate half-life in rats is 5–6 days.

E. **Mechanism of toxicologic damage**

   1. Bromethalin **uncouples oxidative phosphorylation,** leading to **loss of sodium-potassium-adenosine triphosphatase (ATPase).** Inhibition of the sodium pump leads to **intracellular edema, cell swelling,** and **degeneration.**

   2. Bromethalin may induce **cerebral lipid peroxidation.**

F. **Toxicity**

   1. **Acute toxicity** values are given in Table 22-4.

   2. **Chronic toxicity.** Prolonged exposure of rats to 10–20 ppm dietary bromethalin is lethal.

G. **Diagnosis**

   1. **Clinical signs** are **varied** and **dose-dependent.** Cats generally experience a slower onset and more prolonged duration of signs than dogs.
      a. **Acute signs** include **muscle tremors, hyperexcitability, paddling, hyperesthesia,** and **fever.**
      b. **Subacute signs** appear in 2–3 days. They include **posterior paresis, ascending ataxia, reduced conscious proprioception, loss of reflexes, depression, anisocoria,** and **muscle tremors. Vomiting** may or may not occur.

TABLE 22-4. Acute Toxicity Values for Bromethalin

Species	Oral LD_{50}
Cats	1.8 mg/kg
Rats	2.0 mg/kg
Dogs	4.7 mg/kg
Rabbits	13 mg/kg
Guinea pigs	1000 mg/kg

2. **Laboratory diagnosis**
   a. An **electroencephalogram (EEG)** may show spikes and spike-and-wave activity, voltage depression, and an abnormal pattern of high-voltage–slow wave activity.
   b. The **cerebrospinal fluid pressure is increased**.
   c. **Chemical analysis** is not routinely available and interpretation is difficult, but detection of **bromethalin in baits or stomach contents** may help confirm exposure.

3. **Lesions** are minimal, although mild cerebral edema (brain swelling) may be present. Spongy degeneration occurs in the white matter of the brain, spinal cord, and optic nerve.

H. **Treatment, prognosis, and prevention.** Recovery and convalescence are slow (1–2 weeks postexposure).

1. **Treatment**
   a. **Detoxification therapy** is most effective if carried out early.
      (1) **Emetics** should be administered following a small meal to evacuate the stomach.
      (2) **Activated charcoal** should be administered, followed by a saline cathartic. Administration of charcoal (0.5–1 g/kg, three times daily) should continue for 2–3 days to reduce potential enterohepatic recycling of bromethalin and its metabolites.
   b. **Supportive therapy**
      (1) **Cerebral edema must be minimized** to slow the progression of clinical effects.
         (a) **Mannitol** (250 mg/kg every 6 hours) should be administered intravenously to relieve cerebral edema.
         (b) **Dexamethasone** (2 mg/kg every 6 hours) should be administered to minimize brain swelling.
      (2) **Fluid balance should be maintained** with oral fluids.
      (3) **Seizures and hyperexcitability can be controlled with diazepam or phenobarbital.**
      (4) **Hyperventilation therapy** has been recommended for humans, but its effectiveness has not been evaluated in animals.
   c. **Specific antidotes** are not available.

2. **Prognosis** is guarded if signs are severe or advanced.

3. **Prevention.** Treatment of poisoned animals is relatively ineffective; therefore, client education is imperative. It should be stressed that bromethalin exposure is a medical emergency requiring evacuation of the gastrointestinal tract.

VII. YELLOW PHOSPHORUS

A. **Chemical characteristics.** Yellow phosphorus is an **oil-soluble, waxy solid** with a **garlic odor**.

1. It is a **strong oxidizer** and is often stored in oil.

2. **When exposed to moisture,** yellow phosphorus emits a greenish light and white fumes (i.e., **it "glows in the dark"**).

B. **Sources.** Because of its reactivity and the hazards associated with its handling, yellow phosphorus is rarely used as a rodenticide. When it is used, it is concealed in butter or some other type of oil-based bait.

C. **Exposure.** Careless baiting practices most often cause toxicosis.

D. **Toxicokinetics**

1. **Absorption.** Yellow phosphorus is absorbed from the gastrointestinal tract, respiratory tract, and damaged epithelium.

2. **Excretion.** It is excreted in urine and expired air.

E. **Mechanism of toxicologic damage.** Yellow phosphorus is a protoplasmic poison.

1. It causes **extensive fatty degeneration of the liver, kidneys, brain,** and other organs.

2. **Cardiovascular collapse** may result from hypocalcemia or a direct cardiotoxic effect.

3. It is a **strong irritant** and has a **necrotizing effect on the stomach mucosa.**

F. **Toxicity.** Yellow phosphorus is a **highly toxic and dangerous compound.** The **acute LD_{50} in dogs is 2 mg/kg.**

G. **Diagnosis**

1. **Clinical signs**
   a. **Early signs** include **violent vomiting** and **diarrhea,** with **apparent recovery 24–48 hours later.** The **breath** of affected animals has a **characteristic garlic odor.**
   b. The animal then **relapses into profound depression** and **severe shock. Icterus, vomiting,** and **hemorrhagic diarrhea** may return.
   c. **Massive hepatic failure** usually causes death.

2. **Laboratory diagnosis**
   a. **Hepatic enzyme and bilirubin levels** may be elevated.
   b. **Hypoglycemia** may be present.

3. **Lesions** include **severe hepatic and renal fatty change** and **epithelial necrosis of hepatocytes and renal proximal tubule cells.**

H. **Treatment and prognosis**

1. **Detoxification therapy**
   a. A **nonabsorbable oil** (e.g., **mineral oil**) should be administered orally to solubilize phosphorus and prevent absorption.
   b. **Activated charcoal** and a **sorbitol or saline cathartic** may also be useful.

2. **Supportive therapy**
   a. **Acute liver dysfunction must be treated** (see Chapter 8 III D).
   b. **Hypovolemia and acute shock must be treated.**
   c. Measures should be taken to **control pain.**

3. **Antidotal therapy.** Specific antidotes are not available.

4. **Prognosis** is guarded, because of profound vascular dysfunction and severe liver and kidney damage.

VIII. SODIUM FLUOROACETATE (COMPOUND 1080) AND FLUOROACETAMIDE

A. **Chemical structure and characteristics**

1. **Structure** (Figure 22-5). These agents are **fluorinated derivatives of acetic acid,** usually presented as the sodium salt.

2. **Characteristics.** Fluoroacetate and fluoroacetamide are **colorless, odorless, tasteless,** and **water-soluble.**

A

$$FCH_2 - \overset{\overset{\displaystyle O}{\|}}{C} - ONa$$

B

$$FCH_2 - \overset{\overset{\displaystyle O}{\|}}{C} - NH_2$$

FIGURE 22-5. Chemical structures of (*A*) sodium monofluoroacetate and (*B*) 2-fluoroacetamide.

TABLE 22-5. Comparison of Some Older and Less Common Rodenticides

Rodenticide	Availability	Toxicity	Mechanism of Action	Diagnosis	Treatment
Alpha-chlorohydrin (3-chloro-1,2-propanediol)	Available only to exterminators; not widely used in the United States	Rat/mouse LD_{50}: 152–160 mg/kg Dog LD_{50}: 328 mg/kg Cat LD_{50}: 188 mg/kg	Exerts a strong antifertility effect in males, characterized by reduced spermatozoa production and testicular atrophy	Large doses cause depression, anorexia, renal failure, and possible bone marrow suppression	Infertility in dogs is apparently reversible, although no treatment is described
ANTU (alpha naphthyl-thio urea)	Rarely used today	Toxic at 10–50 mg/kg in dogs	Increases capillary permeability of pulmonary vessels; cyanosis leads to death	Clinical signs include vomiting, salivation, gastric pain, lacrimation, urination, severe dyspnea, and air hunger; lesions are massive pulmonary edema and hydrothorax	Treatment is ineffective, although silicone aerosols have been recommended
Alpha-chloralose	Has been used as an anesthetic; rarely used as a rodenticide; old product	Dog LD_{50}: 600 mg/kg Cat LD_{50}: 100 mg/kg Duck LD_{50}: 42 mg/kg	Depresses neurons of the ascending reticular formation	Early signs include excitement followed by depression; severe depression to deep anesthesia develops and may progress to apnea and death; glucuronide is excreted in urine	Restraint of excited animals; diazepam to control seizures; analeptics to correct depression or anesthesia
Barium carbonate	Old rodenticide; rarely used		Soluble salts of barium; block exit channel for K^+ ions, leading to hypokalemia; stimulate both cardiac and smooth muscle	Clinical signs include vomiting, colic, diarrhea, hypertension, ventricular tachycardia, and fibrillation; analysis reveals K^+ in serum and barium in gastric contents or bait	Oral activated charcoal; saline diuresis; intravenous potassium to combat hypokalemia and tachycardia

Name	Description	Toxicity	Mechanism	Clinical signs	Treatment
Crimidine (2-chloro-4-dimethylamino-6-methylpyrimidine)	Old rodenticide; used mainly in Europe	Rodent LD_{50}: 1.2–1.5 mg/kg	Antagonist of vitamin B_6 (pyridoxine)	Acute convulsive seizures 0.5–1 hour after consumption	Animals may recover quickly; pyridoxine HCl (20 mg/kg intravenously); diazepam or barbiturates for seizures
Norbormide	Developed as a "safe" rodenticide against rats; never widely used; not very effective for mice	Rat LD_{50}: 5.3 mg/kg Mouse LD_{50}: 2250 mg/kg Dog/cat LD_{50}: >1000 mg/kg	Causes peripheral vasoconstriction in rats	Rats are ataxic, restless, dyspneic, and weak	Not applicable
Pyriminil (Vacor)	Used in the 1970s, withdrawn from registration	Highly toxic to rats (12 mg/kg) but low toxicity to dogs (500 mg/kg)	Nicotinamide antagonist	Hyperglycemia, nausea, vomiting, depression, miosis, lethargy, possible muscle tremors; dogs may develop night blindness and other visual deficits	Nicotinamide (50–100 mg given intramuscularly) is effective if given early or before signs develop; therapy should be continued for 7–10 days
Red squill (*Urginea maritima*)	Rarely used in the United States	Cat LD_{50}: 100 mg/kg Dog LD_{50}: 145 mg/kg Ruminant LD_{50}: 250 mg/kg	Cardioactive glycoside; unpalatable, strongly emetic	Vomiting and nausea early; bradycardia and cardiac arrest at toxic dosages	Treat hyperkalemia with insulin, glucose, and sodium bicarbonate; atropine or lidocaine for cardiac effects

K^+ = potassium.

B. **Sources.** Fluoroacetate is used to **control rodents and predators**. Because of its extreme toxicity to a variety of domestic animals and wildlife, it is **available only to licensed exterminators** for limited applications.

C. **Exposure**

1. Fluoroacetate may be imported and used illegally in some regions, leading to toxicosis.

2. Accidental exposures occur when baiting is careless or poisoned animals are not picked up and disposed of properly.

3. Secondary (relay) toxicosis may occur in highly susceptible carnivores that consume poisoned rodents.

D. **Toxicokinetics**

1. **Absorption** from the gastrointestinal tract is rapid.

2. **Metabolism.** Fluoroacetate and fluoroacetamide are metabolized to **monofluoroacetic acid** by **hydrolysis**.

E. **Mechanism of toxicologic damage.** Fluoroacetate and fluoroacetamide **replace acetylcoenzyme A** in intermediary metabolism and combine with oxaloacetic acid to **form fluorocitrate**.

1. Fluorocitrate **inhibits aconitase** in the citric acid cycle, blocking completion of the cycle.

2. **Citric acid accumulates, blocking cellular energy production** and **respiration**. The heart and brain are affected first and most severely by the cellular energy deficit.

F. **Toxicity**

1. **Dogs and cats.** Fluoroacetate and fluoroacetamide are highly toxic to carnivores, especially those of the Canidae family.
   a. The **lethal dose** for dogs and cats is **0.05–1.0 mg/kg**.
   b. There is a **narrow margin between toxicosis and death** and few animals survive poisoning with fluoroacetate or fluoroacetamide. Cyanosis, collapse, and death generally occur within 2–12 hours of ingestion of a toxic dosage.

2. **Livestock.** Toxicity in most domestic mammalian livestock is **less than 1 mg/kg**.

3. **Rats and mice.** The **lethal dose** in rats and mice is **5–8 mg/kg**.

4. **Birds,** including raptors, are most resistant, with lethal doses ranging from **1–10 mg/kg**.

G. **Diagnosis**

1. **Clinical signs** have an **acute onset** (0.5–2 hours after ingestion), while fluoroacetate is being converted to fluorocitrate.
   a. **Dogs.** Signs are **most prominent in dogs**.
      (1) **Initial signs** include **restlessness, hyperirritability,** and **vomiting**.
      (2) **Advanced signs** include **repetitive defecation, urination, tenesmus,** and **continuous vomiting**.
         (a) **Dyspnea** and **frothing at the mouth and nostrils** develop.
         (b) The dog periodically experiences **wild running, hysteria,** and **barking**.
         (c) **Intermittent tonic–clonic seizures** occur.
   b. **Cats** exhibit **abnormal vocalization** and **cardiac arrhythmias**.
   c. **Horses and ruminants. Cardiac arrest accompanied by sudden death** is the prominent feature of fluoroacetate toxicosis in horses and ruminants.

2. **Laboratory diagnosis**
   a. **Clinical chemistry studies** generally reveal **hyperglycemia** and **acidosis**.

b. **Citrate levels** are elevated in the blood or renal tissue.

c. **Analysis of suspected bait, stomach contents,** or **vomitus** may reveal residues. Residues are difficult to detect and unreliable in tissues.

3. **Lesions** include an **empty stomach, cyanosis, rapid onset of rigor mortis,** and a **flaccid, pale heart.**

H. | **Treatment and prognosis**

1. **Detoxification therapy**
   a. **Emesis** or **gastric lavage** should be employed **if the animal has not already vomited.**
   b. **Activated charcoal** is helpful if it is administered very early.

2. **Supportive therapy**
   a. **Short-acting barbiturates** can be used to control seizures. They should be used only to effect to avoid respiratory depression.
   b. **Oxygen, artificial respiration,** or **both** should be administered.
   c. **Arrhythmias should be monitored and treated.**

3. **Antidotal therapy**
   a. **Glycerol monoacetate** (0.55 g/kg administered intramuscularly hourly until a total dosage of 2–4 g/kg is reached) may be helpful.
   b. **Ethanol** (50%) and **acetic acid** (5%), 8 ml/kg of each administered orally, supply acetate to reduce the conversion of fluoroacetate to fluorocitrate.

4. **Prognosis** is **guarded to poor** once clinical signs have developed.

IX. **OTHER RODENTICIDES.** Characteristics of some older and less common rodenticides are summarized in Table 22-5.

STUDY QUESTIONS

DIRECTIONS: Each of the numbered items or incomplete statements in this section is followed by answers or by completions of the statement. Select the **one** numbered answer or completion that is **best** in each case.

1. What is the mechanism of action of anti-coagulant rodenticides?

(1) They reverse the final carboxylation of factor VIII.
(2) They antagonize the synthesis of vitamin K in the intestine and colon.
(3) They promote the oxidation of vitamin K to its epoxide.
(4) They prevent the carboxylation of vitamin K.
(5) They inhibit the reduction of vitamin K epoxide to active vitamin K.

DIRECTIONS: Each of the numbered items or incomplete statements in this section is negatively phrased, as indicated by an italicized word such as *not, least,* or *except.* Select the **one** numbered answer or completion that is **best** in each case.

2. All of the following rodenticide active ingredients are currently a likely cause of poisoning in pets *except:*

(1) indanedione.
(2) cholecalciferol.
(3) pyriminil.
(4) strychnine.
(5) zinc phosphide.

3. A client calls his veterinarian at 10 P.M. to report that his dog has just consumed an unknown quantity of a pesticide. The client has no way of getting medical attention for the dog before morning. Which one of the following would be *least* likely to cause clinical signs before the clinic opens at 7 A.M. the next morning?

(1) Brodifacoum
(2) Cholecalciferol
(3) Metaldehyde
(4) Strychnine
(5) Zinc phosphide

DIRECTIONS: The group of items in this section consists of numbered options followed by a set of numbered items. For each item, select the **one** numbered option that is most closely associated with it. Each numbered option may be selected once, more than once, or not at all.

Questions 4–8

Match each toxicosis with the appropriate antidote or therapeutic regimen.

(1) Atropine
(2) Calcitonin
(3) Dexamethasone and mannitol
(4) Phytonadione
(5) Pentobarbital and methocarbamol

4. Bromethalin toxicosis in a dog

5. Cholecalciferol toxicosis in a dog

6. Diphacinone toxicosis in a cat

7. Organophosphate toxicosis in a cow

8. Strychnine toxicosis in a dog

1. The answer is 5 *[II E]*. The precursors of prothrombin and other vitamin K–dependent factors undergo carboxylation to form final, active clotting factors. Vitamin K epoxide reductase reduces vitamin K, which is required for carboxylation. The coumarin and indanedione rodenticides competitively inhibit vitamin K epoxide reductase. Factor VIII is not a vitamin K–dependent clotting factor, so is not affected. Vitamin K acts in the liver, where clotting factors are assembled, not in the intestine, even though considerable vitamin K is synthesized in the colon. Formation of vitamin K epoxide occurs naturally as a consequence of its action in forming clotting factors. Vitamin K is not carboxylated, but participates in carboxylation of the precursors of inactive clotting factors.

2. The answer is 3 *[I B; Table 22-5]*. Pyriminil (Vacor) is a rodenticide of relatively low toxicity to dogs and cats, and has been voluntarily withdrawn from the market because of some potential problems with human exposure. Current evidence supports that the anticoagulant rodenticides (e.g., indanedione derivatives) are the leading cause of toxicosis from rodenticides in pets. Cholecalciferol toxicosis and strychnine toxicosis are also relatively common. Zinc phosphide poisoning is less common, but the phosphides are relatively toxic and hazardous when used.

3. The answer is 1 *[Chapter 22 II G 1, Table 22-2; Chapter 19 VIII]*. Metaldehyde (a molluscacide), strychnine (a rodenticide), and zinc phosphide (a rodenticide) are acute toxicants, and signs often occur within a few hours of ingestion. In addition, the clinical course is violent and often progresses rapidly. Cholecalciferol and brodifacoum have delayed clinical effects, but the probability of signs within 12 hours is greater for cholecalciferol, which can be directly toxic to kidneys, and may have a shortened latent period if the dosage is very high. Brodifacoum is an anti-vitamin K anticoagulant, and the latent period is dependent primarily on the half-life and decay of the coagulation factors already present, a factor which is relatively independent of dosage once an acute toxic dosage is consumed.

4–8. The answers are: 4-3 *[VI H 1 b]*, **5-2** *[III H 2 c]*, **6-4** *[II H 3]*, **7-1** *[Chapter 19 I H 1 b (1)]*, **8-5** *[V H 2]*. Bromethalin uncouples oxidative phosphorylation, promoting energy deficit in the brain followed by cerebral edema and brain swelling. There is no specific antidote for bromethalin toxicosis, but research has demonstrated that using a combination of dexamethasone and an osmotic diuretic (e.g., mannitol) to relieve the brain swelling is of some benefit.

Cholecalciferol causes hypercalcemia. Serum calcium levels above 14 mg/dl may cause shortened Q-T and prolonged P-R intervals, leading to slowing of the heart and death from cardiac failure. Calcitonin reverses the hypercalcemia and promotes elimination of excess calcium. Dexamethasone could be useful for treating early, moderate cases of cholecalciferol toxicosis, but it is not effective for marked, severe toxicosis.

Phytonadione (vitamin K_1) is the antidote for toxicosis from an anticoagulant rodenticide (e.g., diphacinone). Phytonadione supplies additional reduced vitamin K to replace that which is lost when the coumarin and indanedione anticoagulants interfere with vitamin K epoxide reductase in the synthesis of coagulation factors.

Atropine is the classic "antidote" to anticholinesterase (cholinesterase-inhibiting) compounds (e.g., the organophosphate insecticides). Atropine blocks the receptors for acetylcholine (ACh) at cholinergic synapses, thus controlling the signs of excessive cholinergic (parasympathetic) stimulation.

Strychnine is a convulsant toxicant that inhibits the action of the inhibitory neurotransmitter glycine. Therapy is aimed at controlling seizures by inducing central depression (e.g., with pentobarbital) and muscle relaxation (e.g., with methocarbamol). Therapy with pentobarbital alone is effective, but concurrent use of a muscle relaxant reduces the amount of barbiturate needed, thus lessening the possibility of central respiratory depression.

Chapter 23
Prescription Therapeutic Drugs

I. **INTRODUCTION.** This chapter discusses toxicoses resulting from the misuse or unintended use of veterinary prescription drugs in large animals and livestock. Human prescription drugs are rarely encountered as a problem in veterinary medicine.

A. **Toxicosis versus adverse reactions.** Unintentional exposure to a drug in a non-target species is considered a toxicosis, rather than an adverse drug reaction.

B. **Prevention of toxicosis or adverse reactions from therapeutic drugs** is generally the responsibility of the manufacturer seeking approval, the pharmacologist, and the veterinary clinician using, prescribing, or dispensing therapeutic agents. Knowledge of potential problems and prompt access to emergency consultation are invaluable in preventing and dealing with potential or real prescription drug toxicoses.

1. Veterinarians prescribing or dispensing prescription drugs or medicated feeds have a responsibility to inform their clients of the hazards of normal medication and the adverse effects that may occur from unapproved use of the drug. They should request from the manufacturer or wholesaler detailed information about the safety of new or different drugs that they may dispense to clients.

2. The manufacturer or company holding the approved drug label should be readily accessible (e.g., through an emergency number) to answer questions about toxicosis or adverse reactions from their products.

3. Poison control centers maintain extensive computerized indices on the active ingredients and probable clinical toxicology of prescription and over-the-counter drugs. Most of these centers will accept emergency calls from veterinarians. Alternatively, the National Animal Poison Information Center, located at the University of Illinois in Urbana, provides computer-supported telephone consultation on potential acute drug toxicoses for a fee.

C. **Exposure.** Access to prescription items is limited because of controlled distribution, specific instructions from a pharmacist or physician, and the use of childproof caps. Oral exposure (from accidental ingestion of large amounts of tablets, syrups, or elixirs) is most common.

1. Pets gain access to excessive amounts of therapeutic drugs when tablets are spilled or prescription containers are left open. Occasionally, pets will chew the containers, gaining access to their contents.

2. Owners must be cautioned to avoid off-label uses of therapeutic drugs unless there is a valid veterinarian–client–patient relationship.

II. **COMMON PRESCRIPTION DRUGS** that may cause toxicosis when exposure is excessive are summarized in Table 23-1.

TABLE 23-1. Selected Prescription Drugs with Toxicologic Potential in Animals

Therapeutic Agent	Dosage Form	Acute Toxicity	Clinical Effects	Remedial Action
Analgesics				
Hydromorphone	Tablets, suppositories (2-mg, 4-mg)	. . .	Respiratory depression, nausea, vomiting, bradycardia, hypotension	Oral detoxication, artificial ventilation, naloxone
Meperidine	Tablets (50-mg), liquid (10 mg/ml)	. . .	Respiratory depression, coma, apnea, bradycardia, hypotension	See hydromorphone
Methadone	Tablets (5-mg, 10-mg), liquid (1–2 mg/ml)	. . .	Respiratory depression, bradycardia, hypotension	See hydromorphone; effects are long-lasting and may require extended treatment
Oxycodone	Tablets (5-mg)	LD_{50} (dogs): 100 mg/kg	CNS and respiratory depression, intestinal hypoperistalsis	See hydromorphone
Propoxyphene	Tablets (100-mg), liquid (10 mg/ml)	LD_{50} (dogs): 100 mg/kg	CNS and respiratory depression, bradycardia, hypotension	See hydromorphone
Anticoagulants				
Warfarin	Tablets (1-mg, 10-mg)	LD_{50} (dogs): 5–50 mg/kg	See Chapter 22 II G	Transfusion, phytonadione (see Chapter 22 II G)
Antidepressants, Tricyclic				
Imipramine, amitriptyline, nortriptyline	Tablets (10- to 150-mg)	LD_{50} (rats): $\cong$ 300–600 mg/kg	Ventricular tachyarrhythmias, prolonged QRS complex, vomiting, weakness, tremors, depression	Gastric lavage followed by activated charcoal, diazepam to control occasional seizures, sodium bicarbonate for acidosis, phenytoin or lidocaine for arrhythmias
Cardiovascular drugs				
Clonidine	Tablets (0.1-mg, 0.3-mg)	<1 mg: toxic to children	Depression, lethargy, miosis, hypotension, bradycardia	Oral decontamination, atropine for bradycardia, dopamine for hypotension; α-blockers (e.g., yohimbine) reverse effects of clonidine
Guanabenz	Tablets (4-mg, 8-mg)	. . .	Vomiting, miosis, hypotension, bradycardia, hypoventilation	Oral decontamination and administration of pressor drugs have been used to treat human overdosage
Methyldopa	Tablets (125-mg, 500-mg)	10-kg dog: 30 500-mg tablets	Nausea, vomiting, diarrhea, depression, bradycardia, hypotension	Oral decontamination, sympathomimetic drugs (e.g., epinephrine) may be indicated in severe overdosage

Type I antiarrhythmics Quinidine Procainamide Disopyramide	Tablets (300-mg) Tablets (500- to 1000-mg)	LD$_{50}$ (rats): 580 mg/kg (disopyramide)	Arrhythmias, apnea, coma, conduction disturbances, bradycardia, asystole, anticholinergic effects	Human overdosage is treated with oral decontamination, isoproterenol, and dopamine
Type II antiarrhythmics Propranolol			Bradycardia, hypotension, bronchoconstriction	Oral decontamination early after ingestion, atropine for bradycardia, epinephrine for hypotension, aminophylline for bronchoconstriction
Digitoxin/digoxin	Tablets (0.05- to 2.0-mg)	LD$_{50}$: 100–200 mg/kg (500 2-mg tablets in a 10-kg dog)	Vomiting, diarrhea, cardiac arrhythmia, slowed AV conduction, complete heart block	Oral decontamination, atropine for bradycardia, phenytoin to improve AV conduction, oral ion exchange resin to treat hyperkalemia
Hormones Estrogens	Tablets		High concentrations may induce signs of estrus in animals or cause abortion; long-term high estrogen levels (e.g., for 6–12 months) may cause pancytopenia and anemia; signs include pale mucous membranes with petechial hemorrhages, hypothermia, and dark stools; anecdotal reports of pancytopenia in dogs are rare	Fluids, blood transfusion, corticosteroids for shock
Glucocorticoids	Tablets (1- to 10-mg, according to preparation)		Acute exposure: Hyperadrenocorticoid syndrome, sodium and fluid retention, potassium loss, alkalosis, hypertension Chronic exposure: Steroid myopathy, hepatic damage	Oral decontamination following known acute exposures

TABLE 23-1. Continued

Therapeutic Agent	Dosage Form	Acute Toxicity	Clinical Effects	Remedial Action
Levothyroxine	Tablets (25-μg, 300-μg)	· · ·	Nervousness, hyperthermia, cardiac arrhythmias, heat intolerance, diarrhea, elevated serum T_3 and T_4 levels; for moderate dosages, onset of signs may be delayed for several days	Oral decontamination for acute high-dosage exposure; supportive therapy for fever, hypoglycemia, and fluid loss; cardiac glycosides or antiadrenergic agents (e.g., propranolol) to control tachycardia and arrhythmias
Nausea medications Diphenhydramine	Tablets (25-mg, 50-mg)	· · ·	Effects of overdosage vary from depression to stimulation, anticholinergic signs (e.g., dilated pupils, xerostomia, gastrointestinal hypomotility), hypotension	Oral decontamination for acute exposure, vasopressors for clinically serious hypotension
Parasympatholytics Atropine, glycopyrrolate, scopolamine	Tablets (0.025–2 mg, depending on preparation)	· · ·	Dilated pupils, xerostomia, gastrointestinal hypomotility, tachycardia; atropine and scopolamine may cause disorientation and ataxia	Oral decontamination, neostigmine to counteract anticholinergic effects, norepinephrine for severe hypotension, artificial ventilation
Parasympathomimetics Bethanechol chloride	Tablets (5-mg, 50-mg)	· · ·	Similar to those of cholinesterase inhibitor pesticides (e.g., salivation, miosis, vomiting, diarrhea); sedative action of bethanechol may mask nicotinic stimulation	Oral decontamination for excessive acute exposures, atropine for muscarinic signs
Sedatives Barbiturates	Tablets (50-mg, 100-mg)	· · ·	CNS and respiratory depression, areflexia, hypothermia, hypotension, tachycardia, shock, death	Oral decontamination, artificial ventilation or oxygen, fluid therapy to combat shock
Chlorpromazine	Tablets (10-mg, 200-mg)	· · ·	Severe CNS depression, hypotension, extrapyramidal signs	Oral decontamination following acute exposures, stimulants (e.g., amphetamine or caffeine) for severe depression

AV = atrioventricular; CNS = central nervous system; T_3 = triiodothyronine; T_4 = thyroxine.

DIRECTIONS: The numbered item or incomplete statement in this section is followed by answers or by completions of the statement. Select the **one** numbered answer or completion that is **best**.

1. A dog is brought to the veterinarian because he is exhibiting signs of acute hyperthermia, excitement, hyperpnea, and mild diarrhea. The owners state that the animal had been "playing" with a plastic bottle containing one of the drugs listed below, but the label is now destroyed. Based on the signs, which of the following is the most likely source of toxicosis?

(1) Warfarin
(2) Propranolol
(3) Digitoxin
(4) Levothyroxine
(5) Chlorpromazine

DIRECTIONS: The numbered item or incomplete statement in this section is negatively phrased, as indicated by an italicized word such as *not, least,* or *except*. Select the **one** numbered answer or completion that is **best**.

2. All of the following would be a good source of detailed information about the expected clinical response to a prescription drug *except*:

(1) a local pharmacist.
(2) a poison control center run by a local hospital.
(3) the National Animal Poison Control Center.
(4) the manufacturer of the drug.
(5) the prescription label for the drug.

1. The answer is 4 *[Table 23-1]*. Levothyroxine is a thyroid drug that simulates the action of thyroxine (T_4). Excessive amounts of levothyroxine increase the metabolic rate of the animal, leading to fever, hyperactivity followed by weakness, rapid breathing, and, occasionally, diarrhea. The other drugs listed are either depressants (chlorpromazine), anticoagulants (warfarin), or antiarrhythmics (propranolol, digitoxin).

2. The answer is 5 *[I B 1–3]*. Generally, the prescription label contains only the directions for use of the drug, and occasionally information about drugs to avoid because of interactions; therefore, it is not the best source of information concerning the characteristics of adverse reactions or the kind of clinical response expected for a drug overdose. The product insert or the manufacturer's label may contain some of this information. Poison control centers are excellent sources of information concerning drug toxicity (those specializing in human medicine can often assist veterinarians as well). Pharmacists and the drug manufacturer are also able to provide detailed information. Unfortunately, not all manufacturers maintain 24-hour emergency lines to answer questions about drug toxicity. When purchasing a drug for veterinary prescription use, the veterinarian should inquire about the provisions the company has made to provide information quickly.

Chapter 24

Over-the-Counter Drugs and Illicit Drugs of Abuse

I. ACETAMINOPHEN

A. **Chemistry.** Acetaminophen is a **para-amino phenol derivative**. Phenacetin, a related drug, is metabolized to acetaminophen in the liver.

B. **Sources**

1. **Acetaminophen** is a common household analgesic and antipyretic. Regular-strength tablets contain 325-mg acetaminophen/tablet, and extra-strength tablets contain 500-mg acetaminophen/tablet.

2. **Phenacetin** is not commonly used in the United States.

C. **Exposure.** Pets may gain access to acetaminophen by accident, or well-meaning owners may erroneously administer acetaminophen to their pets.

D. **Mechanism of toxicologic damage.** Normally, acetaminophen is biotransformed by hepatic conjugation with glucuronic acid, sulfate, or cysteine and excreted in the urine.

1. Cats are limited in their ability to conjugate drugs as glucuronides and are more likely to be intoxicated by acetaminophen than are most other domestic animals.

2. When the hepatic capacity for protective metabolism by glucuronidation is exceeded, acetaminophen undergoes N-hydroxylation followed by the spontaneous formation of N-acetyl-p-benzoquinone.
   a. Hepatotoxicity. The phase I metabolite, **N-acetyl-p-benzoquinone,** binds covalently to cellular macromolecules, leading to hepatic necrosis.
   b. Methemoglobinemia. Accumulation of oxidizing metabolites produces methemoglobin, which reduces oxygenation of blood.
   c. Heinz body formation. Hemoglobin is denatured and attaches to erythrocyte membranes, forming Heinz bodies. Cats are especially prone to the formation of Heinz bodies and the development of hemolytic anemia. Some moist cat foods may contain from 7%–13% propylene glycol, which may increase the sensitivity of erythrocytes to oxidative stress.

E. **Toxicity**

1. The **feline toxic dosage** is **50–100 mg/kg**. One regular-strength tablet (325 mg) may be toxic to cats, and a second one 24 hours later could be lethal.

2. The **canine toxic dosage** is **600 mg/kg**.
   a. Oral dosages of 500 mg/kg produce methemoglobin levels that exceed 50%.
   b. Three doses within a 24-hour period that total more than 1000 mg/kg cause fulminant hepatic failure. Effects are delayed for approximately 36 hours.

F. **Diagnosis**

1. **Clinical signs**
   a. Cyanosis develops within 4–12 hours of ingestion as a result of methemoglobinemia and anemia. **Hematuria** and **hemoglobinuria** appear when blood methemoglobin levels reach approximately 20%.

   b. **Edema of the face and paws** may occur (especially in cats) and is accompanied by **lacrimation** and **pruritus**.
   c. **Anorexia** and **depression** increase in severity.
   d. **Hemolysis** and **icterus** become apparent within 2–7 days of the toxicosis.

2. **Laboratory diagnosis**
   a. **Methemoglobinemia, depletion of erythrocyte-reduced glutathione, Heinz bodies,** and a **decreased packed cell volume** result from disturbances of hemoglobin and erythrocyte membranes.
   b. **Elevated serum hepatic enzyme levels** and **total** and **direct bilirubin levels** are evidence of hepatic necrosis.

3. **Lesions**
   a. **Gross lesions** include **dark, chocolate-colored blood** and a **mottled liver**.
   b. **Microscopic lesions** include **centrilobular hepatic degeneration** or necrosis, **palpebral conjunctivitis** and **edema,** and **focal lymphoid necrosis**.

G. **Treatment.** Early treatment (within 4 hours of exposure) is most effective; prompt reaction to acetaminophen exposure in cats is very important.

1. **Detoxification.** Early gastrointestinal detoxification using **emesis, activated charcoal,** and **osmotic cathartics** markedly improves the survival rate.

2. **Antidote. Acetylcysteine** replenishes depleted glutathione stores or substitutes for glutathione.
   a. **Principles of administration**
      (1) Acetylcysteine should not be administered within 2 hours of administering activated charcoal, because charcoal may inactivate the antidote.
      (2) Regardless of the time since exposure, acetylcysteine should be administered to cats with clinical signs.
   b. **Dosage.** A loading dose of 140 mg/kg should be administered orally, followed by dosages of 70 mg/kg every 4–6 hours for up to 3 days.

3. **Supportive treatment** to counteract methemoglobinemia and anemia may be helpful.
   a. **Oxygen therapy** is the traditional approach.
   b. **Sodium sulfate** (a 1.6% solution of 50 mg/kg in water) administered intravenously every 4 hours is an effective alternative treatment.
   c. **Methylene blue** in 10% sterile saline given intravenously at a dosage of 1.5 mg/kg is recommended to combat methemoglobinemia in cats. **Ascorbic acid** may also be used.
      (1) The dose may be repeated two or three times without danger of anemia.
      (2) The complete blood count should be monitored for up to 1 week following treatment.
   d. **Corticosteroids** and **antihistamines** are **contraindicated**.

II. ASPIRIN

A. **Chemistry.** Aspirin (acetylsalicylic acid) is a derivative of phenol.

B. **Source.** Aspirin is available as 5- or 7.5-grain (325-mg or 500-mg) tablets.

C. **Exposure**

1. Aspirin may be prescribed by veterinarians.

2. Owners may administer aspirin to pets without consulting a veterinarian.

3. Pets may consume large doses of aspirin after gaining accidental access to it.

D. **Toxicokinetics**

1. **Absorption.** Aspirin, an acidic drug with a low pKa, is un-ionized in the stomach. It is readily absorbed from both the stomach and upper small intestine.

2. **Metabolism and excretion.** Salicylates are conjugated with either glycine or glucuronic acid and excreted in the urine. Cats are at increased risk for toxicity because of their low rate of glucuronide formation.

E. **Mechanism of toxicologic damage**

1. Salicylates **uncouple oxidative phosphorylation** and may cause hyperglycemia and glycosuria.

2. Acetylation of platelet cyclooxygenase **inhibits platelet aggregation,** leading to prolonged bleeding times.

3. High doses of aspirin **inhibit glycolysis,** causing lactic acid to accumulate and leading to metabolic acidosis.

4. Aspirin may severely **restrict focal blood flow to the gastric mucosae,** causing mucosal damage, ulceration, and bleeding.

F. **Toxicity**

1. **Cats**
   a. The **therapeutic dosage** is 25 mg/kg body weight daily.
   b. The **toxic dosage** is 80–120 mg/kg for 10–12 days.

2. **Dogs**
   a. The **therapeutic dosage** that maintains an optimal serum salicylate concentration without producing overt signs of toxicosis is 25–35 mg/kg three times per day.
   b. **Toxic dosage**
      (1) **Acute.** A dosage of 50 mg/kg twice daily causes emesis in dogs. Higher dosages cause depression and fatal metabolic acidosis.
      (2) **Chronic.** A dosage of 100–300 mg/kg per day for 1–4 weeks causes gastric ulceration and hematemesis. Continuation of this dosage for 3–8 weeks can be fatal.

G. **Diagnosis**

1. **Clinical signs** include vomiting, depression, anorexia, fever, hyperventilation (possibly related to acidosis), and signs of toxic hepatitis (see Chapter 8 III C 1 b).

2. **Laboratory diagnosis**
   a. Thrombocytopenia, anemia, and Heinz bodies are evident in cases of chronic exposure (especially in cats).
   b. Serum salicylate levels may confirm exposure, but toxic concentrations are not well defined in veterinary medicine.
   c. Elevated serum sodium and reduced serum potassium concentrations are characteristic but not diagnostic.

3. **Lesions** include **gastric ulceration** and **moderate bone marrow suppression with thrombocyte deficiency.**

H. **Treatment**

1. **Detoxification.** Prompt oral decontamination should be performed within 4 hours of acute exposure, using emesis, gastric lavage, activated charcoal, and osmotic cathartics.

2. **Supportive treatment**
   a. **Intravenous fluids** containing sodium bicarbonate should be administered to treat metabolic acidosis.

      (1) The bicarbonate dosage is 1–3 mEq/L.

      (2) Because fluid therapy may cause pulmonary edema, the animal should be monitored closely. Furosemide is recommended as a diuretic if pulmonary edema develops.

   b. Cooling baths should be used to treat hyperthermia.

   c. Blood transfusion may be indicated if significant anemia or gastric hemorrhage is present.

   d. Sucralfate may be administered to treat gastric ulceration.

   e. Cimetidine and ranitidine, histamine-receptor antagonists, reduce gastric mucosal damage from aspirin in dogs by controlling the acid-secreting capability of the stomach.

III. OTHER NONSTEROIDAL ANTI-INFLAMMATORY DRUGS (NSAIDs)

A. Sources

1. Ibuprofen and **naproxen** are available over-the-counter and are increasingly popular analgesic and anti-inflammatory agents in humans. These agents are also used in veterinary medicine.

   a. Ibuprofen has some clinical applications in dogs, but questions of efficacy and safety have limited its use.

   b. Naproxen is a relatively common anti-inflammatory agent in equine medicine.

2. Phenylbutazone is approved for use in horses and dogs, primarily through veterinary administration or dispensing.

B. Toxicokinetics

1. Absorption is rapid and complete after oral intake.

2. Distribution. The NSAIDs are **highly protein-bound,** so agents that displace them from protein-binding sites (e.g., sulfonamides) may enhance their toxicity.

3. Metabolism and excretion

   a. Ibuprofen is metabolized in the liver to inactive metabolites that are excreted in the urine.

   b. Naproxen undergoes extensive enterohepatic circulation, but does not induce hepatic metabolizing enzymes and is excreted in the urine. It has a plasma half-life of 74 hours in the dog.

   c. Phenylbutazone is biotransformed to an active metabolite, **oxyphenbutazone,** which is excreted in the urine for up to 48 hours following a single dose.

C. Mechanism of toxicologic damage. In high doses, these NSAIDs:

1. Cause a prostaglandin deficiency by inhibiting cyclooxygenase

2. Interfere with circulation and reduce blood flow to critical areas (e.g., the renal medulla and papillae, the gastric mucosa)

3. Impair renin secretion

4. Increase tubular sodium and water resorption

D. Toxicity

1. Ibuprofen

   a. Dogs

      (1) Repeated administration of 50 mg/kg in dogs causes anorexia and mild gastric irritation.

      (2) Dosages of 100 mg/kg cause moderate to severe toxicosis, with primarily gastrointestinal signs, and recovery is likely.

(3) Dosages of 300 mg/kg cause acute toxicosis characterized by renal necrosis (analgesic nephropathy) that may be lethal.

    b. **Cats** are susceptible to dosages of approximately half those that cause toxicosis in dogs.

2. Naproxen

    a. Dosages of 5 mg/kg daily cause significant gastrointestinal damage in dogs.

    b. Dosages of 15 mg/kg are considered toxic.

3. Phenylbutazone

    a. **Dogs.** Dosages of 100 mg/kg twice daily for more than 10 days have caused toxicosis in dogs.

    b. **Cats.** Dosages of 44 mg/kg daily for approximately 2 weeks have been lethal to cats.

E. | Diagnosis

1. Clinical signs

    a. Early signs are **anorexia, nausea, vomiting,** and **abdominal pain**. Affected animals are **depressed** and **drowsy**. **Ataxia** and severe depression or **coma** may follow.

    b. **Dark, tarry stools** result from gastric ulcers.

    c. **Oliguria** and **azotemia** are caused by **acute renal failure** following extremely high dosages.

2. Laboratory diagnosis

    a. **Blood work.** Plasma levels of the drug may help to establish exposure, but methods are not routinely available in veterinary laboratories and interpretation of significant toxic levels may be difficult.

        (1) **Hyperkalemia, azotemia,** and **anemia** are consistent with NSAID toxicosis.

        (2) **Increased bleeding time** can occur.

    b. **Blood gases. Acidosis** is consistent with NSAID toxicosis. **Respiratory alkalosis** may occur from stimulation of the respiratory center by phenylbutazone.

    c. **Radiography** or **gastroscopy** may help to define the extent of damage to the gastric mucosa.

    d. **Urinalysis** may establish exposure.

F. | Treatment

1. Detoxification. Oral decontamination may be helpful if exposure is acute and recent.

2. Supportive treatment

    a. **Assisted ventilation** is necessary when respiratory depression has occurred.

    b. **Sucralfate** and **cimetidine** may be used to treat gastric ulcers.

    c. **Misoprostol,** an **exogenous prostaglandin,** inhibits the development of gastrointestinal toxicity associated with oral administration of NSAIDs.

    d. **Intravenous fluids** should be administered to counteract hypotension.

        (1) It may be necessary to administer **dopamine** if blood pressure and urine output do not respond to fluids.

        (2) **Bicarbonate** may be included in fluid therapy to counteract acidosis and enhance urinary elimination of the NSAID.

    e. **Hyperkalemia must be treated** if oliguria is present (see Chapter 9 IV A 3).

IV. METHYLXANTHINE ALKALOIDS

A. | Chemistry. Caffeine, theophylline, and **theobromine** are methylated xanthines that occur as major alkaloids in coffee, tea, and chocolate, respectively.

B. | Sources include foods and beverages (Table 24-1) and over-the-counter stimulant tablets, which contain 100–200 mg of caffeine/tablet.

TABLE 24-1. Approximate Methylxanthine
Alkaloid Content of Common Food Products

Product	Alkaloid Content
Cacao beans	4–8 g/ounce*
Baking chocolate	400 mg/ounce*
Dark chocolate	150 mg/ounce*
Milk chocolate	50 mg/ounce*
Regular coffee	6–10 mg/ounce

*Approximately 80%–85% theobromine and 15%–20%
caffeine.

C. **Exposure.** Stimulant tablets are a relatively common source of toxicosis in pets. Toxicosis from chocolate is more common around holidays (e.g., Christmas, Valentine's day).

D. **Toxicokinetics**

1. **Absorption and distribution.** Methylxanthines are readily absorbed orally or parenterally, and are widely distributed throughout the body.

2. **Metabolism.** They are metabolized in the liver by microsomal mixed function oxidases (MFOs), N-demethylation, and conjugation.

3. **Excretion.** They are eliminated rapidly in the urine. Methylxanthines are alkaline drugs, thus they are more rapidly excreted when urine is acidified.

E. **Mechanism of action.** Methylxanthines stimulate the central nervous system (CNS) and cardiac muscle, promote diuresis, and induce smooth muscle relaxation. Theobromine is considered a less potent CNS stimulant than either caffeine or theophylline.

1. Methylxanthines inhibit intercellular calcium sequestration, leading to increased activity of skeletal and cardiac muscle.

2. They competitively antagonize cellular adenosine receptors, resulting in CNS stimulation, vasoconstriction, and tachycardia and the accumulation of cyclic nucleotides [especially cyclic adenosine monophosphate (cAMP)].

3. Methylxanthines increase irritability of the sensory cortex, resulting in increased mental alertness. Large doses enhance motor activity and increase the response to normal stimuli.

F. **Toxicity**

1. **Caffeine** and **theobromine.** The acute lethal oral dosage is 100–200 mg/kg in dogs and 80–150 mg/kg in cats.

2. **Theophylline.** The acute lethal oral dosage is 300 mg/kg in dogs and 700 mg/kg in cats.

G. **Diagnosis**

1. **Clinical signs**
   a. **Restlessness, hyperactivity,** and **mild hyperreflexia** occur early (within 1–2 hours of ingestion).
   b. **Urinary incontinence** or **diuresis** may occur.
   c. **Vomiting** and **diarrhea** may occur, especially if chocolate is the source of the toxicosis.
   d. **Excessive hyperactivity, stiffness, muscle twitching, hyperreflexia,** and **tonic to tetanic convulsive seizures** occur late in the clinical course.
   e. **Polypnea** (as evidenced by a respiratory rate of 150–200 breaths/min) and **tachycardia** (with a heart rate reaching 300 beats/min) occur.
   f. **Hyperthermia** is common.

2. **Laboratory evaluation.** The stomach contents, serum, or urine can be analyzed for the presence of alkaloids. The alkaline methylxanthines partition into the acidic stomach, so even washings of an empty stomach may be useful for analysis.

H. **Treatment.** Remedial action and prevention of future incidents may require careful questioning of the pet owner to determine potential sources of methylxanthine alkaloids.

1. **Detoxification.** Rapid oral detoxification via gastric emptying, activated charcoal, and osmotic cathartics should be performed.
   a. Administration of activated charcoal every 3–4 hours may help to reduce the serum half-life of methylxanthines.
   b. Emetics are contraindicated if the animal is experiencing hyperreflexia or seizures, unless the seizures are first controlled using diazepam, phenobarbital, or short-acting barbiturates.

2. **Supportive treatment**
   a. The urine should be acidified to ionize the alkaloid and assist urinary elimination.
   b. Tachycardia must be addressed if it is compromising cardiac function.
      (1) **Lidocaine.** A loading dose of 1–2 mg/kg is administered intravenously, followed by infusion of a 0.1% intravenous solution at a rate of 30 μg/kg/min. **Lidocaine is contraindicated in cats.**
      (2) **Propranolol** (0.1 mg/kg) is effective at controlling tachyarrhythmias, but may slow renal excretion of methylxanthines.
      (3) **Metoprolol** is as effective as propranolol and does not slow methylxanthine excretion. The suggested dosage is 0.04–0.06 mg/kg intravenously, three times daily.
   c. It is necessary to **monitor the animal for hypotension** following treatment with β-blockers.

V. AMPHETAMINE

A. **Chemistry.** Amphetamine is an alkaline drug that is ionized under acidic conditions.

B. **Sources.** Amphetamine is used both legally and illegally to stimulate the CNS, suppress the appetite, and elevate the mood. Amphetamine is available in 5- and 10-mg tablets.

C. **Exposure.** Access to pets is usually accidental, resulting from the careless handling of illicit or prescription amphetamines.

D. **Toxicokinetics**

1. **Absorption.** Amphetamine is well absorbed from the intestinal tract; peak absorption occurs within 2–3 hours.

2. **Metabolism** is by deamination and hydroxylation, primarily to benzoylglucuronide, hippuric acid, norephedrine, and p-hydroxyamphetamine.

3. **Excretion** is pH-dependent, with higher amounts being excreted in acidic urine.

E. **Mechanism of action.** Physiologic effects resulting from the actions of amphetamines include tachycardia, hypertension, mydriasis, polypnea, bronchodilatation, excitement, and agitation.

1. Amphetamine stimulates catecholamine release from adrenergic nerve endings.

2. It inhibits monoamine oxidase (MAO), leading to impaired catecholamine metabolism.

3. It activates cAMP.

4. It stimulates the cerebral cortex, respiratory center, and reticular activating system.

5. Rhabdomyolysis, resulting from violent seizures, may cause secondary renal failure.

F. | **Toxicity.** The approximate oral lethal dose is 10–30 mg/kg.

G. | **Diagnosis**

1. **Clinical signs**
   a. **Hyperexcitability** and **agitation** occur 1–2 hours after ingestion.
   b. **Mydriasis, hyperpnea, tremors, tenseness,** and **hyperactive reflexes** are seen.
   c. **Seizures** are similar to those seen in strychnine toxicosis (i.e., tonic, with rigid musculature). However, the degree of hyperreflexia and hyperesthesia is less than that seen with strychnine toxicosis.
   d. **Trembling** and **shaking** of the entire body may occur.
   e. **Tachycardia, cardiac arrhythmia,** and **hypertension** are seen.
   f. **Lactic acidosis** and **hypoglycemia** are characteristic.

2. **Laboratory diagnosis. Analysis of the stomach contents, plasma,** or **urine** may reveal amphetamines.

3. **Lesions**
   a. The stomach may still contain food or portions of tablets or capsules.
   b. Muscle trauma or hemorrhage can result from violent hyperactivity or seizures.

H. | **Treatment**

1. **Stabilization.** Hyperactivity or convulsions must be controlled first.
   a. **Acetylpromazine** (1 mg/kg) or **diazepam** may be used initially to sedate the animal.
   b. **Haloperidol** (1 mg/kg intravenously) is an alternative to tranquilizers for controlling hyperactivity.
   c. **Barbiturates** should be used only if other means of controlling CNS signs fail.

2. **Detoxification.** Prompt gastrointestinal decontamination with emesis or gastric lavage, activated charcoal, and osmotic cathartics is essential to rapid recovery.

3. **Supportive treatment**
   a. **Acidification of urine** promotes ion trapping and enhances urinary elimination.
   b. **Cooling baths** should be used to control hyperthermia.

VI. MARIJUANA

A. | **Chemistry.** The active ingredient in marijuana is **tetrahydrocannabinol (THC).**

1. The THC content of plants, which may range from 1%–6%, is highest in the leaves and flowering tops of the plants. Plants grown in warm climates have the highest THC content.

2. THC is highly lipophilic.

B. | **Sources**

1. **Marijuana** is the dried leaves and flowers of the hemp plant, *Cannabis sativa.*

2. **Hashish** is the resin extracted from the plant.

C. | **Exposure**

1. Pets may eat butts of marijuana cigarettes or leftover baked products containing *Cannabis.* Because ingestion is the principal route of exposure, dogs are more likely to be exposed than cats.

2. The owner may intentionally give the drug to the pet.

3. Cattle occasionally consume the tops of plants and suffer moderate neurologic signs and gastroenteritis with diarrhea.

D. **Toxicokinetics**

1. **Absorption.** THC is readily absorbed from the gastrointestinal tract, and its smoke is rapidly absorbed via the lungs.

2. **Distribution and metabolism.** Enterohepatic recirculation helps to maintain drug levels and produces a variety of hepatic metabolites.

3. **Elimination.** Prolonged residues are not likely. Most metabolites are excreted in approximately 24 hours.

E. **Mechanism of action.** The actual mechanism of action is not clear. Actions may be related to changes in levels of biogenic amines in the CNS.

F. **Toxicity**

1. The oral LD_{50} in rats is approximately 650 mg/kg.

2. The lethal dosage in dogs is more than 3 g/kg. Death from marijuana exposure is not expected.

G. **Diagnosis** of toxicosis from marijuana (and other illicit drugs) is problematic because histories may be incomplete or misleading.

1. **Clinical signs**
   a. **Ataxia, incoordination,** and **depression** are the most common signs.
   b. **Marked CNS signs,** sometimes alternating between **depression** and **excitement** in dogs, may occur.
   c. Dogs may experience **hallucinations** (evidenced by **barking** and **agitation** for no apparent reason).
   d. Gastrointestinal signs include **vomiting** and **dry mucous membranes**.
   e. **Hyperthermia** and **tachypnea** occasionally occur.

2. **Laboratory diagnosis.** THC can be detected in plasma or urine to confirm recent exposure; however, not all veterinary laboratories routinely offer this analysis.

3. **Lesions** are not usually present.

H. **Treatment.** Most animals recover with detoxification and supportive care.

1. **Detoxification** using emesis, activated charcoal, and cathartics is recommended. Because THC possesses some antiemetic properties, emetics may not always be useful.

2. **Supportive therapy**
   a. **Assisted ventilation** may be necessary if respiratory depression is severe.
   b. Animals should be kept in a **warm, secure place**.
   c. **CNS drugs should not be administered unless they are necessary to save the animal's life. Diazepam** may be used to control excessive excitement or agitation.

VII. COCAINE

A. **Chemistry.** Cocaine is an alkaloid (benzoylmethylecgonine).

B. **Source.** Cocaine is derived from the coca plant, *Erythroxylon coca* or *E. monogynum*.

1. **Freebase** is chemically extracted pure cocaine alkaloid.

2. **Street cocaine** is often "cut" with amphetamine, caffeine, lidocaine, quinine, or even strychnine.

C. **Exposure.** Most pet exposure is the result of accidental access to cocaine used illegally by owners.

D. **Toxicokinetics**

1. **Absorption.** Cocaine is rapidly absorbed from the gastrointestinal tract, mucous membranes, and lungs.

2. **Metabolism.** It is rapidly metabolized to at least six metabolites in the liver and plasma.

3. **Excretion.** The plasma half-life is short (generally less than 3 hours). Both the parent compound and the metabolites are excreted in the urine.

E. **Mechanism of toxicologic damage.** Excessive amounts of cocaine cause cardiac or respiratory arrest. Cocaine inhibits neuronal reuptake of catecholamines and promotes catecholamine release; however, the role of catecholamine changes in the mechanism of toxicosis is unclear.

F. **Toxicity**

1. **Dogs.** The oral LD_{50} is estimated to be 50 mg/kg. The intravenous LD_{50} is approximately one-fourth the oral LD_{50}.

2. **Cats** are of approximately the same susceptibility as dogs.

G. **Diagnosis**

1. **Clinical signs**
   a. Alternate CNS stimulation and profound depression
   b. Hyperesthesia and seizures
   c. Tachycardia and hypertension, tachyarrhythmias, ventricular premature contractions, ventricular tachycardia (in humans)

2. **Laboratory diagnosis**
   a. **Bloodwork.** Hyperglycemia and elevated alanine aminotransferase (ALT) and creatine kinase levels are characteristic but nonspecific changes. Cocaine metabolites may be found in plasma to confirm recent exposure.
   b. **Urinalysis** may confirm recent exposure.

3. **Lesions** are not routinely present, or reliable.

H. **Treatment**

1. **Detoxification** may be relatively ineffective, because cocaine is so rapidly absorbed.

2. **Supportive treatment**
   a. **Respiratory support** may be necessary.
   b. Experimentally, **chlorpromazine** has helped to alleviate the cardiovascular effects of cocaine in dogs, and may aid in preventing seizures.
   c. Hyperthermia should be controlled with **cool-water baths** or **enemas**.
   d. The value of **antiarrhythmic therapy** using propranolol is uncertain, and is not recommended unless the animal's status is critical.

VIII. **PHENCYCLIDINE (PCP)** was introduced in the 1950s as a nonbarbiturate anesthetic, but was removed from the market in 1978 because of undesirable side effects (e.g., delirium, agitation, hallucinations).

A. **Chemistry.** PCP hydrochloride, a chemical analog of ketamine, is an arylcyclohexylamine.

B. **Sources.** PCP is available illegally; common street names are PCP, "angel dust," and "hog."

C. **Toxicokinetics**

1. **Absorption.** PCP is rapidly absorbed from the intestine, but poorly absorbed from the stomach.

2. **Metabolism** takes place in the liver. Enterohepatic recirculation prolongs the plasma half-life of PCP.

3. **Excretion.** Both the parent drug and the metabolites are excreted in urine.

D. **Mechanism of action.** PCP may stimulate α-adrenergic receptors and potentiate the pressor response to epinephrine. There is some evidence that cholinesterase inhibition also plays a role. At high dosages, PCP induces respiratory depression by an unknown mechanism.

E. **Toxicity**

1. **Dogs.** An oral dosage of 25 mg/kg is lethal to most dogs. Clinical toxicosis occurs at dosages of 2.5–10 mg/kg.

2. **Cats.** The toxicity range for cats is similar to that for dogs.

F. **Diagnosis**

1. **Clinical signs** are variable; animals appear to die from respiratory failure complicated by cardiovascular dysfunction.
   a. **CNS signs** include signs alternating between depression and excitation, hypersalivation, mydriasis, tonic–clonic seizures, and champing of the jaws. Hyperactivity and stereotypical circling occur in dogs.
   b. **Cardiovascular signs** include tachycardia, arrhythmias, and hypertension.

2. **Laboratory diagnosis.** Analysis for PCP in veterinary laboratories is not generally available. Forensic or racetrack laboratories could provide such analyses.

3. **Lesions** are not characteristic or consistent. Pulmonary hemorrhage and congestion may occur.

G. **Treatment**

1. **Decontamination** must be rapid. Continued use of activated charcoal (three times daily) may help to prevent enterohepatic recirculation.

2. **Supportive treatment**
   a. Animals should be **kept cool** and **isolated** from external stimuli.
   b. **Diazepam** may be useful to control excitement or seizures.
   c. **Intravenous fluids, acidification of urine,** and **forced diuresis** with **furosemide** may help to promote urinary excretion.

STUDY QUESTIONS

DIRECTIONS: Each of the numbered items or incomplete statements in this section is followed by answers or by completions of the statement. Select the **one** numbered answer or completion that is **best** in each case.

1. Which one of the following mechanisms is responsible for acetaminophen's toxicity in small animals?

(1) Failure of hepatic glutathione to bind to acetaminophen and neutralize its metabolism
(2) Lack of sulfhydryl groups on the erythrocyte membrane
(3) Depletion or deficiency of glucuronyl transferase
(4) Induction of phase II metabolism
(5) Metabolism to cysteine conjugates, which depletes essential sulfur amino acids

2. Which statement is true regarding aspirin toxicosis in dogs?

(1) The acid pKa of aspirin promotes ionization in the stomach, which leads to mucosal damage and ulcers.
(2) Dogs are more susceptible to toxicosis than cats because dogs cannot form glycine or glucuronide conjugates.
(3) Toxicosis is related to the inhibition of prostaglandin synthesis and acetylation of platelet cyclooxygenase.
(4) Metabolic alkalosis develops as a result of impaired gastric acid secretion.

3. Based on clinical signs and mechanism of action, which of the following toxicoses is most similar to methylxanthine toxicosis?

(1) Amphetamine toxicosis
(2) Lead intoxication
(3) Marijuana toxicosis
(4) Metaldehyde toxicosis
(5) Strychnine toxicosis

DIRECTIONS: Each of the numbered items or incomplete statements in this section is negatively phrased, as indicated by an italicized word such as *not, least,* or *except.* Select the **one** numbered answer or completion that is **best** in each case.

4. A syndrome of gastrointestinal bleeding with dark tarry stools, acute renal failure, and increased bleeding time is characteristic of overdose by all of the following *except*:

(1) acetaminophen.
(2) aspirin.
(3) ibuprofen.
(4) naproxen.
(5) phenylbutazone.

5. A client calls the veterinarian because she arrived home from work to find that her cocker spaniel had torn open a bag of gourmet coffee beans as well as some chocolate that was to be used for holiday preparations. Which of the following would be *least* likely to cause toxicosis in a 10-kg dog that had consumed 0.5 kg of the material?

(1) Baking chocolate
(2) Dark chocolate
(3) Milk chocolate
(4) Coffee beans

6. Acute serious signs of methylxanthine toxicosis could be treated with any of the following *except*:

(1) atropine.
(2) diazepam.
(3) lidocaine.
(4) metoprolol.
(5) propranolol.

1. The answer is 3 *[I D]*. Acetaminophen itself is not the toxic agent, but it becomes toxic when metabolized by phase I (cytochrome P-450) reactions to a reactive intermediate, N-acetyl-p-benzoquinone. Acetaminophen is normally metabolized to nontoxic products when phase II metabolism promotes conjugation with glucuronic acid or sulfates. If enzymes to effect this transformation are depleted or deficient (as in cats, which lack glucuronyl transferase), or the dosage of acetaminophen is excessive, then the detoxification pathway is insufficient and the reactive intermediate (N-acetyl-p-benzoquinone) binds with cellular glutathione. Glutathione acts as a second line of defense by forming mercapturic acid derivatives that are excreted in the urine. If glutathione is depleted, the reactive intermediate binds to essential cellular proteins and macromolecules, leading to cell death. In addition, N-acetyl-p-benzoquinone can oxidize hemoglobin, forming both methemoglobin and Heinz bodies.

2. The answer is 3 *[II E 1–2]*. The recognized mechanisms of action for aspirin are inhibition of prostaglandin synthesis and acetylation of platelet cyclooxygenase, combined with inhibition of oxidative phosphorylation and inhibition of oxidative metabolism. Inhibition of glycolysis causes metabolic acidosis, not alkalosis. Aspirin has an acid pKa, which causes it to be un-ionized in the stomach. Cats are more susceptible to toxicosis than dogs because they lack effective glucuronide conjugation. Aspirin does not impair the gastric secretion of acids; in fact, part of the therapy for aspirin toxicosis is administration of histamine-receptor antagonists that help control gastric acid secretion.

3. The answer is 1 *[IV E; V E]*. Both amphetamine and methylxanthines stimulate the cerebral cortex and enhance or increase cyclic adenosine monophosphate (cAMP) activity. Both cause central nervous system (CNS) and cardiovascular effects, leading to tachycardia and arrhythmias, and each has a strong clinical phase of stimulation and hyperactivity, potentially attended by seizures. Marijuana causes bizarre behavior and, possibly, hallucinations, but affected animals are not usually consistently overstimulated. Metaldehyde causes some tremors, but is also accompanied by salivation and vomiting, and generally has little effect on cardiovascular activity. Strychnine is a potent convulsant that acts by facilitating reflex hyperactivity at the level of the spinal cord; in addition, strychnine lacks significant primary cardiovascular effects.

4. The answer is 1 *[I F; II E, G; III E]*. The mechanism of acetaminophen toxicosis is formation of a toxic electrophilic intermediate that binds to cellular macromolecules and oxidizes hemoglobin, resulting in hepatic necrosis, hemolytic anemia, and methemoglobinemia. Aspirin, ibuprofen, naproxen, and phenylbutazone all inhibit cyclooxygenase, leading to reduced prostaglandin synthesis. Reduced prostaglandin synthesis, in turn, may lead to impaired circulation in focal areas of the gastric mucosa, which can lead to the development of ulcers. Large dosages reduce blood flow in critical areas of the renal medulla and papillae, resulting in renal necrosis and the well-known nephropathy associated with excessive nonsteroidal anti-inflammatory drug (NSAID) usage.

5. The answer is 3 *[Table 24-1]*. Chocolate and coffee products contain widely varying concentrations of methylxanthine alkaloids, with coffee beans having the highest concentration (4–8 g/ounce). Baking chocolate contains 400 mg of methylxanthine alkaloids/ounce, dark chocolate contains 150 mg/ounce, and milk chocolate contains 50 mg/ounce. An important part of the anamnesis is determining as accurately as possible the nature and amount of what was consumed. In this case, the owner should be instructed to sweep up the coffee beans and estimate how much of the bag was consumed. In addition, it is important to determine what type of chocolate was consumed by asking the owner or reading the label. If only a small amount of milk chocolate was consumed, treatment is probably not needed, but consumption of a substantial amount of baking chocolate or coffee beans could be a medical emergency.

6. The answer is 1 *[IV H]*. Atropine would be contraindicated in methylxanthine toxicosis because it acts by blocking vagal activity, resulting in a rapid heart rate and ventricular arrhythmias. Diazepam may be useful to control severe hyperactivity and seizures during acute methylxanthine toxicosis. Lidocaine is recommended as initial therapy for tachyarrhythmias. For more severe effects, β-blockers (e.g., propranolol, metoprolol) are helpful.

Chapter 25

Common Household Products

I. INTRODUCTION

A. **Relative risk.** Most household products are relatively safe and largely inaccessible to companion animals. Products available in most homes that present a relatively high risk include automotive radiator antifreeze that contains ethylene glycol and cleaners and disinfectants.

B. **Gathering essential information**

1. **Labels.** The packaging is an invaluable source of information.
   a. It can provide the **trade name** or the **ingredients,** which are necessary in order to evaluate risk and institute therapy or remedial measures.
   b. A standard way of denoting the contents of **fertilizers** has been developed (e.g., 12-12-12 represents 12% **nitrogen,** 12% **phosphorus,** 12% **potassium**).

2. A **human poison control center** can provide valuable information regarding expected clinical effects and appropriate therapy.

3. The **manufacturer** can be contacted for data or suggestions regarding proper response to the exposure.

II. ETHYLENE GLYCOL (ANTIFREEZE)

A. **Chemistry.** Ethylene glycol ($HO—CH_2—CH_2OH$) is a dihydric alcohol (1,2 ethanediol) that is readily soluble in water.

B. **Sources**

1. Ethylene glycol is widely used as a wintertime **antifreeze** solution and a summertime **coolant** for automobile engines.

2. It is also a component of **industrial solvents, rust removers, color film processing fluids,** and **heat exchange fluids**.

C. **Exposure.** Toxicosis from ingesting antifreeze is a relatively common occurrence in dogs and cats, who apparently find the taste acceptable and consume it readily.

1. Swine and poultry have also been affected.

2. The incidence of toxicosis is somewhat seasonal, corresponding to when antifreeze is commonly added or changed (i.e., late fall, early spring).

D. **Toxicokinetics**

1. **Absorption and distribution.** Ethylene glycol is readily absorbed from the gastrointestinal tract and rapidly and evenly distributed to the tissues. The maximal blood concentration from a single ingestion is reached within 1–4 hours of ingestion.

2. **Excretion.** Nearly all of the ethylene glycol is metabolized or excreted within 16–24 hours of ingestion.
   a. The plasma half-life ranges from 2–4 hours.
   b. Much of the absorbed ethylene glycol is excreted unchanged in the urine within 4 hours of consumption.

E. Mechanism of toxicologic damage

1. The intact glycol crosses the blood–brain barrier and exerts narcotic or euphoric effects, such as those seen with ethanol.

2. Metabolism of the glycol to several acidic intermediates (Figure 25-1) causes metabolic acidosis and kidney damage.
   a. Glycolic acid is largely responsible for the severe metabolic acidosis that occurs within 3–4 hours of ingestion.
   b. Oxalate anion binds to plasma calcium to form calcium oxalate crystals in the blood vessels and renal tubules. Renal tubular damage with development of azotemia is observed from 1–3 days after ingestion.

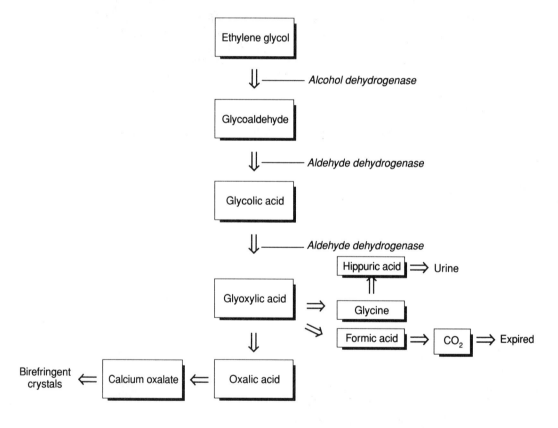

FIGURE 25-1. Pathways of ethylene glycol metabolism. Ethylene glycol is oxidized by alcohol dehydrogenase to glycoaldehyde, which is further metabolized to glycolic acid by aldehyde dehydrogenase. Glycolic acid is largely responsible for the metabolic acidosis associated with ethylene glycol toxicosis. Glycolic acid is converted to glyoxylic acid by aldehyde dehydrogenase. Glyoxylic acid is metabolized to glycine, oxalic acid, and formic acid. Glycine is converted to glycocholic acid or conjugated with benzoic acid to form hippuric acid, which is excreted in urine. There is good correlation between urine glycolic acid (glycolate) levels and prognosis. Oxalic acid can combine with serum calcium to form calcium oxalate, which results in the characteristic birefringent or polarizing crystals seen in blood vessel walls and renal tubules. Formic acid is eventually oxidized to carbon dioxide and excreted via the lungs.

F. **Toxicity.** The margin between a single toxic dose and the lethal dose is relatively narrow (i.e., approximately 1:2).

1. **Cats.** A dosage of **2–4 ml/kg** causes clinical signs and **death** in cats.

2. **Dogs.** The **lethal dosage** in dogs is **4–5 ml/kg.**

3. **Poultry. Intoxication** of poultry occurs at dosages of **7–8 ml/kg.**

G. **Diagnosis**

1. **Clinical signs.** Ethylene glycol poisoning is difficult to diagnose from clinical signs alone.
   a. **First phase.** Early signs (1–4 hours postingestion) include **ataxia, incoordination, tachycardia, polypnea, diuresis, polydipsia,** and **dehydration.** Metabolism of the glycol alleviates the initial central nervous system (CNS) signs.
   b. **Second phase.** The initial signs are followed within 4–6 hours by a second, more serious phase that correlates well with acidosis and the increase of acidic intermediates in the plasma.
      (1) **Anorexia, depression, vomiting, hypothermia,** and **miosis** occur in the second phase of the disease. As the clinical course progresses, the vomiting, depression, ataxia, weakness, and loss of reflexes worsen.
      (2) **Severe depression, increased respiratory rate, coma,** and **death** follow if the toxicosis is untreated.
   c. **Third phase.** In animals that survive the acute acidosis, a third phase consisting of **oliguric renal failure** signals a very poor prognosis.

2. **Laboratory diagnosis**
   a. **Increased osmolality and anion gap.** The anion gap is obtained by subtracting the sum of serum chloride and bicarbonate from the sum of serum sodium and potassium. Normally, this difference is approximately 10–12 mEq/L.
      (1) The anion gap is increased by lower amounts of unmeasured cations or by increased amounts of unmeasured anions. **Lactic acid, glycolate, glyoxalate,** and **oxalate can significantly increase the concentration of unmeasured anions.**
      (2) Anion gaps **greater than 40–50 mEq/L are considered typical** of ethylene glycol.
   b. **Blood pH values less than 7.3** are typical of ethylene glycol toxicosis.
   c. **Characteristic changes in renal function** are caused by advanced ethylene glycol toxicosis with development of oliguric renal failure.
      (1) Blood urea nitrogen (BUN) levels are elevated and the urine specific gravity is low. Urinary phosphorus excretion is reduced and hyperkalemia is seen.
      (2) Urine sediment may contain crystals of calcium oxalate or hippuric acid, as well as erythrocytes, leukocytes, renal epithelial cells, and casts.
   d. **Hyperglycemia** may result from hypocalcemic inhibition of insulin secretion, inhibition of the tricarboxylic acid (TCA) cycle, or both as a result of nicotinamide adenine dinucleotide (NAD) depletion following metabolism of ethylene glycol.
   e. **Residues.** Ethylene glycol, oxalate, and hippurate can be detected in blood, urine, and renal tissue.
      (1) Colorimetric kits allow detection of ethylene glycol within the first 24 hours of exposure.
      (2) Serum glycolic acid may be detectable by standard laboratory analyses for up to 60 hours postingestion.

3. **Lesions**
   a. **Gross lesions**
      (1) Gastric mucosa is hemorrhagic and hyperemic. Gastritis or enteritis in dogs and cats poisoned by ethylene glycol is probably related to azotemia.
      (2) Pulmonary hyperemia and edema occur in ethylene glycol–poisoned animals.
      (3) Kidneys may be pale tan and swollen with intermittent gray or yellow streaks, especially near the corticomedullary junction.

- **b. Microscopic lesions**
    - **(1)** Pale yellow, birefringent, rosette-shaped oxalate crystals are present in and surrounding the convoluted tubules. Birefringent, polarizing crystals may also be seen in the adventitia and perivascular spaces of blood vessels in the brain.
        - **(a)** To view polarizing or birefringent crystals, one polarizing lens is placed above the slide on the microscope stage and another is held below the microscope stage (a lens from a pair of polarized sunglasses works well for this).
        - **(b)** Calcium oxalate crystals are seen as bright rosette-shaped areas on a dark background as one lens is slowly rotated until the light coming through the microscope is obliterated.
    - **(2)** In animals that survive several days, regenerating renal tubules are dilated and lined with flattened tubular epithelium.

H. **Treatment.** Early diagnosis and treatment are essential for a successful outcome.

1. **Detoxification.** Effective oral decontamination with activated charcoal must be performed within 4 hours of ingestion.
2. **Specific antidotes**
    - **a. Ethanol (20%)** is a competitive inhibitor for alcohol dehydrogenase that prevents metabolism of ethylene glycol to its toxic acidic intermediates (see Chapter 6 III H). Unmetabolized ethylene glycol is excreted in the urine.
        - **(1) Recommended dosages** for dogs and cats are given in Table 6-1. The actual ethanol dosage is adjusted so animals are maintained in a depressed or near-comatose state for up to 72 hours.
        - **(2)** If more than 18 hours have passed since the animal ingested the ethylene glycol, ethanol will not be helpful because most of the ethylene glycol has already been metabolized. In fact, **ethanol administered late in the clinical course may harm the animal by causing unnecessary depression and dehydration.**
    - **b. 4-Methylpyrazole (4-MP)** functions similarly but more effectively than ethanol as an ethylene glycol antidote in dogs, but is ineffective in cats (see Chapter 6 III J). 4-MP has fewer side effects than ethanol.
        - **(1)** The **recommended dosage** is given in Table 6-1.
        - **(2)** Because 4-MP is **not available commercially,** it must be purchased from a chemical supplier and mixed to the proper solution strength (see Chapter 6 III J 2).
            - **(a)** Mixing is best done by a registered pharmacist.
            - **(b)** The solution is stable for 1 year if refrigerated.
3. **Supportive therapy**
    - **a. Administration of sodium bicarbonate** to correct acidosis should be based on serial plasma bicarbonate levels (i.e., correlated with the bicarbonate deficit). Alternatively, bicarbonate administration may be adjusted to maintain urine pH at approximately 7.5–8.0. A dosage of 6.2 mEq/kg may be administered every 4–6 hours if plasma bicarbonate values are not known.
    - **b. Fluid therapy** is critical in the successful treatment of ethylene glycol poisoning. Saline (50%) and glucose (5%) may be used to establish urine flow. Potassium-containing fluids should not be used until urine flow is established.
        - **(1)** To avoid pulmonary edema in animals with oliguric renal failure, urine output and the central venous pressure should be monitored.
        - **(2)** Fluid replacement and increased tissue perfusion promote diuresis and help to correct metabolic acidosis.
    - **c. Calcium borogluconate** may be helpful to control seizures resulting from hypocalcemia. A 10% solution (0.25 ml/kg daily) is administered intravenously in three divided doses.
    - **d. Corticosteroids** may be useful to treat shock and pulmonary edema.
    - **e. Peritoneal dialysis** has been used to improve the prognosis for survival in acidotic and oliguric animals.
    - **f.** A **bland, low-protein diet** that does not place undue stress on the kidneys is required by convalescing animals.

I. **Prognosis.** Because antemortem diagnosis of ethylene glycol toxicosis is difficult without a complete history or extensive laboratory assistance, and because by the time clinical signs are apparent, therapy may no longer be effective, the prognosis is **grave**. In advanced cases of ethylene glycol toxicosis, the client must be made aware of the grave prognosis so that he or she is able to make informed decisions about the expensive and intensive therapy that is necessary.

III. COAL TAR- AND PHENOL-BASED PRODUCTS AND THEIR DERIVATIVES

A. **Source.** The destructive distillation of bituminous coal produces a mixture of condensable volatile products, consisting primarily of phenols, cresols, and naphthalene (2%–8%), anthracene oils (16%–20%), and pitch (approximately 50%).

1. **Phenols** are found in **creosote, antiseptics, germicides, household cleaners,** and **disinfectants**.

2. **Pitch. Clay pigeons** used for trap shooting are sometimes encountered accidentally by grazing or foraging animals.

B. **Toxicokinetics**

1. **Absorption.** Most phenols and cresols are readily absorbed from the gastrointestinal tract. Limited absorption may occur through intact skin.

2. **Metabolism** is primarily in the liver via glucuronide conjugation.

3. **Excretion** is primarily via the urine.

C. **Mechanism of toxicologic action**

1. **Direct irritation.** Phenols and cresols are direct protoplasmic toxicants that cause coagulative necrosis.

2. **Accumulation in the liver and kidney.** Absorbed phenols appear to accumulate initially in the liver and kidney, causing renal tubular necrosis.

3. **Stimulation of the respiratory center.** Phenol stimulates the respiratory center, leading to hyperventilation and, possibly, respiratory alkalosis.

D. **Toxicity.** Phenol and cresols have approximately equivalent toxicity.

1. The **oral LD$_{50}$** is approximately **500 mg/kg** for most mammals. **Cats are much more sensitive** to phenols than other mammals because they lack glucuronic acid conjugating ability.

2. The **toxicity of clay pigeons to swine** is estimated at 1 g/kg.

E. **Diagnosis**

1. **Clinical signs**
   a. **Coagulative necrosis, ulceration,** and **white plaques** are caused by direct contact.
   b. **Intense pain** occurs almost immediately after exposure to phenol and some of its congeners.
   c. **Neurologic signs** of tremors, incoordination, and mild muscle fasciculations may develop.
   d. **Icterus** may result from intravascular hemolysis and liver damage.
   e. An **aromatic** or **phenolic odor** may be present on expired air or the skin of recently exposed animals.
   f. **Sudden death** may occur in swine, possibly as a result of massive centrilobular hemorrhagic hepatic necrosis, which is a characteristic effect of clay pigeon poisoning.

2. Laboratory diagnosis
  a. Urinalysis
    (1) Proteinuria, hematuria, and epithelial cells or casts reflect renal damage.
    (2) Phenols and cresols or their metabolites may be detected in urine. Mixing 10 ml of urine with 1 ml of 20% ferric chloride will result in a purple color if phenols are present.
  b. Serum liver enzymes may be elevated because of moderate to massive hepatic necrosis.

3. Lesions
  a. Gross lesions
    (1) Necrosis or ulceration of the skin and upper alimentary tract may be present.
    (2) The kidneys are swollen and pale tan if necrosis has occurred.
    (3) The liver has a mottled appearance and centrilobular hemorrhage is evident as a result of hepatic necrosis.
  b. Microscopic lesions
    (1) Acute pharyngitis, esophagitis, and gastritis with coagulation of the mucosa follow oral exposure.
    (2) Acute multifocal centrilobular hepatic necrosis is typical of clay pigeon poisoning of swine.
    (3) Proximal tubular necrosis with tubular casts reflects renal damage.

F. **Treatment**

1. Detoxification
  a. Oral exposure. Prompt oral decontamination with activated charcoal and a saline cathartic is usually recommended for oral exposure. Administration of egg whites may be indicated to dilute and bind the phenols and to partially protect the gastrointestinal mucosa. Emetics and gastric lavage should be avoided, unless the alimentary tract is not visibly damaged.
  b. Dermal exposure. Phenols, cresols, and asphalt products may be removed by bathing the area with liquid dish soap and applying polyethylene glycol or glycerol.

2. Supportive therapy
  a. Supportive treatment for shock, metabolic acidosis, and liver or kidney failure is important to survival once decontamination is completed.
  b. For large animals exposed to clay pigeons, the only practical solution is preventing further access to the clay pigeons and providing a diet supplemented with B vitamins, vitamin E, and high-quality proteins.

IV. **DETERGENTS**

A. **Types**

1. Anionic detergents include sulfonated or phosphorylated hydrocarbons. Laundry detergents also contain agents to soften the water (e.g., sodium phosphate, sodium carbonate, sodium silicate).

2. Nonionic detergents include alkyl and aryl polyether sulphates, alcohols or sulfonates, polyglycol ethers, polyethylene glycol, and sorbitan monostearate. Nonionic detergents are found in soap and laundry and dishwasher detergents.

3. Cationic detergents (e.g., benzethonium chloride, benzalkonium chloride, methylbenzethonium, cetylpyridinium chloride) are quaternary ammonium compounds that often contain a halogen (e.g., bromide, iodide, chloride).

B. **Sources.** These cleaning and disinfecting agents are commonly available and used in homes and businesses.

C. **Exposure.** The availability and careless use of these agents allow ready access by pets and sometimes livestock. Significant problems develop only when massive exposure has taken place.

D. **Mechanism of toxicologic damage.** Detergents directly irritate the skin and mucous membranes.

E. **Toxicity.** Soaps and detergents are only slightly to moderately toxic, except for automatic dishwashing detergent, which is extremely alkaline.

  1. Nonionic detergents are nearly nontoxic, even following ingestion.

  2. Cationic detergents (quarternary ammonium compounds) at concentrations as low as 1% are irritating and may damage mucous membranes.

F. **Diagnosis**

  1. **Clinical signs**
     a. **Dermal exposure.** Repeated exposure removes natural oils and causes thickening of the skin with **weeping, cracking, scaling,** and **blistering**.
     b. **Ingestion** usually causes **vomiting, nausea, diarrhea,** and **gastrointestinal distention**. Quaternary ammonium compounds may be corrosive to the gastrointestinal tract, causing serious vomiting, diarrhea, shock, and collapse.

  2. **Laboratory diagnosis** is usually not necessary because effects are localized and the presence of the agent is often transient.

  3. **Lesions** consist of mild to moderate, and occasionally severe, irritation, hyperemia, edema, and ulceration of the affected areas.

G. **Therapy**

  1. **First aid.** The owner may feed the animal milk, water, or a weak acid (e.g., vinegar) to dilute and neutralize the alkaline detergent.

  2. **Detoxification**
     a. **Dermal exposure. Soap** is effective to counteract unabsorbed cationic detergents.
     b. **Oral exposure.** Emesis and gastric lavage are contraindicated as for other caustic or corrosive agents. **Milk** or **activated charcoal** may be given orally to help inactivate excessive amounts of detergents.

  3. **Supportive therapy**
     a. **Analgesics, demulcents,** and **gastrointestinal protectants** may be helpful for severe or persistent clinical signs.
     b. Occasionally, for severe exposure to cationic detergents, **respiratory support** and **treatment of shock or seizures** are necessary.

V. **OTHER HOUSEHOLD PRODUCTS.** Tables 25-1 through 25-3 contain clinical toxicology information for common household chemicals, cleaning products, and toiletries, respectively.

TABLE 25-1. Clinical Toxicology of Common Household Chemicals

Chemical	Toxicity Rating*	Ingredients	Clinical Presentation	Treatment
Deicer	4	Approximately 75% ethylene glycol and isopropyl alcohol	Disorientation, ataxia, weakness, depression, irritation of mucous membranes and eyes	Diuresis with furosemide, gastric lavage and/or administration of activated charcoal
Fertilizer	2	Mainly nitrogen (e.g., potassium nitrate, urea), phosphorus, and potassium; may contain small amounts of metals or pesticides	Gastrointestinal irritation, vomiting, diarrhea, methemoglobinemia	Oral decontamination followed by adsorbents and demulcents; intravenous or subcutaneous fluids to counteract the diuretic effect of urea, specific therapy for nitrate/nitrite ammonium, or urea toxicosis
Fuels (cooking fuels, lighter fluid)	3	Petroleum hydrocarbons, kerosene, or methanol	Depression, coma, seizures, vomiting (see Chapter 18 II F)	Activated charcoal or a nonabsorbable oil (see Chapter 18 II G)
Glues	3–4	Carriers include aliphatic or aromatic hydrocarbon solvents (e.g., petroleum solvents, acetone, toluol, toluene, methyl acetate, naphtha)	Direct irritation, depression (see Chapter 18 II F)	Activated charcoal or a nonabsorbable oil (see Chapter 18 II G)
Paint and varnish removers	4	Benzene, acetone, toluene (flammable); methylene chloride, toluene, methanol (nonflammable)	Direct irritation, depression (see Chapter 18 II F)	Respiratory support for inhalation exposure
Radiator cleaners	4	Oxalic acid	Direct irritation of mucous membranes and gastrointestinal tract, muscle twitching, tetany, convulsions, depression, paralysis, renal failure manifested as albuminuria, hematuria, oliguria, and crystals in the urine	Oral soluble calcium salts (lime water, chalk, milk) to precipitate oxalate in the gastrointestinal tract; intravenous calcium gluconate for hypocalcemia, renal supportive therapy
Rust removers	4	Hydrochloric acid, phosphoric acid, hydrofluoric acid, naphtha, and mineral oil	Necrosis	Flush with large amounts of water, sodium bicarbonate paste to neutralize acid on the skin, magnesium hydroxide, water, egg whites, or soap solution (instead of inducing emesis)

Thawing salt	2–3	Calcium chloride, sodium chloride, or potassium chloride	Erythema, exfoliation, ulceration, general irritation of the digestive tract, vomiting, anorexia, diarrhea, direct irritation of footpads, mouth, or pharynx from contaminated water	Flush skin or eyes with cold water, water or egg whites for ingested salts, supportive therapy
Fire extinguisher chemicals	2–4	Chlorobromomethane, methylbromide, or halogenated hydrocarbons consisting of brominated or chlorinated fluoromethanes (100% concentration)	Irritation of skin and eyes, vomiting, CNS signs, hypotension, coma, pulmonary edema	Flush with water or wash with soap and water, supportive therapy for acidosis, pneumonia, renal failure, convulsions
Fireplace colors	3–4 possibly higher	Coke dust, sawdust, heavy metal salts (e.g., copper, chloride, rubidium and cesium compounds, lead, arsenic, selenium, tellurium, barium, molybdenum, antimony, zinc, borates, phosphates)	Severe gastroenteritis, vomiting, and diarrhea, followed by depression, shock, and renal failure	Gastrointestinal decontamination as appropriate
Fireworks	3–4	Fireworks contain oxidizing agents (e.g., potassium nitrate, chlorates); colors are produced by heavy metal salts (e.g., mercury, antimony, copper, strontium, barium, phosphorus)	Vomiting, severe abdominal pain, bloody feces, rapid, shallow breathing, methemoglobinemia, and death from respiratory or cardiac failure; other signs relate to specific effects of toxic heavy metals	Oral decontamination followed by demulcents and adsorbents; supportive treatment for methemoglobinemia
Fluxes	3–4	Zinc chloride; hydrochloric acid (0%–40%); salts of aniline, glutamic, and salicylic acid; aliphatic alcohols; terpenes; hydrocarbons; boric acid and fluorides (silver solder)	Irritation of the mouth, gastrointestinal tract, or skin; nausea, vomiting, and diarrhea; ataxia, delirium, and excitement, progressing to stupor or coma (organic solvents)	Gastrointestinal decontamination should be performed unless severe corrosive damage has occurred, which would contraindicate gastric lavage; methylene blue to treat methemoglobinemia from aniline salts
Matches	2	Potassium chlorate	Methemoglobinemia with cyanosis and hemolysis	Methylene blue or ascorbic acid to treat methemoglobinemia
Photographic developer	4–5	Boric acid, p-methyl aminophenol sulfite, ammonium thiosulfate, potassium thiocyanate, sodium hydroxide	p-Methyl aminophenol sulfite causes methemoglobinemia; corrosive and caustic effects may result from the acids and alkalies	General oral decontamination; methylene blue or ascorbic acid to treat methemoglobinemia

*On a scale of 1–6, where 1 is relatively harmless and 6 is extremely toxic (see Table 1-1).
CNS = central nervous system.

TABLE 25-2. Clinical Toxicology of Household Cleaning Supplies

Product	Toxicity Rating*	Ingredients	Clinical Presentation	Treatment
Bleach	3	Approximately 5% sodium hypochlorite	Acid solutions combined with hypochlorite bleaches can cause release of chlorine gas and hypochlorous acid, presenting an acute inhalation hazard characterized by pain and inflammation of the mouth, pharynx, esophagus, and stomach; oral ingestion results in irritation with edema of the pharynx, glottis, larynx, and lungs	Activated charcoal may minimize damage from hypochlorite; magnesium oxide should be administered to neutralize stomach acids
Drain cleaners		Sodium hydroxide, sodium hypochlorite	Necrosis (coagulative to liquefaction) and ulceration of the oral mucosa and, possibly, the esophagus; sequelae include strictures, laryngeal or glottal edema, asphyxiation, and pneumonia	Flushing with large volumes of water, milk, or dilute vinegar; pain relievers, supportive treatment for shock; liquid diets and surgical intervention if strictures develop
Furniture polish	3	Vehicles include petroleum distillates, mineral spirits, or petroleum hydrocarbons	Depression, coma, seizures, vomiting (see Chapter 18 II F)	Activated charcoal or nonabsorbable oil (see Chapter 18 II G)
Metal cleaners/oven cleaners	3–4	Caustic soda or potash (alkaline cleaners); kerosene, high concentrations of chlorinated ethylenes or 1,1,1-trichloroethane (solvent cleaners); hydrochloric, sulfuric, chromic, or phosphoric acids	Necrosis, vomiting (see Chapter 10 II A–C)	Activated charcoal followed by a moderate dose of saline cathartic
Pine oil disinfectants	3	Both pine oils (terpenes) and phenols may be present, as well as synthetic phenol derivatives (e.g., o-phenyl phenol)	Gastritis, vomiting, and diarrhea are followed by depression, unconsciousness, or mild seizures; phenol causes tissue necrosis, tremors and mild seizures followed by depression and renal tubular necrosis	Decontamination therapy using mineral oil followed by gastric lavage with water, taking precautions to prevent aspiration; demulcents or protectants for gastrointestinal damage; fluids to maintain hydration and maximize urine output if renal function is adequate; artificial respiration or supportive therapy for renal damage
Shoe polish	2	Animal, petroleum, or vegetable waxes and mineral spirits or turpentine; aniline dyes and nitrobenzene or terpenes may also be present	Large amounts could produce methemoglobinemia (typical of petroleum hydrocarbon ingestion)	Activated charcoal or a nonabsorbable oil (see Chapter 18 II G); methylene blue or ascorbic acid for methemoglobinemia

*On a scale of 1–6, where 1 is relatively harmless and 6 is extremely toxic (see Table 1-1).

TABLE 25-3. Clinical Toxicology of Selected Toiletries

Product	Toxicity Rating*	Ingredients	Clinical Presentation	Treatment
Deodorant/ antiperspirant	3	Deodorants contain a cream base and an antibacterial agent; antiperspirants also contain from 15%–20% aluminum salts (e.g., aluminum chlorohydrate, aluminum chloride); less commonly used antiperspirant agents include titanium dioxide, oxyquinoline sulfate, and zirconium salts	Gingival necrosis and hemorrhagic gastroenteritis, sometimes accompanied by incoordination and nephrosis; severe effects are rare unless large amounts of the active ingredient are ingested	Gastrointestinal decontamination with appropriate supportive therapy
Denture cleaners	4	Perborates decompose to form hydrogen peroxide and sodium borate, which are strongly alkaline and very irritating	Salivation, vomiting, early stimulation of the CNS followed by depression, nonspecific liver and kidney damage, hypertrophy of the filiform papillae	Extensive flushing with water, application of demulcents or ointments, gastric lavage (taking care not to aggravate existing damage to the upper alimentary tract), symptomatic treatment for shock
Perfumes	3–4	Alcohol, essential oils (e.g., savin, rue, tansy, apiol, juniper, cedar leaf, cajupute)	Essential oils are often hepatotoxic or nephrotoxic and may irritate the skin, mucous membranes, and lungs, resulting in aspiration, pulmonary edema, and pneumonitis; albuminuria, hematuria, and glycosuria result from renal damage; CNS effects include excitement, ataxia, disorientation, and coma; odor of volatile oils may be present in expired air or in vomitus	Because of the possibility of aspiration pneumonia from volatile hydrocarbons, gastric lavage and emesis should be used cautiously
Rubbing alcohol	2–3	Ethanol or isopropyl alcohol	Disorientation, ataxia, weakness, depression, irritation of mucous membranes	Diuresis with furosemide, gastric lavage and/or administration of activated charcoal

TABLE 25-3. Continued

Product	Toxicity Rating*	Ingredients	Clinical Presentation	Treatment
Shampoos	3	Surfactants, fragrance, sodium lauryl sulfate or triethanolamine dodecyl sulfate; antidandruff shampoos contain one or more metals (e.g., zinc pyridinethione, selenium sulfide) and coal tar derivatives or salicylic acid	Only mild toxicosis is expected in most cases; progressive blindness has been reported in dogs or cats ingesting zinc pyridinethione; lesions include retinal detachment, severe exudative chorioretinitis, and blindness	Emesis or gastric lavage if ingested dosage is large, followed by activated charcoal and a saline cathartic; demulcents or other protectants may be used if vomiting or diarrhea persist
Suntan lotion	2	Alcohol	See "Rubbing alcohol" above	See "Rubbing alcohol" above
Styptic pencil	2	Potassium alum sulfate	Corrosive lesions from sulfuric acid formed during hydrolysis of the salt	Treat for pain and dehydration as indicated; lavage and emetics are not recommended because exposure to acid is involved; neutralizers (e.g., magnesium oxide) may be used; sodium bicarbonate is contraindicated because carbon dioxide gas formation could occur in response to the acid

*On a scale of 1–6, where 1 is relatively harmless and 6 is extremely toxic (see Table 1-1).
CNS = central nervous system.

DIRECTIONS: Each of the numbered items or incomplete statements in this section is followed by answers or by completions of the statement. Select the **one** numbered answer or completion that is **best** in each case.

1. Which one of the following laboratory parameters is decreased in advanced, acute ethylene glycol toxicosis?

(1) Serum anion gap
(2) Blood pH
(3) Urine glycolate
(4) Urinary oxalate crystals
(5) Serum potassium

DIRECTIONS: Each of the numbered items or incomplete statements in this section is negatively phrased, as indicated by an italicized word such as *not, least,* or *except.* Select the **one** numbered answer or completion that is **best** in each case.

---

2. A 4-year-old male cat is diagnosed with ethylene glycol toxicosis. All of the following could be used in the treatment of this cat *except:*

(1) ethanol.
(2) 4-methylpyrazole (4-MP).
(3) sodium bicarbonate.
(4) calcium borogluconate.
(5) corticosteroids.

3. In acute toxicosis caused by consumption of a product with a high phenol content, all of the following treatment measures are indicated *except*:

(1) administration of milk or egg whites.
(2) administration of emetics or gastric lavage.
(3) administration of activated charcoal and a saline cathartic.
(4) pain control.
(5) supportive therapy for shock and hepatic or renal failure.

4. All of the following statements are true about ethylene glycol exposure and toxicosis in small animals *except*:

(1) on a body weight basis, the lethal dosage of ethylene glycol is less in cats than in dogs.
(2) most of the ingested ethylene glycol is excreted unchanged in the urine.
(3) because of charge and polarity, ethylene glycol does not cross the blood–brain barrier.
(4) metabolic products of ethylene glycol include glycoaldehyde, glycolic acid, and glyoxylic acid.
(5) metabolic acidosis caused by ethylene glycol is primarily caused by glycolic acid.

DIRECTIONS: Each group of items in this section consists of numbered options followed by a set of numbered items. For each item, select the **one** numbered option that is most closely associated with it. Each numbered option may be selected once, more than once, or not at all.

Questions 5–8

Match each description with the household chemical it characterizes.

(1) Fertilizers
(2) Glues and adhesives
(3) Bleach
(4) Perfume

5. Contains essential oils that cause central nervous system (CNS) signs; tends to be hepatotoxic or nephrotoxic

6. Highly volatile vehicle is largely responsible for this product's toxicity

7. Ingredients denoted by the formula "n-n-n"

8. Releases highly irritating gas when combined with acid-based cleaning solutions

1. The answer is 2 *[II G 2].* The only laboratory parameter that decreases in ethylene glycol toxicosis is the blood pH, which is driven down by the metabolic acidosis caused by the acid intermediates of ethylene glycol. The serum anion gap increases because of increased osmolality as a result of increased concentrations of small molecules (e.g., the acid intermediates). Many of these metabolites are eventually excreted in urine, including glycolate. Urine glycolate levels correlate well with the severity of toxicosis. Oxalate crystals appear in the urine because the oxalic acid complexes with calcium to form insoluble calcium oxalate, which may precipitate as rosette-shaped birefringent crystals in the blood vessels, renal cortex, and urine.

2. The answer is 2 *[II H].* Although 4-methylpyrazole (4-MP) prevents the formation of acid intermediates in dogs that have ingested ethylene glycol, it has not been shown effective in cats and is not currently recommended as an antidote for this species. Ethanol has been used for many years to reduce the metabolism of ethylene glycol by competing for available alcohol dehydrogenase. Sodium bicarbonate is important to counteract metabolic acidosis. Calcium borogluconate is useful to counteract hypocalcemia, which results from the formation of complexes between oxalate and serum calcium. Corticosteroids are useful in the treatment of shock and pulmonary edema, which are complications of ethylene glycol toxicosis.

3. The answer is 2 *[III F].* Phenols are direct protoplasmic poisons that cause coagulation necrosis and intense pain followed by hepatic and renal damage. Because there is a risk of causing additional damage to the esophagus or gastric mucosa by inducing emesis or applying gastric lavage, these procedures are not recommended. Instead, first aid consisting of administration of a bland material that contains protein (e.g., egg white, milk) dilutes the phenol and provides additional protein for it to bind to. The use of activated charcoal and a saline cathartic is also recommended to adsorb any remaining phenols. Supportive therapy for shock and hepatic or renal failure is advised.

4. The answer is 3 *[II D 1–2, E 1–2, F].* Ethylene glycol is a small, uncharged molecule that readily passes the blood–brain barrier, causing transient inebriation before the metabolites form that lead to metabolic acidosis. Ethylene glycol is only mildly toxic until it undergoes biotransformation. The major metabolites are glycoaldehyde, glycolic acid, and glyoxylic acid, with glycolic acid being most important in the development of metabolic acidosis. Although it has toxic metabolites, most ingested and absorbed ethylene glycol is excreted rapidly and unchanged in the urine.

5–8. The answers are: 5-4 *[Table 25-3],* **6-2** *[Table 25-1],* **7-1** *[I B 1 b],* **8-3** *[Table 25-2].* Perfumes are carried in either water or alcohol vehicles and contain a variety of essential oils extracted from natural sources. Early effects from their ingestion include inebriation, ataxia, or disorientation; liver or kidney necrosis develops later. Ingestion of essential oils requires prompt detoxification therapy; however, their volatile nature may preclude emesis or gastric lavage.

Many questions arise from owners regarding the nature of animals chewing or ingesting products that contain adhesives. The volatile compounds in fresh adhesives (e.g., hydrocarbon solvents, naphtha) are often quite toxic to the central nervous system (CNS) and respiratory tract and present an inhalation hazard. Once the carriers have volatilized and the product has hardened or polymerized, it is nearly inert, unaffected by digestive processes, and, therefore, essentially nontoxic.

The conventional formula used to denote the ingredients in fertilizer states the percentage of nitrogen, phosphate, and potassium. Therefore, 10-6-6 would indicate 10% nitrogen, 6% phosphate, and 6% potassium. Knowledge of this notation allows quick determination of the major ingredients in a fertilizer.

Sodium hypochlorite, the most common ingredient in laundry bleach, is usually found in concentrations of 5%. Combination of sodium hypochlorite with an acid causes the release of chlorine gas, which presents an acute inhalation hazard. Characteristic signs include acute conjunctivitis and inflammation of the nasal passages, larynx, trachea, and, possibly, the lungs. Edema of the pharynx, larynx, glottis, and lungs is potentially life-threatening.

Chapter 26

Feed-Related Toxicoses

I. INTRODUCTION

A. **Feed** is any edible material prepared for and offered to livestock, exclusive of growing forages, silage, and cured hay.

B. **Sources of feed-related toxicoses**

1. **Additives.** Toxicoses may be related to additives that are mixed or formulated into the basic feedstuffs. For example:
   a. **Antibiotics** and antibacterials (e.g., sulfonamides, nitrofurans, lincomycin)
   b. **Antiparasitic drugs** (e.g., coccidiostats, phenothiazine)
   c. **Growth or performance enhancers** (e.g., ionophores, organic iodine)
   d. **Metals** (e.g., copper, molybdenum, arsenic, selenium; see Chapter 17)

2. **Excessive or improper use of nutrients** may cause toxicosis.
   a. **Nonprotein nitrogen (NPN) products** (e.g., urea, ammonium salts)
   b. **Ammoniation of dietary carbohydrates**
   c. **Raw soybeans**
   d. **Gossypol**

3. **Alterations in feedstuffs** as a result of harvest or storage can produce toxicosis. For example:
   a. **Wilted forages** can cause the release of free cyanide. Conversion of nitrate to nitrite is discussed in Chapter 28 VIII D 1.
   b. **Mycotoxins** are discussed in Chapter 29.

C. **General characteristics of feed-related toxicoses**

1. **Distribution of toxicant.** Toxic ingredients may be mixed uniformly in the feed, favoring relatively equivalent delivery of toxicant to the entire herd. Therefore:
   a. Highly toxic chemicals carry a relatively high morbidity (attack) rate.
   b. Differences in response are caused by animal or environmental factors, rather than differences in dosage.
   c. If only a portion of the herd is affected, the potential for residues exists in the remainder, because of the wide distribution of the toxicant to the unaffected members of the herd.
   d. Animals often are affected similarly within a relatively narrow time frame, due to consistent availability and dosage.

2. **Differential susceptibility.** Any herd has differential susceptibility to the same dose, according to the laws of normal distribution. Except when there are very high concentrations of toxicant in the feed, a range of responses may be seen. Some animals may be seriously poisoned and die, others may be moderately or mildly affected, and some may remain unaffected.

3. **Probable cause.** A recent change in the source or mixing of feed, or addition of new ingredients, is often the cause of toxicosis. However, a change in feed or ingredients without other supporting documentation is not sufficient evidence to confirm a toxicosis.

4. **Liability issues.** Feed-related toxicoses are often followed by questions of liability for damages and assessment of blame.

  a. Potential feed-related cases should be well documented (in writing) by the attending veterinarian.
  b. Representative samples of feed as actually fed to animals should be collected, identified, labelled, and properly stored. Legal claims may arise months or even years after the event.

II. ANTIBIOTICS AND ANTIBACTERIALS

A. Lincomycin

1. Pharmacology
  a. Chemistry. Lincosamide antibiotics are monobasic derivatives of an amino acid- and sulfur-containing octose.
  b. Mechanism of action. Lincomycin binds to 50S subunits of bacterial ribosomes and inhibits protein synthesis.
  c. Pharmacokinetics. Lincomycin is absorbed from the gastrointestinal tract, metabolized in the liver, and excreted in bile and urine.
  d. Pharmacologic effects. Lincomycin and a closely related human antibiotic, clindamycin, are generally inhibitory to gram-positive cocci, but not to gram-negative bacteria. Of the *Clostridia, Clostridium difficile* is usually resistant.
  e. Normal dosage. Feed concentration for swine is 20–200 ppm (g/ton). For chickens, it is 2–4 ppm, for both preventive and therapeutic purposes.
  f. Adverse effects. Swine may develop diarrhea, swelling of the anus, or both within 2 days of beginning treatment. Rarely, reddening of the skin and irritability may occur in swine. These conditions resolve within 5–8 days without treatment.

2. Toxicology. Horses, guinea pigs, hamsters, and rabbits appear uniquely sensitive to lincomycin, and, if exposed to generally acceptable feed levels for swine, may experience severe gastrointestinal hemorrhage and necrosis. Similar effects in these species are caused by tetracyclines.
  a. Exposure. Accidental access to feeds containing lincomycin is the most common cause of feed-related toxicosis from lincomycin, and horses are most commonly affected.
  b. Mechanism of toxicologic damage. Apparently, toxins from proliferation of *C. difficile* are the cause of toxicosis.
  c. Clinical signs are similar to those of "colitis X" in horses, and include acute necrotizing colitis, colic, diarrhea, dehydration, and shock.
  d. Treatment is only nonspecific and supportive; the mortality rate in clinical cases is very high.

B. Nitrofurans are mainly of historical importance; their use is currently restricted or prohibited in food animals.

1. Pharmacology
  a. Preparations and therapeutic uses. Nitrofurans are yellow-colored synthetic antibacterials formerly used as bacteriostats and coccidiostats. They are powders or crystals that are generally sparingly soluble in water.
  (1) Nitrofurazone was used as a feed additive to treat swine enteritis (dosage, 500 ppm) and poultry coccidiosis (dosage, 50–150 ppm).
  (2) Nitrofurantoin has been used to treat chronic respiratory and urinary tract infections in horses and small animals.
  (3) Furazolidone was used to treat bacterial enteritis in swine (dosage, 100–300 ppm) and as a coccidiostat for chickens, turkeys, and rabbits. It is currently used for turkeys and swine at dosages of 110 ppm and 220 ppm, respectively, to prevent and treat bacterial diseases.

b. Mechanism of action. Nitrofurans inhibit the enzymes of the tricarboxylic acid (TCA) cycle, interfering with aerobic oxidation of glucose. Metabolically active tissues highly dependent on aerobic metabolism (e.g., brain, testes, kidney, liver) are most susceptible to nitrofuran toxicosis.

2. Toxicology

a. Exposure. Misuse of remaining supplies of nitrofurans by individuals could result in toxicosis.

b. Mechanism of toxicologic damage. Furazolidone toxicosis may be mediated by action on the TCA cycle. Pyruvate and lactate are increased, possibly indicating a decreased conversion of pyruvate to acetyl coenzyme A.

c. Toxicity and clinical signs

(1) Nitrofurazone

(a) Rats. The oral LD_{50} in rats is approximately 500 mg/kg. Clinical signs are mainly neurologic, including irritability, tremors, weakness, convulsions, and apnea.

(b) Dogs. In dogs, hepatitis, depression, diarrhea, and vomiting occur when the dosage exceeds 2.0 mg/kg by IV injection. Oral dosages of 50 mg/kg cause neurologic signs.

(c) Poultry. Single oral doses of 150–200 mg/kg cause either depression or seizures in young chicks.

(d) Calves

(i) Nitrofurazone causes death in calves dosed daily for 5 days at 30 mg/kg.

(ii) Dosages of 15 mg/kg produce seizures within approximately 20 days, and further exposure may cause death.

(iii) Dairy calves given nitrofurazone in water at > 30 mg/kg body weight develop acute clinical signs within 24–48 hours of the initial treatment. Clinical signs include opisthotonus, tremors, circling, and intermittent seizures.

(2) Furazolidone

(a) Poultry

(i) Continued use of 200 ppm in feed may reduce the hatchability of eggs and delay the onset of egg production in hens or reproduction in cockerels.

(ii) Furazolidone at 400 ppm in the diet of broilers, when fed with amprolium, causes abnormal posture and ataxia.

(iii) Concentrations of furazolidone above 500 ppm reduce growth in poultry.

(iv) Cardiomyopathy occurs at dosages of 500–700 ppm. Cardiac hypertrophy in poultry is known as "round heart disease," and is characterized by increased moisture content and cardiac glycogen deposition. Mortality in turkeys and chicks appears correlated with increased heart:body weight ratio.

(b) Swine. High dosages (i.e., greater than 600 ppm) cause mild ataxia with paresis of the hind limbs in a syndrome similar to that of arsanilic acid toxicosis. When combined with arsanilic acid feed additive, furazolidone concentrations of 400 ppm may be neurotoxic to swine.

(i) The gait includes hypermetria (goose stepping) or posterior weakness.

(ii) Clinical signs are worse when swine are excited.

d. Diagnosis. Chemical analysis of the diet will confirm if overdosage in the feed occurred. Nitrofurans are rapidly metabolized and excreted; therefore, analysis of tissues may not be helpful.

e. Treatment

   (1) **Supportive therapy** is necessary to correct renal insufficiency, dehydration, or malnutrition.

   (2) **Good nursing care** may be important to recovery.

C. Sulfonamides

1. Pharmacology

  a. Preparations. Water medication or feed additive sulfonamides include sulfathiazole, sulfamethazine, sulfamerazine, and sulfachlorpyridazine.

  b. Pharmacokinetics. Sulfonamides are usually metabolized by conjugation or acetylation and excreted in the urine.

  c. Adverse effects

   (1) Long-term administration of sulfonamides at therapeutic dosages can inhibit iodine metabolism, resulting in goiters and thyroid hyperplasia.

   (2) Agranulocytosis and hypoprothrombinemia are reported, especially from sulfaquinoxaline use in poultry.

   (3) Sulfaquinoxaline causes a vitamin K–responsive coagulopathy in poultry and dogs, apparently by interfering with vitamin K–dependent synthesis of coagulation factors.

   (4) Peripheral neuritis and reduced egg production may occur in poultry.

2. Toxicology

  a. Exposure. Sulfonamide toxicosis can occur through individual dosing or therapeutic applications in feed. Most cases result from overdosing animals individually, or from feeding sulfonamides to animals that have limited water supplies or high fluid losses as a result of diarrhea.

  b. Mechanisms of toxicologic damage

   (1) **"Drug shock."** Rapid intravenous injection causes an acute "drug shock" with collapse and possible death.

   (2) **Uremia.** Renal tubules may become obstructed by sulfonamide crystals after 5–7 days of sulfonamide exposure if the dosage is excessive or adequate water is not available.

    (a) Sulfonamides are insoluble in acid aqueous solutions and increase in solubility as urine pH increases. Renal tubule crystalluria occurs mainly in cats and dogs, which produce an acid urine.

    (b) Renal tubular crystal formation occurs when renal excretion is high. Dehydration and low urine output predispose to chronic renal toxicosis.

   (3) **Hypersensitivity.** A hypersensitivity reaction (sometimes known as "drug fever") similar to an anaphylactoid reaction may result after repeated exposure. Respiratory difficulty and urticaria are the major clinical signs. Anaphylactoid reactions are nonspecific.

  c. Diagnosis

   (1) **Acute toxicosis.** Diagnosis of the acute "drug shock" phenomenon is based largely on history and symptomatology, and the cause usually is evident enough to warrant a diagnosis. **Clinical signs** of acute toxicosis include salivation, vomiting, diarrhea, and polypnea; weakness, ataxia, and spastic rigidity are relatively rare.

   (2) **Chronic uremic toxicosis**

    (a) **Clinical signs** of the uremic form include anorexia, depression, with hematuria, albuminuria, and oliguria. Sulfonamide crystals are visible on preputial or vulvar hair.

    (b) **Laboratory diagnosis.** Increased blood urea nitrogen (BUN) levels and plasma sulfonamide levels above 15 mg/100 ml is supportive of a diagnosis.

    (c) **Lesions.** Microscopic examination reveals sulfonamide crystals in the renal tubules and renal pelvis. The kidney sample must be fixed in acidified formalin solution or absolute ethanol to preserve the crystals.

(3) Chronic toxicosis in poultry and dogs. Bone marrow depression with granulocytopenia, anemia, and hypoprothrombinemia suggest sulfaquinoxaline toxicosis in poultry or dogs. Analysis of muscle, kidney, or liver tissue reveals sulfonamide concentrations above 20 ppm.

d. Treatment
    (1) Restoration of renal function is necessary.
    (2) Rehydration. Normal saline and bicarbonate may be administered intravenously, along with oral electrolytes and water.
    (3) Epinephrine and **antihistamines** are used as needed to treat hypersensitivity reactions.

D. Tiamulin

1. Pharmacology
    a. Pharmacokinetics. Tiamulin is readily absorbed from dietary sources.
    b. Therapeutic uses. Tiamulin fumarate acts against gram-positive bacteria, *Mycoplasma,* and *Serpulina hyodysenteriae.*

2. Toxicology
    a. Mechanism of toxicologic damage. Concurrent use of tiamulin and monensin in swine or poultry has caused ionophore toxicosis (see IV A 2), myonecrosis, and death. Tiamulin itself is of low toxicity, but it interferes with the metabolism and elimination of polyether ionophores (e.g., monensin, salinomycin, lasalocid, narasin).
    b. Prevention. Adequate or elevated selenium and vitamin E appear somewhat protective against the toxic interaction of tiamulin and ionophores.

III. ANTIPARASITIC DRUGS

A. Phenothiazine (PTZ)

1. Pharmacology
    a. Therapeutic uses
        (1) PTZ has been used as an **anthelmintic** since the 1930s, primarily **in ruminants and horses.** Relatively high toxicity has limited or prevented its use in swine, dogs, and cats.
        (2) PTZ has been used in low-level prophylactic feeding programs to **reduce parasite egg production,** but this has largely been supplanted by safer and more effective anthelmintics.
    b. Pharmacokinetics. Metabolism of PTZ to **phenothiazine sulfoxide** in the gastrointestinal mucosa is followed by oxidation in the liver to form leucophenothiazine and leucothionol, which are excreted in the urine. Upon exposure to sunlight, these urinary metabolites are further oxidized to reddish-brown dyes (phenothiazine and thionol) that color the urine and milk a red to red-brown color for several days after treatment.

2. Toxicology
    a. Mechanism of toxicologic damage. Toxicosis results from **excessive amounts of phenothiazine sulfoxide**.
        (1) Phenothiazine sulfoxide may permeate the ocular fluids and dermis, producing **photophobia** and **photosensitization**.
        (2) Excess phenothiazine causes **hemolytic anemia, icterus, hemoglobinuria, anorexia, colic, fever,** and **oliguria.**
    b. Toxicity. Doses of more than 30–50 g per adult horse have been toxic, depending on the initial condition of the animal. Anemic and debilitated animals are more susceptible to toxicosis from overdosage or continuous exposure in feed.
    c. Diagnosis of suspected toxicosis may be confirmed by analysis of the urine for phenothiazine or its metabolites, correlated with a history of exposure and typical clinical signs.

    d. Treatment involves supportive therapy for anemia and photosensitization and symptomatic therapy.

B. **Amprolium** is a competitive antagonist of thiamine **used as a coccidiostat in poultry and cattle.**

    1. Feeding concentrations of two to ten times the recommended concentration for 3 weeks or more has caused **polyneuritis in poultry.**

    2. Extremely excessive dosages (i.e., 50 times greater than the recommended dosage) have been associated with **polioencephalomalacia in preruminant calves and lambs.** However, this is unlikely to occur under most conditions of use.

IV. GROWTH AND PERFORMANCE ENHANCERS

A. **Ionophores** include monensin, lasalocid, salinomycin, and narasin.

    1. Pharmacology
        a. Chemistry. Ionophores are biologically active compounds produced by **Streptomyces cinnamonensis.** They are classified as **polyethers.**
        b. Uses
            (1) Initially, ionophores were developed as **poultry coccidiostats** and used at 100 g/ton of feed.
            (2) In ruminants, ionophores enhance propionic acid production by altering rumen fermentation. They are used in **feedlot cattle** at 5–30 ppm of finished ration **to improve feed efficiency** by 10%–20%.
        c. Mechanism of action. Because of their ability to transport specific alkali metal cations across cell membranes, ionophores are antibiotic. They selectively transport sodium and potassium ions between extracellular and intracellular spaces.
        d. Pharmacokinetics
            (1) **Absorption** is low at recommended feeding levels.
            (2) **Liver metabolism** converts the parent compound to several polar metabolites.
            (3) **Excretion** is primarily via feces; most of the drug is not absorbed at all.

    2. Toxicology
        a. Mechanisms of toxicologic damage
            (1) **Interference with potassium transport.** Ionophores interact with the carrier mechanism that regulates potassium transport across mitochondrial membranes, inhibiting adenosine triphosphate (ATP) hydrolysis and diminishing cellular energy production. Electron micrographs have confirmed that monensin causes severe mitochondrial damage.
            (2) **Interference with calcium transport.** Some evidence indicates that ionophores may alter calcium transport by changing the sodium component of the sodium–calcium exchange diffusion carrier in cell membranes, leading to the accumulation of calcium in the cells and mitochondria and possibly causing cell death.
        b. Toxicity (Table 26-1). Acute or subacute poisoning is of most concern. Horses are at greatest risk.
            (1) **Horses** can be poisoned by feed containing 100 ppm monensin (i.e., the poultry feeding level) and have been killed by eating feed containing 300 ppm (i.e., the premix level).
            (2) **Cattle.** Clinical signs have been observed at 3–5 times the recommended feeding level in cattle. Apparent field cases of toxicosis and experimental trials are not in agreement regarding toxicity in cattle.
                (a) Field cases of toxicosis in cattle have been associated with feed containing 50–160 ppm monensin offered at approximately 1.6% of body weight.

TABLE 26-1. LD$_{50}$ Values for Ionophore Toxicosis

Species	Monensin	Lasalocid	Salinomycin
Horses	2–3 mg/kg	21.5 mg/kg	0.6 mg/kg
Dogs	20 mg/kg		
Rats	35 mg/kg		
Cattle	22 mg/kg		
Mice	125 mg/kg		
Chickens	200 mg/kg		

*Single dose by gavage.

     (b) Studies of monensin given to cattle at 300 ppm indicate feed consumption reduced by 90% within 3 days. No mortality was observed.

c. Diagnosis

  (1) Clinical signs

    (a) Horses

       (i) Initial signs include partial to complete anorexia, uneasiness, and profuse, intermittent sweating. Fever is variable. Polyuria occurs early, followed by a terminal oliguria.

      (ii) Intermediate signs include progressive ataxia (12–36 hours postexposure) followed by colic and stiffness ("tying up"). Posterior paresis and intermittent recumbency and standing occur as signs progress.

     (iii) Advanced signs. Tachycardia, hypotension, hyperventilation, and dyspnea are terminal, indicating a grave prognosis.

    (b) Cattle

       (i) Signs of acute toxicosis include anorexia (24–36 hours postexposure), depression, weakness, ataxia, dyspnea, and diarrhea (36–48 hours postexposure). Cattle recovered from acute toxicosis may experience collapse and death during periods of exertion or high environmental temperatures.

      (ii) Signs of subacute toxicosis are indicative of reduced cardiac function and congestive heart failure.

  (2) Laboratory diagnosis

    (a) Serum alkaline phosphatase (AP) is increased moderately to markedly, and isoenzyme distribution is associated with bone AP.

    (b) Bilirubin levels increase after 24 hours as a result of unconjugated bilirubin.

    (c) BUN levels are elevated early, and may return to normal.

    (d) Serum calcium is moderately reduced (e.g., by 10%–15%) for 12–18 hours.

    (e) Creatine kinase levels are from three to one hundred times greater than normal as a result of skeletal muscle necrosis.

    (f) Serum creatinine increases within 24–36 hours, and may return to normal.

    (g) Hematocrit is elevated.

    (h) Lactate dehydrogenase (LDH) levels increase for 36 hours, mainly from myocardial and erythrocyte sources.

    (i) Serum potassium is decreased after 24 hours, but may recover in survivors.

    (j) Aspartate transaminase (AST) levels increase.

    (k) Feed analysis is most commonly used to establish exposure. **Tissue analysis** is difficult to perform and the results are difficult to interpret; most laboratories do not offer this service.

  (3) Lesions

    (a) Gross lesions are mild hemopericardium, epicardial hemorrhages, and a pale myocardium. Hydrothorax, ascites, and pulmonary edema may be present in cattle.

(b) Microscopic lesions include pale cardiac myofibers, loss of muscle cross-striations, multifocal vacuolar degeneration of cardiac muscle, and scattered areas of myocardial necrosis along with attempts at myocardial regeneration and replacement with fibrous tissue. Toxic nephrosis, tubular hydropic degeneration, and toxic hepatitis may also occur.

d. Treatment
    (1) Detoxification. Prompt gastrointestinal decontamination should be performed using activated charcoal and a saline cathartic.
    (2) Supportive treatment
        (a) Fluids and electrolytes should be administered to correct changes in the hematocrit, serum potassium, and serum calcium.
        (b) Early administration of selenium and vitamin E may lessen the severity of muscle damage.

B. **Organic iodine**

1. Pharmacology
    a. Source. Iodine is a trace element that occurs at 1 part/15 million in the earth's crust. Major sources include **seaweed** and the **nitrate-bearing Chilean caliche rock.**
    b. Preparations and therapeutic uses
        (1) Potassium iodide is used to treat *Actinobacillus* and *Fusobacterium* infections.
        (2) Ethylenediamine dihydriodide (EDDI)
            (a) EDDI was used as a feed additive for **prevention of foot rot** and **lumpy jaw** and as a **mild expectorant,** but it is no longer cleared for these uses.
            (b) Nutritional supplement. EDDI is added to the rations of cattle to correct iodine deficiency. Cattle require 0.5–1 mg/day iodine.
                (i) EDDI is prohibited in dairy cattle.
                (ii) The Northeast and Northwest United States are areas of endemic goiter.

2. Toxicology
    a. Toxicity. Acute toxicosis is rare; subacute or chronic effects are more likely. The minimal toxicologic response occurs at dosages of 250–1250 mg/day.
    b. Diagnosis
        (1) Clinical signs
            (a) Dosages of 1000 mg EDDI/day for 1 week produce mild expectorant action and serous nasal discharge. The clinical signs subside 2–3 days after EDDI is removed from the diet.
            (b) Dosages of 250–1250 mg EDDI/day produce a dose-related response (characterized by coughing, mucopurulent nasal secretions, seromucous ocular discharge, and excess salivation) within 30 days. After approximately 30 days, calves develop hyperkeratosis, rough hair, exfoliative dermatosis, and alopecia. Changes are prominent on the dorsum of the animal and in the periorbital region.
            (c) At dosages of 1250 mg EDDI/day, signs persist for 2–3 months. At 250 mg/day, signs diminish after 6 weeks.
            (d) High doses of iodine appear to interfere with titers to some antigens, reduce lymphoblastogenesis, decrease phagocytosis, and lower leukocyte counts. Impaired humoral and cellular immunity may be responsible for the increased occurrence of infectious disease and the decreased response to therapy.
        (2) Laboratory diagnosis
            (a) Total serum iodine increases according to the iodine dose: Dosages of 50 mg/day produce serum iodine levels of 300 ng/ml; dosages of 1000 mg/day produce serum iodine levels of 1400 ng/ml.
            (b) At dosages of 1250 mg EDDI/day, **serum triiodothyronine (T_3)** and **thyroxine (T_4)** decrease by 50% within 3 to 7 weeks. Levels of less than 250 mg/day do not affect thyroid function.

(3) Lesions
  (a) Gross lesions include focal dermal exfoliation, congested conjunctiva, excessive nasal discharge, bronchopneumonia with consolidation of the apical and cardiac lobes, enlarged mediastinal lymph nodes, congestion of the tracheal mucosa, and serous to mucopurulent tracheal exudate.
  (b) Microscopic lesions
    (i) Tracheal lesions include mucosal ulceration and congestion, necrotic areas, squamous metaplasia, and lymphocytic and neutrophilic multiple focal tracheitis.
    (ii) Lung lesions are typical of fibrinous or purulent bronchoalveolar pneumonia.
    (iii) Thyroid lesions. Flat or low columnar epithelium, pale granular colloid, and degenerative follicular nuclei are present.

V. NONPROTEIN NITROGEN (NPN) PRODUCTS are added to the feed of ruminants to provide up to 40% of their protein nitrogen requirements.

A. Introduction

1. **Products.** NPN products and the nitrogen they provide are summarized in Table 26-2. **Major ingredients** used today are **urea** or **urea phosphate**. The structure of urea is shown in Figure 26-1.

2. **Delivery forms**
   a. **Feed.** NPN products are available as **dry supplements** for mixing or blending into rations.
   b. **Range blocks** and **range cubes** can contain urea or ammonium salts.
   c. **Lick tanks,** used in pasture and range conditions, contain **liquid supplements** (molasses–NPN combinations).

3. **Calculations**
   a. **Protein equivalent of NPN product.** The protein equivalent is the protein value gained from a given amount of urea. The protein equivalent can be determined from the nitrogen content.
   (1) Protein is approximately 16% nitrogen. Therefore:

$$PE = N \times \frac{100}{16}$$

$$N \times 6.25, \text{ where}$$

PE = protein equivalent and N = nitrogen content

   (2) Example. Feed-grade urea contains 45% nitrogen; therefore, the protein equivalent = 45% × 6.25 = 281%.

TABLE 26-2. Nonprotein Nitrogen (NPN) Products

Source	Nitrogen (%)
Feed-grade urea	45%
Feed-grade biuret*	37%
Diammonium phosphate†	17%
Ammonium polyphosphate solution	9%
Ammonium sulfate	21%
Monoammonium phosphate	9%

*Biuret is a product produced by condensing two urea molecules.
†Ammonium phosphates are used primarily as phosphorus sources.

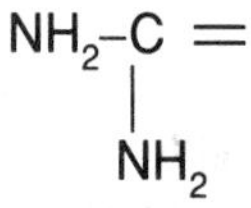

$$NH_2-C = O$$
$$|$$
$$NH_2$$

FIGURE 26-1. Structure of urea.

    b. NPN content of feed. The NPN content of feed is calculated by dividing the amount of crude protein in the feed by the protein equivalent provided by the pure NPN source. Feed tags list the amount of crude protein supplied by the feed. Therefore, a supplement with 28% crude protein from feed-grade urea would contain 10% urea:

$$\text{NPN content} = \frac{28}{281} = 0.10$$

4. The **normal feeding rate** for NPN products is 3% of the grain ration or 1% of the total ration.

5. Poor performance of animals fed urea may be a management problem, as opposed to a toxicologic problem. "Chronic" urea poisoning is not commonly recognized.

    a. Inconsistent feeding results in an inability of animals to adapt to the utilization of urea. Weather, movement, and sickness may affect supplement intake. Consequently, the ammonia release rate and ruminal pH are poorly controlled.

    b. Nutrient imbalance or deficiency
        (1) If high-energy feeds are not provided, full utilization of ammonia is not obtained.
        (2) If natural proteins are not fed, phosphorus, vitamins, and sulfur may be deficient.

    c. Immature animals (i.e., those weighing less than 250 kg) may not fully utilize urea due to a lack of ruminal competency.

B. **Toxicology.** Urea or NPN poisoning is an **acute condition** that is mainly a practical problem to ruminants.

1. Mechanism of toxicologic damage. Toxicosis usually occurs as a result of variability or excesses in urea intake and lack of ruminal adaptation to NPN.

    a. The **major metabolite of urea** is **ammonia.** The release of ammonia is stimulated by ruminal microflora and urease. Ammonia is a short-lived product in blood and is rapidly converted in the urea cycle and excreted unless blood ammonia is excessive.

    b. Ruminant microflora must adapt to the amount of ammonia that is released in order to assimilate ammonia into a bacterial protein that can be digested by the abomasum and intestines. Adaptation requires several days; therefore, rapid access to urea or other NPN products without adequate ruminal adaptation increases susceptibility to poisoning.

    c. The release of excessive ammonia in the rumen leads to **hyperammonemia.**
        (1) Excess ammonia released rapidly by urease is not utilized by the microbial population of the rumen and is absorbed by the bloodstream via the ruminoreticular wall.
        (2) Excess ammonia is toxic to enzymes of the TCA cycle, resulting in **metabolic acidosis.**

    d. Death probably results from **lactic acidemia** and **hyperkalemic heart failure.**

2. Predisposing factors for urea toxicosis

    a. Fasting, which causes a loss of the energy needed by ruminal microbes to metabolize urea

    b. High-roughage (i.e., **low-energy**) **diets**

    c. High ruminal pH, which promotes ammonia in an un-ionized form and increases absorption

    d. Dehydration or **low water intake**

    e. Hepatic insufficiency, causing an inability to metabolize urea in the urea–ammonia cycle

    f. Lack of natural protein, which may be required in small amounts for rumen microbes to utilize ammonia

TABLE 26-3. Nonprotein Nitrogen (NPN) Toxicity Values by Species

Species	NPN Product	Toxic Dosage (g/kg)	Lethal Dosage (g/kg)
Ruminants	Urea	0.3–0.5	1–1.5
	Urea phosphate	1	—
	Ammonium salts	1–2	—
	Biuret	8	—
Horses	Urea	—	4
Monogastrics	Urea	Nearly nontoxic	—
	Ammonium salts	1.5	—

3. **Toxicity**
   a. **Toxicity values** by species are given in Table 26-3.
   b. **Factors that enhance toxicity**
      (1) **Plant urease** (e.g., from raw soybeans) may enhance the hydrolysis of urea.
      (2) **Alkaline conditions in the rumen** enhance urea toxicity. At a ruminal pH below 6.2, ammonia is in the form of ammonium ions, which are not absorbed significantly through the rumen wall.
         (a) Urease ureolysis is stimulated and ruminal absorption of ammonia is increased.
         (b) Urea phosphate or other salts that maintain a lower rumen pH (e.g., ammonium sulfate) reduce absorption of ammonia.

4. **Diagnosis.** The clinical course of toxicosis ranges from 0.5–6 hours. Toxic manifestations occur when rumen ammonia levels exceed 80 mg/dl or blood ammonia levels exceed 1 mg/dl.
   a. **Clinical signs.** The acute onset of signs usually occurs from 0.5–4 hours after ingestion.
      (1) Early signs are frothy salivation, grinding of the teeth, abdominal pain, and polyuria.
      (2) Muscle tremors, blepharospasm, incoordination, and weakness follow rapidly.
      (3) Recumbency, often forequarters first, indicates advanced toxicosis. Polypnea, bloat, and regurgitation of the rumen contents are serious effects in advanced toxicosis.
      (4) Hyperthermia, anuria, and cyanosis may occur prior to death.
   b. **Laboratory evaluation.** High blood ammonia levels are responsible for the major toxic effects.
      (1) **Decreased blood pH (metabolic acidosis)** is characteristic of toxicosis.
      (2) **Elevations** occur in **blood glucose, blood lactic acid, BUN, AST, serum potassium, blood ammonia levels,** and **rumen pH**.
      (3) **Diagnostic values**
         (a) **Blood ammonia:** 1–4 mg/100 ml
         (b) **Rumen ammonia:** > 80 mg/100 ml (rumen liquor composite sample)
         (c) **Rumen pH:** pH > 7.5
      (4) **Specimen collection and preservation.** Autolysis and warm temperatures cause further ammonia release and proteolysis, leading to false–positive results. Therefore, **preservation is imperative**.
         (a) **Freezing.** Specimens should be frozen if tests cannot be performed within 1 hour, because spontaneous release may change the ammonia concentration.
         (b) **Mercuric chloride** (1%–3% of a saturated solution) may be used as a preservative if samples cannot be frozen.
   c. **Lesions** include rapid antemortem or postmortem bloat, fresh rumen contents with an ammonia odor, and pulmonary and tracheal congestion.

5. **Treatment**
   a. **Ruminal infusion** of cold water and acetic acid should be repeated every 6 hours for up to 48 hours. Best results are obtained if the animal is still ambulatory.

(1) **Cold water** (3–10 gallons per animal for cattle) may dilute the urea and lower ruminal temperature.

(2) **Acetic acid (5%)** or **vinegar** (2–8 liters per animal) may lower rumen pH and reduce absorption of ammonia.

b. **Ruminal intubation** should be used to relieve bloat.

c. **Intravenous administration of normal saline** with **bicarbonate or lactate** may help to combat metabolic acidosis.

d. **Rumenotomy.** If animals will tolerate surgery, rumenotomy may be helpful to remove excessive amounts of contaminated feed.

VI. 4-METHYLIMIDAZOLE

A. **Sources.** Ammoniated molasses, wheat straw, and hay are fed to cattle. 4-Methylimidazole, a by-product formed from ammoniation of carbohydrates, results from interaction of reducing sugars with ammonia. Toxicosis is reported mainly in Kentucky, Texas, and Oklahoma.

B. **Diagnosis.** The clinical syndrome is known as **"bovine bonkers" syndrome.**

1. **Clinical signs.** Central nervous system (CNS) signs (e.g., stampeding, ear twitching, trembling, champing, salivating, convulsions) occur in cows and their nursing calves within 24–36 hours of consumption.

a. Convulsive episodes last up to 30 seconds and may be repeated at 5- to 10-minute intervals.

b. Clinical signs have been mistaken for chlorinated hydrocarbon insecticide poisoning, urea toxicosis, organophosphate poisoning, and grass tetany.

2. **Laboratory diagnosis**

a. Blood urea and ammonia levels are normal.

b. Preferred samples for testing are suspect forage or molasses or rumen contents. Relatively few laboratories perform this analysis.

C. **Treatment**

1. **Pentobarbital** and **acepromazine** are helpful for controlling clinical signs, but their effect on survival is not documented.

2. **Thiamine** (1–2 g intravenously or intramuscularly) has been used as nonspecific neurologic supportive therapy.

VII. RAW SOYBEANS

A. **Exposure.** Accidental access to raw soybeans occasionally causes acute toxicosis.

B. **Mechanism of action.** Soybeans have high concentrations of both carbohydrates and proteins, as well as active urease enzyme. Overconsumption of soybeans by ruminants can cause acute carbohydrate fermentation and excessive ammonia release. The condition is presumed to be a combination of **ammonia toxicosis** and **lactic acidosis.**

C. **Diagnosis**

1. **Clinical signs.** Affected cattle or sheep have ruminal engorgement, with development of a gray, pasty diarrhea. Neurologic signs include ataxia, weakness, muscle tremors, and recumbency.

2. **Lesions.** Necropsy often reveals whole soybeans in the rumen, along with heavy, pasty, gray ruminal contents. Ruminal contents are slightly alkaline, presumably due to proteolysis of soy protein.

D. **Treatment** is often unsuccessful, although early rumenotomy may prevent full development of toxicosis.

VIII. GOSSYPOL

A. **Sources.** Gossypol is a polyphenolic pigment found in the pigment glands of cottonseed.

1. Gossypol **content varies** with species of plant and may range from 0.002% to more than 6%.

2. It occurs in cottonseed as both a **bound form** and a **free form**. The **free form is toxic,** but the bound form is nontoxic because of protein binding.

B. **Exposure**

1. The addition of excessive cottonseed meal to the diet of swine or young ruminants lacking a fully functional rumen can cause toxicosis.
   a. Use in swine and poultry diets is restricted because of potential toxicity to monogastric animals.
   b. The gossypol content of swine feeds is regulated; diets must contain less than 0.01% (100 ppm).

2. Accidental access in the environment may occur if animals gain access to whole cottonseed or to cottonseed by-products.

C. **Toxicokinetics**

1. Gossypol is lipid-soluble and readily absorbed from the digestive tract.

2. Gossypol binds strongly to proteins (including the amino acid lysine) and to iron salts (e.g., ferrous sulfate), which may inactivate the gossypol. Dietary iron fed at a 1:1 ratio with gossypol can markedly reduce susceptibility to toxicosis.

3. Metabolism and conjugation of gossypol result in limited excretion of metabolites in the urine. However, most gossypol is eliminated in the feces.

D. **Mechanism of toxicologic damage.** Toxic effects usually occur only after weeks or months of exposure to gossypol.

1. **Heart damage.** Cardiac necrosis causes congestive heart failure to develop. Animals that die suddenly with no cardiac lesions are believed to experience a form of cardiac conduction failure similar to hyperkalemic heart failure.

2. **Kidney damage.** Renal-associated hypokalemia may occur.

3. **Hepatic damage.** Gossypol inhibits glutathione-S-transferase, which impairs the liver's ability to metabolize xenobiotics. Hepatic necrosis may be a sequela of congestive heart failure.

4. **Protein malnutrition** and **reduced weight gain** may occur as a result of protein binding, which interferes with the use of amino acids (especially lysine and methionine).

5. **Reproductive effects**
   a. Gossypol inhibits enzymes necessary for steroid synthesis in testicular Leydig cells, as well as LDH. The result is spermatozoal abnormalities and infertility.
   b. Gossypol appears to interrupt pregnancy by exerting a luteolytic action on the ovary.

E. Toxicity

1. **Acute toxicity** from gossypol is not likely, because exposure is primarily in the diet and cumulative effects require long-term exposure.

2. **Subacute** to **chronic toxicity** is somewhat age- and species-dependent, and is influenced by the amount of dietary iron.
   a. **Horses** are relatively resistant.
   b. **Swine** and **poultry** are affected by dietary concentrations above 100 ppm and 200–400 ppm, respectively.
   c. **Ruminants**
      (1) **Mature** ruminants usually tolerate up to 1000 ppm dietary gossypol, but concentrations of 1500 ppm may cause mild to moderate toxicosis (e.g., anemia and reduced growth or milk production).
      (2) **Young** ruminants (i.e., less than 6 months of age) should not receive more than 100 ppm dietary free gossypol.

F. Diagnosis

1. **Clinical signs**
   a. **Swine** show early signs of increasing anorexia, reduced weight gain, and lower feed efficiency. As the disease progresses, weakness, dyspnea (which, when pronounced, is referred to as "thumping"), cyanosis, and death occur.
   b. **Poultry.** Discoloration of egg yolks is a mild side effect of gossypol in hens. Anorexia, weight loss, and reduced hatchability are typical signs of advanced toxicosis in poultry.
   c. **Cattle** exhibit mild anemia and erythrocyte fragility (hemolysis). More advanced signs include dyspnea, weakness, edema of the brisket, depression, and death.

2. **Laboratory diagnosis**
   a. Distinctive hematologic or clinical chemistry changes include elevated serum liver enzymes [i.e., sorbitol dehydrogenase (SDH), γ-glutamyl transpeptidase (GGT), AST, LDH], mild anemia, increased erythrocyte fragility, and elevated cholecystokinin.
   b. Analysis for elevated dietary levels of free gossypol confirms excessive exposure.
      (1) Analysis of feed must be correlated with typical clinical signs and lesions.
      (2) The feed that initiated the cumulative toxicosis may no longer be available for analysis.
      (3) Gossypol analysis is available at a limited number of laboratories.

3. **Lesions** in most animals include:
   a. Straw-colored to red-tinged fluids in the thorax and abdomen
   b. Cardiac dilatation, pale myocardial streaking, and enlarged and dilated ventricles
   c. Interstitial pulmonary edema with markedly edematous interlobular septa
   d. Enlarged, congested, and friable liver with accentuated lobules and, sometimes, generalized icterus
   e. Histopathologic lesions of cardiomyopathy or cardiac necrosis with attempts at regeneration, centrilobular hepatic congestion and necrosis, and mild renal tubular nephrosis

G. Treatment

1. **Detoxification** is primarily by removal of excessive gossypol from the diet.
   a. Because exposure is chronic, adsorbents and cathartics are usually of little value.
   b. Addition of iron to the diet (1:1 with free gossypol) helps to inactivate free gossypol.

2. **Supportive therapy** includes a high-quality diet supplemented with lysine, methionine, and fat-soluble vitamins.

H. Prognosis

Prognosis for recovery is limited, because exposure is usually chronic and lesions may be serious and advanced before diagnosis is confirmed.

STUDY QUESTIONS

DIRECTIONS: Each of the numbered items or incomplete statements in this section is followed by answers or by completions of the statement. Select the **one** numbered answer or completion that is **best** in each case.

1. Shortly after a new batch of feed is delivered, it is fed to a group of ten yearling colts. Within the next 12 hours, eight of the colts experience moderate to severe colic, and four of them develop severe diarrhea accompanied by dehydration and shock. Within 24 hours, all four have died. The most likely cause of the acute syndrome in these animals is:

(1) *Clostridium botulinum* contamination and growth in the feed.
(2) accidental mixing of ammonium phosphate in the feed.
(3) accidental mixing of urea in the feed.
(4) contamination of the feed with a swine premix containing lincomycin or tetracyclines.
(5) accidental inclusion of 100 ppm organic iodine in the feed.

2. Which one of the following feed additives causes acute neurologic signs (seizures, hyper-irritability) when given to dairy calves?

(1) Amprolium
(2) Clindamycin
(3) Ethylenediamine dihydriodide (EDDI)
(4) Monensin
(5) Nitrofurazone

3. Necropsy of several swine reveals pulmonary congestion and bronchopneumonia, dehydration, and pale yellow streaks in the renal cortex and medulla. A feed toxicosis is suspected. A sample of the kidney for histopathology should be fixed in:

(1) absolute alcohol.
(2) mercuric chloride.
(3) neutral buffered formalin.
(4) polyethylene glycol.

4. A relatively new antibiotic compound that potentiates the toxic action of monensin by delaying its metabolism and elimination is

(1) albamycin.
(2) clindamycin.
(3) lincomycin.
(4) tiamulin.
(5) tylosin.

5. Which one of the following animals is most likely poisoned by monensin at a concentration of 100 ppm in feed?

(1) Chicken
(2) Cow
(3) Horse
(4) Pig
(5) Turkey

6. Which of the following serum components is most likely elevated to high levels in a horse or cow suffering from monensin or lasalocid toxicosis?

(1) Calcium
(2) Creatine kinase
(3) Lactate dehydrogenase (LDH)
(4) Potassium
(5) Alkaline phosphatase (AP)

7. Gossypol toxicosis is most strongly interfered with by which one of the following minerals?

(1) Calcium
(2) Iron
(3) Magnesium
(4) Phosphorus
(5) Selenium

DIRECTIONS: The numbered item or incomplete statement in this section is negatively phrased, as indicated by an italicized word such as *not, least,* or *except.* Select the **one** numbered answer or completion that is **best**.

8. All of the following are differential diagnoses for 4-methylimidazole toxicosis *except:*

(1) ammonia toxicosis.
(2) grass tetany.
(3) organophosphate toxicosis.
(4) polioencephalomalacia.
(5) nitrofurazone toxicosis.

DIRECTIONS: The group of items in this section consists of numbered options followed by a set of numbered items. For each item, select the **one** numbered option that is most closely associated with it. Each numbered option may be selected once, more than once, or not at all.

Questions 9–14

Match each description with the appropriate feed-related toxicant.

(1) Lincomycin
(2) Monensin
(3) Urea
(4) Gossypol
(5) Sulfaquinoxaline

9. Causes hemorrhage and vitamin K–responsive coagulopathy in dogs

10. Causes male spermatozoal abnormalities and infertility

11. Ruminal enzymes and raw soybeans increase toxicity

12. Affects transmembrane movement of sodium and calcium

13. Strongly binds to proteins, especially those containing lysine

14. Clinical effects in the horse appear similar to those of acute inorganic arsenic toxicosis

ANSWERS AND EXPLANATIONS

1. The answer is 4 *[II A 2]*. Lincomycin is well known to induce acute necrotizing colitis in animals that depend on cecal microbial action for digestion (e.g., horses, rabbits, guinea pigs, hamsters). *Clostridium difficile* has been implicated in this acute toxicosis, and it is known that *C. difficile* is relatively resistant to lincomycin compared to other gram-positive bacteria in the colon and cecum. *C. botulinum* is highly toxic to horses, but clinical signs are slower to develop and are primarily neuroparalytic rather than alimentary. High concentrations of ammonium phosphate and urea could release ammonia, causing ammonia toxicosis. Although ammonia toxicosis occurs rapidly, it is associated with metabolic acidosis and neurologic signs rather than prominent gastrointestinal signs. Organic iodine causes lacrimation, a moist cough, fever, weight loss, and scaling of skin.

2. The answer is 5 *[II B 2 c (1) (d) (i)]*. Nitrofurazone interferes with enzymes of the tricarboxylic acid (TCA) cycle, limiting the availability of energy metabolism in the central nervous system (CNS). The resultant anoxia causes acute neurologic signs of seizures and hyperirritability in calves. Amprolium is a thiamin antagonist which is only toxic at dosages of 50 times the recommended level for several weeks or more. Clindamycin is a human antibiotic, similar to lincomycin, that affects the colon and cecum. Ethylenediamine dihydriodide (EDDI) causes lacrimation, nasal discharge, fever, and scaling of skin. It does not cause seizures or an acute response. Monensin is a feed additive ionophore that primarily affects the mitochondria of striated muscles. Monensin may cause muscle weakness and trembling, but is not associated with seizures or primary CNS activity.

3. The answer is 1 *[II C 2 c (2) (c)]*. Because the swine have pulmonary congestion and bronchopneumonia, they likely had respiratory signs and could have been treated with an antibacterial. Sulfonamides, which are commonly used for this purpose, can cause renal toxicosis with precipitation of sulfonamide crystals in the urine. If sulfonamide toxicosis is suspected, either the kidneys can be analyzed chemically for sulfonamides, or morphologic evidence can be obtained by histopathology. Either acidified formalin (acid conditions reduce solubility of the sulfonamide) or absolute alcohol is required to preserve the

kidney and maintain the sulfonamide crystals for examination by a pathologist. Neutral buffered formalin is likely to dissolve the crystals.

4. The answer is 4 *[II D 2]*. Tiamulin itself has low toxicity, but it interferes with the metabolism and elimination of ionophores, allowing cellular accumulation and toxicosis to develop. This interaction is clearly noted on labels and package inserts, and should not be ignored by clinicians or livestock producers.

5. The answer is 3 *[IV A 2 b; Table 26-1]*. Horses are highly sensitive to monensin—the LD_{50} in horses is nearly 10 times less in horses than in cattle. Feeding studies have shown that horses can be severely poisoned by feed levels of 100 ppm, whereas the same dosage produces only mild toxicosis and anorexia in cattle. The experimental LD_{50} value for chickens is 200 mg/kg, as opposed to 2–3 mg/kg in horses.

6. The answer is 2 *[IV A 2 c (2) (e)]*. Muscle necrosis induced by ionophore toxicosis causes the moderate to massive release of creatine kinase, a muscle enzyme. Levels of the other enzymes [lactate dehydrogenase (LDH) and alkaline phosphatase (AP)] may be moderately or mildly elevated. Serum calcium and potassium levels actually decrease transiently because of the substantial changes in cation transport caused by ionophores.

7. The answer is 2 *[VIII C 2]*. Experimental and feeding studies have shown that iron (e.g., ferrous sulfate) binds strongly to the polyphenolic entities of gossypol and limits its absorption, thereby reducing the potential for toxicosis. This interaction is used for both therapy and prevention of gossypol toxicosis. There is no evidence that calcium, magnesium, phosphorus, or selenium bind to gossypol.

8. The answer is 4 *[VI B 1 b]*. Polioencephalomalacia is primarily a neurologic disease of cattle, characterized by brain swelling and cerebrocortical necrosis resulting in blindness, depression, somnolence, anorexia, coma, and death. (Recovery is rare.) The acute hyperexcitability, trembling, champing, and seizures characteristic of 4-methylimidazole toxicosis are similar to signs seen in ammonia toxicosis, grass tetany, organophosphate toxicosis, and nitrofurazone toxicosis.

9–14. The answers are: 9-5 *[II C 1 c (3)],*
10-4 *[VIII D 5 a],* **11-3** *[V B 1, 3 b],*
12-2 *[IV A 1 c, 2 a],* **13-4** *[VIII C 2],*
14-1 *[II A 2 c].* Sulfaquinoxaline interferes with
vitamin K reduction after epoxidation during
the final carboxylation step in synthesis of
prothrombin and other vitamin K–dependent
clotting factors. In addition, thrombocyte
inhibition may exacerbate bleeding tendency,
especially in poultry and dogs.

Gossypol inhibits enzymes needed for steroid
synthesis in testicular Leydig cells, resulting in
abnormally formed spermatozoa and infertility.

Urea is naturally present in rumen micro-
flora and in raw soybeans. The urease activity
in ruminants is sufficient to quickly hydrolyze
urea to ammonia, but the bacteria necessary to
synthesize protein from urea require several
days to adapt to increased ammonia synthesis.
Until adaptation takes place, the animal is at
increased susceptibility to urea/ammonia
toxicosis.

By definition, the ionophores facilitate
movement of monovalent and divalent cations
through appropriate channels in the cell membranes. Excessive promotion of this transport
can lead to imbalances, especially of calcium.
Calcium imbalance may lead to the inhibition
of energy metabolism in mitochondria and cell
death.

Gossypol has numerous phenolic groups
and strong protein-binding properties, especially to lysine. This binding can interfere with
adequate utilization of both lysine and methionine, leading to protein malnutrition, reduced
weight gain, and cardiomyopathy.

Lincomycin causes acute necrotizing colitis
that is often described as similar to "colitis X"
in the horse. Acute arsenical toxicosis also
causes acute, fluid diarrhea, mucosal necrosis,
dehydration, shock, and death. However, postmortem examination reveals that arsenic
causes lesions in the stomach, duodenum,
jejunum, and ileum, with some effects in the
colon and cecum, whereas lincomycin causes
lesions primarily in the colon and cecum.

Chapter 27
Water-Related Toxicoses

I. **INTRODUCTION.** Water is the earth's most abundant and most often neglected nutrient. There are 273 liters of water for every square centimeter of the earth's surface.

A. **Distribution of the earth's water supply.** Less than 1% of the world's water is available for irrigation, livestock consumption, and human use.

1. Oceans (97%)

2. Polar caps and glaciers (2.29%)

3. Underground (0.68%)

4. Surface (0.01%)

5. Atmosphere (0.001%)

B. **Implications for husbandry and agriculture**

1. Livestock require approximately two billion gallons of water per day.

2. Except for precipitation, 75% of the water used in agriculture comes from surface supplies, and 25% comes from wells and springs. The remainder is from streams, lakes, and reservoirs.

II. **WATER QUALITY**

A. **Total dissolved solids (TDS)** refers to all of the constituents dissolved in water. The term "TDS" is often used interchangeably with the term "salinity" (see II B 4). Water is often described in terms of its TDS (Table 27-1).

1. **Constituents.** Ten elements constitute approximately 99% of the mineral compounds in water: hydrogen, oxygen, sodium, potassium, magnesium, calcium, silicon, chlorine, sulfur, and carbon.
   a. **Major constituents** (10–1000 mg/L) include calcium, magnesium, sodium, bicarbonate, chlorine, silicate, and sulfate.
   b. **Secondary constituents** (0.1–10 mg/L) include boron, iron, potassium, strontium, fluoride, nitrate, and phosphate.

TABLE 27-1. Classification of Water According to TDS Content

Description	TDS Content (mg/L)
Fresh	< 1000
Brackish	1000–10,000
Salty	10,000–100,000
Brine	> 100,000

TDS = total dissolved solids. (Borrowed with permission from National Academy of Sciences Subcommittee on Nutrient and Toxic Elements in Water: *Nutrient and Toxic Substances in Water for Livestock and Poultry.* Washington, D.C., 1974.)

TABLE 27-2. Use of Saline Waters for Livestock and Poultry

TDS Content (mg/L)	Acceptability as a Water Source
< 1000	Presents little or no hazard to livestock or poultry
1000–2999	Acceptable for all classes of livestock and poultry; may cause transient diarrhea
3000–4999	May cause transient diarrhea or reduced water intake in unaccustomed animals; poultry are most susceptible to increased mortality, diarrhea, and decreased growth
5000–6999	Relatively safe for dairy and beef cattle, sheep, swine, and horses; higher levels should be avoided for pregnant or lactating animals; not acceptable for poultry
7000–10,000	Unfit for poultry, swine, pregnant or lactating cows, horses, sheep, or the young of these species, or any animals subjected to heavy heat stress or water loss; older ruminants and horses may tolerate these concentrations if not stressed

TDS = total dissolved solids. (Borrowed with permission from National Academy of Sciences Subcommittee on Nutrient and Toxic Elements in Water: *Nutrient and Toxic Substances in Water for Livestock and Poultry.* Washington, D.C., 1974.)

    c. Minor constituents (less than 0.1 mg/L) include arsenic, cadmium, copper, lead, molybdenum, and zinc.

  2. Effect on potability. As the amount of soluble salts in the water increases slightly, intake increases, whereas animals reduce intake or refuse to drink water of extreme salinity (Table 27-2). Depressed feed intake often accompanies decreased water intake.

B. **Characteristics**

  1. Acidity (pH) usually ranges from 6–9.

  2. Hardness is the calcium carbonate equivalent of calcium and magnesium salts.
    a. Water is generally classified as "soft" or "hard" based on the amount of calcium and magnesium salts (Table 27-3).
    b. Hardness may also be expressed as grains per gallon: 1 grain/gallon is equivalent to 17 mg calcium and magnesium/L.

  3. Sediment, undissolved material carried in suspension in water, settles to the bottom if the water loses velocity.
    a. Sediment cations may contribute to TDS.
    b. Sediment may adsorb or transport a variety of organic or inorganic toxicants that are not soluble in water (e.g., pesticides, heavy metals).

  4. Salinity is the TDS in water after all carbonates are equilibrated or expressed as oxides, all bromide and iodide are expressed as chloride, and all organic matter has been oxidized.

  5. Conductivity is a numerical expression of the ability of water to carry an electric current.
    a. Conductivity depends on the ions present and the temperature.
    b. The conductivity of potable waters in the United States is generally 50–1500 µohm/cm.

TABLE 27-3. Classification of Water According to Calcium and Magnesium Salt Content

Grains of Hardness/Gallon	Calcium and Magnesium Salt Content (mg/L)	Description
0–4	0–60	Soft
7–10	120–180	Hard
> 10	> 180	Very hard

C. Analysis

1. **Ammonia content.** Elevated ammonia increases pH and may be highly toxic to fish.
   a. **Source.** Ammonia is formed by the decomposition of organic nitrogen accompanied by increasing oxidation (nitrification):

   $$\text{Organic N} \Rightarrow NH_3\text{—N} \Rightarrow NO_2N \Rightarrow NO_3\text{—N}$$

   Nitrification places a large oxygen demand on waters.
   b. **Sampling.** A fresh sample is best; alternatively, the sample can be preserved for a maximum of 24 hours with 1 ml/L concentrated sulfuric acid (H_2SO_4).
   c. **Acceptable levels.** Recommended limits are less than 0.5 mg/L. Heavily polluted water, fresh domestic sewage, or treated effluents may contain 1–10 mg/L ammonia nitrogen.

2. **Nitrate or nitrite content**
   a. **Source.** Nitrogen in waters tends to occur in the nitrate (NO_3) oxidation state. Nitrates are associated with decaying organic matter, animal wastes, feces, and fertilizers. If nitrate-reducing bacteria are present, nitrite may be formed. Algae and plant growth often lower the nitrate concentration of impounded waters.
   b. **Sampling**
      (1) Bacterial conversion of nitrate to nitrite can occur if water samples are not properly preserved by refrigeration or acidification (see II C 1 b).
      (2) Expression of nitrogen in water varies among laboratories. Common expressions are nitrate, nitrate nitrogen, and potassium nitrate.
         (a) **Nitrate nitrogen** is the actual nitrogen in the nitrate ion and is equal to the nitrate concentration divided by 4.4 (i.e., $NO_3/4.4 = NO_3$—N).
         (b) **Potassium nitrate** is 7.2 times the nitrate nitrogen (i.e., $KNO_3/7.2 = NO_3$—N).
   c. **Acceptable limits**
      (1) For swine and other monogastrics, nitrite is considered approximately ten times more toxic than nitrate.
      (2) Based on both field and experimental evidence, less than 300 ppm nitrate in water is medically and economically acceptable.
         (a) Acute toxicity (e.g, methemoglobinemia) occurs in ruminants when ingestion of nitrate exceeds 500 mg/kg body weight. Toxic levels of nitrate in water for ruminants range from 1500–3000 mg/L.
         (b) Tolerance depends in part on the animal's total nitrate intake (i.e., in diet and water).

3. **Sulfide content**
   a. **Source.** Sulfide is a toxic by-product of anaerobic decomposition. It may occur as free sulfide or dissolved hydrogen sulfide (H_2S). Concentrations greater than or equal to 1 ppm cause a rotten egg odor.
   b. **Sampling** must involve minimal aeration. Fresh samples should be analyzed within 3 minutes of collection. Water to be analyzed for sulfide content only can be preserved using 2 ml zinc acetate per liter.
   c. **Acceptable levels** have not been established for animals.

4. **Sulfate content**
   a. **Source**
      (1) Sulfates often occur in conjunction with highly saline waters in the western United States.
      (2) Industrial processes or pyrite oxidation (associated with acid mine drainage) may produce sulfates.
      (3) Sulfide is oxidized to sulfate.
   b. **Sampling.** Certain bacteria in organic matter reduce sulfate to sulfide. Samples for analysis should be stored at a low temperature or preserved with formaldehyde.
   c. **Acceptable levels.** Sulfates as a component of saline waters are associated with a purging or diarrheic effect similar to the effects from saline cathartics (e.g., sodium or magnesium sulfate). The response to saline-sulfate waters is usually transient; animals adapt to the high sulfate intake after 3–7 days.

(1) Field observations have led to recommendations that waters containing more than 1000 ppm sulfates be used cautiously, especially in weanling pigs.

(2) Experimentally, swine have tolerated 2000–3000 ppm added sulfate in water with minimal effects (e.g., soft feces). Levels of 3000 ppm have not been shown to interfere with gain, feed efficiency, or reproduction in swine.

d. Removal of sulfates from water. Sulfates can be removed from water by ion-exchange resin systems that are available commercially. These systems are expensive, especially for high-volume water use; therefore, one should be convinced that a water supply is intolerable before taking such measures.

5. TDS content

a. Quantification may be accomplished by:

(1) Weighing the residue remaining following evaporation of a filtered water sample

(2) Evaluating the electrical conductivity of water, which is proportional to the TDS (stated in μohms)

b. Acceptable limits. High concentrations often relate to performance impairment in livestock (see Table 27-2). Whenever total salts are greater than 3000 mg/L, then alkalinity and nitrate levels should also be considered.

(1) Water containing alkaline ions in excess of 2000 mg/L is not recommended for consumption.

(2) The degree of harm varies with the form of alkaline anion, with OH being more harmful than CO_3, which is more harmful than HCO_3.

6. Iron content

a. Source. Iron usually is present as Fe^{2+} in ground waters, but it is readily oxidized to Fe^{3+}, which is insoluble.

b. Acceptable limits. Iron is primarily an aesthetic consideration. The mucilaginous secretions of "iron bacteria" contain hydrated ferric hydroxide, which turns plumbing fixtures brown.

(1) Iron causes a bitter (astringent) taste at 0.1–0.2 mg/L.

(2) Very high levels (i.e., greater than or equal to 5000 ppm) are required to affect animal nutrition.

7. Manganese content. Manganese is relatively soluble; therefore, it is a good general indicator of pollution. Like iron, manganese is primarily an aesthetic consideration.

8. Total organic carbon (TOC) measures all carbon compounds regardless of degradation rate. When evaluated in conjunction with the biological oxygen demand (BOD), TOC may provide evidence of nondegradable organic products. TOC is measured via the catalytic conversion of organic carbon to carbon dioxide.

9. Total organic halides (TOX) measure the gross quantity of halogenated hydrocarbons (e.g., pesticides, solvents, halogenated organics) in water.

a. The minimum sample size for analysis is 500 ml.

b. The sample should be stored at 4°C in an amber glass bottle with a Teflon or foil lid liner. The bottle should be filled to the top without allowing any head space.

c. For chlorinated samples, 1 ml of 0.1 sodium sulfite per liter should be added.

10. Bacterial content. Coliform indicator organisms (e.g., *Escherichia coli*), which generally indicate contamination of well water with bacteria of soil or fecal origin, are a common laboratory measure of water quality. Fecal streptococci and fecal coliforms are more specific indicators of fecal contamination.

a. Sampling

(1) The outlet is sterilized with a flame and the water is allowed to run for a minimum of 5 minutes before collection.

(2) Sterile containers are used to collect the sample, and then they are capped and sealed.

(3) Samples are refrigerated until the sample is cultured; bacterial numbers may change if held at higher temperatures.

(4) The **standard plate count** is the number of bacteria multiplying at 35°C; it is used to judge the efficacy of water treatment processes.

    b. Acceptable limits. The value of coliform counts in animals exposed to surface waters and animal wastes is questionable, because coliforms are not necessarily pathogens, and the counts are always high. Generally, coliform levels greater than or equal to 5000/100 ml should be avoided.

11. **Toxicity to fish.** Fish are sensitive indicator species to many toxicants and water quality problems.
    a. The selection of species, numbers, and test methods may depend on the alleged problems.
    b. Fish exposed to pesticides in water often die at concentrations 10 times less than those that would be toxic to livestock. Thus, fish kills are very sensitive biomarkers for animal safety.

III. TOXICOSES RESULTING FROM SODIUM–WATER IMBALANCE. Both water deprivation (sodium ion) toxicosis and water intoxication involve an imbalance of intracellular sodium and water.

A. | **Water requirements**

1. **Physiologic conditions**
    a. Lactation. Water consumption may double in lactating cows or sows.
    b. Renal disease (i.e., a lack of concentrating ability) increases urination and water intake (i.e., causes polyuria and polydipsia).
    c. High salt intake increases water requirements in order to aid sodium excretion.
    d. High protein intake increases metabolic water needs.

2. **Species requirements.** Most species require 2–3 liters of water per kilogram of dry feed consumed.

3. **Environmental conditions.** The water requirement varies according to the ambient temperature, relative humidity, and exercise.

B. | **Water deprivation (sodium ion) toxicosis** occurs most frequently in swine, cattle, and poultry. Rarely, it occurs in dogs.

1. **Causes of water deprivation (sodium ion) toxicosis**
    a. Mechanical problems with watering troughs
    b. Neglect
    c. Unpalatable water (e.g., from the addition of medication)
    d. Freezing (e.g., in open water troughs or because of faulty automatic water heaters)
    e. Overcrowding animals, leading to a lack of sufficient water space
    f. Placing animals in an unfamiliar place where the water supply is not known
    g. Unusual husbandry practices (e.g., feeding garbage, whey, or kitchen waste without increasing water intake)

2. **Mechanism of toxicologic damage**
    a. Normal physiology. Normal blood plasma and cerebrospinal fluid (CSF) sodium levels are 135–145 mEq/L and 130–140 mEq/L, respectively. Sodium enters the brain by passive diffusion and is removed by active transport, which requires energy.
    b. Pathophysiology. With limited water intake or dehydration, blood plasma sodium levels increase to 150–190 mEq/L, while those in the central nervous system (CNS) increase to 145–185 mEq/L.
        (1) High levels of sodium in the brain inhibit anaerobic glycolysis, so that no energy is available for the active transport of sodium out of the CNS.
        (2) As water intake and renal excretion of sodium increase, blood levels of sodium return to normal. However, brain levels remain high because the lack of energy precludes active transport out of the CNS.

(3) The combined effect of increased water intake and increased cerebral sodium levels creates an osmotic gradient between the blood and brain. Water moves from the blood to the brain, causing cerebral edema.

3. Toxicity

  a. A diet containing from 0.5%–1% salt is normally acceptable, but can become toxic if water is withheld or water intake is reduced.

  b. More than 10% of the diet may be salt if adequate water is available. Increased urination will occur, but not toxicosis.

4. Diagnosis

  a. Clinical signs. In a group of animals, not all signs may be seen at any one time because of the varied progression of the syndrome in individual animals.

  (1) Initially, animals exhibit **thirst** and **constipation,** but this sign may not be noticed.

  (2) Intermittent convulsive seizures develop suddenly, especially in swine following reaccess to water.

   (a) Seizures last from 30 seconds to 2–3 minutes.

   (b) The interval between seizures lasts approximately 2 hours, decreasing to 3 minutes as the clinical course progresses.

   (c) Seizures may be interrupted by other signs, such as depression, standing in a corner, pivoting around on one foot, and head-pressing.

   (d) Affected animals become oblivious to their environment, and seizures cannot be elicited by external stimulation.

  (3) As the syndrome develops, **convulsive seizures, circling, severe CNS depression, blindness,** and **head-pressing** may be seen. Terminal signs include **lateral recumbency** accompanied by **paddling motions** of all limbs.

  (4) Poultry may show only **depression, collapse,** and **ascites**.

  b. Laboratory diagnosis

  (1) Serum and CSF sodium values that exceed 160 mEq/L support a tentative diagnosis. CSF values are often higher than serum values.

  (2) Brain sodium values above 2000 ppm are considered supportive of sodium toxicosis.

  (3) Ocular fluid is an alternative tissue for postmortem analysis.

  c. Lesions

  (1) Gross lesions are not pathognomonic.

   (a) Inflammation of the gastric mucosa may be seen, but occurs in normal pigs as well.

   (b) More significant is the presence of **pinpoint ulcers filled with clotted blood** in the **gastric mucosa**.

  (2) Microscopic lesions. Lesions in the deep layer of the cerebral cortex and the adjacent white matter are the most important criteria for establishing a diagnosis.

   (a) Eosinophilic meningoencephalitis (i.e., eosinophilic perivascular cuffing of blood vessels in the meninges and parenchyma of the cortex) is prominent if the animal dies early in the clinical course.

   (b) There is an increase in vascularity because of **endothelial proliferation** in the deep layers of cortex and adjacent white matter.

   (c) There is an **increase in histiocytes (macrophages)** in the white matter adjacent to the deep layers of the cortex.

   (d) In pigs that die during the first 12 hours, **eosinophils are present in the brain;** they disappear after 24–36 hours.

   (e) Edema and **necrosis** or **malacia** of the **cerebral cortex** may occur 3–6 days after initial signs begin.

5. Treatment is nonspecific and may be of limited value. The mortality rate is often 50% regardless of treatment.

  a. Small amounts of water may be given at frequent intervals to gradually establish correct osmotic balance. Quantities equalling approximately 0.5% of body weight can be given every 60 minutes. Animals may recover in 4–5 days.

    b. Diuretics (e.g., mannitol) and **anticonvulsants** may be of some use in small animals, but their value has not been documented. Administration to swine or cattle is not always practical. Upon rehydration, rebound cerebral edema may occur after mannitol treatment.

C. **Water intoxication** occurs when cerebral edema is induced by sudden access to large amounts of fresh water.

    1. Circumstances of intoxication. Intoxication can occur when an animal has limited fluid intake (e.g., milk only) and then is permitted sudden access to large amounts of water (e.g., following weaning). **Calves that are bucket- or bottle-fed milk are most susceptible.**

    2. The **mechanism of toxicologic damage** and **clinical signs** of water intoxication in calves appear similar to those of water deprivation (sodium ion) toxicosis in swine (see III B 2, 4).

IV. TOXICOSES RESULTING FROM SEWAGE SLUDGE

A. **Sludge** is the solids removed from wastewater at sewage treatment plants. It is generally odor-free if stabilized by aerobic or anaerobic digestion or extended lagooning and usually contains fewer pathogens than raw sewage. Sludge may contain:

    1. Chemical compounds from businesses, industries, and homes
        a. Organochlorine compounds have been detected in some municipal sludges in past years, but current levels are low.
        b. Polynuclear aromatic hydrocarbons are found in some sludges. Two of these (benzo[a]pyrene and benzofluoroanthene) are carcinogens.

    2. Heavy metals, which can accumulate in soil

    3. Bacteria (e.g., *Staphylococcus, Clostridium, Mycobacterium, Klebsiella, Enterobacteriaceae, Salmonella*), **poliovirus,** and **other enteroviruses**

B. **Toxic organics**

    1. Polychlorinated biphenyls (PCBs) in soils are reported to cause plant contamination, animal residues, or both.
        a. Plants do not translocate PCBs, but may be contaminated via volatilization from the soil.
        b. Contamination also occurs during rainfall, which splashes soil on plants.
        c. Soil is ingested by animals during normal forage consumption.

    2. Insecticides in sludge bind to organic constituents.
        a. Accumulation of insecticides is greatest in the root zone and lower stems, and lowest in the leaves and seeds.
        b. Pesticides degrade in microbiologically active soils over time, but degradation varies according to pesticide type.

C. **Inorganic toxicants (metals)**

    1. Factors that alter the availability of metals to crops
        a. Industrial pretreatment reduces metal effluents.
        b. Sludge application rate. As application rates increase, soil availability and uptake by plants increase.
        c. Soil pH. Acid soil generally favors the uptake of problematic metals.
        d. Crop selection. Generally, leafy crops accumulate more metals than do grain crops.

    2. Low-hazard metals (e.g., manganese, iron, aluminum, chromium, mercury, arsenic, selenium, antimony, lead) either have low solubility in slightly acid or neutral soils, or they are present in low levels in soils.

3. Hazardous metals

a. Cadmium (see also Chapter 17 X A). Crops may contain undesirable cadmium levels without exhibiting signs of plant toxicity. Factors influencing crop uptake include:

   (1) Soil pH. Uptake is reduced when the soil pH is higher than 6.5.

   (2) Crop selection. Crops vary in cadmium content and distribution. Corn grain is lower in cadmium than wheat, oats, soybeans, or sorghum.

   (3) Other metals. Copper may increase the cadmium content of crop foliage, grain, or both, whereas zinc, selenium, or molybdenum may decrease the cadmium content.

b. Copper (see also Chapter 17 III) is found in all soils at levels of 10–80 ppm. The normal range in plants is 5–20 ppm; the copper content of plants may reach 20–50 ppm before plant toxicity occurs.

   (1) Plants high in copper may be hazardous to sheep if molybdenum and sulfate intake are not adjusted.

   (2) The addition of copper to surface waters as an algicide may also present a risk to sheep.

c. Molybdenum (see also Chapter 17 VII). Sludge contains 5–40 ppm molybdenum, and plants tolerate high levels (i.e., several hundred ppm) of the metal. Maximum sorption to soil occurs at a pH of 4.2; availability increases as the soil pH increases. At maximum levels, repeated application of sludge to non-leaching, high-pH soils could pose a threat to sensitive species (e.g., cattle).

d. Nickel. Sludges may contain from 2000–3500 ppm nickel. Nickel is normally present at levels of 10–100 ppm in soils. Livestock tolerance to dietary nickel is approximately 50 ppm, the same level at which nickel becomes toxic to plant tissues.

e. Zinc (see also Chapter 17 IX). The availability of zinc is reduced by liming, the presence of organic matter, and the presence of iron in the soil. Animals generally tolerate up to 500 ppm without adverse effects.

STUDY QUESTIONS

DIRECTIONS: Each of the numbered items or incomplete statements in this section is followed by answers or by completions of the statement. Select the **one** numbered answer or completion that is **best** in each case.

1. In a normal water supply, the element likely to be present in lowest concentration is:

(1) arsenic.
(2) calcium.
(3) fluoride.
(4) nitrate.
(5) phosphate.

2. What is the finding of coliform bacteria in water indicative of?

(1) Serious contamination by enteropathogenic organisms that are associated with diarrhea in animals
(2) Contamination by animal fecal matter
(3) Potential soil or fecal contamination
(4) Nothing of significance

3. The laboratory reports 100 ppm nitrate nitrogen in a well water sample. What is the equivalent amount of nitrate?

(1) 23 ppm
(2) 100 ppm
(3) 440 ppm
(4) 720 ppm
(5) None of the above

DIRECTIONS: Each of the numbered items or incomplete statements in this section is negatively phrased, as indicated by an italicized word such as *not, least,* or *except.* Select the **one** numbered answer or completion that is **best** in each case.

4. All of the following are suitable specimens for diagnostic confirmation of water deprivation (sodium ion) toxicosis in swine *except:*

(1) fresh brain tissue.
(2) formalin-fixed brain tissue.
(3) cerebrospinal fluid.
(4) hepatic tissue.
(5) ocular fluid.

5. If municipal sewage sludge is consistently used to fertilize crops, which one of the following would be *least* likely to accumulate in forage or crop plants grown on that soil?

(1) Cadmium
(2) Copper
(3) Lead
(4) Molybdenum
(5) Nickel

ANSWERS AND EXPLANATIONS

1. The answer is 1 *[II A 1].* Arsenic is a minor constituent of the water supply, present at levels less than 0.1 mg/L. Fluoride, nitrate, and phosphate are secondary constituents (i.e., they are found at concentrations that range from 0.1–10 mg/L). Calcium is a major constituent, present at levels that range from 10–1000 mg/L. The most highly toxic elements are generally not present in normal water supplies, and would be expected only in circumstances involving industrial waste pollution.

2. The answer is 3 *[II C 10].* Coliform bacteria may originate in either soil or water, and their presence shows only that a soil or fecal contamination of the water has occurred. To indicate fecal contamination, specific *Streptococci* or fecal coliforms must be cultured. Coliforms are not necessarily enteropathogenic. Coliform contamination is more likely in surface waters, which are directly exposed to runoff and animal wastes that contain high populations of coliform bacteria. Coliform contamination of well water usually suggests a breach in the cover or casing of the well near the surface, because deep water supplies are not generally contaminated with coliforms.

3. The answer is 3 *[II C 2 b (2)].* Nitrate (NO_3) has a molecular weight of 62 (N = 14, O = 16). Therefore, 14 of the 62 parts of the molecule are nitrogen. If 62 divided by 14 is 4.4, then the nitrate equivalent is 4.4 times that of the nitrogen. Thus, for 100 ppm nitrate nitrogen, the nitrate content is 440 ppm. This distinction is important to remember when reading laboratory reports or research or tolerance data, to avoid misinterpretation of information.

4. The answer is 4 *[III B 4 b].* Of the choices, only the liver is not measurably affected by changes in sodium and water balance. Water deprivation (sodium ion) toxicosis is caused by reduced water intake leading to high concentration of sodium in the central nervous system (CNS). High sodium levels may inhibit anaerobic glycolysis, limiting the energy available to the brain to maintain the sodium-potassium-ATPase pump that effects the removal of intracellular sodium. When anaerobic glycolysis is inhibited, sodium accumulates in the brain and exerts an osmotic effect, pulling water into the brain and resulting in cerebral edema. Sodium levels increase in the plasma, cerebrospinal fluid, and the brain parenchyma. Ocular fluids reflect the sodium concentration of plasma; therefore, they are also useful for diagnosing water deprivation (sodium ion) toxicosis. In pigs, the response triggers the perivascular accumulation of eosinophils known as eosinophilic meningoencephalitis, a classic lesion of water deprivation (sodium ion) toxicosis detectable by histopathologic examination of formalin-fixed tissues.

5. The answer is 3 *[IV C 3].* From experience and experimental work with sewage sludge, consistently higher values are obtained in plant tissues for cadmium, copper, molybdenum, and nickel than for lead. The first four metals are usually found in relatively high levels in sludge, and can accumulate in plant tissues to detrimental levels for animals before damage is done to the plant. Lead requires rather strong acid conditions for solubilization, and may be retarded by calcium content of the soil as well. All available evidence indicates that lead is not readily absorbed from the soil. However, one should remember that all metals can contaminate plants by direct contact through dust, splashing of soil by rain, or by flooding and contamination with silt.

Chapter 28
Plant-Related Toxicoses

I. **INTRODUCTION.** The plants covered in this chapter are those most commonly considered to be a problem by authorities from several geographic regions of North America.

A. **Characteristics of plant toxins**

1. Plant toxins are **secondary products of plant metabolism** (i.e., they are not essential to plant growth or reproduction).

2. Toxins appear to have evolved as an adjunct mechanism of plant survival. **Many plant toxins are bitter or induce strong physiologic reactions** that reduce foraging or the survival of plant predators (e.g., ruminants).

3. Plant toxicants **vary widely in structure and chemical properties.** Many toxins with similar chemical characteristics (e.g., alkaloids, glycosides, saponins) occur across a variety of plant genera or species. Characteristics of major classes of plant toxicants are described in Table 28-1.

B. **Factors favoring plant-related toxicosis**

1. **Adverse climatic conditions** may influence plant metabolism, increasing the production of secondary plant metabolites. For example, the production of cyanogenic glycosides is influenced by the ambient temperature.

2. **Agricultural practices** (e.g., fertilization, treatment with herbicides) may alter plant metabolism and increase secondary metabolites.

3. **Animal management practices** may place animals at risk to toxic plants in their environment. Many toxic plants are relatively unpalatable and not readily consumed unless animals are forced to them by hunger or management changes.
   a. **Nutrient deficiencies** (e.g., salt hunger) may induce abnormal appetites (pica) in animals, leading to consumption of unusual or toxic plants.
   b. **Overgrazing** causes inadequate forages, leading animals to consume toxic plants. In addition, overgrazing can lead to a relative increase in the number of weeds, many of which can be toxic, in the pasture.
   c. **Placement of thirsty or hungry animals in an unaccustomed location** following shipment or trailing can lead to the consumption of toxic plants.
   d. **Confinement** may lead to the consumption of toxic plants by pets as a result of curiosity or boredom.

C. **Recognition of plant-related toxicosis.** Accurate recognition of poisonous plant problems depends on:

1. **Familiarity with indigenous toxic plants,** including common outdoor garden and indoor ornamental plants

2. **Knowledge of seasonal variations in the concentration of toxic principles** in plants

3. **Access to other resources**
   a. Herbalists, botanists, horticulturalists, extension agents, garden store managers, and college or university professors can assist in identifying suspected toxic plants.
   b. Plant identification manuals appropriate to the type and range of toxic plants in a local practice area are available from state agricultural colleges or agricultural extension services, governmental agencies, and private publishing companies.

TABLE 28-1. Toxic Principles in Major Poisonous Plants

Toxicity Category	Characteristics
Alkaloids	Alkaloids are basic (pH > 7) compounds that form salts with acids. They are insoluble or sparingly soluble in water. They contain nitrogen, usually in a heterocyclic or aromatic ring structure. Thousands of alkaloids are known; however, many are not known to be toxic. Most toxic alkaloids are characterized by a bitter taste that may be important in prevention of plant predation.
Diterpene (phorbol) esters	Diterpene esters are tricyclic compounds often containing a combination of five-, six-, and seven-membered rings and a variety of phenolic or alkyl side chains or esters. They are soluble in water and other polar solvents.
Glycosides	Glycoside is a generic term describing the ester linkage between an organic compound or toxin (the aglycone) and a sugar. Glycosides are bitter, colorless, and noncrystalline. Glycosides are widespread; most are not known to be toxic. The aglycone often is not considered toxic until after hydrolysis releases it from the sugar.
Cyanogenic glycosides	Cyanogenic glycosides yield hydrogen cyanide upon hydrolysis. Ruminants are highly susceptible because the rumen contains large amounts of β-glucosidase, which hydrolyzes the glycoside.
Cardiac glycosides	Cardiac glycosides are steroid-like structures with 23 or 24 carbons and sugar molecules esterified to the number 3 carbon. The 23-carbon glycosides, known as cardenolides, are most important in veterinary medicine.
Goitrogens	Goitrogens prevent the accumulation of organic iodide, thus inhibiting the formation of thyroxine.
Isothiocyanates	Irritant oil glycosides, most commonly allyl isothiocyanate, are found primarily in the Cruciferae (mustard) family.
Protoanemonin	The glycoside ranunculin yields a lactone known as protoanemonin upon hydrolysis. Protoanemonin is a volatile yellow oil that combines with sulfhydryl groups and produces a strong vesicant and irritant action on skin and mucous membranes.
Saponins	Saponins are large molecules that form a colloidal suspension and produce a soapy froth when shaken with water. They are usually chemically similar to steroids or triterpenoids.
Grayanotoxins	Grayanotoxins are diterpenoid molecules found primarily in *Rhododendron* and *Kalmia* species. They are crystalline and soluble in hot water, and toxicity depends on hydroxyl groups at specific points on the molecule.
Nitrates	Nitrates are water-soluble toxicants that are naturally present in plants as part of the nitrogen cycle.
Oxalates	
Calcium oxalate	Calcium oxalate occurs as insoluble needle-like crystals or spicules in the tissues of many plants, especially those grown indoors as ornamentals.
Soluble oxalates	Soluble oxalates occur as sodium or potassium salts in plant tissues.
Tannins	Tannins were formerly considered the toxic principle in oak leaves and acorns. Currently, the toxin is believed to be several polyhydroxyphenolic compounds known collectively as gallotannins. Tannins precipitate proteins under alkaline conditions.
Toxalbumins (phytotoxins)	Toxalbumins are large molecules classified chemically as glycoproteins. They are considered highly toxic, but are not well absorbed from the gastrointestinal tract, and parenteral toxicity is much greater than oral toxicity. Many animal cells contain receptors for certain toxalbumins, the best known of which are ricin and abrin. Seeds are the most concentrated source of the toxin.

D. **Diagnosis of plant-related toxicosis.** Hundreds of plants are considered toxic based on anecdotal reports, clinical associations, or research verification. However, the number of plants that present a great risk within a specific geographic location (e.g., a local veterinary practice) is relatively small. Many times, the important clinical issue is determining whether toxic plants were actually consumed by affected animals.

1. The **history** should be consistent with the opportunity for plant consumption.
   a. Considerations such as the time of year, expected range and habitat of toxic plants, availability of specific toxic portions of plants, and the conditions that favor toxin accumulation can help the clinician to estimate the probability that plant toxicosis has occurred. For example, if only the seeds of a plant are toxic, and if only imma- ture plants are available, poisoning is unlikely.
   b. Other factors to consider include:
      (1) Changes in pasture or forage offered
      (2) Recent melting of snow cover, or plant growth following flooding
      (3) The potential for overgrazing

2. **Examination** of the **environment** or **ingesta** should confirm that available toxic plants have actually been consumed.

3. **Clinical signs** and **lesions** should be compatible with the known effects of the suspect toxic plants.

4. **Laboratory diagnosis.** Toxic principles in plants are often not detected by routinely available tests in diagnostic or chemical laboratories. It is necessary to know the avail- ability of confirmatory chemical testing for important plants of interest in a specific veterinary practice.

5. **Identification of toxic plants** is easiest if the entire plant is supplied, including flower- ing parts. A good history of where the plant was collected (e.g., woodlands, swamp, prairie) is essential.
   a. Green plants can be preserved for several days by sealing them in a plastic bag and refrigerating them.
   b. If plants must be dried before identification is possible, they should be pressed between two flat surfaces (e.g., two sheets of heavy cardboard) and several layers of absorbent paper. The press should be placed over a warm, dry area for 1–3 days to promote drying.

E. **General treatment and prevention of plant-related toxicosis**

1. **Treatment**
   a. **Reducing exposure.** Animals should be prevented from accessing toxic plants and provided with adequate water and an alternative feed source.
   b. **Detoxification.** Prompt oral detoxification using emesis or gastric lavage followed by activated charcoal and osmotic cathartics is rational therapy unless specifically contraindicated.

2. **Prevention.** Specific antidotes are not available for many plant toxins; therefore, general preventive measures are of utmost importance.
   a. When introducing forage-consuming animals to pasture or range containing toxic plants, a period of acclimation should be allowed, and animals should be provided with alternative feeds to limit initial consumption of toxic plants.
   b. Overgrazing and withholding of water should be avoided.
   c. Animals should be prevented from accessing areas recently sprayed with herbicides. Some herbicides, especially the phenoxy acetic acid derivatives (e.g., 2,4-D) may enhance the palatability of some toxic plants.
   d. Animals should not be fed chopped or ground forages known to contain poisonous plants, because the animals will not be able to sort unwanted plants from good forages.
   e. Close confinement of pets should be minimized.

II. NEUROTOXICANTS

A. Seizures and increased central nervous system (CNS) activity

1. *Asclepias* (milkweed)
   a. **Description.** Plants of the "milkweed" family exude a white, milky juice from broken or cut surfaces. Both narrow-leafed (whorled) and broad-leafed species exist; the narrow-leafed variety is most toxic. The fruit is a follicle (i.e., a capsule filled with numerous seeds); a silky tuft aids spread of seeds by the wind.
   b. **Geographic range.** Milkweeds are found throughout the United States in open, sunny areas that may be either dry or swampy.
   c. **Toxic principle**
      (1) The primary toxic principle, **galitoxin,** is of the **resinoid** class. Galitoxin is found **in all vegetative parts of the plant**.
      (2) In addition, a group of toxicants known as **cardenolides** may be responsible for digitalis-like signs that cause or contribute to death.
   d. **Toxicity**
      (1) Dosages of whorled milkweed as low as 0.1%–0.5% of the animal's body weight may cause toxicosis and, possibly, death.
      (2) Cattle, sheep, and horses are most susceptible.
   e. **Diagnosis**
      (1) **Clinical signs** include profuse salivation, incoordination, violent seizures, bloating in ruminants, and colic in horses. Early signs are followed by bradycardia or tachycardia, arrhythmias, hypotension, and hypothermia. Death may occur from 1–3 days after ingestion of the milkweed.
      (2) **Lesions** are few and unreliable for diagnosis.
   f. **Treatment** includes gastrointestinal detoxification, sedation or tranquilization, and medical treatment to counteract cardiac glycoside effects (see VI B 5).

2. *Cicuta maculata* and *C. douglasii* (water hemlock)
   a. **Description.** Water hemlock, a member of the Umbelliferae family, is characterized by large terminal inflorescences that radiate from a central point, hollow, purple-streaked stems, and leaves with veins that end in the notches of the serrations. The bundle of roots somewhat resembles a cluster of small sweet potatoes.
   b. **Geographic range.** The plant grows throughout North America and is found near streams or in swampy or wetland areas.
   c. The **toxic principle** is a **resinoid** known as **cicutoxin.** Cicutoxin is present mainly in the **roots** and **base of the stem**. Roots are readily pulled out of the soil by grazing animals when the soil is soft and damp.
   d. **Toxicity.** As little as 8 ounces of water hemlock may be lethal to cattle or horses.
   e. **Diagnosis**
      (1) **Clinical signs.** Water hemlock toxicosis is characterized by the acute onset of violent tetanic seizures that resemble strychnine poisoning. Salivation is followed by muscle twitching that rapidly progresses to seizures, champing of the jaws, coma, and death.
      (2) **Lesions** are indistinctive.
   f. **Treatment** is usually of little value because of the rapid course and extreme toxicity of water hemlock.

3. *Corydalis* (fitweed)
   a. **Description.** *Corydalis* is a fleshy, herbaceous biennial shrub that can grow up to 3 feet tall. It has long (3-inch) racemes of creamy white flowers that have spurs and are sometimes purple at the tips.
   b. **Geographic range.** *Corydalis* is found primarily in the hilly or mountainous regions of the Western or Appalachian states, usually in rocky or sandy soils that have a high pH.
   c. The **toxic principle** is an **isoquinoline alkaloid,** which is present in all plant parts.

d. Toxicity. Consumption of dosages as low as 2% of the body weight causes clinical signs; dosages equaling 5% of the body weight may cause death.

e. Diagnosis
  (1) Clinical signs occur in ruminants, especially sheep, and include acute onset of polypnea, tremors, and ataxia followed by periodic seizures, facial twitching, and champing of the jaws. Death or recovery occurs within 24 hours.
  (2) Lesions. Characteristic lesions are not present.

f. Treatment is general and symptomatic, but death or recovery may occur before treatment can be instituted.

4. *Dicentra culcullaria* (Dutchman's breeches)
  a. Geographic range. *D. culcullaria* is primarily a wildflower of shaded gardens and woods. Related species are grown as a potted plant (e.g., bleeding heart).
  b. Toxic principle. Isoquinoline alkaloids are present in **leaves** and **roots**.
  c. Dosages of 2%–4% of body weight are toxic.
  d. Diagnosis
    (1) Small animals. Vomiting, diarrhea, convulsions, and paralysis may occur in small animals, but poisoning is rare.
    (2) Large animals. Clinical effects in large animals are similar to those caused by *Corydalis* (see II A 3).
  e. Treatment involves administration of fluids and medication to control seizures.

5. *Gelsemium sempervirens* (yellow jessamine)
  a. Description. This evergreen vine has fragrant, yellow, trumpet-shaped flowers approximately 1 inch in length.
  b. Geographic range. *G. sempervirens* is found primarily in the southeastern United States, where it favors damp soils in or at the edge of woods. Is may also be found as an ornamental vine on porches or trellises.
  c. Toxic principle. Gelsemine, gelseminine, and related **indole alkaloids** are structurally similar to strychnine. **All parts of the plant, including honey** made from the plant, are toxic.
  d. Diagnosis
    (1) Clinical signs. Abdominal pain, slow respiration, muscle weakness, convulsions, hypothermia, and signs of colic may progress to death in 24–48 hours.
    (2) Lesions are absent or nonspecific.
  e. Treatment. Controlled ventilation and vascular support may be helpful. The stomach should be evacuated, and activated charcoal and intravenous fluids should be administered.

B. | Incoordination, depression, bizarre behavior, agitation

1. *Aesculus glabra* (Ohio buckeye, horse chestnut)
  a. Description. *A. glabra* is characterized by palmate leaves consisting of five to seven leaflets, each 4 to 6 inches in length. Three fruits (nuts) are encased in a capsule with blunt spines. When mature, the shiny brown fruit is 3–4 cm in diameter and has a pale tan surface patch that measures approximately 1 cm in diameter. Foliage appears in early spring, well before that of many other deciduous trees.
  b. Geographic range. *A. glabra* grows wild in temperate to subtropical areas of the eastern United States. It is also grown as a landscape tree.
  c. Toxic principle. Aesculin (a mixture of **saponin glycosides**) is the toxic principle. The **nuts, bark,** and **leaves** are toxic.
  d. Toxicity. Clinical toxicosis is caused by intake of dosages equaling 0.5%–1% of the animal's body weight. Cattle and horses are most susceptible.
  e. Diagnosis
    (1) Clinical signs
      (a) Neurologic. Incoordination, staggering, hypermetria, weakness, and falling are characteristic. Some animals may be injured by falling over cliffs or drowning in ponds or rivers.

(b) **Gastrointestinal.** Severe gastroenteritis, excessive fluid loss, and electrolyte imbalance sometimes accompany the neurologic signs.

(2) **Lesions.** Hepatic and renal congestion are nonspecific lesions.

f. **Treatment**

(1) **Detoxification** is useful, but difficult in large animals.

(2) **Supportive treatment**

(a) Animals should be segregated and protected from self-inflicted injury.

(b) Fluid and electrolyte replacement and demulcents may be useful for gastroenteritis.

2. *Astragalus* (locoweed)

a. **Description.** More than 200 species of locoweeds are recognized, although not all are toxic. Species identification usually requires a trained specialist.

(1) **Fruit.** Locoweeds are perennials of the Leguminosae family, which is characterized by an asymmetrical flower consisting of five petals and a fruit (i.e., the **legume,** an elongated pod with a longitudinal groove that contains from five to fifteen seeds, such as a pea pod).

(2) **Leaves** of locoweeds are pinnately compound and the flowers are usually white or purple.

(3) **Roots.** The plants grow in tufts or clumps from large taproots.

b. **Geographic range.** Locoweeds are found from the Great Plains to the Rocky Mountains, primarily in dry, alkaline soils.

c. **Toxic principle.** Locoweeds contain one of three toxic fractions.

(1) **Miserotoxin,** a **glycoside,** is hydrolyzed in ruminants to a toxic form known as **3-nitropropanol**.

(a) Toxicity may be due, in part, to nitrite released from the 3-nitropropanol, or to an unknown neurotoxic principle.

(b) *A. emoryanus* and *A. miser* are species with high concentrations of miserotoxin.

(2) **Swainsonine,** an **alkaloid** found in many locoweeds, inhibits α-mannosidase.

(a) Inhibition of a-mannosidase leads to increased lysosomal accumulation of oligosaccharides, resulting in neuronal swelling and vacuolization.

(b) Examples of swainsonine-containing locoweeds include *A. lambertii, A. mollisimus, A. lentigenosus,* and *Oxytropis.*

(3) **Selenium.** Some species of *Astragalus* and *Oxytropis* are selenium accumulators (see "alkali disease," Chapter 17 VIII B 1).

d. **Toxicity**

(1) Fresh plants are toxic. The toxicity is gradually lost as the plant dries, except for that of selenium accumulators, which are not affected by drying.

(2) Swainsonine poisoning occurs after 2 weeks or more of ingestion. Cattle and horses may become habituated to locoweed and seek it out, even when good forages are available. Swainsonine may be passed in the milk.

e. **Clinical signs**

(1) **Miserotoxin**

(a) **Neurologic signs.** Demyelination of the posterior spinal cord causes incoordination, hypermetria, ataxia, and clicking of the dewclaws (a condition known as "cracker heels").

(b) **Respiratory signs** include emphysema (primarily in sheep), dyspnea, and cyanosis. Sudden collapse and death may occur within 4–24 hours in animals poisoned by large doses.

(2) **Swainsonine**

(a) **Neurologic signs.** Affected animals exhibit ataxia, emaciation, staggering, and proprioceptive deficits. Horses may become belligerent or startle violently from inconsequential stimuli.

(b) Vision may be impaired by decreased lacrimation and retinal degeneration.

(c) Immunosuppression of the cellular immune system can occur.

(d) Abortions are common in mid- to late pregnancy, and teratogenic effects (e.g., contracted tendon) also occur.

(e) Male infertility with reduced spermatogenesis is reported.

f. Lesions

  (1) **Gross lesions** include emaciation, increased incidence of congestive right heart failure (high mountain disease), pulmonary emphysema, and congestion of the lungs and liver.

  (2) **Microscopic lesions** include myelin degeneration and neuronal vacuolation. Lesions of alkali disease are described in Chapter 17 VIII G 2.

g. Treatment of chronically affected animals is rarely effective.

  (1) **Reducing exposure.** Animals should be removed from ranges infested with locoweed, and measures should be taken to reduce range infestation (e.g., by pasture management, appropriate herbicides).

  (2) **Supportive treatment**

    (a) Methemoglobinemia and selenium poisoning should be treated (see Chapter 16 III D 3; Chapter 17 VIII H).

    (b) Reserpine administration to horses may reduce severity of locoism. Owners should be advised that "locoed" horses may not be safe to ride.

3. *Centaurea solstitialis* **and** *C. repens* **(yellow star thistle, Russian knapweed)**

  a. Description. *Centaurea* is a member of the Composite (sunflower) family. It is an annual weed that grows to approximately 1 foot in height. The leaves are covered with fine hairs. The early flower resembles a dandelion, but later matures and develops a spiny base.

  b. Geographic range

    (1) **Yellow star thistle** grows primarily in the dry regions west of the Rocky Mountains.

    (2) **Russian knapweed** grows west of the Missouri River.

  c. The **toxic principle** is unknown; however, it causes ischemic necrosis of the substantia nigra and globus pallidus.

  d. Toxicity

    (1) Toxicosis develops only after more than 100 kg of plant material have been ingested (e.g., such as would occur following consumption of plants for more than 30 days).

    (2) Dried plants are toxic.

    (3) Horses appear most susceptible.

  e. Diagnosis

    (1) **Clinical signs** reflect necrosis of major nuclei in the brain. There is hypertonicity of facial muscles, partial to complete paralysis of the tongue, chewing motions without swallowing, and an inability to eat or drink normally that leads to emaciation. Facial signs may be unilateral.

    (2) **Lesions.** The classic lesion is nigropallidal encephalomalacia with **ischemia** and **necrosis** of the **globus pallidus** and **substantia nigra**.

  f. Treatment of this permanent neurologic lesion is ineffective.

4. *Ipomea* **(Morning glory)**

  a. Description. *Ipomea* has heart-shaped leaves and showy, trumpet-shaped, white, blue, or violet flowers. It exhibits a vining growth pattern (i.e., it climbs naturally on fences and trellises).

  b. Geographic range. *Ipomea* is grown as a garden or potted plant throughout the United States.

  c. Toxic principles include **lysergic acid** and other **indole alkaloids. Seeds** are the major source of toxin, containing as much as .035% of the alkaloids. Seeds are often soaked in water prior to planting, which may increase the risk of consumption by pets.

  d. Clinical signs. Nausea, mydriasis, hallucinations, decreased reflexes, diarrhea, and hypotension are the major clinical signs. Bizarre behavior, barking, and disorientation may occur.

  e. Treatment. Activated charcoal may be administered after clearing the gastrointestinal tract. Tranquilizers or sedatives may be necessary to keep animals quiet.

C. **CNS depression**

1. *Cannabis sativa* (**marijuana, hemp**) is discussed in Chapter 24 VI.

2. *Eupatorium rugosum* (**white snakeroot**)
   a. **Description.** The plant is 2–3 feet tall, with dark green opposite and acuminate leaves with serrated margins. The brilliant white flowers appear in clusters at the top of the plant during September or October.
   b. **Geographic range.** White snakeroot is a member of the Composite family and grows throughout the east central and northeastern United States. It occurs primarily in rich, well-shaded forest soils or at the interface between forests and croplands.
   c. The **toxic principle** was originally named **trematol,** a crude fraction that includes the ketone, **trematone.** Although trematone is believed to be a significant toxic fraction, the true toxic principle is not clearly identified.
   d. **Toxicity**
      (1) The **vegetative parts of the plant** are toxic, both in the fresh and dried state. A cumulative dosage of 1%–10% of body weight is toxic or lethal.
      (2) The toxin is readily passed in milk and may poison nursing animals or babies. Early settlers in the eastern United States died as a result of "milk sickness" caused by white snakeroot.
   e. **Diagnosis**
      (1) **Clinical signs**
         (a) **Horses** develop depression, weakness, and signs of congestive heart failure (e.g., ventral swelling, jugular pulse, tachycardia), tremors, and posterior weakness. The signs appear after several days of ingesting the plant and death can occur within 3–14 days.
         (b) **Cattle** become depressed, unsteady, and ataxic. Muscle tremors are prominent about the face, neck, flank, and hind quarters, but convulsive seizures are not seen. Coma and death develop within 3–10 days. Additional signs may include constipation, salivation, and the odor of ketone or acetone on the breath.
      (2) **Laboratory diagnosis.** The toxin is reliably detected by chemical analysis. Serum clinical chemistry changes include large increases in creatine phosphokinase and alkaline phosphatase (AP), and moderate elevations of aspartate transaminase (AST) and alanine aminotransferase (ALT).
      (3) **Lesions**
         (a) **Horses.** Lesions confirm congestive heart failure with myocardial degeneration, necrosis, and fibrosis. Hepatic necrosis and lipidosis may also be present.
         (b) **Cattle.** Postmortem lesions include hepatic congestion and lipidosis and variable cardiac hemorrhages. Myocardial necrosis has not been observed in cattle.
   f. **Treatment**
      (1) **Detoxification** may be helpful in reducing further exposure.
      (2) **Supportive treatment** of congestive heart failure (in horses) and liver insufficiency (in all species) may be helpful.

3. *Isocoma wrightii* (**rayless goldenrod**)
   a. **Description.** The plant is 2–3 feet tall with narrow, pointed leaves and clusters of yellow flowers at the tips of the branches.
   b. **Geographic range.** *I. wrightii,* formerly known as *Haplopappus heterophyllus,* ranges throughout the southwestern United States as far east as Texas. It grows best in low, moist areas.
   c. **Toxic principle.** Like white snakeroot, the toxic principle is **trematol** or **trematone.**
   d. **Toxicity.** Toxicosis is associated with a cumulative dosage of 1%–2% of body weight.
   e. **Clinical signs** are identical to those of white snakeroot (see II C 2 e), although myocardial lesions in horses have not been described.
   f. **Treatment** considerations are the same as for white snakeroot (see II C 2 f).

4. *Stipa robusta* (**sleepy grass**)
   a. **Description.** Sleepy grass is a perennial grass, 2–4 feet tall, with relatively broad leaves. The grass has a distinctive twisted awn on the flowers and seeds.
   b. **Geographic range.** Sleepy grass is limited to the southwestern United States.
   c. A **toxic principle** is not described, but neurologic depression is the main toxic effect.
   d. **Toxicity.** Cattle are relatively resistant. Poisoning occurs mainly in horses.
   e. **Clinical signs.** Moderate to severe CNS depression may progress to recumbency.
   f. **Treatment** is general and supportive; there is no antidote.

D. **Anticholinergic effects**

1. *Atropa belladonna* (**belladonna, deadly nightshade**)
   a. **Description.** Belladonna, a member of the nightshade family (Solanaceae), is a coarse herb with large (6-inch), ovoid, pointed leaves. Its flowers are approximately 1 inch long, five-pointed, and purple. Berries change from green to purple or black as they ripen.
   b. **Geographic range.** Belladonna occurs in the United States primarily as a cultivated garden plant. Access is limited principally to small animals.
   c. The **toxic principle** is **atropine**. **All plant parts** may be toxic, but the green berries are most likely to be ingested by small animals.
   d. **Toxicity.** Poisoning is uncommon.
   e. **Clinical signs** are similar to effects of overdosage by atropine or poisoning by Jimson weed (see *Datura stramonium*, II D 2). They include thirst, visual disturbances, and delirium with hallucinations.
   f. **Treatment.** Parasympathomimetic drugs to stimulate cholinergic secretions and activity may be helpful, in addition to general gastrointestinal detoxification.

2. *Datura stramonium* and *D. metel* (**Jimson weed, angel's trumpet**)
   a. **Description.** The plant is large (achieving heights of 2–4 feet) and has irregular, simple alternated leaves 5–9 inches in length. The stems are smooth and brown to purple. Flowers are trumpet-shaped, white, and 2–3 inches long. The fruit is a spiny capsule containing numerous dark, wrinkled seeds.
   b. **Geographic range.** *Datura* occurs as a weed in gardens, crop fields, and dry lots. Some varieties are also cultivated as an ornamental. It ranges throughout the entire United States, but is most prominent in the eastern United States and grows best in fertile soils.
   c. The **toxic principle** is a group of toxins known as **belladonna alkaloids** (i.e., **atropine, hyoscyamine, hyoscine**). The toxin is present in the **entire plant,** but is most **concentrated in seeds**.
   d. **Exposure**
      (1) Seed that heavily contaminates small grains may be a greater hazard than the green plants, which are relatively unpalatable and rarely consumed except by hungry animals.
      (2) Jimson weed seeds are sometimes taken as a drug of abuse for their potential hallucinogenic effects, and small animals may accidentally gain access to the seeds or teas prepared from the seeds.
   e. **Diagnosis and treatment.** Clinical signs and therapeutic approaches are identical to those for *Atropa belladonna* poisoning (see II D 1 e, f).

3. *Solanum tuberosum* (**potato**) and *S. nigrum* (**black nightshade**)
   a. **Description.** Both are members of the nightshade family, which generally have fused, five-petaled, white to purple flowers and alternate irregular or entire leaves. The fruit may be a capsule or berry. The berries are green and turn to purple or black when ripe.
   b. **Geographic range.** Potatoes are cultivated in gardens for their edible tubers, but the foliage may be toxic. Black nightshade occurs most commonly in moist, well-drained fertile soils, often as an invading annual weed of crop fields or hay.

    c. Toxic principle. Potatoes and black nightshade contain a substantial amount of **tropane alkaloids** with activity similar to atropine. The clinical response may be complicated by the effects of steroidal glycoalkaloids (e.g., solanine, solanidine), which may cause gastroenteritis. The **vines, green skin, sprouts,** and **green berries** are toxic. Ripe berries are nontoxic.

    d. Clinical signs. Colic, diarrhea, salivation, ataxia, weakness, bradycardia, hypotension, and paralysis may occur.

    e. Treatment should include general gastrointestinal detoxification, monitoring for the cardiac effects of atropine, and administration of cholinergic drugs (e.g., physostigmine) if needed.

E.   **Anticholinesterase effects.** The **Solanaceae (nightshade) family** includes weeds, food plants, ornamental plants, and medicinal plants.

    1. Description. *Lycopersicon* species (tomato), *Physalis* species (ground cherry), and *Solanum* species are most often implicated; selected members of *Solanum* are described in Table 28-2.

        a. Flowers are five-petaled and often fused at the base to form a tubular flower with a central, two-part fused pistil and five stamens.

        b. Leaves are often dark green and smooth to shiny with irregular margins.

        c. Fruits are either a capsule or berry, and the green berry ripens to a red, purple, or black color.

    2. Geographic range. The nightshade family is a large and widespread family, occurring over large portions of the United States.

    3. The **toxic principle** is **solanine,** a **glycoside** that is hydrolyzed to yield the sugar moiety and **solanidine,** an active principle characterized as a **steroidal alkaloid**.

    4. Toxicity. Usually the ripe fruit is considered nontoxic, but the water-soluble, heat-stable toxic principle is present in **leaves** and **green berries** and is stable when dried.

        a. Toxicity ranges from 0.1%–1.0% of animal body weight consumed as green plant.

        b. *S. eliagnifolium* (silverleaf nightshade) is extremely toxic, with toxicity established at dosages of 0.1% of body weight.

    5. Diagnosis

        a. Clinical signs. The clinical course is rapid; affected animals may succumb or recover within 24–38 hours.

            (1) CNS signs include depression, incoordination, tremors, posterior weakness, and prostration. The pupillary response to light may be altered. Unconsciousness, paralysis, shock, and coma are terminal signs.

TABLE 28-2. *Solanum* Species with Anticholinesterase Effects

Name	Description	Geographic Range
S. nigrum (black nightshade)	Leaves often perforated by insect foraging	Gardens, croplands, and the edges of woodlands
S. eleagnifolium (silverleaf nightshade)	Perennial with prickly spines and hairy leaves	Southern United States
S. carolinense (horsenettle, bullnettle)	Short, flowers are five-petaled with prominent yellow stamens, leaves are irregular with spines, berries are large, amber or yellow when ripe	Eastern two-thirds of the United States
S. dulcamara (European bittersweet)	Vining plant, sometimes maintained as an ornamental	Entire United States; more common in moist, temperate zones
S. rostratum (buffalo bur)	Short with irregular leaves and yellow flowers, leaves and stems covered with sharp spines up to 2 cm in length	Entire United States, except deserts and mountains

      (2) Gastrointestinal signs are anorexia, salivation, vomiting, and diarrhea. Large dosages may be associated with intestinal atony and constipation.

    b. Lesions are usually limited or absent. The gastroenteritis is mucoid or, occasionally, hemorrhagic. Renal lesions reported for swine are very rarely, if ever, present.

6. Treatment. General detoxification measures should be followed by supportive therapy for vomiting and diarrhea, fluid losses, and serious neurologic signs.

F. | **Neuromuscular (nicotinic) effects**

1. *Conium maculatum* **(poison hemlock)**

    a. Description. Poison hemlock is a perennial member of the Umbelliferae (parsley) family. The plants are up to 6 feet tall with smooth, hollow stems covered with purple spots. Leaves are finely divided, resembling those of parsley or carrots. Crushed leaves have a mouse-like odor. The plant is sometimes confused with wild carrot (*Daucus carota*, Queen Anne's lace). There is a large white to pale yellow taproot.

    b. Geographic range. Poison hemlock grows on fertile, moist soils across the United States in locations such as woodlots, fencerows, and waste areas.

    c. Toxic principle. Coniine and related **pyridine-type alkaloids** are present in the **root, young plants,** and **seeds.** As plants mature, the foliage loses alkaloid content, but the seeds accumulate the alkaloid.

    d. Toxicity. The whole green plant is toxic at dosages of approximately 1% of body weight.

    e. Diagnosis

      (1) Clinical signs. The clinical course is rapid, and animals may be found dead or die within a few hours.

        (a) Initial consumption may cause a burning sensation in the mouth, salivation, emesis, and diarrhea.

        (b) Rapidly developing neurologic signs include muscle tremors, muscular weakness, dim vision, convulsions, and coma. Death results from respiratory failure.

        (c) Frequent urination and defecation may also occur.

        (d) The pyridine alkaloids are teratogenic and may cause crooked limbs, cleft palate, and crooked tails in calves or pigs exposed in utero during mid-gestation (i.e., 40–72 days in cattle and 30–60 days in swine).

      (2) Laboratory diagnosis. The alkaloid may be detected in the stomach contents and urine.

      (3) Lesions are not present in poisoned animals.

    f. Treatment. The stomach should be evacuated, and activated charcoal administered. Respiratory support by mechanical ventilation may be life-saving in small animals.

2. *Delphinium* **(larkspur)** is a major cause of cattle losses in some portions of the Great Plains and Rocky Mountains.

    a. Description. The plants, which belong to the Ranunculaceae family, are erect and range from 0.3–1.5 meters in height. The alternate leaves are palmately lobed and veined, similar in appearance to buttercup leaves (also members of the Ranunculaceae family). The striking blue flowers with a prominent "spur" are borne on a terminal stem.

    b. Geographic range

      (1) Tall larkspurs (*D. barbeyi, D. occidentale, D. glaucum*) grow primarily at high altitudes (6000–11,000 feet) in moist areas, often under or near stands of aspen.

      (2) Low larkspurs (*D. bicolor, D. gyeri, D. nelsonii*) grow at lower elevations in open areas and grasslands.

      (3) Horticultural varieties are widely grown as ornamental garden plants.

    c. Toxic principle. Polycyclic diterpene alkaloids, neuromuscular blocking agents that affect cholinergic and nicotinic receptors, are the toxic principle in larkspurs.

    d. Toxicity. The plant is toxic during the entire growing period. Dosages as low as 0.5%–1.5% of body weight may be toxic or lethal to cattle, and mortality is relatively high among poisoned animals. Cattle are considered much more susceptible than sheep or horses.

    e. Diagnosis depends on knowledge of circumstances and a history of typical clinical signs.

      (1) Clinical signs appear suddenly.

        (a) Initial signs include excitability, disorientation, muscle tremors, stiffness, and paresis. Affected animals may bloat or attempt to vomit, which can cause aspiration pneumonia. Cardiac arrhythmia may be present.

        (b) Signs progress to severe weakness, prostration, and seizures. Death may result from respiratory paralysis.

      (2) Laboratory diagnosis is not routinely available.

      (3) Lesions. Congestion of major organs and bloat are the only lesions expected.

    f. Treatment

      (1) Prompt gastrointestinal detoxification using activated charcoal and osmotic cathartics is necessary.

      (2) Relief of bloat may be essential as an early life-saving procedure.

      (3) Physostigmine (approximately 0.06 mg/kg intravenously) has been helpful in overcoming the neuromuscular blockade.

3. *Laburnum anagyroides* (goldenchain)

    a. Description. *L. anagyroides* is a landscape tree with distinctive long chains of yellow flowers.

    b. The **toxic principle is cytisine**.

    c. Toxicity. The entire plant is toxic, but the attractive flowers or resultant seeds may be most dangerous. Small animals kept near or under the trees are most susceptible.

    d. Clinical signs include emesis, drowsiness, weakness, incoordination, sweating, headache, mydriasis, and tachycardia.

    e. Treatment. An oral slurry of activated charcoal should be administered following evacuation of the stomach.

4. *Lobelia* (cardinal flower, giant lobelia)

    a. Description. Plants may be tall (up to 4 feet) with blue, white, or red flowers.

    b. Geographic range. Several species of *Lobelia* occur as wild plants or cultivated ornamentals. They are found primarily in the eastern United States, as far west as Colorado. They grow best in damp to wet soils in open areas or near the edge of woodlands.

    c. The **toxic principle** is a **pyridine alkaloid** known as **lobeline,** which acts similarly to nicotine.

    d. Toxicity. The entire plant is toxic, but consumption of quantities significant enough to cause toxicosis is rare.

    e. Clinical signs mimic the effects of nicotine and include nausea, vomiting, mydriasis, muscle tremors, weakness, paralysis, and death.

    f. Treatment. Gastrointestinal detoxification and supportive therapy are recommended.

5. *Lupinus* (lupine, bluebonnet)

    a. Description. Lupines are in the Legume family, which is characterized by irregular, five-petaled flowers with a central "keel."

      (1) Flowers are blue; occasionally white, red, or yellow varieties are seen.

      (2) Leaves. The leaf, a palmately compound leaf with five to seven elongated, ovoid leaflets, is somewhat distinctive.

    b. Geographic range. Both cultivated garden lupines and native lupines of the western rangelands are toxic. In rangelands, they occur from the dry, open ranges of the Great Plains to the Rocky Mountains.

    c. Toxic principle. Lupinine, a **quinolizidine alkaloid,** induces nicotinic effects in animals.

      (1) Leaves, seeds, and **fruits** all contain lupinine, which is retained in dried plants.

      (2) Pods may concentrate the toxin, becoming a source of poisoning during the winter season when livestock are moved through infested areas or contaminated hay is fed.

    d. Toxicity. Lupines are a major toxic problem in range sheep. Lupines are toxic at 1% or less of body weight.

e. Clinical signs

    (1) Salivation, ataxia, seizures, and dyspnea are major acute clinical signs and are more common in sheep than in cattle.

    (2) Head-pressing and excitement may also be seen.

    (3) Effects not related to the nervous system include the "crooked calf syndrome" (i.e., carpal flexure, torticollis, and scoliosis in calves exposed in utero during days 40–70 of gestation). The toxic principle for this effect is the alkaloid anagyrine.

f. Treatment. Oral detoxication and control of seizures in severely affected animals is the only recourse. Prevention through correct range management is preferred.

6. *Sophora secundiflora* **(mescal bean)**

a. Description. Mescal bean is a woody evergreen shrub or small tree. Its alternate pinnately compound leaves are slightly hairy on the underside and yellow-green on the upper side.

b. Geographic range. Mescal bean is a legume of the southwestern United States. Plants do well in arid, alkaline soils.

c. The **toxic principle** is **cytisine** or other quinolizidine alkaloids.

d. Toxicity

    (1) Leaves and seed pods contain the toxin. **Seed pods** are most dangerous; 0.5 g/kg body weight is considered a lethal dose.

    (2) Cattle, sheep and goats are susceptible, and human toxicoses have been reported following use of the seeds as a hallucinogen.

e. Clinical effects

    (1) Neurologic signs include salivation, tremors, excitement, muscle rigidity, delirium, paralysis, coma, and death.

    (2) Gastrointestinal signs of nausea, vomiting, and diarrhea accompany the neurologic signs.

f. Treatment is as described in Chapter 19 I H. Surviving animals may appear somnolent for up to 3 days.

G. Weakness or paralysis

1. Of primarily neurologic origin

a. *Acacia berlandieri* **(guajillo)**

    (1) Description. *A. berlandieri* is a legume that can serve as an alternative forage plant for grazing animals. The plant is a shrub or small tree with alternate bipinnately compound leaves and leaflets 4–6 mm in length. The flowers are white to yellow, typical irregular legume flowers.

    (2) Geographic distribution. Guajillo is of limited geographic distribution, occurring mainly in Texas with related species in the alkaline areas of Arizona.

    (3) The **toxic principle** is believed to be **sympathomimetic amines, tyramine, N-methyl tyramine,** and **N-methyl-β-phenylethylamine,** which are monoamine oxidase (MAO) inhibitors. The toxin is present in the **leaves.**

    (4) Toxicity

        (a) The oral lethal dosage ranges from 0.5–5.0 g/kg body weight (about 0.05%–0.5% body weight).

        (b) If most of the diet is consumed as guajillo for more than 6 months, chronic toxicosis develops.

        (c) Goats are at risk because of their habit of browsing heavily on trees and shrubs.

    (5) Clinical signs develop slowly after extended intake of the plant.

        (a) Early signs are posterior ataxia and weakness that is sometimes called "limberleg."

        (b) Excitement and exercise may exacerbate the condition. Paresis is ascending in nature, and eventually animals become recumbent. Recumbent animals remain alert and retain their appetite.

        (c) Death usually results from starvation, thirst, or predation.

    (6) Treatment. Animals should be prevented access to the plants, and good nursing care is necessary until animals recover, which may require several months.

  b. *Karwinskia humboldtiana* **(coyotillo)**

    (1) Description. Coyotillo is a shrub or small tree with ovate to elliptical opposite leaves 4–8 centimeters long. Flowers are small and yellow-green, occurring in the leaf axils. They have five petals and five prominent sepals.

    (2) Geographic range. Coyotillo is limited to southwestern Texas, southern California, and other limited areas of the desert southwest.

    (3) The **toxic principle** is not known, but is speculated to be a polyphenolic compound. The mechanism of action is unknown, but the plant appears to induce segmental demyelination of the peripheral nerves and degeneration of the ventral horn cells of the spinal cord.

    (4) Toxicity. Consumption of seeds at 0.1%–0.3% of body weight may be toxic, whereas toxicosis from green foliage requires dosages equalling 10%–20% of body weight.

    (5) Diagnosis

      (a) Clinical signs suggest an ascending paresis and paralysis that may appear from 3 days to 3 weeks after consumption of the plant. Early signs of muscle tremors and ataxia progress to incoordination, weakness, dyspnea, and prostration.

      (b) Lesions

        (i) Segmental demyelination with splitting of myelin lamellae precedes axonal degeneration.

        (ii) Degeneration and chromatolysis of ventral horn cells in the spinal cord follow as a result of the peripheral neuropathy.

    (6) Treatment. Thiamine is sometimes recommended for general supportive therapy, but is of limited benefit. Because of the permanent nature of the neurologic lesion, recovery is unlikely.

  c. *Lathyrus* **(vetchling, wild pea, singletary pea)**

    (1) Geographic range. Several toxic species occur throughout the United States.

      (a) *L. hirsutus* and *L. pusillus* are grown as cover crops or forage.

      (b) *L. incanus* ranges throughout the Great Plains.

      (c) *L. sylvestris* grows wild in the southeastern United States.

    (2) The **toxic principle,** occurring at different concentrations in various *Lathyrus* species, is β-amino propionitrile (BAP). BAP is concentrated primarily in the **seeds**. It may be resistant to drying but is heat-labile and destroyed by cooking.

    (3) Toxicity. Toxicosis is only likely if large quantities of *Lathyrus* are consumed over substantial periods of time.

    (4) Clinical signs

      (a) Acute signs include slowness, weakness, and shifting of weight from one limb to another. Neurologic effects may progress to apparent stiffness or a stilted gait, or both. Horses may be affected more severely than cattle.

      (b) Osteolathyrism is a second syndrome, affecting mainly cattle, that produces lameness that may appear to be caused by a neurologic deficit. Evidence for this problem in the United States is primarily anecdotal and very limited.

    (5) Treatment is generalized and supportive.

  d. *Sorghum* **(sorghum, Sudan grass, milo, Johnson grass).** *Sorghum* species are both valuable crop plants (Sudan grass, milo) and weeds (Johnson grass).

    (1) Description. Plants are tall (up to 2 meters) with coarse, dull green leaves and a terminal inflorescence of green to greenish-yellow florets. Seeds are dark brown to purple or black, plump, shiny, and 0.3 centimeters long.

    (2) Geographic range. *Sorghum* species grow throughout the temperate regions of North America, and are readily adapted to the dry, hot conditions of the area south of the Great Plains to Texas.

    (3) The **toxic principle** that affects the nervous system is believed to be β-cyano alanine, which is similar to the toxic principle in *Lathyrus* species. Cyanogenic glycosides have also been suspected as potential agents in the neurologic effects of sorghums.

(4) Toxicity. Toxicosis is associated with grazing of the foliage, not with consumption of the seeds. Some forage *Sorghums* contain a warning label against grazing by horses.

(5) Diagnosis

(a) Clinical signs. Equine sorghum cystitis–ataxia syndrome is characteristic.

(i) Urinary incontinence and dribbling of the urine are common in both mares and males, predisposing the horse to **cystitis** in the prolonged presence of clinical signs and urine stasis. In mares, periodic opening and closing of the vulva occurs as well. Urinary irritation may contribute to the appearance that mares are in estrus.

(ii) Horses develop **posterior ataxia** and **incoordination** after grazing for several days on rapidly growing *Sorghum* forages. Forced exercise may cause affected horses to stumble or drop to the ground momentarily.

(b) Laboratory diagnosis. Epithelial cells, bacteria, and inflammatory cells may be present in the urine sediment.

(c) Lesions include inflammatory cystitis, pyelonephritis, and axonal degeneration of spinal cord neurons.

(6) Treatment. Animals should be removed from the pasture and the cystitis should be treated with antibiotics. If ataxia has developed, recovery may not be complete.

2. Of muscular origin. *Cassia occidentalis, C. tora* **(coffee senna, sicklepod)** causes muscle damage, leading to weakness and paralysis.

a. Description. *Cassia,* a member of the Legume family, is a coarse annual with pinnately compound leaves containing four to eight leaflets. The leaflets are 3–5 cm in length. The flowers are yellow and irregular. The pods are narrow and elongated (approximately 10–20 cm in length).

b. Geographic range. *Cassia* grows throughout the southeastern United States, and is especially prominent in the sandy soils of the coastal plain, in crop fields, waste areas, and open pine forests.

c. The **toxic principle** is unknown, but the plant causes mild to extensive myodegeneration and necrosis of skeletal and cardiac muscle. The toxin is present in the **seeds, leaves,** and **stems** of both fresh and dried plants.

d. Toxicity. Toxicosis is induced by dosages of 1% of body weight daily for approximately 1 week. Cattle are most susceptible.

e. Diagnosis

(1) Clinical signs reflect muscle damage.

(a) A slow gait, ataxia, muscle tremors, and weakness are early signs. Affected animals become progressively weaker and finally recumbent, although there is no loss of appetite and the animal remains alert.

(b) Tachycardia and respiratory difficulty are concurrent with muscle weakness. Death may result from hyperkalemic heart failure.

(c) Gastroenteritis, as evidenced by diarrhea, may be caused by anthraquinone glycosides in the plant.

(2) Laboratory analysis

(a) Myoglobinuria signals significant muscle necrosis.

(b) Elevated AST and **creatine phosphokinase** confirm muscle necrosis and indicate moderate liver or kidney damage, which may also occur.

(c) Hyperkalemia may also be seen.

(3) Lesions include pale cardiac and skeletal musculature, myodegeneration and necrosis, and mild to moderate hepatic lipidosis and necrosis. Degeneration of renal tubules may be related to myoglobinuria.

f. Treatment involves supportive therapy for muscle necrosis and myoglobinuria. Selenium and vitamin E may be helpful, but are not highly effective.

III. PLANTS CAUSING GASTROINTESTINAL TOXICITY

A. Stinging, inflammation, and swelling of the oral mucosa

1. Plants commonly associated with physical damage to the digestive tract are summarized in Table 28-3.

2. Some plants elicit a chemical response in addition to directly irritating the oral mucosa.
   a. **Urtica (nettle, stinging nettle)**
      (1) **Description.** Members of the *Urtica* species are perennials that reproduce from seeds and spread from underground rootstocks; therefore, they tend to occur in contiguous patches. The plants may grow as tall as 1.5 meters, and the opposite leaves and stems are covered with stinging hairs that release acetylcholine (ACh), histamine, serotonin, and formic acid.
      (2) **Clinical signs.** Contact results in pain, salivation, vomiting, nasal and oral irritation, weakness, and, occasionally, death.
      (3) **Treatment.** Atropine, antihistamines, and supportive therapy may help to reduce the clinical effects.
   b. **Calcium oxalate crystal-containing plants.** The plants listed in Table 28-4 contain calcium oxalate crystals, which irritate the oropharynx.
      (1) **Description.** Most of these plants have some form of broad green or variegated green leaves. Flowers are often inconspicuous or absent.
      (2) **Geographic range.** These plants are found generally in woods, gardens, and as indoor ornamental plants.
      (3) **Mechanism of toxicologic damage.** Calcium oxalate crystals form needle-like spicules (raphides) that are believed to penetrate the tongue and pharynx. Some plants (e.g., *Dieffenbachia*) are also known to contain proteolytic enzymes, which trigger the release of kinins and histamines to cause a rapid inflammatory response.

TABLE 28-3. Plants that Cause Physical Damage to the Mouth and Skin

Name	Description	Geographic Range
Arctium (burdock)	Coarse biennial herb with large burs ending in small hooks	
Bromus (wild brome grass)		Throughout the United States in pastures and waste areas
Cacti	Spines of various shapes, lengths	Texas, Oklahoma, desert southwest
Cenchrus (sand bur)	Prostrate growth habit, 0.5-cm spiny burs	Dry to moist soils throughout the United States
Hordeum (wild barley)	Cool season annual grass	Pastures and disturbed prairie areas over much of the United States
Setaria (foxtail)*	Annual grass with erect stems and hairless leaves, light green flowers borne in a dense panicle at the tip of the stem, small seeds with one or two awns	
Stipa (needle grasses)*	Perennial grass, grows in clumps, up to 1 meter tall, seeds have long, twisted awn	Southwestern United States
Tribulus terrestris (goathead, puncture vine)	Recumbent vine with trailing branches, small yellow flowers, bur with two strong spines	Pastures, waste areas, roadsides, cultivated fields west of the Missouri River

*Dermal irritation only.

TABLE 28-4. Plants Containing Calcium Oxalate Crystals

Alocasia (alocasia)	*Dieffenbachia* (dieffenbachia, dumbcane)
Arisaema triphyllum (jack-in-the-pulpit)	*Monstera* (split leaf philodendron)
Calla (wild calla)	*Philodendron* (philodendron)
Colocasia (colocasia)	*Symplocarpus foetidus* (skunk cabbage)

    (4) Toxicity. All parts of these plants are considered toxic. Small animals are most often at risk because of access to house or garden plants.

    (5) Clinical signs include a burning sensation on the lips and in the mouth and throat, inflammation, edema, and salivation. Severe poisoning may cause choking and respiratory difficulty or death.

    (6) Treatment. The animal's mouth should be rinsed with large amounts of water. Cool liquids or demulcents placed in the mouth may bring relief, and antihistamines are recommended. Signs may persist for several hours or more after treatment.

B. **Vomiting, diarrhea.** The following plants directly irritate the gastric and intestinal mucosa, leading to vomiting, diarrhea, or both.

  1. *Abrus precatorius* (**rosary pea, precatory bean**)
    a. Description. The bright red seeds with a dark scar are attractive to children and possibly pets or pet birds.
    b. Geographic range. *A. precatorius* is native to the Caribbean islands, but the seeds have been imported to the United States.
    c. Toxic principle. Abrin, a plant phytotoxin, is concentrated in the seeds.
    d. Toxicity. Broken seeds are highly toxic—one seed approximately 0.5 cm in diameter can kill a small child or medium-sized dog.
    e. Diagnosis
      (1) Clinical signs
        (a) An initial latent period of up to 24 hours is followed by nausea, vomiting, diarrhea, and, occasionally, ulcerative lesions in the mouth and esophagus.
        (b) Trembling, tachycardia, incoordination, and paralysis may follow.
        (c) Body temperature may be elevated 3–4 degrees.
      (2) Lesions include mucosal and serosal gastric hemorrhages and increased fluids in the lumen of the intestine.
    f. Treatment. Emesis or lavage should be followed with charcoal, demulcents, fluids, and electrolytes. Prognosis is guarded to grave.

  2. *Agrostemma githago* (**corn cockle**)
    a. Description. Corn cockle, a member of the carnation family, is recognized by its five partially fused pink or purple petals. Prominent, long, narrow sepals extend well beyond the petals. The leaves are opposite, long and narrow, and pubescent.
    b. Geographic range. Corn cockle grows across the eastern and southern United States.
    c. The **toxic principle** is a **saponin** called **githagenin.** The toxin is concentrated mainly in the **seeds,** which may contaminate small grains (e.g., wheat, rye).
    d. Toxicity
      (1) Ingestion of as little as 0.1% of body weight as seeds may be toxic to livestock, and seeds are more toxic when they are ground.
      (2) Toxicosis has been reported in birds, horses, and cattle.
    e. Clinical signs include vomiting, gastroenteritis, diarrhea, and purgation.
    f. Treatment. The gastrointestinal tract should be evacuated, and activated charcoal should be administered. Gastroenteritis can be treated with demulcents.

  3. *Amanita phalloides* (**deadly amanita, death angel**) is characterized by an initial gastrointestinal phase; however, because its toxic principle is a hepatocellular toxin, *A. phalloides* is discussed in IV A 1.

4. *Brassica* **(mustards),** annual plants of the Mustard family, include forage crops (e.g., rape, kale). Plants appear and flower early in the spring and may be the first green plants available.

  a. Description. The stems are tipped with small yellow or white four-petaled flowers. Leaves are mainly simple, alternate, and variously lobed. The small dark brown to black seeds may contaminate small grains.

  b. The **toxic principle** is a variety of **glucosinolates,** which are glycosides that hydrolyze to yield aglycones that include **isothiocyanate** and **thiocyanate**. Some species (e.g., *Rape*) contain **goitrogens** (L-5-vinyl-2-thiooxazolidone). Toxic principles are present in **all plant parts,** but are most **concentrated in the seeds**.

  c. Clinical signs. Gastrointestinal signs (e.g., anorexia, fluid to hemorrhagic diarrhea, dehydration) are nonspecific but may be severe. Death occasionally occurs.

  d. Treatment involves gastrointestinal detoxification followed by supportive therapy to alleviate diarrhea and restore fluids and electrolytes.

5. *Colchicum autumnale* **(autumn crocus)**

  a. Geographic range. Autumn crocus is often grown as a house or garden plant. Bulbs set on window ledges or counter tops are accessible to dogs and cats.

  b. Toxic principle. Colchicine, a toxic alkaloid, acts as an antimetabolite or spindle poison during mitosis. The toxin is present throughout the entire plant, but is most **concentrated in the bulbs**.

  c. Toxicity. Dogs are most susceptible because of the canine habit of promiscuous ingestion.

  d. Clinical signs include a burning sensation in the mouth and throat, thirst, nausea, diarrhea, weakness, and circulatory failure.

  e. Treatment. Gastrointestinal decontamination should reduce the severity and duration of signs if accomplished soon after ingestion. Fluids, analgesics, and atropine may help to alleviate colic and diarrhea.

6. *Daphne mezereum* **(daphne)**

  a. Description. Daphne is a small, woody landscape shrub with lanceolate green leaves and small pink or white tubular flowers. Bright red or yellow seeds appear to be directly attached to the stem.

  b. Toxic principle. Daphnetoxin and **mezerein, diterpene esters,** appear to cause both gastroenteritis and renal damage.

  c. Toxicity. Toxin is present in the entire plant. The berries are most often consumed because they are accessible and noticeable.

  d. Clinical signs. Initial signs include vesication and edema of the lips, oral cavity, and oropharynx. Salivation is followed by thirst, abdominal pain, emesis, and bloody diarrhea.

  e. Treatment. Gastrointestinal decontamination with activated charcoal and cathartics may reduce toxicosis if performed early. Fluids and electrolytes must be restored to compensate for vomiting and diarrhea.

7. *Euphorbia.* The most common toxic varieties are listed in Table 28-5. There are at least two dozen toxic varieties.

  a. Description

   (1) Flowers may be much reduced or prominent, and in some cases the sepals rather than the petals are prominent (e.g., poinsettias).

   (2) The **fruit** is a rounded, three-seeded capsule.

TABLE 28-5. Common Toxic Varieties of *Euphorbia*

E. corollata	(flowering spurge)
E. cyparissias	(cypress spurge)
E. maculata	(milk spurge)
E. marginata	(snow-on-the-mountain)
E. pulcherima	(poinsettia)

(3) The **leaves** may be opposite or alternate. For some species, the cut or broken stem or leaf petiole may exude a white sap similar in appearance to that of milkweed.

b. Geographic range. *Euphorbia* species, of the family Euphorbiaceae, are known as "spurges" and may occur as garden or indoor ornamental plants or weeds. They are found worldwide and range widely over the United States. Both annuals and perennials comprise the family.

c. Toxic principle. Complex diterpene or phorbol esters (**ingenol, phorbol, daphane**) activate protein kinase C, which indirectly affects enzyme function and may cause cytoskeletal damage.

d. Toxicity
(1) The sap is toxic in fresh and dried plants.
(2) Ingestion of plant material in excess of approximately 1% of the body weight may cause clinical signs.

e. Clinical signs include direct irritation and vesiculation of the skin and mucosa, salivation, vomiting, diarrhea, and dermatitis.

f. Treatment. Gastrointestinal decontamination including activated charcoal, should be followed with fluids and electrolytes to prevent dehydration. Local inflammation and necrosis can be treated with careful washing of the skin and administration of analgesics and demulcents.

8. *Hedera helix* (English ivy)
a. Description. The leaves, which are similar in appearance to maple leaves, are dark green or variegated, smooth, and three- to five-lobed. Small white to greenish flowers produce a dark berry approximately 0.3 cm in diameter.

b. Geographic range. English ivy is a commonly cultivated vine and house plant grown throughout the United States.

c. Toxic principles. Hederagenin, a saponin, and **falcarinol,** a polyacetylene, are the reported toxic principles. The **berries** and **leaves** are toxic.

d. Clinical signs. Salivation, thirst, emesis, gastroenteritis, diarrhea, and skin irritation are major signs. Excitement, dyspnea, and seizures may occur.

e. Treatment. Dermal irritation can be treated with corticosteroids. Symptomatic treatment for the gastroenteric signs is recommended.

9. *Helenium* (sneezeweed)
a. Description. *Helenium*, which is a member of the Composite family, produces flowers that are yellow and daisy-like with both disk flowers (the "head" of the daisy) and ray flowers (the "petals" of the daisy). Leaves may be lanceolate to finely divided. Plants may be either annuals or perennials.

b. Geographic range. *Helenium* grows at high elevations (5000–10,000 feet) in moist, well-drained mountain meadows of the western mountain states from Montana south to New Mexico and west to California.

c. Toxic principles include **sesquiterpene lactones** (**helenalin** and **tenulin**) and a **glycoside** called **dugaldin.** Toxins, which are present throughout the plant, may bind to sulfhydryl groups and inactivate enzymes or glutathione.

d. Toxicity. Poisoning occurs mainly in sheep during late summer or fall when good forages may be scarce. Depending on species, dosages from 0.3%–1.0% of body weight may be fatal, especially if consumption has taken place over several days.

e. Clinical signs
(1) **Acute.** Vomiting or spewing of rumen contents is characteristic. Severe diarrhea may develop within 24 hours. Neurologic signs of seizures and head-pressing occasionally are observed.
(2) **Chronic.** Vomiting, muscle weakness, and emaciation result from several weeks of ingestion. Animals are anorectic and depressed.

f. Treatment. Individual animal treatment in large flocks may not be practical. Good quality alternative feeds should be offered, and the weed should be controlled with herbicides. Improved pasture management (e.g., by alternative species grazing or seasonal grazing control) can also help control weed growth.

10. *Helleborus niger* (**Christmas rose**)
    a. **Geographic range.** Christmas rose is a common garden perennial and house plant.
    b. **Toxic principles. Hellebrin, helleborin,** and **helleborein** (cardiac glycosides) and **protoanemonin** act as cathartics. The **entire plant** is toxic.
    c. **Clinical signs.** Major signs are pain in the mouth and abdomen, nausea, emesis, colic, and diarrhea. Arrhythmia and hypotension may occur in advanced cases.
    d. **Treatment.** Gastric lavage or induced emesis followed by activated charcoal or saline cathartics may be helpful.

11. *Hydrangea* (**hydrangea**)
    a. **Description.** Hydrangeas are ornamental shrubs with large (15-cm), serrated, dull, dark green leaves and large, showy clusters of white, pink, or blue flowers.
    b. **Toxic principle.** Hydrangeas may contain hydrogen cyanide, but the clinical effects of gastroenteritis are not related to cyanide.
    c. **Toxicity.** Presumably, all parts of the plant are toxic, but poisoning is rare and occurs mainly following consumption of the leaves.
    d. **Clinical signs.** Severe gastroenteritis and mucoid to hemorrhagic diarrhea are associated with *Hydrangea* toxicosis.
    e. **Treatment** is supportive.

12. *Hymenoxys odorata* (**bitterweed**)
    a. **Description.** Bitterweed, a member of the Composite family, has daisy-like yellow flowers and finely cut or divided leaves.
    b. **Geographic range.** Bitterweed is found primarily in western Texas, western Oklahoma, Arizona, and New Mexico.
    c. The **toxic principle, hymenoxon,** is a **sesquiterpene lactone** that appears to inactivate sulfhydryl groups of enzymes and, possibly, glutathione. The toxin is present in **all parts of the plant** and is resistant to drying.
    d. **Toxicity.** Bitterweed toxicosis is a major problem in sheep, as opposed to cattle. Poisoning is most likely in late winter or early spring. The toxic range for ingestion is 0.5%–1.5% of the body weight.
    e. **Clinical signs**
        (1) **Acute** poisoning may cause ruminants to vomit and cough. Rumen stasis and bloat are also prominent. Acute signs may lead to death within 2–3 days.
        (2) **Chronic.** Affected animals are depressed and anorectic, lose weight, and develop weakness and ataxia.
    f. **Treatment** is the same as that for sneezeweed toxicosis (see III B 9 f).

13. *Ilex* (**holly**)
    a. **Description.** Dark, shiny evergreen leaves are broadly oval but with distinctive lobes that end in sharp spines. The fruit is a showy red berry often used as an ornamental during holiday seasons.
    b. **Geographic range.** Holly grows wild in mild and damp locations and is also cultivated as a landscape plant.
    c. **Toxic principle. Saponins are contained in the berry.**
    d. **Clinical signs.** Nausea, vomiting, and diarrhea may be prolonged and severe.
    e. **Treatment.** Gastrointestinal decontamination should be accompanied by symptomatic and supportive therapy, including administration of replacement fluids for diarrhea.

14. *Ligustrum vulgare* (**privet**)
    a. **Description.** Privet is a landscape shrub grown extensively for hedges and screening. Shiny, dark green leaves are lanceolate. White flowers yield dark blue to black berries.
    b. The **toxic principle,** which causes severe gastroenteritis, is not identified. Toxic portions of the plant include the **leaves** and **berries**.
    c. **Clinical signs** are nonspecific vomiting, colic, diarrhea, shock, and, occasionally, renal damage (possibly resulting from shock).
    d. **Treatment** entails standard detoxification and supportive measures.

15. *Narcissus* (daffodil, jonquil)
    a. **Description.** *Narcissus* is grown primarily as an ornamental garden plant that flowers early in the spring.
    b. **Toxic principles. Lycorine** and other alkaloids have an irritant and purgative effect. **Bulbs** contain the highest concentration of toxin.
    c. **Toxicity.** A portion of one bulb may be toxic or lethal to small animals.
    d. **Clinical signs.** Nausea, emesis, hypotension, and diarrhea may be complicated by tremors and seizures.
    e. **Treatment** entails gastric lavage, administration of activated charcoal, and fluid replacement therapy.

16. *Phoradendron* (mistletoe)
    a. **Description.** Simple oblong and oval shaped leaves are 1–3 cm long. The fruit is comprised of small white berries.
    b. **Geographic range.** Mistletoe is an evergreen plant that parasitizes deciduous trees in the eastern half of the United States and along the West Coast.
    c. The **toxic principle** is a **phytotoxin** or **toxalbumin** and is similar to that of castor bean and rosary pea. The **leaves** and **berries** contain the toxin, but the berries are most often ingested by pets or small children.
    d. **Clinical signs.** Severe gastroenteritis and violent purgation occur 18–24 hours after ingestion of only a few berries. Shock, polyuria, dyspnea, and bradycardia are advanced signs.
    e. **Treatment.** Decontamination and the administration of activated charcoal should be followed by supportive therapy (e.g., atropine, treatment of cardiovascular dysfunction that is similar to digitalis toxicosis).

17. *Phytolacca americana* (pokeweed)
    a. **Description.** Pokeweed is a coarse perennial herb. The stems are large, smooth, and dark purple. The leaves are ovate and the white flowers occur in loose racemes. The flattened, dark purple berries form clusters.
    b. **Geographic range.** Pokeweed grows up to 1.5 meters tall and occurs widely across the eastern United States and lower Midwest, especially in the rich, moist soil of waste areas near shaded or wooded areas.
    c. **Toxic principle. Saponins** and **alkaloids (phytolaccin)** are the reported toxic principles. Although all parts of the plant are toxic, the large **taproot** contains the greatest concentration of toxin.
    d. **Toxicity.** The relatively unpalatable plant is unlikely to be eaten, except by hungry or starved animals.
    e. **Diagnosis**
       (1) **Clinical signs**
          (a) Pokeweed, a strong gastrointestinal irritant, causes oral irritation, vomiting, and severe watery diarrhea.
          (b) Tremors, seizures, and impaired vision are also reported.
       (2) **Lesions.** Severe ulcerative or hemorrhagic gastroenteritis may be evident at autopsy.
    f. **Treatment.** Detoxification and supportive therapy for gastroenteritis are recommended.

18. *Podophyllum peltatum* (mayapple, mandrake)
    a. **Description.** The plants are typically 0.25 meters tall with a smooth, green stem and two large (15- to 25-cm) peltate leaves. Up to two white or cream-colored flowers in the angle of the two leaves yield a 3- to 5-cm greenish fruit that ripens to dull yellow in late April or early May.
    b. **Geographic range.** Mayapple is a woodland plant that tends to grow in patches in rich, moist forest soils.
    c. The **toxic principle** is reported to be **podophyllin,** a resinous substance that irritates the mucous membranes and may have antimitotic effects. The **root, green fruit,** and **leaves** are considered toxic.
    d. **Clinical signs.** Severe gastroenteritis with vomiting and marked fluid diarrhea may be accompanied by salivation and some degree of agitation or excitement.
    e. **Treatment.** General detoxification and supportive therapy are recommended.

19. *Ranunculus* (buttercup) and *Caltha palustris* (marsh marigold)
   a. **Description.** Leaves grow low on the stem. The prominent flowering stalk contains yellow five-petaled flowers and a central compound pistil.
   b. **Geographic range.** Buttercups and marsh marigolds favor wet, swampy areas throughout the temperate United States.
   c. The **toxic principle** is **protoanemonin, an irritant oil glycoside.** The **bulbous roots** are a concentrated source of the toxin.
   d. **Exposure and toxicity.** Grazing animals may pull up the roots from damp, soft soils, but poisoning is rarely reported.
   e. **Clinical signs** include pain and inflammation of mouth, salivation, diarrhea, dizziness, skin irritation and CNS depression.
   f. **Treatment.** Detoxification, demulcents, corticosteroids, and antibiotics may reduce the clinical effects.

20. *Ricinus communis* (castor bean)
   a. **Description.** Castor bean is an ornamental garden annual plant that grows up to 2 meters tall.
      (1) It has distinctive, large (25-cm) alternate palmately veined leaves and a large stem that appears jointed.
      (2) The fruits develop in a red or orange spiny capsule. The seeds are 0.5 cm in diameter, ovoid, and dark brown with multiple light patches (scars).
   b. The **toxic principle** is **ricin** (toxalbumin), a plant lectin or protein. The **seeds** are the most concentrated source of the toxin.
   c. **Toxicity.** Ingestion of only one seed can kill a medium-sized dog, especially if the seed is chewed.
   d. **Clinical signs.** Following a latent period of up to 24 hours, colic, emesis, diarrhea, and thirst develop. Renal damage may also occur.
   e. **Treatment.** Emesis, detoxification using charcoal, and administration of fluids and electrolytes is indicated.

21. *Robinia pseudoacacia* (black locust)
   a. **Description.** The pinnately compound leaves have oval leaflets 2–5 cm in length. Fragrant white or cream-colored legume flowers develop into large brown leathery pods containing five to nine seeds. The black locust typically has short (1- to 2-cm) thorns.
   b. **Geographic range.** Several species of locust trees are naturalized in the woods of the eastern half of the United States. They are also grown as landscape trees.
   c. **Toxic principle. Robin,** a plant phytotoxin, is similar to the toxic principles found in castor bean and rosary pea. The **bark, seeds,** and **leaves** contain the toxin.
   d. **Toxicity.** Consumption of as little as 0.04% of body weight is toxic to horses; cattle may be affected by consumption of approximately 0.5% body weight.
   e. **Clinical signs.** Nausea, emesis, diarrhea, and renal failure may be accompanied by weakness, dyspnea, tachycardia, and depression.
   f. **Treatment** is of limited value, but should include detoxification and supportive therapy.

22. *Saponaria officinalis* (soapweed, bouncing bet)
   a. **Description.** Plants have opposite leaves attached directly to the stem without an apparent petiole. The flowers are pale red or white to pink, and the lower portions of the petals are enclosed in a tubular calyx.
   b. **Geographic range.** *S. officinalis* grows across the eastern half of the United States.
   c. The **toxic principle** is a **saponin.** The highest concentration of toxin is in the **seeds,** which may contaminate small grains.
   d. **Toxicity.** Toxic or lethal effects may occur from consumption of the vegetative portion of the plant in amounts equalling 3% of body weight.
   e. **Clinical signs** include gastroenteritis, vomiting, and diarrhea.
   f. **Treatment** includes gastrointestinal protectants and activated charcoal.

23. **Sesbania drummondii (rattlebox, senna bean), S. punicea (coffee bean, daubentonia), and S. vesicaria (bladderpod, bagpod)**
    a. **Description.** Leaves are alternate, pinnately compound, and 2–4 centimeters long. The flowers range from yellow to red, depending on species, and the fruit is a legume.
    b. **Geographic range.** *Sesbania* species are indigenous to the southern half of the United States. Members of the Legume family, they occur in moist, rich soils as a shrub or small tree.
    c. The **toxic principle**, a **saponin**, is concentrated in **green seeds**. It is present to a lesser extent in mature seeds.
    d. **Toxicity.** Consumption of amounts equalling 0.1% of the body weight produces clinical signs in cattle and sheep. Poultry may be affected by dosages equalling 1% of body weight.
    e. **Clinical signs.** Anorexia, diarrhea, prostration, coma, and death may occur. Severe hemorrhagic to necrotic enteritis develops.
    f. **Treatment.** Detoxification and supportive therapy are recommended.

IV. PLANTS CAUSING HEPATOXICITY

A. Hepatocellular degeneration

1. **Amanita phalloides (deadly amanita, death angel) and Galerina.** The genus Amanita, which also includes *A. verna* and *A. virosa*, comprises the most dangerous group of mushrooms in North America.
   a. **Description.** The cap is usually white or a pale color, and the gills on the underside of the cap are white and not physically attached to the stem. A ring around the stalk (the annulus) and a cup-shaped structure (the volva) at the bottom of the stem are structural features of *Amanita*, but positive identification usually requires a trained specialist.
   b. **Geographic range.** *Amanita* grows primarily in moist, woodland soils along the east and west coasts of the United States.
   c. **Toxic principle**
      (1) **Amanita toxins (amatoxins)** are cyclic octapeptides that reduce protein synthesis by inhibiting ribonucleic acid (RNA) polymerase and transcription.
      (2) **Heptapeptide phallotoxins** affect the hepatic cytocavitary network.
      (3) Toxins are present in **all parts of the fungus** and are stable to heat and drying. The amatoxins are relatively more toxic than the phallotoxins.
   d. **Diagnosis**
      (1) **Clinical signs**
         (a) **Gastrointestinal phase.** Following a latent period of 8–36 hours, abdominal pain, vomiting (sometimes bloody), and acute, severe fluid to hemorrhagic diarrhea occur.
         (b) **Hepatic phase.** Apparent recovery from the gastrointestinal phase is followed in 1–3 days by severe hepatic failure with hepatic necrosis, icterus, and coagulopathy.
      (2) **Laboratory diagnosis**
         (a) Serum clinical chemistry shows elevated serum hepatocellular enzymes and hyperbilirubinemia.
         (b) The toxin can be identified by thin-layer chromatography and radioimmunoassay, but analysis is not routinely available in veterinary diagnostic laboratories.
      (3) **Lesions** at postmortem include acute massive liver necrosis, icterus, and variable gastroenteritis.
   e. **Treatment.** Prompt, rigorous gastrointestinal decontamination, activated charcoal, and catharsis are necessary. Once clinical signs have developed, the prognosis is guarded. There is no effective antidote, but supportive therapy for diarrhea, shock, and liver failure may increase the survival rate.

2. *Cycas* (false sago palm) and *Zamia* (cycads)
   a. **Description.** The leaves are fern-like or palm-like and the stem is thick.
   b. **Geographic range.** Growth of these plants is limited to tropical and subtropical areas in the United States, such as Florida (*Zamia*) and Texas (*Cycas*).
   c. **Toxic principle.** Glycosides, including **cycasin, macrozamin,** and **α-amino β-methyl aminopropionic acid,** cause both hepatotoxicosis and neurotoxicosis. The toxin appears to concentrate in the **seeds;** lower concentrations are found in the **leaves.**
   d. **Diagnosis.** Poisoned livestock may show neurologic signs as well as those of hepatotoxicosis.
      (1) **Clinical signs.** Vomiting and gastroenteritis are followed by icterus and coagulopathy.
      (2) **Laboratory diagnosis.** Laboratory findings are typical of hepatic failure (see Chapter 8 III C 2).
      (3) **Lesions.** Centrilobular necrosis, bile retention, icterus, and ecchymotic hemorrhages are seen at postmortem.
   e. **Treatment** is supportive. No effective antidote is available.

3. *Microcystis aeruginosa* (blue-green algae)
   a. **Description.** *Microcystis* is a one-celled algal organism that tends to colonize in clusters of small coccoid cells held together by a mucinous secretion. During conditions favorable to rapid growth, "bloom" may occur: the algae may begin to deteriorate and die, rising to the surface of lakes or ponds where they are concentrated by prevailing winds.
   b. **Geographic range.** *Microcystis* is one of several toxic blue-green algae that can occur across North America in stagnant waters during drought periods or in late summer or early fall.
   c. **Toxic principle**
      (1) **Microcystin** is a cyclic peptide produced during an algal bloom. Toxin production may be variable during the bloom.
         (a) Microcystin causes dysfunctional phosphorylation of cellular keratins, leading to disruption of normal cytoskeletal structure.
         (b) Disruption of the cytoskeletal structure leads to a "rounding up" of the hepatocyte, disruption of hepatic sinusoids, separation of hepatocytes, and excessive apoptosis, resulting in liver failure.
      (2) **Lipopolysaccharide endotoxins** may be present in algal cell walls.
      (3) *Clostridium botulinum* may use algal bloom as a growth medium. *C. botulinum* is highly toxic to waterfowl and certain livestock (e.g., horses).
   d. **Diagnosis**
      (1) **Clinical signs**
         (a) **Gastrointestinal.** Microcystin causes acute gastroenteritis with vomiting and hemorrhagic diarrhea.
         (b) **Hepatic.** Icterus and other secondary effects of acute liver failure occur. Hepatogenous photosensitization may occur.
      (2) **Laboratory identification**
         (a) Algae can be identified after fixing fresh samples in a 1:10 dilution of formalin.
         (b) Frozen water samples can be evaluated for lethality using a mouse bioassay.
      (3) **Lesions** include acute gastroenteritis, a swollen, congested liver, centrilobular necrosis, and edema of the gall bladder.
   e. **Treatment** involves detoxification and supportive treatment for diarrhea, dehydration, shock, and hepatic insufficiency.

4. *Xanthium strumarium* (cocklebur)
   a. **Description.** The mature plant is coarse, 1–1.5 meters tall, with brown to purple stems and large, shovel-shaped leaves with irregular margins.
   b. **Geographic range.** Cocklebur is a ubiquitous plant in the United States It is an annual that germinates readily from the spiny 1.5-centimeter bur in floodplains or moist rich soils.

c. The **toxic principle** is **carboxyatractyloside,** a glycoside that appears to inhibit adenosine triphosphatase (ATP) transport into mitochondria. However, this mechanism may not explain the predilection for hepatic damage.

   (1) The toxin is present in the **seeds** and in the **recently germinated cotyledons** or "seed leaves."

   (2) Toxicity is retained after drying.

d. **Toxicity.** Ingestion of less than 1% of body weight of the cotyledons is lethal. Burs eaten by cattle have also caused toxicosis.

e. **Diagnosis** depends primarily on history of consumption of cocklebur and presence of lesions.

   (1) **Clinical signs** may be acute and include depression, abdominal pain, anorexia, vomiting, weakness, coma, and death. The clinical course may last as long as 48 hours.

   (2) **Laboratory diagnosis.** Although not routinely available, chemical analysis can detect the toxin in rumen contents.

   (3) **Lesions.** Postmortem lesions include gastroenteritis, subserosal hemorrhages, hepatic centrilobular hemorrhage, and necrosis. Mild to moderate tubular degeneration may also occur.

B. **Pyrrolizidine alkaloid (PA) toxicosis** is a serious livestock poisoning problem in some regions of the United States.

1. **Sources**
   a. *Amsinckia intermedia* **(fiddleneck)**

      (1) **Description.** Fiddleneck is a member of the family Boraginaceae, and is recognized by its hairy leaves and tubular flowers, which form a curved floral structure that looks like a shepherd's crook or the head and neck of a violin.

      (2) **Geographic distribution.** Fiddleneck is primarily distributed in grain fields of the northwestern United States, and may be more prominent in drought years. Seed contamination of small grains is the major route of toxicosis.

   b. *Crotalaria* **(crotalaria)**

      (1) **Description.** The pea-like flowers are yellow and form the typical legume or pea-type of pod. Unlike many legumes, *Crotalaria* has simple leaves.

      (2) **Geographic range.** *Crotalaria* is an annual legume that primarily grows as a contaminant of grain fields in the southeastern United States.

   c. *Cynoglossum officinale* **(hound's tongue)** is the only known PA-containing plant that ranges into the midwest, where it grows in pastures, waste areas, and by the roadside.

   d. *Eichium* **(viper's bugloss)** and *Helioptropium europaeum.* Heliotropes are found only rarely in the United States (usually in the eastern or southeastern states) and are not documented to have caused toxicosis in this country, although they cause significant problems in other countries.

   e. *Senecio* **(tansy ragwort, groundsel)** is a major source of PA toxicosis.

      (1) **Description.** *Senecio* is a member of the Composite family. Varieties have yellow-headed flowers and green sepals. Plants are biennials with basal growth the first year, turning into tall (0.5–1 meter), erect, flowering plants the second year.

      (2) **Geographic range.** *Senecio* occurs primarily in the Pacific Northwest and California. They commonly invade pastures and hayfields and may be grazed by horses or cattle.

   f. *Symphytum* **(comfrey)** is used to make a herbal tea. It presents little risk to animals, but overuse in humans has been associated with PA toxicosis.

2. **Chemistry.** The PA alkaloids are cyclic alkaloid compounds that contain two five-membered rings and a nitrogen atom as part of the ring structure.

3. **Mechanism of toxicologic damage.** The pyrrole metabolites that result from dehydrogenation of the PA appear to bind to deoxyribonucleic acid (DNA), resulting in impaired cell division.

a. High dosages may cause cellular necrosis, whereas moderate exposure inhibits cell division, leading to hepatic megalocytosis and eventual degeneration of the hepatocyte with liver failure.

b. Bile duct hyperplasia occurs in response to cellular degeneration and necrosis.

c. PAs are also considered to be carcinogens and present a potential public health problem because they are excreted in milk.

4. Toxicity

a. Flowers are most toxic, followed by leaves and stems. Roots are not toxic.

b. Toxicosis most commonly occurs from **long-term consumption,** leading to the development of chronic liver failure.

c. Sheep are more resistant than horses and cattle, partially because their rumen flora detoxify the PA.

5. Diagnosis

a. Clinical signs

(1) Chronic PA toxicosis is characterized by **icterus, depression,** and **anorexia.**

(2) Often there are **manifestations of hepatic encephalopathy** [e.g., aimless wandering ("walking disease"), head-pressing, and excitement or disorientation]. CNS signs seem to be more common in horses than in cattle.

(3) **Secondary (hepatogenous) photosensitization** may occur.

b. Laboratory diagnosis. Pyrrolic metabolites may be detected by the Erlich reaction (a generalized response) or by thin-layer chromatography, but few veterinary laboratories offer routine analysis of tissues for PA content.

c. Lesions are primarily in the liver and consist of portal fibrosis, megalocytosis, hepatocellular necrosis, bile duct hyperplasia, bile stasis, and nodular hyperplasia.

6. Treatment is often futile because serious damage has already occurred by the time the animals are recognized as ill. Animals should be given supportive care and managed for hepatic failure.

7. Prevention. Control of PA-containing plants with herbicides and pasture management and cleaning of contaminated grain is the best approach.

C. **Secondary (hepatogenous) photosensitization**

1. Sources

a. *Agave lechiguilla* **(Agave)**

(1) **Description.** Agave is a perennial with thick, fleshy leaves that are elongated, broad at the base, and tapered to a point. The plants grow in a clump, and the stalk rises 1–2 meters with a terminal panicle that bears white or cream-colored flowers. The plant blooms only after 10–15 years of growth.

(2) **Geographic range.** Agave is limited primarily to western Texas and New Mexico. Some varieties may be grown as an ornamental.

b. *Kochia scoparia* **(kochia, fireweed, burning bush)** is a palatable plant that is readily grazed by cattle or sheep.

(1) **Description.** The plant is 1–2 meters tall, erect, with medium green leaves that are lanceolate to linear and lack petioles. Flowers are inconspicuous and greenish and occur in the axil of the upper leaves.

(2) **Geographic range.** Kochia occurs as an annual weed of waste areas, fence rows, and crop fields, and is also cultivated as a forage. Kochia ranges across almost the entire United States, but appears to grow best under relatively dry and alkaline conditions.

(3) The **toxic principles** include oxalates, a factor (possibly sulfate) associated with polioencephalomalacia, and an unidentified principle associated with hepatotoxicity.

c. *Lantana camara* **(lantana)**

(1) **Description.** Lantana is a perennial shrub that may grow to 1–2 meters in height. Leaves are oval and serrated with prominent veins. The showy red and yellow flowers are clustered at the tip of the stems and they yield dark blue to black berries that are approximately 1 centimeter in diameter.

    (2) Geographic range. Lantana naturally occurs in tropical to subtropical areas, but it is cultivated as an ornamental in northern areas of the United States.

    (3) The **toxic principle** is a **polycyclic triterpene**.

  d. *Nolina texana* **(bunchgrass, sachuiste)**

    (1) Description. *N. texana* is a perennial that grows in large clumps. It has narrow leaves up to 1 meter in length that are triangular in cross-section.

    (2) Geographic range. *N. texana* is limited to the rangelands of the southwestern United States.

    (3) The **toxic principle** is a **saponin**.

  e. *Panicum* **(panic grass)**

    (1) Description. *Panicum* is a warm season perennial bunchgrass with bluish-green leaves. Growth is from underground rhizomes and the plant may exceed 1 meter in height. The flowering head is a large, open panicle.

    (2) Geographic range. The usual range is Texas and small portions of nearby states.

    (3) The **toxic principle** is a **saponin**.

  f. *Tetradymia glabrata* **(horsebrush) and** *T. canescens* **(littleleaf horsebrush)** are browsed primarily by sheep, which are the main susceptible species.

    (1) Description. The plants are coarse woody shrubs up to 1 meter in height with numerous branches and stems that vary in color from light green to gray. Leaves are small and linear with sharp, pointed tips. Flowers are yellow and of the Composite family.

    (2) Geographic range. These plants are native to the Rocky Mountain states, growing primarily in arid regions.

    (3) The **toxic principle** is a **sesquiterpene**.

  g. *Tribulus terrestris* **(puncture vine;** see Table 28-3)

2. The **mechanism of toxicologic damage** is discussed in Chapter 13 III D 3 c (2).

3. Toxicity. Consumption of hepatotoxic plants that coincides with the intake of significant amounts of chlorophyll-containing forages causes photosensitization within 1–3 days.

4. Clinical signs are discussed in Chapter 13 III D 3 b.

5. Treatment is nonspecific.

  a. Once signs appear, gastrointestinal detoxification is usually ineffective.

  b. Treating liver damage and dressing the skin or eye lesions (using antibiotics for secondary bacterial infections if necessary) is rational supportive therapy.

V. PLANTS CAUSING NEPHROTOXICITY

A. **Oxalate toxicosis**

1. Sources

  a. *Beta vulgaris* **(beet)** is grown as a garden vegetable. The tops are high in soluble oxalates and can cause oxalate toxicosis if fed to ruminants or other herbivores.

  b. *Chenopodium album* **(lamb's quarters)**

    (1) Description. The plant is erect and up to 1.5 meters tall with simple alternate leaves that are ovate to broadly lanceolate and 2–5 centimeters long. The leaves are dull green on top but silvery gray on the underside. Flowers are inconspicuous, small, green, and located at the tips of the stems.

    (2) Geographic range. Lamb's quarters is a common annual weed throughout much of the United States. It grows in crop fields and hay or pasture and is adaptable to both moist, rich soils and dry alkaline conditions.

    (3) Toxic principle. Lamb's quarters contains both soluble oxalates and high concentrations of nitrates. It is not unpalatable and may be readily grazed or eaten in hay.

  c. *Halogeton glomeratus* **(halogeton)**

    (1) Description. The plant is low-growing and succulent, with fleshy, round leaves that taper to a point with a small hair at the tip.

(2) Geographic range. Halogeton is an introduced naturalized annual that has spread widely over arid and desert regions such as the western intermountain region. It tolerates high-saline soils and grows readily along roads, in waste areas, and in overgrazed, disturbed, or burned areas.

(3) Toxic principle. Peak oxalate content occurs in the fall and persists in the plant throughout the winter.

d. *Rheum rhaponticum* (rhubarb)

(1) Description. Rhubarb is a perennial garden plant with edible, tart, leaf petioles. The leaf petiole is reddish-brown to purple and the plant emerges early in the spring.

(2) Toxic principle. The **leaves** contain **anthroquinone glycosides** and large quantities of **soluble oxalates**. Ingestion of rhubarb leaves has caused death in both humans and animals.

e. *Sarcobatus vermiculatus* (greasewood)

(1) Description. The bark is smooth and white and the branches are spiny with thick, narrow, pale gray-green leaves and small white flowers.

(2) Geographic range. Greasewood is a large perennial shrub of the Chenopodiaceae family. It is found in the western range states in flood plains and other areas where soils are somewhat moist.

(3) Toxic principle. The oxalates are present throughout the plant and become more concentrated as the plant matures.

2. **Mechanism of toxicologic damage.** Soluble oxalates form a **complex with serum calcium** to form **calcium oxalate**.

a. The formation of calcium oxalate depletes ionized calcium and causes functional **hypocalcemia**.

b. Calcium oxalate may crystallize in renal tubules, forming polarizing, rosette-shaped crystals that are associated with **fatal renal tubular toxicosis**.

3. **Toxicity.** Vegetative parts of the plants are concentrated sources of oxalates. One-time consumption of oxalates is sufficient to cause acute toxicosis.

4. **Clinical signs**

a. Early clinical signs of oxalate-induced hypocalcemia include muscle twitching, mild seizures, prostration, and possibly death.

b. Renal tubular necrosis from calcium oxalate crystals results in oliguria, depression, vomiting, azotemia, depression, hyperkalemia, and cardiac failure. Animals that do not die from acute hyperkalemia may develop chronic tubular nephrosis with polyuria and hyposthenuria.

5. **Treatment**

a. **Detoxification** to reduce acute absorption is recommended, followed by oral activated charcoal or limewater (calcium hydroxide) to precipitate oxalate in the intestinal tract.

b. **Supportive treatment** of hypocalcemia or supportive therapy for nephrosis may aid survival, but advanced clinical signs signal a poor prognosis.

B. **Cholecalciferol (vitamin D) toxicosis** is discussed in Chapter 22 III. Plants known to contain toxic concentrations of vitamin D include:

1. *Cestrum diurnum* (night-blooming jessamine)

a. **Description.** Night-blooming jessamine is a woody perennial vine with lanceolate evergreen leaves and prominent yellow flowers.

b. **Geographic range.** The plant grows in the southern and southeastern United States and ranges from open fencerows to woodlands.

c. **Toxicity.** Approximately 20% of the diet as *Cestrum* leaves for several days may cause toxicosis.

2. *Solanum malacoxylon*

a. **Geographic range.** *S. malacoxylon*, a member of the Nightshade family, is found in Hawaii and South America.

b. Toxicity. Grazing cattle have been poisoned by this plant, which contains 1,25 dihydroxycholecalciferol.

C. Oak poisoning

1. **Source.** Various species of *Quercus* can cause oak poisoning.
   a. **Description.** Oaks range in size from shrubs to tall trees. They have simple, alternate leaves with irregularly rounded lobes. Flowers appear as pendulant racemes or catkins and the fruit (known as an acorn) is a smooth nut with a basal cap.
   b. **Geographic range.** Oaks have a wide geographic distribution.

2. The **toxic principle** in oak buds and acorns is **gallotannin, a polyhydroxyphenolic moiety**. Both **leaves** and **acorns,** especially sprouted acorns, contain the toxin, and toxicity is not diminished by freezing or drying.

3. **Toxicity.** Oak poisoning is most common in cattle and calves, much less so in sheep and horses.

4. **Diagnosis**
   a. **Clinical signs**
      (1) Early signs are anorexia, dullness, rumen atony, and constipation. Feces may be dark, solid, and covered with a film of mucus, but can become black with a tarry or fluid consistency as a result of hemorrhagic enteritis.
      (2) Poisoned animals become weak and prostrate 3–7 days after exposure, and mortality may be high.
      (3) Icterus, hematuria, dehydration, polyuria, and hyposthenuria are often present in advanced stages of the disease. Pregnant animals may abort.
   b. **Laboratory diagnosis.** Urine may contain blood and granular and hyaline casts.
   c. **Lesions**
      (1) Gastroenteritis, ascites, and hydrothorax may be seen.
      (2) Subserosal petechial or ecchymotic hemorrhages are distributed over the surface of the gastrointestinal tract.
      (3) Acorns may be found in the rumen.
      (4) Gelatinous, blood-tinged edema occurs around the kidneys. Kidneys are enlarged, pale, and hemorrhagic with coagulative necrosis of the proximal convoluted tubules and pink-staining casts of epithelial cells and protein.
   d. **Treatment**
      (1) Animals should be removed from further access to oak and given activated charcoal, oils, or ruminatorics.
      (2) Parenteral fluids to correct dehydration and acidosis are helpful.
      (3) A ration of 10%–15% calcium hydroxide in grain has been fed to aid precipitation of oak tannins and reduce mortality in cattle unavoidably grazing with access to oak trees.

D. Kidney failure

1. *Amaranthus retroflexus* (redroot pigweed)
   a. **Description.** The tall (1- to 1.5-meter), coarse, erect stem has rough alternate leaves and a large, rough, green inflorescence. The lower stem and root are deep pink to red. *A. hybridus* (smooth pigweed) is similar in appearance to redroot pigweed, except the leaves are smaller and the entire plant is smooth.
   b. **Geographic distribution.** Pigweed grows in rich, moist, disturbed soils and is found in fencerows, gardens, row crops, and waste areas throughout the United States.
   c. **Toxic principle.** Varieties of *Amaranthus* may have oxalate contents as high as 30% on a dry-weight basis and are known nitrate accumulators, but neither of these principles appears to cause the nephrosis that affects swine and cattle.
   d. **Toxicity.** Approximately 25%–50% of the total daily diet as pigweed can cause acute clinical signs within 3 days of ingestion. The dried plant is toxic, but less so than the fresh material.

e. Diagnosis
  (1) Swine
    (a) Clinical signs appear 5–10 days after pigs begin eating pigweed. Early signs of weakness, trembling, and incoordination progress to knuckling of the pastern joints, paralysis of the hind limbs, coma, and death.
    (b) Laboratory diagnosis
      (i) Elevated blood urea nitrogen (BUN), creatinine, and serum potassium confirm serious renal toxicosis.
      (ii) The electrocardiogram (EKG) of affected swine shows bradycardia and the effects of hyperkalemic heart failure.
    (c) Lesions
      (i) Renal tubular cloudy swelling and hyaline degeneration is followed by coagulative tubular necrosis. Sloughing of necrotic cells forms eosinophilic granular casts and gross lesions of perirenal retroperitoneal edema.
      (ii) Kidneys from animals that survive acute *A. retroflexus* toxicosis often have chronic lesions of interstitial fibrosis and dilated tubules with flattened tubular epithelium. Many such swine appear clinically normal.
  (2) Cattle. Clinical signs and lesions in cattle are similar to those seen in oak poisoning (see V C 3).
f. Treatment
  (1) Removal of affected animals from access to pigweed is the initial management recommendation.
  (2) Management of hyperkalemia and renal failure could improve survival, but the cost of intensive treatment for swine may not be economically justifiable.
g. Prevention. Pigs raised in confinement should not be allowed free access to pastures containing heavy growth of *A. retroflexus*.

2. *Hemerocallis* **(daylily) and** *Lilium* **(lilies)**
  a. Description. Plants usually have smooth, linear, leathery, green leaves that grow in a basal clump or arise along a tall stem. The attractive white, yellow, or orange flowers are present for long periods during the summer.
  b. Geographic range. Both daylilies and other varieties of lilies (e.g., Easter lily, tiger lily) are common garden ornamentals that sometimes escape from cultivation and become naturalized around old farmsteads or along roadsides.
  c. Toxic principle. An unidentified toxic principle has been associated with renal toxicosis in cats. All parts of the plant are nephrotoxic.
  d. Diagnosis
    (1) Clinical signs in cats include anorexia, depression, and anuria.
    (2) Lesions. Acute renal tubular necrosis is observed in postmortem specimens.
  e. Treatment. Prevention of toxicosis is important, because no effective antidote or treatment is available.
    (1) Ingestion of lily plants by cats (and perhaps by dogs) should be considered a **medical emergency,** because the resultant acute renal failure carries a high mortality rate.
    (2) Following **gastrointestinal detoxification** and the administration of activated charcoal and osmotic cathartics, **fluid diuresis** should be instituted for 24 hours.

VI. PLANTS CAUSING CARDIOTOXICITY

A. Andromedotoxicosis (grayanotoxicosis)

1. Sources
  a. *Kalmia* **(laurel, lambkill, calfkill)**
    (1) Description. *Kalmia* is a large shrub or small tree with smooth, elliptical alternate or whorled leaves. Showy white or pink flowers with fused petals arise in

the leaf axils of the upper stems. The plant has green leaves all year in moderate climates and is primarily a threat to browsing animals like sheep, goats, and, less commonly, cattle and horses.

    (2) Geographic range. *Kalmia* grows wild in the woods and mountain foothills of the southeastern, Appalachian, and mid-Atlantic coastal states. Some species are found in the Pacific coastal states and in temperate areas along the Pacific Coast north to Alaska.

  b. *Rhododendron* **(rhododendron, azalea)**

    (1) Description. *Rhododendron* are large shrubs or small trees with evergreen lanceolate to elliptical leaves and terminal clusters of large, attractive pink to purple flowers.

    (2) Geographic range. Accidental exposure of foraging animals or pets can occur over much of the United States. The plant does best in well-drained, sandy or rocky soils at elevations above 3000 feet.

      (a) Some species of this genus are grown as garden or landscape plants (e.g., azaleas), whereas others range wild in the woods and mountain foothills of the southeastern and Appalachian states. Plants generally do not survive in the northern states with very cold winters.

      (b) Rhododendron also grow in the Pacific coastal states and western British Columbia.

      (c) Ornamental varieties may be grown extensively in the Midwest.

  c. *Pieris japonica* **(Japanese pieris)**

    (1) Description. Japanese pieris is a shrub or small tree with oval to lanceolate leaves with finely serrated margins. Small white flowers are borne on a terminal panicle.

    (2) Geographic range. Japanese pieris grows in a range and habitat similar to that of rhododendrons and azaleas, but it is less common.

2. Toxic principle. Andromedotoxins (grayanotoxins) are water-soluble **diterpenoid compounds. Leaves** and **flower nectar** (including honey made from plant nectar) are sources of the toxin.

3. Mechanism of toxicologic damage. Andromedotoxins bind to and modify the sodium channels of cell membranes, leading to **prolonged depolarization** and **excitation.** Modification of the sodium channels favors calcium movement into cells and results in a **positive inotropic effect** similar to that of digitalis.

4. Toxicity. As little as 3 ml nectar/kg body weight or 0.2% of the body weight as leaves may be toxic or lethal.

5. Clinical signs

  a. Salivation and a burning sensation in the mouth are followed by emesis, diarrhea, muscular weakness, and impaired vision.

  b. Bradycardia, hypotension (caused by vasodilation), and atrioventricular block are serious cardiovascular effects that may be lethal.

  c. Dyspnea, depression, and prostration develop, and death may occur within 1–2 days.

6. Treatment

  a. Detoxification. Emesis is used where appropriate. Activated charcoal should be administered repeatedly the first day.

  b. Supportive therapy

    (1) Fluid replacement therapy and **respiratory support** may be necessary.

    (2) Atropine is recommended for severe bradycardia.

    (3) Isoproterenol or **sodium channel blockers** (e.g., **quinidine**) may be used to treat heart block.

B. | **Digitalis glycoside poisoning**

1. Sources

  a. *Apocynum* **(dogbane)**

    (1) Description. Dogbane is an erect perennial that can grow up to 1.5 meters tall. It has dark reddish to purple stems and milky sap. Leaves are opposite, ovate, and medium green with smooth margins. Flowers are white to cream to greenish and occur in terminal, flat-topped clusters. Seeds occur in paired, pencil-shaped "pods."

    (2) **Geographic range.** Dogbane ranges throughout the United States at the edges of woods, along roadsides, and in pastures and waste areas. Because they spread from underground rootstalks, plants often occur in well-defined patches.

b. *Convallaria majalis* (**lily-of-the-valley**)

    (1) **Description.** Lily-of-the-valley is short with slightly cupped, spear-shaped green leaves and white bell-like, drooping flowers that grow on one side of the flowering stem.

    (2) **Geographic range.** Lily-of-the-valley is usually found as a cultivated garden ornamental. Moist, rich soils and shaded locations favor growth.

    (3) **Toxic principle.** The toxin is present in the **flowers, leaves,** and **seeds,** but not the fleshy berries. Small animals are most at risk because of the accessibility of the plants.

c. *Digitalis purpurea* (**foxglove**) is the plant of origin for natural medicinal digitalis.

    (1) **Description.** Foxglove is tall, with broadly lanceolate, dark green, hairy leaves that are low on the erect, flowering stalk. Trumpet-shaped flowers of several colors are profuse along the upper flowering stalk.

    (2) **Geographic range.** Foxglove is grown as a cultivated garden ornamental because of its distinctive foliage and flowers.

    (3) **Toxic principle. Digitalis glycosides** and some **saponins** are present in **all parts** of the plant.

d. *Nerium oleander* (**oleander**)

    (1) **Description.** Oleander is a shrub measuring 1–4 meters tall. It has smooth, green bark and dark green, leathery leaves. The leaves are opposite near the bottom of the plant but whorled near the top. Attractive flowers of several colors may be present nearly all year.

    (2) **Geographic range.** Oleander, a member of the dogbane family, is widely grown as an ornamental in mild and subtropical climates of the United States. It has become naturalized in some parts of the country.

    (3) **Toxicity.** Oleander is highly toxic; a few ounces may be sufficient to kill a horse.

2. Mechanism of toxicologic damage. When cardioactive glycosides are excessive, normal electrical conductivity in the myocardium is lost, resulting in conduction block and eventual asystole.

3. Toxicokinetics. Toxins are readily absorbed from the gastrointestinal tract, and enterohepatic cycling may contribute to persistence of the toxin.

4. Clinical signs

  a. Gastrointestinal signs are prominent initially, following acute exposure to cardioactive glycosides. Vomiting and abdominal pain are followed by moderate to severe diarrhea (sometimes hemorrhagic).

  b. Cardiovascular signs. The slowed heart rate can progress to arrhythmias, ventricular premature systoles, and paroxysmal tachycardia followed by complete heart block and asystole. Affected animals become weak, depressed, and comatose prior to death as a result of cardiac insufficiency.

5. Treatment

  a. Detoxification. Early and active gastrointestinal decontamination should be followed by the administration of activated charcoal and osmotic cathartics.

  b. Supportive treatment

    (1) Serum potassium should be monitored and hyperkalemia treated as necessary.

    (2) Phenytoin may be used to assist atrioventricular conduction and increase heart rate.

    (3) For severe clinical toxicosis, use of antidigitalis antibody fragments (FAB) may be necessary.

C. **Digitalis-like glycoside poisoning**

1. *Aconitum napellum* (monkshood)
   a. **Description.** Monkshood, a member of the Ranunculaceae (buttercup) family, is a cultivated garden plant with dark green opposite leaves that are deeply cut and sharply lobed. The flowers are dark blue, purple, or yellow racemes on the tops of erect flowering stalks and are characterized by a distinctive cap or "monk's hood."
   b. The **toxic principle** is **aconitine** and **related alkaloids**. The toxin is present in the entire plant.
   c. **Clinical signs** include oral and pharyngeal inflammation, salivation, nausea, emesis, and blurred vision. Hypotension, cardiac arrhythmia, and weakness occur in advanced cases prior to death.
   d. **Treatment** as for cardioactive glycoside overdose is recommended (see VI B 5).

2. *Asclepias* (**milkweed**) is discussed in II A 1.

D. **Miscellaneous cardiac effects**

1. *Cassia occidentalis* (**coffee senna**) can cause hyperkalemic heart failure (see II G 2).

2. *Eupatorium rugosum* (**white snakeroot**) causes signs of congestive heart failure (see II C 2).

3. *Taxus cuspidata* (**Japanese yew**) and *T. baccata* (**English yew**)
   a. **Description.** These plants are landscape shrubs with small, narrow, strap-like evergreen leaves that are two-ranked along the stem. The leaves taper bluntly to a point. The fleshy fruit (known as an aril) turns red when ripe.
   b. **Exposure.** Animals gain access when trimmed hedges or shrubs are carelessly cast into pastures, or when animals escape into landscaped areas.
   c. **Toxic principle.** Taxine alkaloids (A and B) are believed to inhibit depolarization in the heart. The **whole plant, except for the red aril** (fruit), is toxic.
   d. **Toxicity.** This plant is highly toxic to herbivores. As little as 6–8 ounces of fresh yew may kill an adult cow or horse.
   e. **Diagnosis.** Acute onset and sudden death are common. Often animals are found dead with no premonitory signs.
      (1) **Clinical signs**
         (a) Trembling, muscle weakness, dyspnea, and collapse are cardinal clinical signs.
         (b) Arrhythmia, bradycardia, and diastolic heart block appear to be the cause of death.
      (2) **Lesions.** Diagnosis often depends on finding evidence of yew leaves in the rumen or stomach contents.
   f. **Treatment**
      (1) Assisted respiratory and vascular support may be helpful.
      (2) Detoxification measures, including activated charcoal and catharsis, should be promptly taken.
      (3) Atropine may be helpful to combat the cardiodepressant effect of taxine, but must be given early in the course of the disease.

4. *Zygadenus* (**death camas**)
   a. **Description.** Death camas emerges from a bulb in early spring and is one of the first green plants available. The gently curving, linear leaves are grass-like in appearance. They emerge directly from the bulb at soil level. A flowering stalk arises from the center of several leaves and bears yellowish-white flowers at the top of the stalk.
   b. **Geographic range.** Several varieties of death camas are important toxic plants of the Great Plains and Rocky Mountain states. The plant grows well in dry, sandy or rocky soils at elevations below 8000 feet.
   c. The **toxic principle** is a **steroidal alkaloid** known as **zygadenine** or **zygacine** that causes arteriolar dilatation and hypotension. **All parts of the plant** contain toxin at all stages of growth.

d. Diagnosis
  (1) Clinical signs include salivation, nausea and vomiting, rapid pulse, stiffness, trembling, ataxia, weakness, recumbency, coma, and death. The course is rapid.
  (2) Lesions are minimal and may include only generalized congestion of the gastrointestinal tract and liver.
e. Treatment. Under field conditions, treatment is usually ineffective and impractical. Grazing management and control of plants with herbicides may be useful preventive approaches.

E. | **Altered peripheral circulation**

1. *Berteroa incana* **(hoary alyssum)**
  a. Description. Hoary alyssum is a member of the mustard family (Cruciferae). It has hairy stems and leaves and white, four-petaled flowers.
  b. Geographic range. Hoary alyssum is a plant of the central United States and upper midwest, found mainly in pastures, hay fields and waste areas.
  c. The **toxic principle** is unknown.
  d. Toxicity. Acute consumption of more than 25% of the diet as hoary alyssum is usually required to produce toxicosis.
  e. Clinical signs include moderate to severe **laminitis** in up to 50% of horses consuming large amounts of the plant. There may be **edema** of the lower limbs.
  f. Treatment. Detoxification and symptomatic treatment of laminitis and edema are recommended.

2. *Festuca arundinacea* **(Kentucky 31 tall fescue)**
  a. Description. Fescue is a coarse grass with leaves that have fine linear striations and feel "sandpapery" when touched. It is a "bunchgrass" (i.e., it grows in clumps). The open panicle produces seeds in late May to early June.
  b. Geographic range. Tall fescue is a major forage grass in the southeastern United States.
  c. Toxic principle. Early plantings of fescue contained an endophytic fungus, *Acremonium coenophialum*, which was transmitted to other plants through infected fescue seed. **Ergopeptide alkaloids** (especially **ergovaline**) found in endophyte-infected fescue are associated with the fescue toxicosis. The fungus and ergot alkaloids are found in **leaves** and **seeds;** however, endophyte-free strains of fescue are currently available.
  d. Clinical syndromes
    (1) Fescue foot is a dry gangrene of the extremities, affecting primarily the feet, tail, and ears.
      (a) Temperature and blood flow in the distal portion of the limbs are reduced, leading to lameness, separation of the hoof at the coronary band, and dry gangrene very similar to classical gangrenous ergotism.
      (b) Cold weather accentuates the severity of clinical signs and may increase the incidence of peripheral necrosis.
      (c) Lameness is commonly observed to begin in the rear limbs of cattle.
    (2) Bovine fat necrosis is reported in the southeastern United States and is associated with nearly pure stands of fescue that have been heavily fertilized with nitrogen or poultry litter. The lesion consists of large masses of hardened fat in the abdominal cavity. Necrotic fat is calcified and higher than normal fat in ash, calcium, magnesium, and cholesterol.
    (3) "Summer syndrome" or **"summer slump"** is the most economically damaging of the fescue problems. Animals grazing infected pastures during periods of high ambient temperatures commonly spend less time grazing.
      (a) Clinical signs include lower weight gains, reduced milk production, and heat intolerance. Cows have reduced reproductive performance and fertility, indicated by increased postpartum intervals and reduced pregnancy rates.

        (i) Poor weight gains can following grazing endophyte-infected pastures during cool weather as well.

        (ii) In severe cases, agalactia may occur.

        (iii) Signs of heat intolerance include increased respiratory rate, higher body temperatures, and more time spent in shade or water. Some affected animals show increased salivation.

     (b) Laboratory diagnosis. Endophyte toxins may reduce prolactin synthesis and release; therefore, laboratory analysis may show reduced serum prolactin levels.

  e. Treatment and prevention

     (1) Treatment. Currently, there are no antidotes for fescue toxicosis. Cattle with dry gangrene should be protected from stress and treated for pain and secondary bacterial infection. They may be marketed after an appropriate withdrawal period.

     (2) Prevention. Infected pastures are a greater problem if stockpiled for winter grazing. Mowing to reduce the accumulation of seed heads seems to reduce the incidence and severity of the lesion. Reseeding with uninfected fescue seed is possible, but may not be economically feasible.

        (a) Fescue foot. Grazing of fescue that is known to be infected should be limited or prevented during cold weather.

        (b) Summer toxicosis may by prevented by alternative grazing or minimized by providing shade and water for cooling.

3. *Juglans nigra* (black walnut)

  a. Description. Walnut trees are 50–100 meters tall and have dark, deeply furrowed bark, alternate pinnately compound leaves with approximately 20 leaflets, and a spherical fruit 3–7 centimeters in diameter. A thick green husk breaks open to reveal a hard, brown, furrowed nut.

  b. Geographic range. Black walnut trees range widely throughout the eastern United States as far west as the Missouri river. They prefer the moist, rich soils of bottomlands.

  c. Exposure. Shavings or sawdust from walnut trees is occasionally used as animal bedding. Horses are most at risk.

  d. The **toxic principle** is unknown. A compound known as **juglone** has been suspected to be the toxin, but efforts to document this have been inconclusive.

  e. Clinical signs in horses occur within 24 hours of exposure to walnut shavings and include rapid onset of laminitis, a digital pulse, distal edema of the limbs, polypnea, and elevated temperature. Necrosis of the dorsal laminae may occur and complicate recovery.

  f. Treatment

     (1) The source of the walnut should be removed, and gastrointestinal detoxification carried out using mineral oil or activated charcoal and a mild cathartic.

     (2) The legs and feet should be washed.

     (3) Phenylbutazone or acepromazine can be used to treat laminitis.

VII. PLANTS CAUSING PULMONARY TOXICOSIS

A. Sources

1. *Brassica* (rape, canola) is discussed in III B 4. Rape seed and canola meal are used as alternative sources of oil and protein, especially in the northern United States and Canada, where their cold tolerance and rapid maturation rate are suited to the climate.

2. *Ipomea batata* (sweet potato) is grown for human consumption. Waste or lower-quality sweet potatoes may be used as livestock feed.

3. *Perilla frutescens* **(purple mint, beefsteak plant)** is an annual weed of the mint family.
    a. **Description.** Purple mint is characterized by square stems that bear alternate lanceo-late and serrated leaves that are green on the upper surface and pale violet to purple on the lower surface. Flowers are small and white and arise from the leaf axils or from terminal stems.
    b. **Description.** The plant occurs throughout the southern United States, in moist soils of pastures, fields, and waste areas.

B. Toxic principles

1. **Rapeseed** and **canola** may contain **glucosinolates,** which are glycosides that yield **isothiocyanates** following hydrolysis in the stomach or rumen.

2. **Sweet potatoes.** *Fusarium solani* can infest sweet potatoes, producing **ipomeanol,** a 3-substituted furan mycotoxin that causes acute pulmonary emphysema in cattle.

3. *Perilla frutescens.* **Perilla ketone,** produced by Perilla frutescens, is a 3-substituted furan similar to ipomeanol.

C. **Mechanism of toxicologic damage.** Mixed function oxidases (MFOs) appear to bioactivate the substituted furans, which bind covalently to proteins.

1. Type I epithelial cells are destroyed, causing emphysema and edema.

2. Type II alveolar cells proliferate to replace the Type I epithelium, leading to less effec-tive pulmonary air exchange.

D. Diagnosis

1. **Clinical signs** include dyspnea and cyanosis resulting from anoxia.
    a. Affected cattle stand with their heads extended and exhibit open-mouthed breathing, excessive salivation, and an audible expiratory grunt.
    b. As cyanosis and anoxia progress, animals may show some disorientation and bel-ligerence, presumably as a result of cerebral anoxia.
    c. Affected animals may be come recumbent and die within a few hours or 1–2 days.

2. **Lesions**
    a. **Gross lesions** include massive pulmonary emphysema with air trapped in large bul-lae, especially in the interlobular septa. If emphysema is extensive, air may infiltrate the subcutaneous areas over the thorax and behind the scapulae. Tissues may be cyanotic and congested.
    b. **Microscopic lesions.** Type I cells are absent or necrotic. Mild to moderate interstitial edema may be present. In advanced cases (i.e., those lasting longer than 2 days), extensive replacement of alveolar epithelium by cuboidal Type II cells gives the lungs a characteristic glandular appearance referred to as "adenomatosis."

E. **Treatment.** No antidote is available. Stress should be minimized. Supportive treatments (e.g., antibiotics, antihistamines, corticosteroids, anti-prostaglandins) have been tried, but are relatively ineffective.

VIII. PLANTS THAT AFFECT THE BLOOD

A. **Hematopoietic depression.** *Pteridium aquilinum* **(bracken fern)** depresses hematopoiesis in cattle.

1. **Description.** Bracken is a true fern that grows in large, dense patches and spreads by means of underground rhizomes. Bracken is large, with large bipinnately lobed leaves that are shaped like an elongated triangle.

2. **Geographic range.** The plant is found in forested areas of the northern United States, and is quite common in the Pacific Northwest. Cattle may graze fronds that invade pastures near the edge of woodlands.

3. **Toxic principle.** A lactone molecule, **ptaquiloside,** is considered responsible for bone marrow suppression and anemia caused by bracken fern. **All parts** of the plant, including the fronds and rhizomes, are toxic.

4. **Toxicity**
   a. **Cattle.** Bone marrow depression causes aplastic anemia, granulocytopenia, and thrombocytopenia. Urinary bladder neoplasms are reported in cattle consuming bracken for long periods of time.
   b. **Horses.** In horses, the plant has thiaminase activity, resulting in chronic ataxia, weakness, and paralysis. Bracken is not associated with anemia in horses.

5. **Diagnosis**
   a. **Clinical signs.** Hemorrhage, anemia, hematuria, and ventral edema occur after 4–6 weeks of continuous exposure in cattle.
   b. **Lesions** in cattle include anemia, pale bone marrow, and petechial and ecchymotic hemorrhages of the mucous membranes.

6. **Treatment**
   a. The **classic antidote** for bovine bracken fern toxicosis, **DL batyl alcohol** (1 g per adult bovine), is of limited value, especially in clinically advanced cases.
   b. Animals should be removed from contaminated areas and provided blood transfusions and high-quality diets to aid convalescence. Thiamine injections may be helpful for horses.

7. **Prognosis** for recovery in advanced cases is poor.

B. | **Hemolysis**

1. *Acer rubrum* (**red maple**)
   a. **Description.** Red maple is a typical maple with opposite simple leaves. The leaves are broad and have three to five lobes with palmately arranged veins. The fruit is a two-winged, two-seeded structure; the wings form a "V", and the two seeds lie at the bottom of the V.
   b. **Geographic range.** Red maple ranges naturally over the entire eastern United States and grows well on well-drained or moist, swampy soils. It may be a pest species in cut-over areas such as utility rights-of-way or deforested pasture lands. It is also grown as a cultivated ornamental tree.
   c. The **toxic principle** has not been identified, but it causes acute hemolysis.
   d. **Toxicity.** Fresh, wilted, and dried leaves are toxic, and as little as 0.3 % of the body weight as leaves is toxic to horses.
   e. **Diagnosis**
      (1) **Clinical signs** are typical of acute hemolytic disease: depression, icterus, anemia, hemoglobinemia, and hemoglobinuria. Polypnea and tachycardia may result from severe anemia, and cyanosis may also be present.
      (2) **Laboratory diagnosis** of blood reveals a low packed cell volume (PCV), mild methemoglobinemia, Heinz bodies, hyperbilirubinemia, and, sometimes, increased creatine phosphokinase.
   f. **Treatment** is completely supportive, because there is no antidote.
      (1) A whole blood transfusion may be life-saving.
      (2) Intravenous fluids and diuresis to reduce the probability of hemoglobin nephrosis may be helpful.

2. *Allium* (**onions, garlic**)
   a. **Description.** Onions and garlic are cultivated garden plants. The edible portion is a modified expanded leaf that resembles a bulb.

    b. The **toxic principle** is **N-propyl disulfide,** which denatures hemoglobin, leading to the formation of Heinz bodies and acute hemolysis. The toxicant is present in the edible **"bulb."**

    c. Toxicity. Cattle may be more susceptible than other species, but dogs, horses, and rabbits are also susceptible. Ingestion of a large number of onions at one time may cause toxicosis.

    d. Clinical signs are characteristic of acute hemolytic crisis (i.e., weakness, polypnea, icterus, hemoglobinuria, and cyanosis).

    e. Treatment is similar to that for red maple toxicosis (see VIII B 1 f).

  3. *Brassica*

    a. Description. Rape is described in III B 4.

    b. Toxic principle. S-methyl cysteine sulfoxide, which is present in rapeseed, is reduced to **dimethyl disulfide.** Dimethyl disulfide oxidizes hemoglobin, resulting in Heinz body hemolytic anemia. In most livestock diets using rapeseed, hemolytic anemia would not be expected unless use was excessive or prolonged.

    c. Clinical signs and **treatment** are similar to those for red maple and onions.

C. | **Hemorrhage**

  1. Sources

    a. *Lespedeza sericea* **(lespedeza)** is a perennial legume grown as a minor hay or forage crop.

    b. *Melilotus officinalis* **and** *M. alba* **(sweetclover)** is a legume forage or cover crop with white or yellow flowers in racemes. The leaves are compound, composed of three leaflets that are oblong and rounded at the tips. The vegetative portion can be distinguished from alfalfa by the presence of serrations along the entire margin of the leaf and by the longer petiole of the central leaflet.

  2. Toxic principle. Coumarin glycosides in the plants are dimerized by the metabolic activity of molds (e.g., *Penicillium, Humicolor, Mucor, Aspergillus*) that invade plants that are improperly cured for hay or in molded silage. The toxic agent, **dicoumarol,** interferes with the final carboxylation of prothrombin (factor II) or other clotting factors by competitively inhibiting vitamin K epoxide reductase.

  3. Toxicity. Cattle are most often poisoned because of their relatively common exposure to legume hays.

    a. Dicoumarol concentrations exceeding 20–30 ppm may cause toxicosis after exposure for 3 months.

    b. Concentrations greater than 60 ppm may cause poisoning within 2–3 weeks.

  4. Clinical signs are similar to those caused by anticoagulant rodenticides and include acute blood loss, subcutaneous hematomata, anemia, epistaxis, hemorrhagic diarrhea, and abortion resulting from placental hemorrhage.

  5. Treatment measures are the same as those taken for anticoagulant rodenticide toxicosis (see Chapter 22 II H).

D. | **Methemoglobinemia** can result from nitrate-containing plants (Table 28-6).

  1. Nitrogen, nitrite, and **nitrate.** Atmospheric nitrogen (N) used by nitrogen-fixing bacteria is converted to nitrate (NO_3), which can be reduced to nitrite (NO_2). The nitrite is used by plants to form vegetable protein.

    a. Nitrate reductase activity prevents nitrate accumulation in plants.

    b. Nitrates accumulate in vegetative tissue (e.g., stalks, leaves), not in fruits or grain.

TABLE 28-6. Nitrate-Containing Plants

Amaranthus retroflexus (redroot pigweed)	*Chenopodium album* (lamb's quarters)
Avena sativa (oats)	*Sorghum* (Johnson grass, Sudan grass, milo)
Beta vulgaris (beets)	*Zea mays* (corn, maize)

2. **Factors affecting nitrate content of plants**
   a. **Plant species.** Some species more readily accumulate nitrates.
   b. **Chemical form of nitrogen.** Nitrate and ammonia supply nitrate readily to plants.
   c. **Moisture content of soil.** Adequate moisture is necessary for nitrate uptake and movement from stems to leaves.
   d. **Soil pH.** Acid soils favor nitrate absorption.
   e. **Nitrate reductase activity**
      (1) Molybdenum, sulfur, phosphorus, and adequate light are necessary for nitrate reductase activity.
      (2) Frost damage interferes with nitrate reductase activity for several days after the freeze.
      (3) Drought conditions reduce nitrate reductase activity and prevent adequate nitrate translocation in the plant.
   f. **Presence of herbicides. Phenoxy acetic herbicides** are plant hormones that increase the growth rate and nitrate accumulation in early stages. Nitrate concentrations tend to be highest 3–5 days after herbicide application.
   g. **Plant phase.** Nitrate levels are highest prior to flowering and drop off rapidly after pollination.
   h. **Ensiling.** Anaerobic fermentation in silages reduces nitrate to nitrite and then to ammonia, with the majority of the nitrate lost. Oxides of nitrogen, known as "silo gases," are formed during the ensiling process and may accumulate in sufficient concentration to kill livestock within a few hours of ensiling.

3. **Toxicity**
   a. Forage nitrates exceeding 1% nitrate (dry-weight basis) may cause acute toxicosis. Higher levels of nitrates are tolerated when the dosage is spread throughout the feeding period or mixed in the diet.
      (1) The LD_{50} of nitrate in cattle is approximately 1 g/kg.
      (2) The LD_{50} for ruminants is approximately 0.5 g/kg body weight.
   b. Ruminants can adapt to higher nitrate concentrations with time, and tolerance to nitrate is increased by high-quality diets with readily available carbohydrate.

4. **Mechanism of toxicologic damage.** Nitrite ion oxidizes the ferrous iron in hemoglobin to the ferric state, forming methemoglobin, which is incapable of oxygen transport.
   a. Methemoglobin levels of 30%–40% cause clinical toxicosis, and death occurs when methemoglobin reaches 80%–90%.
   b. Methemoglobin in pregnant females results in abortions within 2–3 days as a result of fetal death from anoxia.

5. **Diagnosis.** Poisoning occurs within 4 hours of ingestion of plants with a high nitrate content.
   a. **Clinical signs** are anxiety, polypnea, dyspnea, and a rapid, weak pulse. Weakness, ataxia, and low exercise tolerance occur in severe cases.
   b. **Laboratory diagnosis**
      (1) Forage, hay, and water can be analyzed for nitrate.
      (2) Methemoglobin concentration can allow estimation of the severity of poisoning, but sample stability must be ensured through proper preservation techniques. One part blood to twenty parts of a phosphate buffer (pH 6.6) will preserve methemoglobin for later analysis.
   c. **Lesions**
      (1) **Physical lesions** include dark brown blood with staining of tissues and cyanosis. Petechial and ecchymotic hemorrhages may be observed on serous surfaces.
      (2) **Laboratory findings.** Nitrite and methemoglobin disappear rapidly from the blood and nitrate is quickly lost from the rumen contents after death as a result of continued microbial nitrate reduction.
         (a) Urine, plasma, serum, and rumen contents are rather unstable after death and may not be useful for nitrate analysis.
         (b) Ocular fluids appear to maintain nitrate stability and are a useful specimen for analysis. Concentrations above 30 ppm indicate excessive nitrate exposure.

6. Treatment

a. Methylene blue (see Table 6-1) is the recommended reducing agent for ruminants and monogastrics (except for cats). Methylene blue may need to be repeated several times because nitrite continues to be formed in the rumen.

b. Activated charcoal, ruminal lavage with cold water, or **large oral doses of antibiotics** may inhibit ruminal reduction of nitrate to nitrite.

E. Cyanide toxicosis

1. Factors influencing cyanide accumulation in plants

a. Species. The species and variety of plant influence the cyanogenic glycoside content.

(1) **Pitted fruits** (e.g., peaches, apricots, cherries, almonds)

(2) **Pome fruits** (e.g., apples, pears)

(3) **Grasses** (e.g., Johnson grass, sorghums, corn)

(4) **Elderberry**

(5) **Legumes** (e.g., birdsfoot trefoil, white clover, vetch)

b. Portion of plant. Cyanogenic glycosides concentrate in the seeds, leaves, bark, stems, and fruit (in order from greatest to least).

c. Phase of plant growth. Young, rapidly growing plants or plants undergoing regrowth are usually highest in glycoside content.

d. Environmental factors

(1) **Stresses** (e.g., wilting, frost, drought) may cause glycoside formation to increase. Damage to the cell walls causes the release of β-glucosidase, which liberates free cyanide.

(2) **Soil conditions.** High nitrogen or low phosphorus contents may favor an increase in cyanogenic glycoside formation.

(3) **Temperature, light,** and **soil pH** have an effect on the rate of plant growth and cyanide accumulation.

2. Mechanism of toxicologic damage. Cyanide combines with iron in cytochrome oxidase, preventing electron transfer and blocking cellular respiration.

3. Toxicity

a. Forage levels greater than 200 ppm are significant.

b. The enzyme rhodanese provides a natural detoxification system; therefore, small amounts in forage are tolerable.

(1) Cyanide + Thiosulfate + Rhodanese → Thiocyanate

(2) The thiocyanate is eliminated in the urine. Detoxification is dependent on thiosulfate availability.

c. Factors affecting toxicity

(1) **Size and species of animal.** Ruminants are more susceptible, because the rumen contains large amounts of β-glucosidase.

(2) **Speed of ingestion.** Natural detoxification protects the animal if ingestion is slow.

4. Diagnosis

a. Clinical signs. Acute or peracute onset is typical.

(1) Initial excitement and muscle tremors may occur within 30 minutes of ingesting a toxic dose.

(2) The blood and tissues are a characteristic cherry red, because the blood is oxygenated but cannot release oxygen to the cells. Polypnea, dyspnea, chronic convulsions, coma, and death occur as a result of cellular anoxia.

b. Laboratory diagnosis. Samples must be frozen if it is necessary to delay analysis.

(1) Suspect plants may be analyzed for cyanide.

(2) Urinary thiocyanate levels are elevated.

(3) Many veterinarians use a quick, qualitative test using picric acid–impregnated paper.

c. Lesions

(1) The hyperoxygenated blood clots slowly, or not at all.

(2) Subendocardial and subepicardial hemorrhages are present.

(3) The abomasum and intestine may be congested and contain petechial hemorrhages.

(4) The rumen may exude a "bitter almond" smell.

5. **Treatment.** The goal of treatment is to break the cyanide–cytochrome oxidase bond.
   a. The **recommended therapeutic regimen** is 10–20 mg/kg of sodium nitrite administered intravenously in a 20% solution, along with up to 600 mg/kg of 20% sodium thiosulfate.
      (1) Administering **sodium nitrite** causes cyanmethemoglobin to form, releasing cytochrome oxidase from the cyanide.
      (2) Administration of **thiosulfate** assists natural detoxification.
   b. **Cobalt salts** have also been recommended, but generally have not been used.

IX. PLANTS THAT AFFECT REPRODUCTION

A. Abortion

1. *Astragalus* (see II B 2). Exposure to locoweed during mid- to late pregnancy commonly causes abortion. Teratogenic effects (e.g., contracted tendon) and reduced spermatogenesis leading to male infertility also occur.

2. *Iva augustifolia* (**sumpweed**) grows in moist areas of the southwestern United States.
   a. Cattle are affected by plants in the seedling stage.
   b. Abortions are reported in the last half of the gestation period, following several weeks of consumption by the pregnant cow.

3. *Pinus ponderosa* (**Western yellow pine, ponderosa pine**) and *P. taeda* (**loblolly pine**)
   a. **Description.** Pines are evergreen trees with narrow needles in bunches of two or three. Seeds are borne in a characteristic "cone."
   b. **Geographic range.** Ponderosa pine ranges in the mountains of the northwestern United States. Loblolly pine is found in the eastern and southeastern United States.
   c. **Toxic principle.** An unidentified, water-soluble agent **in fresh** and **dried pine needles** causes abortion in cattle.
   d. **Toxicity.** Substantial intake of pine needles for several days is associated with abortions.
   e. **Clinical presentation.** Abortion is common in the last trimester of pregnancy and is often accompanied by edema of the udder and vulva in the dam. Retained placentas and metritis often are part of "pine needle abortion syndrome."
   f. **Prevention.** Measures include providing supplemental feed to reduce pine needle consumption and restricting access of pregnant cattle to pine needles.

4. *Xanthocephalum* (**Western broomweed**)
   a. **Description.** The plant is woody and branched. It grows to 0.75 meters in height and produces small, yellow flowers.
   b. **Geographic range.** Western broomweed is a perennial member of the Composite family that grows in the southwestern United States from Texas to California and north to Idaho.
   c. The **toxic principle** is considered to be a saponin.
   d. **Toxicity.** Ruminants, swine, and rabbits are susceptible.
   e. **Clinical signs**
      (1) **Acute toxicosis** is characterized by depression, anorexia, nasal discharge, and diarrhea.
      (2) **Chronic toxicosis.** Abortion occurs in cattle during the first two-thirds of gestation. Aborted calves are small and the dam usually has a retained placenta.

B. Clinical estrogenism. Clinical effects and documented infertility in the United States as a result of estrogen-containing plants appears rare, and is often suspected but not proven.

1. **Sources**
   a. *Trifolium repens* (subterranean clover), a classic high-estrogen clover, is grown in Europe and New Zealand.

TABLE 28-7. Teratogenic Plants

Plant	Toxic Principle	Susceptible Species	Period of Susceptibility	Effects
Astragalus lentiginosus, A. pubentissimus (locoweed)	Possibly swainsonine	Sheep	Early to mid-gestation	Arthrogryposis, contracted tendon, excessive carpal flexure, increased incidence of abortion
Conium maculatum (poison hemlock)	γ-Coniceine	Cattle, swine	Days 40–70	Arthrogryposis, scoliosis cleft palate
Lupinus (lupine, bluebonnet)	Anagyrine	Cattle	Days 40–70	"Crooked calf" disease (i.e., torticollis, scoliosis, cleft palate, twisted or bowed limbs)
Nicotiana tabacum (tobacco)	Anabasine	Swine	Days 10–30+	Arthrogryposis, twisting and dorsal flexure of the forelimbs and hindlimbs
Veratrum californicum (veratrum, false hellebore)	Cyclopamine	Sheep	Day 14 (cyclopian malformations)	Single or double fused ocular orbit, brachygnathia, large lambs as a result of prolonged gestation

    b. *T. subterraneum,* grown in Australia and the Pacific Northwest, is also high in natural estrogens. Other *Trifolium* species grown in the United States contain relatively low levels of estrogens and rarely cause problems.

    c. *Medicago sativa* (alfalfa), grown in the United States, produces coumestrol, which is weakly to moderately estrogenic and suspected of causing infertility.

  2. Toxic principle. The **isoflavone estrogens, genistein** and **formononetin,** are responsible for causing clinical estrogenism associated with *Trifolium.* Formononetin is non-estrogenic but is metabolized to an estrogenic compound, **equol.**

  3. Mechanism of toxicologic damage. Excessive levels of natural estrogens interfere with transport and fertility of ova, cause cystic hyperplasia of the cervix, and induce feminization and reduced libido in males.

C. **Teratogenic effects.** Plants associated with teratogenic effects are summarized in Table 28-7.

D. **Agalactia.** *Claviceps purpurea* **(ergot;** see Chapter 29 V) and *Festuca arundinacea* **(Kentucky 31 tall fescue;** see VI E 2) can cause agalactia.

X. PLANTS THAT AFFECT THE SKIN

A. **Primary photosensitization** (see also Chapter 13 III D 3)

  1. *Cymopterus watsonii* **(spring parsley)** is a low-growing desert plant of Arizona and Utah. The furanocoumarin compounds **xanthotoxin** and **bergapten** are phototoxic and have been isolated from the plant.

  2. *Fagopyrum esculentum* **(buckwheat)**

    a. Description. Buckwheat is an annual plant grown for its seed, which is commonly used in pancake flour. Leaves are triangular to heart-shaped.

    b. Toxic principle. The alleged toxic principle is **fagopyrin.** Both green and dry plant parts cause photosensitization.

3. *Hypericum perforatum* (St. Johnswort)
   a. **Description.** St. Johnswort is an erect, multiple-branched perennial with narrow, triangular leaves that are attached directly to the stem. The leaves contain numerous small spots that are nearly clear. Flowers are yellow with many small black spots on the petals.
   b. **Geographic range.** The plant ranges throughout the United States, but is found most commonly east of the Mississippi River in waste areas, pastures, and roadsides.
   c. **Toxic principle.** St. Johnswort contains a photodynamic red pigment known as **hypericin**.
   d. **Toxicity.** Cattle are apparently more susceptible than sheep, but both species have been affected.

B. **Physical damage.** Plants that cause physical damage to the skin are summarized in Table 28-3.

DIRECTIONS: Each of the numbered items or incomplete statements in this section is followed by answers or by completions of the statement. Select the **one** lettered answer or completion that is **best** in each case.

1. Which statement is true regarding secondary metabolites?

(1) They provide structural and reproductive capabilities for the plant.
(2) They are attractive compounds that promote contact with vectors (e.g., insects) to promote dissemination of seeds.
(3) They are only activated following consumption by animals or insects.
(4) They appear to have evolved as a mechanism to aid plant survival.
(5) The toxic secondary compounds are unique to individual species of plants and serve as a "chemical fingerprint."

2. The most dangerous portion of *Cicuta maculata* is the:

(1) seed.
(2) leaf.
(3) upper stem.
(4) flower.
(5) root.

3. What one specimen would be most useful to collect from a horse that had accidentally eaten rhubarb leaves and died 2 days later?

(1) Myocardial tissue
(2) Hepatic tissue
(3) Renal tissue
(4) Brain tissue
(5) Stomach contents

4. The characteristic fruit and seeds of locoweed are housed in which type of structure?

(1) Flat wings arranged in a "V"
(2) A large, spiny capsule that splits open to discharge 50–100 small, black seeds
(3) A flattened pod that contains 5–15 seeds
(4) A large, tapered capsule that contains small dark seeds and is topped with a white tuft
(5) A capsule with blunt spines that breaks open to reveal three, large, shiny, brown fruits

5. Nitrate accumulation during drought is most likely in which part of a plant?

(1) Flowers
(2) Seeds
(3) Leaves
(4) Stems
(5) All parts

6. A dog ingests a toxic dose of *Datura* tea. Which one of the following drugs would be most useful for counteracting the toxicosis?

(1) Atropine
(2) Calcium gluconate
(3) Corticosteroids
(4) Digitalis
(5) Physostigmine

7. Which pair of plants causes the most similar microscopic lesion?

(1) *Astragalus* (locoweed) and *Senecio* (tansy ragwort, groundsel)
(2) *Senecio* and *Acer rubrum* (red maple)
(3) *Acer rubrum* and *Quercus* (oak)
(4) *Quercus* and *Amaranthus retroflexus* (redroot pigweed)
(5) *Amaranthus retroflexus* and *Astragalus*

8. Which one of the following animals is most likely to experience toxic effects from black walnut?

(1) Cat
(2) Cow
(3) Dog
(4) Horse
(5) Pig

9. Which one of the following toxic principles is most likely to cause hepatomegalocytosis and bile duct hyperplasia?

(1) Pyrrolizidine alkaloids (PAs)
(2) Gallotannins
(3) Oxalates
(4) Nitrates
(5) Swainsonine

DIRECTIONS: Each of the numbered items or incomplete statements in this section is negatively phrased, as indicated by an italicized word such as *not, least,* or *except.* Select the **one** numbered answer or completion that is **best** in each case.

10. *Astragalus* plants contain several toxic principles that present a risk to cattle and horses. Which one of the following is *least* likely to be found at toxic quantities in *Astragalus*?

(1) Miserotoxin
(2) Nitrite
(3) Oxalate
(4) Selenium
(5) Swainsonine

11. Most neurotoxicants cause bilateral, symmetrical effects. Which one of the following neurotoxicants is the *exception* to this general rule?

(1) *Aesculus glabra* (Ohio buckeye)
(2) *Centaurea solstitialis* (yellow star thistle)
(3) *Dicentra culcullaria* (Dutchman's breeches)
(4) *Eupatorium rugosum* (white snakeroot)
(5) *Isocoma wrightii* (rayless goldenrod)

12. All of the following are associated with oral irritation, choking, salivation, and edema of the pharynx and glottis *except:*

(1) *Alocasia* (alocasia)
(2) *Cassia occidentalis* (coffee senna or sicklepod)
(3) *Dieffenbachia* (dieffenbachia, dumbcane)
(4) *Arisaema triphyllum* (jack-in-the-pulpit)
(5) *Philodendron* (philodendron)

13. All of the following plants target the same organ *except:*

(1) *Amsinckia intermedia* (fiddleneck)
(2) *Crotalaria* (crotalaria)
(3) *Perilla frutescens* (purple mint, beefsteak plant)
(4) *Senecio* (tansy ragwort, groundsel)
(5) *Xanthium strumarium* (cocklebur)

1. The answer is 4 *[I A]*. Evidence strongly suggests that plant toxins, secondary products of plant metabolism, have evolved to protect plants from predation by a variety of foraging species, ranging from insects to elephants. The secondary compounds are not essential for normal growth and reproduction; in fact, they are usually quite complex compared with the basic molecules needed for structural and reproductive processes. Toxic secondary metabolites vary widely in chemical structure and properties and occur across a variety of plant species.

2. The answer is 5 *[II A 2 c]*. The resinoid toxin, cicutoxin, is concentrated in the bundled roots and lower stem of *Cicuta maculata* (water hemlock). These plants grow in wet, swampy areas and grazing animals may pull them up by the roots, making this most toxic portion available for consumption.

3. The answer is 3 *[V A 1 d, 2, 4]*. Rhubarb leaves contain soluble oxalates that combine with ionized calcium to form calcium oxalate crystals. Following renal filtration, these crystals precipitate in the kidneys, where they are associated with fatal renal tubular nephrosis. Findings of a high concentration of oxalates in the kidneys at a postmortem performed 2 days after rhubarb ingestion is likely. Stomach contents would not be expected to contain oxalates from a toxic ingestion, because of the 2-day time lapse between ingestion and death. *Rheum rhaponticum* toxicosis is not associated with hepatic, cardiac, or cerebral lesions.

4. The answer is 3 *[II B 2]*. Locoweeds are members of the Leguminosae family, which also contains many important forage crops (e.g., alfalfa, clover, lespedeza) and food crops (e.g., soybeans, peanuts). The fruit is commonly referred to as a "pod" because it resembles a pea pod, although, technically, it is known as a legume. Maple trees produce a two-seeded fruit with flat wings arranged in a "V." Jimson weed is characterized by a large, spiny capsule that splits open to discharge small black seeds. Milkweed has a large, tapered capsule with a white tuft, which helps disperse the small, dark seeds contained in the capsule. Ohio buckeye has a capsule with blunt spines that breaks open to reveal three, large, shiny, brown fruits.

5. The answer is 4 *[VIII D 1 b, 2 c]*. Nitrate absorbed from the soil is transported from roots to stems to leaves for processing into ammonia and then to plant protein. The vascular system of the stems carries the nitrate to the leaves, where it is reduced by nitrate reductase. Because the stem lacks nitrate reductase, accumulation is more likely in this poriton of the plant. Numerous tests have shown that nitrate accumulation is highest in lower stems and that the probability of poisoning can be reduced by avoiding harvest of that portion of the plant.

6. The answer is 5 *[II D 2 d (2), e]*. *Datura* (Jimson weed or angel's trumpet) contains belladonna alkaloids, which have an action similar to atropine. The suggested physiologic antidote to belladonna alkaloids is a parasympathomimetic drug (e.g., physostigmine). Atropine would actually be harmful and contraindicated. Calcium deficiency and inflammation are not associated problems; therefore, calcium gluconate and corticosteroids would be of no therapeutic value. The action of digitalis on the cardiac muscle might be somewhat antagonistic to the action of atropine, but administration of physostigmine is the recommended approach.

7. The answer is 4 *[V C 4 c, D 1 e (2)]*. Both *Quercus* (oak) and *Amaranthus retroflexus* (redroot pigweed) cause acute to subacute tubular necrosis (nephrosis) characterized by a prominent coagulative necrosis and hyaline tubular casts. *Astragalus* (locoweed) is a neurotoxicant that causes neuronal vacuolation. *Senecio* (tansy ragwort, groundsel) contains pyrrolizidine alkaloids (PAs) and causes liver damage. *Acer rubrum* (red maple) contains an unidentified toxin that causes Heinz body hemolytic anemia.

8. The answer is 4 *[VI E 3]*. Black walnut shavings are occasionally used as animal bedding; however, this practice has been associated circumstantially and experimentally with laminitis and lameness in horses. The toxic principle is unknown. No other animals are known to be affected.

9. The answer is 1 *[IV B 3, 5 c]*. The pyrrolizidine alkaloids (PAs) bind to deoxyribonucleic acid (DNA), causing cellular necrosis and interruption of the cell cycle. These effects produce enlarged, undividing cells and bile duct hyperplasia. Gallotannins are nephrotoxins associated with oak toxicosis. Oxalates are also nephrotoxins. Nitrates are responsible for the oxidation of hemoglobin to the ferric state, resulting in methemoglobinemia. Swainsonine inhibits a-mannosidase and results in vacuolation of neurons.

10. The answer is 3 *[II B 2 c]*. Oxalates are not found at toxic concentrations in *Astragalus* (locoweed). Oxalate-containing plants in the same geographic range as *Astragalus* include *Halogeton glomeratus* (halogeton) and *Sarcobatus vermiculatus* (greasewood). Miserotoxin is a glycoside formed from the aglycone 3-nitropropanol, which can release a neurotoxic principle and nitrite. Swainsonine is the toxic principle found in locoweed that is responsible for the clinical signs of "loco." Many of the *Astragalus* species are known selenium accumulators, and some are actually selenium-dependent.

11. The answer is 2 *[II B 3 e]*. Yellow star thistle (*Centaurea solstitialis*) causes an asymmetric ischemic necrosis of the globus pallidus and substantia nigra. Because the necrosis may affect different regions of the nuclei or may not be complete, facial signs may be unilateral and asymmetrical. *Aesculus glabra* (Ohio buckeye), *Dicentra culcullaria* (Dutchman's breeches), *Eupatorium rugosum* (white snakeroot), and

Isocoma wrightii (rayless goldenrod) cause systemic neurologic effects that are generalized and symmetrical. Another exception to the rule is the mycotoxin fumonisin B1 (FB1), which causes leukoencephalomalacia and may affect the two hemispheres differentially.

12. The answer is 2 *[II G 2; III A 2 b; Table 28-4]*. Coffee senna (*Cassia occidentalis*) is a southern weed that causes myodegeneration and necrosis of the skeletal and cardiac muscles. Animals become weak or paralyzed; the gastrointestinal tract is not affected. Alocasia, dieffenbachia, jack-in-the-pulpit, and philodendron are all members of the Araceae family and are associated with oral irritation and pharyngeal edema. These effects are caused by penetration of the oral mucosa by calcium oxalate spicules (raphides) and possibly by the release of kinins that stimulate inflammatory response.

13. The answer is 3 *[IV A 4, B 1 a, b, e; VI A 3, C]*. All but *Perilla frutescens* (purple mint, beefsteak plant) are hepatotoxins. *P. frutescens* contains substituted furans that produce severe pulmonary emphysema and edema. *Amsinckia* (fiddleneck), *Crotalaria* (crotalaria), and *Senecio* (tansy ragwort, groundsel) contain pyrrolizidine alkaloids (PAs). *Xanthium strumarium* (cocklebur) contains carboxyatractyloside, a hepatocellular toxin.

Chapter 29
Mycotoxins

I. **INTRODUCTION.** Mycotoxins are **secondary metabolites of fungi** that are recognized as toxic to other life forms. Although more than 250 mycotoxins have been detected chemically, the biologic and veterinary medical impact of many mycotoxins has not yet been defined. Common mycotoxins are summarized in Table 29-1.

A. Fungal growth and mycotoxin production

1. **Fungal growth** is influenced by a variety of plant and environmental factors. These factors may also influence whether a mycotoxin is produced.
   a. **Field fungi** grow under conditions occurring **prior to harvest**. Major genera are *Alternaria, Cladosporium, Fusarium, Helminthosporium,* and *Pullaria*. Of these, only **Fusarium** is commonly recognized as a toxin producer.
      (1) **Growth conditions.** Field fungi usually require relative humidity above 80% and a grain moisture content that exceeds 22%. They usually do not grow after harvest because storage conditions do not meet their critical moisture needs.
      (2) **Effects on plants.** Field fungi are primary invaders of seeds on field plants. They often cause death of ovules, shriveling of seeds or kernels, and weakening or death of plant embryos. The grading term for this effect is "weathering."
      (3) **Effects of storage.** Under usual storage conditions, *Fusarium* may die within a few months. They do not generally persist in or reinvade grains that have been dried and remoistened.
   b. **Storage fungi** belong to various genera (including *Aspergillus* and *Penicillium*). They normally do not invade intact grain prior to harvest.
      (1) **Growth conditions**
         (a) **Moisture** (relative humidity at 70% and grain moisture content of 14%–24%) supports fungal growth.
         (b) **Temperature** optima vary with the fungus, and mycotoxin production may occur at temperatures different from those optimal for fungal growth (Figure 29-1).
         (c) **Conditions that damage the seed coat** (e.g., insects, drought stress, mechanical harvest, hot air drying) may enhance fungal invasion by making substrate at the interior of the seed more accessible.
      (2) *Aspergillus flavus* may produce aflatoxin in the field under appropriate conditions, although it is classified as a storage fungus.

2. **Mycotoxin production** often occurs sporadically under poorly defined growth conditions (usually those that create fungal stress). Production is often related to climate, weather patterns, insect damage, or production practices.
   a. Aflatoxins occur most commonly in warm, humid regions of the southeastern United States, and in subtropical or tropical regions worldwide.
   b. Zearalenone, a common estrogenic mycotoxin, is most likely in the north-central United States and in Canada.
   c. Trichothecenes are reported most frequently in cool, temperate regions (e.g., the northern United States, Canada, Russia, northern Europe).

TABLE 29-1. Fungi and Substrates Commonly Associated with Mycotoxin Production

Toxin	Chemical Structure	Fungus	Common Substrates
Aflatoxins		*Aspergillus flavus* *Aspergillus parasiticus*	Corn, cottonseed, peanuts, milo
Fumonisins		*Fusarium moniliforme* *Fusarium proliferatum*	Corn
Ochratoxin A		*Aspergillus ochraceus* *Penicillium viridicatum*	Corn, barley, wheat, rye
Citrinin		*Penicillium citrinum* *Penicillium viridicatum*	Wheat, barley, rye, oats

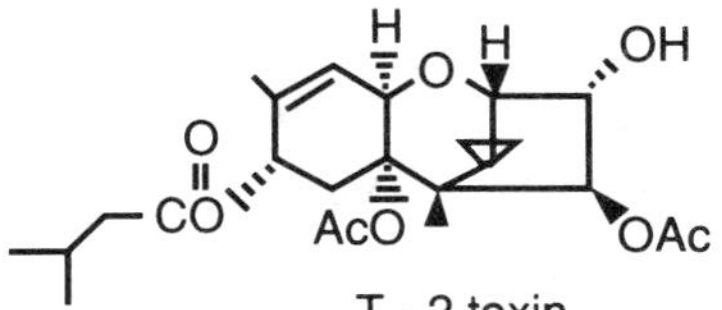 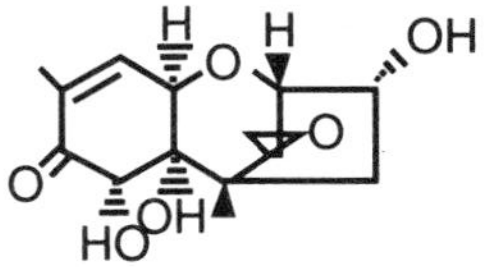 Trichothecenes	*Fusarium sporotrichioides* *Fusarium poae* *Fusarium graminareum* *Fusarium culmorum* *Fusarium roseum*	Corn, barley, rye, wheat, milo
Zearalenone, zearalenol	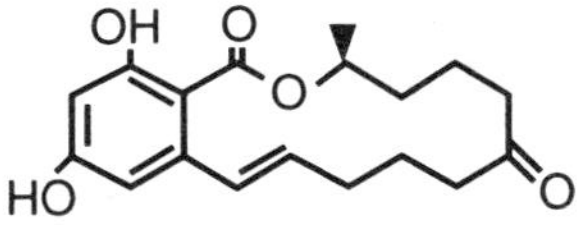 *Fusarium roseum* *Fusarium moniliforme*	Corn, wheat, barley, milo
Slaframine	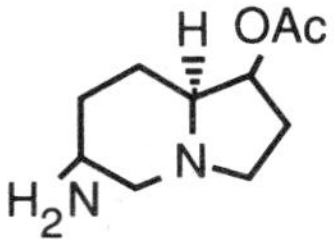 *Rhizoctonia leguminicola*	Red clover, ladino clover, alfalfa
Penitrem A	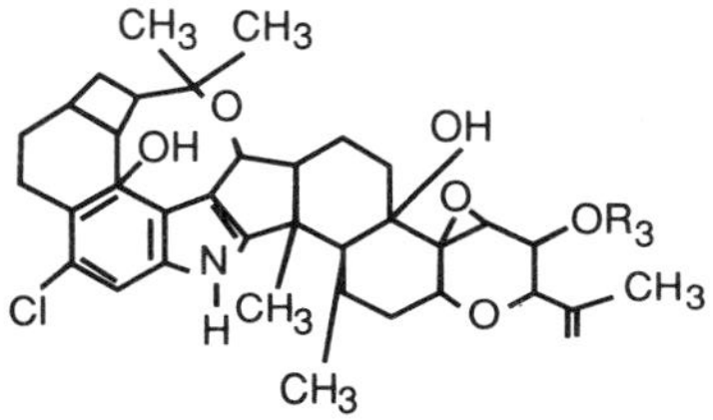 *Penicillium cyclopium* *Penicillium palitans* *Penicillium crustosum* *Penicillin puberulum*	Corn, peanuts, pecans, walnuts, cream cheese

T - 2 toxin

Dioxynivalenol

TABLE 29-1. (Continued)

Toxin	Chemical Structure	Fungus	Common Substrates
Lolitrem-B		*Acremonium lolii*	Perennial ryegrass (*Lolium perenne*)
Paspalitrem A and B		*Calviceps paspali*	Dallis grass (*Paspalum dilatatum*)
Ergot alkaloids Ergotamine	R = CH₂	*Claviceps purpurea*	Rye, wheat, oats, barley, grass forages

Ergovaline

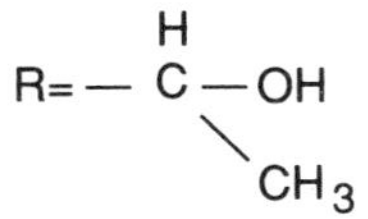

$$R = -\underset{\underset{CH_3}{|}}{\overset{\overset{H}{|}}{C}} - OH$$

Dicoumarol

Acremonium
coenophialum

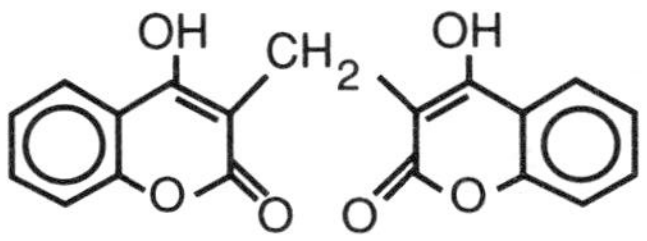

Penicillium
Mucor
Humicolor

Fescue forages (*Festuca
arundinaceae*)

Sweet clover (*Melilotus*)

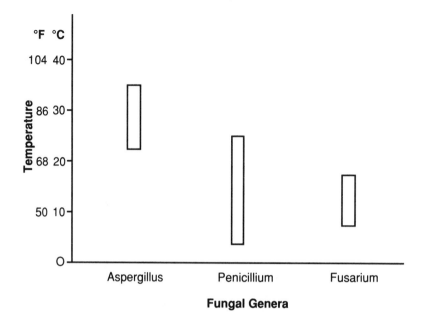

FIGURE 29-1. Temperature ranges favoring growth of mycotoxin-producing fungi and the production of mycotoxins.

B. **Characteristics of mycotoxin-induced disease**

1. Disease is **not transmitted among animals;** rather, it is only associated with the consumption of contaminated feeds or forages.

2. **Pharmaceutical treatment does not alter the course** of the disease.

3. Mycotoxicosis most often presents as a **vague, subacute** or **chronic condition,** although acute clinical effects have been described for each of the major mycotoxins affecting animals.
   a. The important toxicologic principle of "dose and response" is difficult to apply in the diagnosis of mycotoxin-related disease, because of the chronic nature of the disorder, the uneven distribution of the toxin in the feed, and other factors, such as nutritional status, that affect animal response.
   b. The clinical response is often separated chronologically from the known or initial exposure to a moldy feed, so obvious association between clinical effects and change to a mycotoxin-contaminated feed is not readily apparent.
   c. Because a major effect of many moldy grains is feed refusal, sample palatability must be considered. Drastically reduced consumption may limit the toxic effects if animals refuse to eat the feed.
   d. Heat, chemicals, and sunlight all have the potential for altering the structure and activity of mycotoxins.

C. **Diagnosis of mycotoxin-induced disease**

1. **Correlation with molds.** Because not all secondary metabolites are toxic, the presence of mycotoxins cannot be predicted by the presence of a specific fungus or verified by mold spore counts.
   a. Mold spores are common in feedstuffs, and only when conditions are proper for their growth and toxin production do they produce mycotoxins.
   b. Mycotoxicosis is less likely from heterogenous mold populations, as opposed to when only one toxin-producing species and strain is present.

2. Confirmation of the diagnosis. A mycotoxin diagnosis can be confirmed either by:
   a. Test feeding the suspected ration and observing reproduction of a characteristic mycotoxic disease
   b. Identifying a known mycotoxin in the diet or animal tissues. The mycotoxin isolated must be known to produce disease typical of the field problem observed.
      (1) Suspected feeds or grains may have evidence of mold growth; processing such as heating, solvent extraction, or pelleting can kill fungi and mask the signs of fungal invasion.
      (2) Representative samples are essential for mycotoxin identification in feed or grain.

3. Sampling and analysis of feed or forages
   a. Accuracy of sampling. Sampling for mycotoxins does not always result in an accurate assessment of the toxicologic status of the feedstuff.
      (1) Uneven distribution of the toxin within the feedstuff places heavy responsibility on proper and thorough sampling (see I C 3 b).
      (2) The responsible feed may have been consumed and unavailable for testing before substantial clinical signs became apparent.
   b. Sampling. Because contamination can vary widely within the same storage unit, or even among kernels on the same ear of corn, thorough sampling is required.
      (1) Principles
         (a) Samples of feed or forage for analysis or feeding trials **should reflect all the sources of feed available at the time the problem occurred**.
         (b) Whenever possible, **samples should be taken after particulate size has been reduced** (e.g., by shelling or grinding). If blending has recently occurred (as in harvesting, loading, or grinding), reducing particulate size permits a more representative sample to be obtained.
      (2) Methods are illustrated in Figure 29-2.

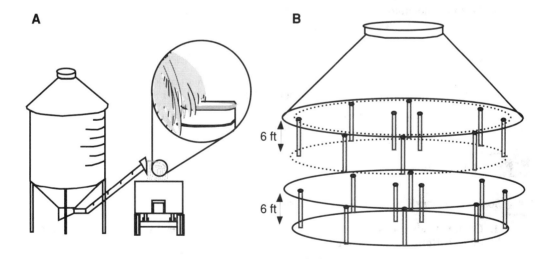

FIGURE 29-2. Sampling techniques. (*A*) The "moving stream" method. A cup is periodically passed through a moving stream of grain over a periof of 15–30 minutes. The collected subsamples are then combined and mixed thoroughly and a 5- to 10-lb sample is taken for analysis. (*B*) Probe sampling is less reliable than sampling via the moving stream method because microenvironments within the storage facility can cause area of mold or mycotoxin concentration. Multiple probe samples are taken at a depth of 6 feet, both at the perimeter and the center of the bin. The subsamples are then combined and sampled as described in (*A*).

    c. **Sample analysis**
       (1) **On-site analysis.** Economical and reliable methods of on-site mycotoxin analysis are being developed. Cross-reactivity with similar toxins in feeds and interference by other chemicals or natural molecules in mixed feeds can reduce the accuracy of these tests.
       (2) **Storage and transport of samples**
         (a) **Drying.** Dry samples are preferred for transport and storage.
           (i) Samples can be oven-dried at 176°F–194°F (80°C–90°C) for 3 hours to reduce moisture to 12%–13%.
           (ii) For mold cultures, samples should be dried at 140°F (60°C) for 6–12 hours to preserve fungal viability.
         (b) **Containers.** Paper or cloth bags should be used to store and transport dried samples.
           (i) Plastic bags may promote moisture condensation, leading to molding of the grain in transit.
           (ii) Samples with a high moisture content can be held in plastic bags if refrigeration, freezing, or mold inhibitors are used to retard mold growth.
       (3) **Long-term storage.** For long-term storage, samples should be dried to less than 12% moisture and stored sealed in moisture-proof containers.

D. Treatment of mycotoxin-induced disease

1. For most mycotoxins, there is no specific treatment or antidote.

2. Supplementation with vitamins and selenium may be helpful, and provision of adequate high-quality protein is advisable after animals have consumed mycotoxins.

E. Prevention of mycotoxin-induced disease

1. **Avoiding** grain that is known to be moldy is the best management strategy.

2. **Diluting** contaminated grain with clean grain reduces the initial mycotoxin level.

3. **Cleaning** the grain often markedly reduces the mycotoxin load, because many mycotoxins are associated with low-quality, small, cracked, or broken seeds.

4. **Testing** of suspect molded feeds and grains may be helpful to rule out the presence of known mycotoxins.

5. **Drying** grain and feed to a moisture level of 13%–15% may prevent recontamination during storage. Storage bins and feeders should be kept dry and clean.

6. **Adding** organic acids will prevent mold growth, but will not destroy preformed toxins.

II. AFLATOXIN

A. Sources. *Aspergillus flavus* and *A. parasiticus* produce aflatoxins.

1. **Common substrates.** Aflatoxins occur most commonly in **feed grains,** especially **corn, milo, cottonseed,** and **peanuts**.

2. **Factors favoring production of aflatoxins**
    a. **Environmental conditions**
       (1) **Temperature.** The optimum temperature range for aflatoxin formation is a sustained temperature of 78°F–90°F (25°C–32°C), although temperatures as low as 55°F for 2 or more days can support aflatoxin formation.
       (2) **Drought stress** enhances *A. flavus* aflatoxin production by prolonging the survival of fungal spores and reducing host mechanical barriers (e.g., ear husks).

(3) High relative humidity or **grain moisture** supports fungal growth and enhances the potential for aflatoxin formation. *A. flavus* can produce aflatoxin at a grain moisture content of 16%–28%.

   (a) In storage, *Aspergillus*-infected grain may continue to produce aflatoxins if grain is not dried to a moisture content of less than 15%.

   (b) Continued fungal respiration uses oxygen and carbohydrates to form carbon dioxide and water, thus providing additional free ("unbound") water to support additional fungal growth.

b. Physical characteristics

   (1) Corn ears with shortened husks maturing in an upward position appear to be more susceptible than ears covered by husks that mature in a downward position.

   (2) Insect damage or scarification during harvest damage the seed coat, allowing *Aspergillus* to access the carbohydrate (endosperm) within the seed, providing a substrate for fungal growth.

B. **Chemical characteristics.** Aflatoxins are **polycyclic furan compounds**.

1. Aflatoxins **exhibit** intense **blue** or **green fluorescence under ultraviolet light**. The four major natural aflatoxins, **aflatoxins B1, B2, G1,** and **G2,** are grouped according to their chromatographic and fluorescence characteristics. Aflatoxin B1 (AFB1) is the most abundant.

2. **Aflatoxin M1** is a **metabolite of AFB1** found in animal urine, milk, or tissues.

C. **Toxicokinetics.** AFB1 is metabolized by hepatic microsomal mixed function oxidases (MFOs) to form **at least seven metabolites,** each with different biological activity. One major metabolite of AFB1 is a **highly reactive electrophilic epoxide** that forms covalent adducts with deoxyribonucleic acid (DNA), ribonucleic acid (RNA), and protein.

D. **Mechanism of toxicologic damage.** Aflatoxin inhibits protein synthesis by modifying the DNA template and depressing messenger RNA synthesis, interfering with transcription. **Impaired protein synthesis** interferes with the formation of enzymes necessary for energy metabolism and fat mobilization. The liver is most affected (Figure 29-3).

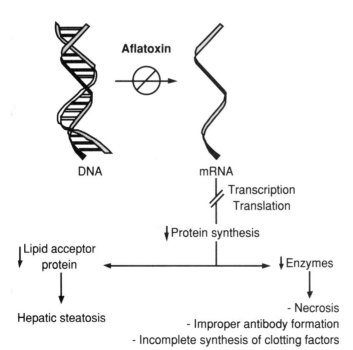

FIGURE 29-3. Pathogenesis of aflatoxicosis. Aflatoxin binds to guanine in deoxyribonucleic acid (*DNA*), inhibiting the signal for the formation of messenger ribonucleic acid (*RNA*). Interruption of protein synthesis leads to deficiencies of structural proteins, enzymes, and lipid acceptor protein. The long-term effects of impaired protein synthesis include hepatic steatosis and a variety of metabolic and function derangements.

1. **Loss of enzymes** results in reduced formation of structural proteins, improper antibody formation, reduced fat digestion, and incomplete synthesis of clotting factors.

2. **Lack of formation of lipid acceptor protein** in the liver leads to hepatic steatosis.

3. **Decreased cellulose digestion, reduced volatile fatty acid formation,** and **inhibition of proteolysis** have been observed in artificial rumen systems.

4. **Necrosis** results from lack of key enzymes that support essential metabolic reactions.

E. **Toxicity** (Table 29-2). Cattle, sheep, and other ruminants appear less susceptible than monogastric animals or poultry.

1. Young animals of most species are more susceptible to aflatoxins than mature animals.

2. Nutritional deficiencies, especially protein, selenium, and vitamin E deficiencies, increase susceptibility to aflatoxins.

TABLE 29-2. Relative Response of Animals to Dietary Aflatoxins*

Concentration (ppb)	Species	Violative residues	Decreased performance	Impaired immunity	Hepatic lesions	Clinical illness
50	Dairy cattle	+	−	−	−	−
100	Broiler chicks	−	−	−	−	−
	Feedlot cattle	−	−	−	−	−
	Piglets	−	−	−	−	−
	Adult swine	−	−	−	−	−
200	Broiler chicks	−	−	−	−	−
	Calves	−	±	−	−	−
	Feedlot cattle	−	−	−	−	−
	Piglets	−	±	±	±	−
	Adult swine	−	−	−	−	−
	Turkey poults	−	+	+	++	−
400	Broiler chicks	±	±	+	+	−
	Calves	−	±	−	−	−
	Feedlot cattle	+	−	−	−	−
	Piglets	+	±	±	+	−
	Adult swine	+	±	±	+	−
	Turkey poults	+	+	+	++	+
500	Broiler chicks	+	+	+	+	−
	Calves	+	+	±	+	±
	Feedlot cattle	+	−	−	±	−
	Piglets	+	++	+	++	−
	Adult swine	+	+	±	±	−
	Turkey poults	+	+	+	++	−
750	Broiler chicks	+	+	+	++	±
	Calves	+	+	+	+	±
	Feedlot cattle	+	±	±	+	−
	Piglets	+	++	+	++	±
	Adult swine	+	+	±	+	−
	Turkey poults	+	+	+	++	+
1000	All	+	+	+	++	+

*Estimates are based on extended feeding times (more than 2 weeks)
− = no effect; ± = variable effect; + = affected; ++ = severely affected.

F. **Diagnosis**

1. **Clinical signs**
   a. **Acute.** Major acute clinical effects in most animals include depression, anorexia, reduced gain or milk production, and subnormal body temperature.
   b. **Chronic**
      (1) **Poultry.** Chronic signs in poultry include a **decreased growth rate** and **reduced feed efficiency,** as well as **steatorrhea** resulting from impaired fat digestion. Increased capillary fragility in poultry has been associated with **bruising** or loss of tissue strength, which may result in carcass condemnations at slaughter.
      (2) **Swine.** Major chronic disease manifestations include **anorexia, unthriftiness, slow growth, icterus, mild anemia, ascites,** and increased **susceptibility to infectious diseases**.
      (3) **Cattle.** Aflatoxin at high concentrations (1–4 ppm) may reduce rumen motility for 24–48 hours.

2. **Laboratory diagnosis**
   a. **Bloodwork**
      (1) **Mild anemia** is nonspecific.
      (2) **Serum liver enzymes** are elevated, including aspartate transaminase (AST), alanine aminotransaminase (ALT), alkaline phosphatase (AP), ornithine carbamyl transferase, and isocitric dehydrogenase.
      (3) **Serum bile acids** may be elevated early in aflatoxicosis. Hyperbilirubinemia develops in chronic toxicosis.
      (4) **Serum albumin** and the albumin:globulin ratio are decreased.
      (5) **Prothrombin** activity may be reduced as a result of poor synthesis of coagulation factors.
   b. **Tissue analysis and urinalysis**
      (1) **Milk and urine.** Aflatoxin M1 can be detected in milk or urine for several days after aflatoxin exposure stops.
      (2) **Liver and kidney.** Most aflatoxin is excreted 72–96 hours after exposure stops; however, the liver and kidney appear to retain measurable residues of aflatoxin longer than other tissues. (These residues also dissipate after 2 weeks.)
   c. **Analysis of grains or feeds**
      (1) **"Black light" test.** Bright greenish-yellow fluorescence (BGYF) is seen in contaminated grain viewed under ultraviolet light.
         (a) BGYF is the result of a **marker fungal product, kojic acid,** produced under similar conditions as aflatoxin. Therefore, BGYF is only a presumptive indicator for aflatoxin.
         (b) Fluorescence is **best seen in broken or damaged grains** where mold growth has invaded the endosperm.
      (2) Additional specific testing by **thin-layer chromatography, gas–liquid chromatography, mass spectrometry,** or other instrumental methods is needed to confirm the presence of aflatoxin.

3. **Lesions**
   a. **Acute aflatoxicosis** causes centrilobular hemorrhagic hepatic necrosis, hemorrhage, and ascites.
   b. **Subacute aflatoxicosis**
      (1) **Gross lesions** include hepatic fatty change, a pale, soft, clay-colored liver, mild anemia, icterus, and ascites.
      (2) **Microscopic lesions** include:
         (a) Hepatocyte degeneration and necrosis, regeneration of liver cells, fatty change, and proliferation of bile duct epithelium, progressing to hepatic interlobular fibroplasia and extensive bile duct proliferation
         (b) Karyomegaly, atypical nuclei, multiple nucleoli, hepatocyte vacuolization, and bile retention

G. **Treatment and prevention**

1. **Treatment**
   a. **Detoxification. Hydrated sodium calcium aluminosilicate (HSCAS)** has a high affinity for aflatoxin and can **adsorb** aflatoxins, reducing their absorption from the gastrointestinal tract.
      (1) HSCAS reduces aflatoxin M1 residues in the milk of dairy cows fed AFB1.
      (2) HSCAS corrects impaired growth rate and liver lesions induced by aflatoxins in swine.
   b. **Supportive treatment.** Supplemental **vitamin E** and **selenium** have been used with variable success to ameliorate the effects of aflatoxins.

2. **Prevention**
   a. **Mold inhibitors** may prevent further growth and toxin formation of *A. flavus* in prepared feeds, but they will not destroy preformed toxins.
   b. **Treatment of grain with anhydrous ammonia** for 10–14 days reduces its aflatoxin content, but because uncertainty regarding the breakdown products exists, the Food and Drug Administration (FDA) has not yet cleared this detoxication method.

H. **Public health considerations.** Because aflatoxin has proven to be a carcinogen in laboratory animals, milk is routinely monitored for aflatoxins. The FDA considers aflatoxin in milk to be a serious regulatory violation.

1. Although estimates vary, aflatoxin in milk appears at approximately 1% of the dietary concentration.

2. Milk from dairy cattle fed feed containing more than 20 ppb aflatoxin may contain residues in excess of the current FDA action level (0.5 ppb).

III. ZEARALENONE

A. **Sources.** Zearalenone is produced by *Fusarium roseum* (*F. graminearum*), the conidial stage of *Giberella zea*, and by some isolates of *F. moniliforme*.

1. **Common substrates** are **corn, wheat, barley,** and **milo;** zearalenone is also occasionally produced in **oats**.
   a. Fungal infections of corn and wheat are commonly known as **"pink ear rot"** and **"scab,"** respectively.
   b. In the United States, zearalenone concentration in grain rarely exceeds 3 ppm and rarely, if ever, occurs in hay.

2. **Factors favoring production of zearalenone**
   a. **High moisture** (grain moisture content of 22%–25%). Stored corn is unlikely to produce zearalenone unless it is stored as ear corn or the moisture content exceeds 22%.
   b. **Alternating high and low temperatures** [45°F–70°F (7°C–21°C)] during the maturing and harvesting stage, such as occur in the midwestern United States and Canada

B. **Chemical characteristics.** Zearalenone is a **substituted resorcyclic acid lactone** that is structurally similar to the anabolic agent zearalenol. It can be isolated as a white crystalline compound with a molecular weight of 318.

C. **Toxicokinetics**

1. **Absorption.** Zearalenone is readily absorbed from the gastrointestinal tract.

2. **Metabolism and excretion.** Zearalenone is metabolized to α and β zearalenol and excreted in bile and feces as well as the urine.
   a. Enterohepatic cycling promotes prolonged retention of zearalenone after consumption stops.
   b. Limited amounts of zearalenone are secreted in the milk.

D. Mechanism of toxicologic damage

1. Zearalenone **binds to cytosolic receptors for estradiol-17β**. The zearalenone–receptor complex migrates to the nucleus and binds to estradiol sites on DNA, initiating specific RNA synthesis.

2. Physiologically, zearalenone **functions as a weak estrogen** with a potency two to four times less than that of estradiol. It inhibits secretion and release of follicle-stimulating hormone (FSH), which inhibits preovulatory ovarian follicle maturation.

E. Toxicity

1. Toxicity is **low** for all effects except reproductive function. Adverse effects are usually related to the concentration of zearalenone in the *ad lib* diet of domestic animals (Table 29-3).

2. **Age** and **species** influence the response to zearalenone.
   a. Swine are the most susceptible domestic species to the reproductive effects of zearalenone. Zearalenone given to pregnant sows 7–10 days postmating causes failure of implantation, and embryos do not survive beyond 21 days (i.e., early embryonic death occurs).
   b. Infertility in cattle as a result of zearalenone has generally been of very low clinical incidence and is not prolonged beyond exposure to zearalenone.

F. Diagnosis

1. **Clinical signs** vary according to the animal's species, age, and reproductive status.
   a. Swine
      (1) Prepubertal females (gilts) exhibit a **syndrome of hyperestrogenism** characterized by behavioral estrus, swelling and edema of the vulva, enlargement of the mammary glands, tenesmus, and, often, vaginal and rectal prolapse. Clinical signs appear 2–7 days after exposure and subside 4–10 days postexposure.
      (2) Mature sows may experience either nymphomania or anestrus and pseudopregnancy.
         (a) Nymphomania. Zearalenone exposure early in the estrus cycle of nongravid sows prevents follicular development, causing suppression of ovulation and physiologic signs of estrus, which may be severe and prolonged.
         (b) Anestrus and pseudopregnancy. Exposure to zearalenone in the middle of the estrus cycle (days 11–14) has a luteotropic effect, resulting in retained corpora lutea and anestrus.
            (i) Retention of functional, progesterone-secreting corpora lutea may persist for 60–80 days, causing a period of anestrus often called "pseudopregnancy."
            (ii) Signs of anestrus and pseudopregnancy can persist for 40–60 days after zearalenone has been removed from the diet.

TABLE 29-3. Effects of Zearalenone in Domestic Mammals

Dietary Zearalenone (ppm)	Susceptible Species/ Class of Animal	Clinical Effects
1–3	Prepubertal gilts	Hyperestrogenism, vulvovaginitis, tenesmus, vaginal and rectal prolapse
3–10	Sexually mature sows	Anestrus and pseudopregnancy with retention of corpora lutea for 40–60 days
> 10	Virgin heifers	Infertility, reduced conception rate, repeat breeding
> 15	Bred sows 7–10 days postmating	Early embryonic death, prolonged interestrus intervals
> 20	Young boars	Loss of libido, preputial enlargement, possible infertility
> 25	Mature cows	Infertility, reduced conception rate, repeat breeding

(3) **Castrated males** may develop **enlargement** of the **prepuce** and **nipples.**
(4) **Immature boars** experience **reduced libido** and **retarded testicular develop-ment,** whereas **mature boars are not affected** by dietary zearalenone levels below 200 ppm.

  b. **Cattle**
  (1) **Vaginitis** may occur, and **vaginal secretions** may be increased.
  (2) **Mammary enlargement** may occur in virgin heifers.

2. **Laboratory diagnosis**
  a. **Bloodwork.** In sexually mature sows, plasma progesterone may confirm the presence of functional corpora lutea.
  b. **Tissue analysis and urinalysis.** Zearalenone exposure is not readily detected by analysis of body fluids or tissues.
  c. **Chemical analysis of grains or feeds** is the most useful means of confirming signifi-cant exposures. However, because effects may only be apparent long after consump-tion of the responsible feed has stopped, planned retention and dating of samples from all diets fed aids identification of the responsible feed or grain.

3. **Lesions** are present only in the reproductive system.
  a. **Prepubertal gilts** exhibit swelling and edema of the vulva, mammary enlargement, and vaginal or rectal prolapse. The uterus is enlarged and edematous with cellular proliferation and hypertrophy. Microscopic lesions of uterine and vaginal metaplasia and follicular atresia are characteristic.
  b. **Mature sows** with anestrus exhibit retained and functional corpora lutea, uterine edema, mammary alveolar development, and ductular squamous metaplasia.

4. **Differential diagnoses.** Other plants (e.g., legumes) contain estrogens that could mimic some effects of zearalenone; therefore, the diet should be checked for other sources of estrogens.

G. **Treatment.** Signs of hyperestrogenism should resolve within 1–2 weeks of changing the source of grain.

1. **Detoxification**
  a. Activated charcoal binds zearalenone in the gastrointestinal tract and helps to pre-vent enterohepatic recycling.
  b. Alfalfa and alfalfa meal fed to swine may reduce absorption and increase fecal excre-tion of zearalenone. However, alfalfa meal must comprise approximately 25% of the diet, and this is not considered practical.

2. **Supportive treatment**
  a. Vaginal or rectal prolapse and physical damage to the external genitalia must be treated.
  b. Administration of one 10-mg dose of **prostaglandin F$_{2\alpha}$,** or two 5-mg doses on suc-cessive days usually resolves retained corpora lutea and corrects anestrus in sows.
  c. **Bentonite** added to contaminated diets has been claimed helpful in controlling zear-alenone effects.

IV. **TRICHOTHECENES.** There are over 140 known metabolites in the trichothecene class. Best known and of greatest concern in North America are **T-2 toxin, diacetoxyscirpenol (DAS)** and **dioxynivalenol (vomitoxin, DON).**

A. **Sources.** Toxins of concern are produced primarily by field fungi, including *Fusarium sporotrichioides* (T-2 toxin and DAS) and *Fusarium roseum* (DON).

1. **Common substrates** for the trichothecene-producing *Fusaria* include corn, milo, wheat, rye, barley, and other cereal crops.
  a. Production of the major trichothecenes in hay is rarely reported.
  b. *Stachybotrys atra* is reported to produce the toxic trichothecene satratoxin in molded forage in eastern Europe.

2. Factors favoring production of trichothecenes
   a. Mold growth and toxin production are favored by **alternating cool and warm temperatures,** ranging from 41°F–59°F (5°C–15°C).
   b. Toxin production may occur in **late-harvested** or **overwintered grain**. Widespread outbreaks of alimental toxic aleukia occurred in humans in Russia during World War II; the outbreak was believed to result from the production of T-2 toxin in over-wintered cereal crops.

B. **Chemical characteristics.** Trichothecenes belong to a class of **sesquiterpene lactones** known as **12, 13-epoxytrichothecenes**. Toxicological properties depend, in part, on the presence of a 12,13 epoxy group; loss of the epoxide function markedly reduces toxicity.

1. Four types of trichothecenes are recognized.
   a. Type A trichothecenes contain a **nonketone functional group at C-8**. T-2 toxin and DAS are type A trichothecenes.
   b. Type B trichothecenes have a **carbonyl function at C-8**. DON and nivalenol are type B trichothecenes.
   c. Type C and **D** trichothecenes currently contain no mycotoxins of major veterinary clinical interest.

2. The toxin is **stable in the environment,** and **resistant to the heat and pressure of cooking, feed milling,** and **processing**.

C. **Mechanism of toxicologic damage**

1. Trichothecenes are **potent inhibitors of protein synthesis** in mammalian cells, reportedly by degrading polyribosomes and inhibiting the initiation phase of protein synthesis. T-2 toxin has a high affinity for 60S ribosomal subunits, which may explain its effects on protein synthesis.

2. Trichothecene mycotoxins **inhibit DNA and RNA nucleic acid synthesis**. Higher dosages are required to inhibit nucleic acid synthesis than to inhibit protein synthesis, implying that a different mechanism may be operative for each effect.

3. Low dosages of trichothecenes **inhibit membrane transfer of glucose, calcium,** and **some amino acids** in vitro. These effects are independent of the inhibition of protein synthesis.

4. Trichothecenes are **directly cytotoxic** to a variety of cells in vitro. The mechanism is unclear, but direct cytotoxicity may explain the dermonecrotic effects reported for trichothecenes.

5. Trichothecenes **affect immunity,** increasing susceptibility to certain infectious diseases.
   a. Antibody formation is suppressed.
   b. Delayed hypersensitivity reactions are enhanced in association with inhibition of suppressor T cells.
   c. Mitogen-induced lymphocyte blastogenesis is impaired.

D. **Toxicity.** Voluntary feed refusal often prevents full expression of oral toxicosis from contaminated feeds. However, dosing studies using parenteral injection and oral administration reveal that trichothecenes are potent toxicants.

1. Mice are more resistant than rats, guinea pigs, swine, and chickens.

2. Cats appear more sensitive to T-2 toxin than other domestic species.

E. **Diagnosis**

1. Clinical signs
   a. Dermal and **oral irritation** and **necrosis** occur in animals following direct contact with contaminated feed.
      (1) Epithelial necrosis appears on the **feet** or **underline of animals** where they touch contaminated feed, or at the **commissures of the mouth** or **beak** following consumption of T-2–contaminated feed.

(2) Labial or **glossal epithelial necrosis** with ulceration and exudation of serum occurs after several days.

(3) Erosion and **loss of ruminal papillae** may occur after consumption of contaminated rations by ruminants.

b. Gastroenteritis with vomiting and diarrhea, sometimes hemorrhagic, are reported, especially in animals initially consuming or gavaged with high dosages of trichothecenes.

c. Hemorrhaging has been occasionally reported in association with exposure to T-2 toxin, but this effect is uncommon and poorly documented. Both hypoprothrombinemia and platelet suppression have been offered as causes.

d. Feed refusal is the most common response of *ad lib* access to trichothecene-containing feeds. **Secondary effects** of weight loss, anemia, hypoproteinemia, and weakness may follow prolonged feed refusal.

(1) A **dose-related** reduction of feed intake is apparent within 12 hours following consumption of contaminated feed (Figure 29-4). Concentrations of T-2 or DON ranging from 5–10 ppm can induce nausea or vomiting.

(2) Feed refusal is a **learned response,** known as **taste aversion;** therefore, flavoring agents do not prevent subsequent feed refusal.

(3) Thresholds for reduced feed intake in common domestic animals are 1 ppm in swine, 10–20 ppm in ruminants, and 100 ppm in poultry.

e. Neurologic effects (e.g., ataxia, abnormal postures) have been observed in poultry.

f. Abnormal feathering has been associated with broilers receiving high dosages of T-2 toxin.

2. Laboratory diagnosis

a. Bloodwork

(1) A **complete blood count** may reveal mild anemia, leukopenia, and reduced platelet numbers.

(2) Increased clotting and **prothrombin times** have occasionally been reported in experimentally-induced T-2 toxicosis.

b. Tissue analysis and urinalysis. Trichothecenes are rapidly metabolized and excreted as hydroxylated metabolites in the bile and urine, so diagnostic confirmation by chemical analysis is difficult or impossible.

c. Analysis of grains or feeds. Trichothecenes can be readily detected and quantified in representative grains and feeds using **thin-layer chromatography, gas–liquid chromatography** and **ELISA techniques.**

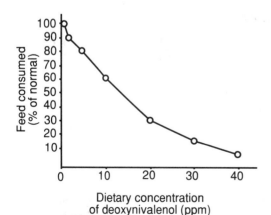

FIGURE 29-4. Correlation between feed refusal and doxynivalenol (vomitoxin, DON) content of the feed in swine.

3. Lesions
   a. Acute, high-level exposure to type A trichothecenes (i.e., T-2, DAS) is associated with gastrointestinal ulceration, hemorrhagic enteritis and necrosis, and ulceration of lymphoid follicles. Erythema, ulceration, and serum exudation of the exposed oral mucosa are seen.
   b. Chronic exposure to type A trichothecenes causes lymphoid depletion in the thymus, spleen, bursa of Fabricius (in chickens), and lymphoid follicles of the intestinal tract. Small and misshapen feathers appear in chickens exposed to T-2 toxin.

F. **Treatment**

1. **Supportive treatment** may be needed to correct the effects of diarrhea, dehydration, coagulopathy, and oral or dermal necrosis.

2. **Stress and exposure to animals with potential infectious diseases should be avoided** to prevent potentially immunocompromised animals from becoming infected.

G. **Public health considerations.** Residues in edible animal tissues are not a practical problem because trichothecenes are rapidly metabolized and excreted.

V. ERGOT

A. **Source.** Ergot alkaloids are produced by sclerotia of ***Claviceps purpurea,*** which invades the ovary of the grass flower during its maturation and formation. Frequently produced ergot alkaloids include **ergotamine** and **ergonovine**. Recently, tall fescue (***Festuca arundinaceae***) that has been invaded by the endophytic fungus *Acremonium coenophialum* has also been shown to contain the ergot alkaloid **ergovaline**.

1. **Common substrates.** Ergot sclerotia are most often found in small grains, including rye, barley, wheat, and oats. Grain is considered unfit for sale as feed when the ergot sclerotia content exceeds 0.3%.

2. **Factors favoring production of ergot.** Warm, humid conditions favor growth of the ergot fungus.

B. **Chemical characteristics.** Ergot alkaloids are **derivatives of lysergic acid;** more than 40 derivatives are known. Autoclaving, exposure to high temperatures (i.e., greater than 150°C), or application of a 1% chlorine solution markedly reduces the toxicity of ergot alkaloids.

C. **Mechanism of toxicologic damage**

1. Ergot alkaloids are **potent initiators of contraction in smooth muscle,** such as the uterus and the medial layer of the small arteries. Uterine contractions are initiated in the sensitized uterus in late pregnancy, but solid evidence for abortion is limited.

2. Ergot alkaloids **mimic the action of dopamine** in the central nervous system (CNS).

D. **Diagnosis**

1. **Clinical signs**
   a. High concentrations of ergot alkaloids cause prolonged constriction of the arteries, which leads to ischemia and **dry gangrene** that is exacerbated in cold weather. **Lameness, swelling of the feet and fetlocks,** and development of **sharply demarcated necrosis** of the **feet, ears,** and **tail** are characteristic. In severe cases, the hooves or feet and tail may slough.

    b. Increased temperature, increased pulse and **respiration rates,** and **anorexia** are also seen.

    c. Female swine, cattle, and horses in late pregnancy have little or no udder development and give birth to normal young, but **lactation does not occur** as a result of ergot-induced inhibition of prolactin secretion. As a result, the neonate dies from starvation.

    d. Occasionally, clinical signs include **hyperexcitability, hypermetria,** and **tremors** that are enhanced by stress or excitement. Signs usually subside markedly when animals are left alone to rest.

    e. Ergot alkaloids may be responsible for **heat intolerance in cattle** when consumption occurs in warm weather. Affected animals seek shade and water holes, eat less, may be depressed, and have elevated rectal temperatures.

2. Laboratory diagnosis

    a. Analysis of body tissues and fluids. Tests to detect ergot alkaloids in body fluids and tissues are not routinely available or reliably interpreted.

    b. Analysis of grains and feeds. Ergot alkaloids can be identified using thin-layer or gas chromatography or mass spectrometry.

3. Lesions

    a. Gross lesions. Mammary glands of females in late pregnancy are small and flaccid, and there is no evidence of lacteal secretion.

    b. Microscopic lesions associated with gangrene include endothelial damage, thrombosis, and coagulative necrosis.

E. Treatment

1. Contaminated feed should be replaced, and the animals should be provided with a warm, clean, stress-free environment.

2. Secondary bacterial infections in gangrenous areas must be controlled with antibiotics.

3. Colostrum and supplemental milk feeding are necessary for neonatal animals until lactation commences (usually 5–7 days after ergot alkaloids are removed from the diet).

VI. OCHRATOXIN AND CITRININ. At least nine ochratoxins are identified, but ochratoxin A is most common and has the greatest toxicological significance. Conditions for citrinin formation are similar to those for ochratoxin A, which may occur as a co-contaminant with citrinin.

A. Sources. Fungi that commonly produce ochratoxins include *Aspergillus ochraceus* and *Penicillium viridicatum.* Citrinin is produced by *P. viridicatum* and *P. citrinum.*

1. Common substrates for ochratoxin production most often are corn, barley, wheat, and rye, and the highest levels are usually found in cereal grains. Toxin production can continue during long-term storage of grains.

2. Factors favoring production of ochratoxin and citrinin

    a. A grain moisture content greater than 16% and an equilibrium relative humidity greater than 85% favor fungal growth and toxin production.

    b. The optimal temperature range for toxin formation is 54°F–77°F (12°C–25°C), although toxin production may occur at temperatures as low as 4°C. *P. viridicatum* is more likely to produce ochratoxins in the lower temperature ranges, such as occur in northern Europe, the northern United States, and Canada.

B. Chemical characteristics

1. Ochratoxins are **isocoumarin compounds** synthesized from phenylalanine. They are **stable** and unlikely to be affected by storage.

2. Citrinin is a **quinone** similar in structure to unsubstituted ochratoxin.

C. **Toxicokinetics.** Ochratoxin is converted to active metabolites by microsomal MFOs. Metabolites of ochratoxin A include ochratoxin-a and phenylalanine.

D. **Mechanism of toxicologic damage.** Ochratoxin and citrinin target the **renal proximal tubule,** decreasing metabolite clearance and urine concentrating ability, inhibiting anion transport, and causing the release of renal brush border enzymes (e.g., leucine amino peptidase). On a cellular level, ochratoxin and citrinin:

1. Bind strongly to proteins (e.g., albumin)
2. Interfere with synthesis of transfer RNA and messenger RNA
3. Interfere with protein synthesis
4. Disrupt carbohydrate metabolism
5. Increase the generation of free radicals (via cytochrome P-450 reductase metabolism)

E. **Toxicity.** Ruminants are more resistant than swine and poultry.

1. **Acute toxicity.** The acute oral toxic range for swine and poultry is 1–5 ppm. Signs may appear within 3–7 days. Citrinin causes effects similar to those caused by ochratoxin, but dietary levels ranging from 100–200 ppm may be required to produce toxicosis.

2. **Chronic toxicity.** Concentrations greater than 0.3 ppm for 2–6 weeks can cause tubular nephrosis and fibrosis in swine and poultry.

F. **Diagnosis**

1. **Clinical signs**
   a. **Acute signs,** which are relatively rare, include anorexia, vomiting, diarrhea, dehydration, and depression.
   b. **Subacute to chronic signs** are more common and include weight loss, reduced feed efficiency, polyuria, polydipsia, and dehydration. Immunosuppression, teratogenicity, carcinogenesis, and hemorrhages are occasionally reported in cases of natural or experimental ochratoxicosis.

2. **Laboratory diagnosis**
   a. **Bloodwork.** The blood urea nitrogen (BUN) level and serum creatinine are elevated.
   b. **Urinalysis** reveals hyposthenuria and increased numbers of epithelial cells and casts in the urine.
   c. **Tissue analysis.** Ochratoxin A can be detected in renal, hepatic, and adipose tissue.
      (1) Residues in the part-per-billion range may be detected by immunoassay techniques.
      (2) Detectable residues may be present for 2–4 weeks after exposure stops.
   d. **Chemical analysis of grains and feeds** using thin-layer chromatography or high-pressure liquid chromatography will reveal ochratoxin A.

3. **Lesions**
   a. **Renal lesions** predominate.
      (1) **Gross lesions.** Subacute to chronic cases present pale, enlarged kidneys with a rough irregular surface. The cut surface of the renal cortex reveals pale cortical streaking and multiple small cystic areas typical of fibroplasia. Dilated and regenerating renal tubules are also visible.
      (2) **Microscopic lesions** include renal tubular swelling, loss of the epithelial brush border, degeneration of mitochondria and the endoplasmic reticulum, and necrosis. Interstitial fibrosis and dilated tubules with flattened renal tubular epithelium are characteristic of chronic lesions. Thickened basement membranes and sclerosis of glomeruli may be present.
   b. **Hepatic lesions.** High concentrations of ochratoxin A may also cause hepatic necrosis and lymphoid depletion.
   c. **Species-specific lesions**
      (1) Gastric ulcers are common in swine.
      (2) Visceral gout and endochondral bone loss are seen in poultry.

G. **Treatment and prevention**

1. **Treatment**
   a. **Detoxification.** Activated charcoal reduces absorption, but usually is not practical in cases of chronic exposure.
   b. **Supportive treatment.** Because surviving or convalescent animals usually suffer from chronic renal insufficiency, limitations should be placed on protein intake and appropriate supportive therapy is necessary.

2. **Prevention** is most important.
   a. Proper harvesting and drying for storage are essential.
   b. Questionable grain supplies should be tested for ochratoxin contamination.

H. **Public health considerations.** European countries routinely test for ochratoxin in slaughter swine.

VII. SLAFRAMINE

A. **Sources**

1. **Common substrates.** The fungus *Rhizoctonia leguminicola* infests red clover (*Trifolium praetense*) and, occasionally, other legumes, causing the disease commonly known as "black patch." Concentrations in natural infestations may range from one to several hundred parts per million.

2. **Factors favoring production of slaframine** include cool, wet weather, especially during the regrowth period of forages (i.e., mid- to late summer).

B. **Chemical characteristics.** Slaframine is an **indolizidine alkaloid**.

1. It is chemically similar to the alkaloid swainsonine, which occurs in other plants [e.g., Darling pea (*Swainsona canescens*) and spotted locoweed (*Astragalus lentigenosus*)].

2. Slaframine is stable and **persists** in **dried** and **sun-cured forages**.

C. **Toxicokinetics.** Slaframine is bioactivated by microsomal MFOs.

D. **Mechanism of toxicologic damage.** Slaframine has **parasympathomimetic** properties and **mimics the action of acetylcholine (ACh)**, binding to Ach receptors.

E. **Toxicity**

1. The toxic dose is not well-defined, and experience with purified toxin is limited. Based on limited experience, concentrations in hay above 10 ppm may be associated with clinical signs.

2. Cattle, horses, sheep, and goats are highly susceptible. Swine are occasionally affected.

F. **Diagnosis.** Identification of "black patch" disease by a plant pathologist correlated with clinical signs and lesions may be the most useful approach to diagnosis.

1. **Clinical signs** develop rapidly, often within 1–3 hours of consumption of contaminated forage. Signs generally subside 48–72 hours after consumption of contaminated forage stops, but will reappear if animals are reexposed to contaminated hay or forage.
   a. Early onset of **profuse salivation** is the characteristic clinical response.
   b. **Mild lacrimation, frequent urination,** and **diarrhea** are seen.
   c. **Bloat, stiffness,** and **cessation of milk production** may follow if signs persist more than 24 hours.

2. **Laboratory diagnosis.** There are no distinctive or characteristic laboratory findings in affected animals. Chemical analysis of suspect hay or forage can be performed, but this type of testing is not routinely offered by diagnostic laboratories.

3. **Lesions** are few.
   a. Severe cases may present with dilated, fluid- filled intestines.
   b. Swainsonine, which may be present in contaminated clover along with slaframine, is known to cause vacuolation of neurons and other cells, but this effect is not documented in naturally occurring slaframine toxicosis.

G. **Treatment and prevention**

1. **Treatment.** Once exposure stops, recovery is usually rapid and uneventful.
   a. Atropine may provide symptomatic relief of salivation and diarrhea.
   b. Observation and general supportive care for dehydration and respiratory difficulty is necessary.

2. **Prevention.** Animal owners should be educated regarding the possible effects of contaminated red clover forages. Cautious test feeding is advisable when a new source of red clover hay is used.

VIII. **TREMORGENS**

A. **Sources**

1. The endophytic fungus, **Acremonium lolii,** produces **lolitrem-B.**
   a. **Common substrates.** *A. lolii* commonly infects **perennial ryegrass** (*Lolium perenne*). Toxicosis produces the condition known as "ryegrass staggers."
      (1) Increasing levels of infestation are correlated with higher concentrations of the toxins.
      (2) Concentration of the endophyte and toxin are greatest in the lower leaves and stems of toxic pastures.
   b. **Factors favoring production of lolitrem-B.** Lolitrem B production is often associated with overgrazed ryegrass pastures under warm, dry conditions (e.g., during late summer or early fall). Overgrazing may favor infection of grass from the soil.

2. *Claviceps paspali* is a pale tan, globoid, roughened ergot that produces **paspalitrem A** and **B, paspalanine,** and **lysergic acid.**
   a. **Common substrates.** *C. paspali* parasitizes **Dallis grass** (*Paspalum dilatatum*).
   b. **Factors favoring production of paspalitrems.** Paspalitrems are usually associated with warm, humid climates, which are the natural range of Dallis grass.

3. *Penicillium crustosum, P. cyclopium, P. palitans,* and *P. puberulum* produce **penitrem A.** Penitrem A is often associated with molded walnuts, especially in the warm, dry regions of California. In addition, toxin may be produced on moldy produce, cream cheese, or other commodities.

B. **Chemical characteristics.** These mycotoxins are characterized by an **indole moiety** that is part of a **complex ring structure** that includes **lysergic acid.**

C. **Mechanism of toxicologic damage**

1. The various derivatives of lysergic acid, including the tremorgenic mycotoxins, are associated with **reduced** concentration or function of the **inhibitory amino acids** [e.g., **γ-aminobutyric acid (GABA), glycine**].
   a. Increased presynaptic neurotransmitter release and prolonged depolarization may occur.
   b. Synaptic transmission at the motor end-plate is facilitated.

2. A second potential mechanism is the **vasoconstriction of cerebral vasculature,** which may lead to cerebral anoxia.

D. **Toxicity** of these toxins is not well-defined for domestic animals. Ruminants are most commonly affected by contaminated ryegrass or Dallis grass pastures, whereas dogs are intoxicated by eating moldy walnuts and various refrigerated foods.

E. **Diagnosis**

1. **Clinical signs** are typically mild and subtle when animals are at rest, but excitement or exercise causes exaggerated and severe signs.
   a. Early effects include fine tremors about the head and neck.
   b. Stiffness, ataxia, hypermetria, tremors, opisthotonus, and seizures develop within a few minutes, but may subside quickly if animals are left undisturbed.
   c. Some animals may become belligerent, injuring themselves or others. Occasionally, drowning occurs when affected animals fall into bodies of water.

2. **Laboratory diagnosis**
   a. A mouse bioassay has been used to aid detection. Suspect materials are ground and suspended in saline, then administered orally at dosages of approximately 0.5 ml/mouse. Signs of tremors and seizures appear within 10–30 minutes.
   b. The endophyte *A. lolii* may be detected by microscopic examination of infected ryegrass.
   c. The ergot sclerotia of *C. paspali* are visible by macroscopic examination of seed heads of infected Dallis grass.

3. **Lesions.** No characteristic neurologic or muscle lesions are produced by the tremorgenic mycotoxins.

F. **Treatment.** Morbidity is typically high (greater than 50%), but mortality in uncomplicated cases is low (less than 10%).

1. Affected animals should be removed from the suspect forage and kept separated from the herd in a quiet, secure place. Recovery usually occurs within 3–7 days.

2. **Detoxification.** Activated charcoal and saline cathartics for oral decontamination are helpful, but may be difficult to administer on a herd basis.

3. **Supportive treatment**
   a. Animals should be protected from the sun and provided with fluids to prevent dehydration during recovery. Affected or recumbent animals often will eat and drink on their own accord.
   b. Medications that increase the central nervous system (CNS) concentration of glycine (e.g., mephenesin, nalorphine) have reduced tremorgenic mycotoxin effects in mice.

G. **Public health considerations.** Residues are not considered a problem; the alkaloids apparently do not accumulate in edible tissues or fat.

IX. FUMONISINS

A. **Sources.** *Fusarium moniliforme* and *F. proliferatum* are isolated from field cases of fumonisin toxicosis.

1. **Common substrates** include both white and yellow corn worldwide.

2. **Factors favoring production of fumonisins** have not been clearly defined.
   a. Current information suggests that a period of drought during the growing season, followed by cool, wet conditions during pollination and development of the corn favors toxin production.
   b. Highest concentrations of the fumonisins are found in corn screenings (i.e., damaged kernels).

B. | **Chemical characteristics**

1. The toxin is characterized chemically as an **aliphatic hydrocarbon** with a **terminal amine group** and **two tricarboxylic acid (TCA) side chains**. Toxins are classified as **fumonisin B1 (FB1), fumonisin B2 (FB2),** or **fumonisin B3 (FB3)** according to the number and position of the hydroxyl groups.

2. The fumonisins are unique among mycotoxins because they are **water-soluble,** as well as **heat-stable** and **resistant to** the **alkali** treatments used to inactivate many other common mycotoxins.

C. | **Mechanism of toxicologic damage.** Fumonisins inhibit the enzyme-mediated conversion of sphinganine to sphingosine. The interference of fumonisins in sphingolipid synthesis is currently presumed to be a significant factor in their toxicity and carcinogenicity.

D. | **Toxicity.** Current evidence suggests that FB1 and FB2 are of approximately equal toxicity, but FB3 is much less toxic. Feed concentrations are used to compare the toxic potential for domestic animals.

1. **Swine**
   a. Dietary fumonisins greater than 100 ppm produce acute pulmonary toxicosis and hepatic toxicosis in swine after 5–10 days of feeding.
   b. Dietary fumonisins of 50 ppm cause mild liver lesions in swine within 7–10 days, but concentrations of 25 ppm or less cause no apparent clinical effects.

2. **Cattle** and **sheep** are mildly affected by dietary concentrations greater than 100 ppm, but fatalities do not occur.

3. **Horses** appear to be the **most sensitive** of the domestic animals; dietary concentrations as low as 10 ppm for more than 30 days may cause fatal leukoencephalomalacia.

E. | **Diagnosis**

1. **Clinical signs** are distinctive among species.
   a. **Horses** develop a rapidly progressing neurotoxicosis characterized by depression, blindness, ataxia, aimless wandering, facial paralysis, coma, and death.
      (1) The condition, known as **equine leukoencephalomalacia,** is fatal in essentially all affected animals.
      (2) Death may occur as early as 24 hours after the onset of clinical signs, or as late as 1 week after the onset of signs.
   b. **Swine**
      (1) Swine receiving **high dosages** of fumonisins develop a rapidly progressing syndrome characterized by dyspnea, cyanosis, and weakness, within 4–7 days of fumonisin consumption. **Death** usually occurs within 4 hours of the onset of the **respiratory syndrome.**
      (2) Swine receiving dosages of fumonisins below the pulmonary toxic level develop icterus, reduced feed intake, weight loss, and, occasionally, diarrhea.
   c. **Ruminants** fed diets containing up to 200 ppm fumonisins display anorexia and mild weight loss but few other significant or persistent signs.
   d. **Poultry** appear more resistant than mammals to fumonisins. Clinical effects develop at dosages of 200–400 ppm and may include inappetence and skeletal abnormalities.

2. **Laboratory diagnosis**
   a. All animals have some **evidence of hepatic dysfunction.** The following serum enzymes and constituents are increased in animals with fumonisin toxicosis:
      (1) Cholesterol
      (2) Lactic dehydrogenase (LDH)
      (3) AST
      (4) ALT
      (5) γ-glutamyl transpeptidase (GGT)
      (6) Bilirubin

b. The **serum sphinganine:sphingosine ratio** is increased and may be the most sensitive indicator of fumonisin exposure in most species. However, most clinical laboratories do not offer this analysis.

3. Lesions
a. Horses. Massive softening and liquefaction of the cerebral white matter, which may range from discrete focal areas to large cavitations and inward collapse of the cortical gray matter, is characteristic of leukoencephalomalacia. Hemorrhages are prominent, and microscopically there is liquefaction and proliferation of macrophages in response to the necrosis.

b. Swine

(1) Pulmonary lesions. Acute pulmonary edema in swine is characterized by marked to massive intralobular pulmonary edema and marked hydrothorax. The lungs are distended and turgid and the thoracic cavity is filled with straw-colored proteinaceous fluid. Microscopically, the edema is primarily interstitial and interlobular in nature.

(2) Extrapulmonary lesions in swine include multiple areas of focal pancreatic necrosis and hepatic lesions characterized by disorganization of hepatocyte organization, increased mitotic figures, necrosis of single hepatocytes, and mild bile retention. Pigs with advanced hepatic lesions are icteric.

F. Treatment and prevention

1. Treatment
a. Detoxification. Because of the time lag before the onset of clinical signs and the chronic nature of the toxicosis, oral decontamination is usually not helpful.

b. Supportive treatment. Animals with liver damage should be provided appropriate supportive care.

2. Prevention.
Suspect corn can be analyzed for fumonisins and cleaned if necessary. The grain is then analyzed to confirm the removal of toxic levels of residues.

G. Public health considerations.
Although residues are currently not considered a significant problem in food animals because fumonisins appear to be excreted rapidly in both bile and urine, fumonisins are potential carcinogens and regulation of the fumonisin content of foodstuffs seems likely in the future.

DIRECTIONS: Each of the numbered items or incomplete statements in this section is followed by answers or by completions of the statement. Select the **one** numbered answer or completion that is **best** in each case.

1. Which one of the following statements regarding molds known as "field fungi" is true?

(1) They include the genus *Aspergillus*.
(2) They readily grow and produce mycotoxins at a grain moisture content of 15%.
(3) They often cause death of ovules and shriveling of seeds.
(4) They are not associated with mycotoxins of significance to animals.
(5) They often reoccur in storage as a result of reinvasion of dried grain.

2. Which combination of conditions favors aflatoxin production under field conditions?

(1) Ambient temperatures greater than 75°F, drought, and insect damage
(2) Ambient temperatures ranging from 45°F–65°F and persistent light rainfall
(3) Alternating low and high temperatures on overwintered grain
(4) Wheat and barley crops deficient in soil nitrogen and phosphorus
(5) Anaerobic conditions

3. Microsomal mixed function oxidases (MFOs) are known to bioactivate and increase toxicity of which one of the following?

(1) Aflatoxin
(2) Deoxynivalenol (DON, vomitoxin)
(3) Ergot alkaloids
(4) Fumonisins
(5) T-2 toxin

4. A material effective for adsorption of aflatoxin, but not other mycotoxins, is:

(1) activated charcoal.
(2) anhydrous ammonia.
(3) bentonite.
(4) fuller's earth.
(5) hydrated sodium calcium aluminosilicate (HSCAS).

5. If a herd of dairy cows were inadvertently exposed to a load of feed containing 300 ppb aflatoxin, what would be the best advice regarding marketing of the milk?

(1) Stop marketing the milk until the source of aflatoxin is removed, withhold milk for up to 2 weeks, contact regulatory officials, and test the milk to determine when marketing can resume
(2) Stop marketing the milk immediately, notify regulatory officials, and make plans to dispose of the cows because of persistent aflatoxin contamination
(3) Stop marketing the milk until the source of aflatoxin is removed, add aluminosilicates to the feed, contact regulatory officials, and test the milk to determine when marketing can resume
(4) Contact regulatory officials, but continue to market the milk because 300 ppb is below the threshold for contamination
(5) Add aluminosilicate to the feed and continue marketing the milk, because the aluminosilicate is highly effective for removing aflatoxin residues

6. Which combination of laboratory findings is most characteristic of damage by aflatoxins?

(1) Increased blood urea nitrogen (BUN), creatinine, and serum potassium and hyposthenuria
(2) Hypercholesterolemia, hyperbilirubinemia, and increased sphinganine:sphingosine ratios in plasma
(3) Elevated serum progesterone in females or decreased testosterone in males
(4) Hypoproteinemia, elevated serum bile acids, increased serum aspartate transaminase (AST), hyperbilirubinemia, and mild anemia
(5) Leukopenia, thrombocytopenia, normal AST, and elevated one-stage prothrombin time

433

DIRECTIONS: Each of the numbered items or incomplete statements in this section is negatively phrased, as indicated by an italicized word such as *not, least,* or *except.* Select the **one** numbered answer or completion that is **best** in each case.

---

7. Propionic acid mold inhibitors do all of the following *except*:

(1) lower the pH of grain.
(2) reduce fungal growth.
(3) prevent mycotoxin formation.
(4) destroy mycotoxins.
(5) provide a source of nutrients to ruminants.

DIRECTIONS: Each group of items in this section consists of numbered options followed by a set of numbered items. For each item, select the **one** numbered option that is most closely associated with it. Each numbered option may be selected once, more than once, or not at all.

Questions 8–17

Match the clinical syndrome or diagnostic information with the appropriate mycotoxin.

(1) Aflatoxin
(2) Deoxynivalenol (vomitoxin, DON)
(3) Fumonisins
(4) Ochratoxin A
(5) Zearalenone

8. Slow growth, icterus, anemia, and elevated serum liver enzymes including alanine aminotransaminase (AST), lactic dehydrogenase (LDH), and sorbital dehydrogenase

9. Vomiting, feed refusal, weight loss, and normal kidney and liver function tests

10. Equine blindness, ataxia, depression, stumbling, hypotonicity of facial muscles and lips, icterus, and moderate elevation of γ-glutamyl transpeptidase (GGT) and AST

11. Weight loss, polyuria, and polydipsia in a herd of swine; necropsy reveals pale tan to white kidneys and gastric ulcers

12. Centrilobular fatty change and hepatocellular necrosis accompanied by moderate interlobular fibrosis and bile duct hyperplasia in swine

13. Viewing grain under untraviolet (UV) light discloses a yellow-green fluorescence in approximately 8% of the grain

14. Young boars develop a feminizing syndrome when fed contaminated grain for approximately 6 weeks

15. Sixty percent of a herd of feeder pigs develop acute dyspnea, cyanosis, and weakness followed by death consuming contaminated grain for approximately 5 days

16. Following exposure 2 weeks after normal estrus, sows became anestrus for approximately 2 months

17. Broilers fed this grain for 5 weeks had soft, greasy feces and bruised easily when handled

1. The answer is 3 *[I A 1 a]*. Field fungi are often associated with damage to grain in the form of shriveled seeds, which may be pale and smaller than normal. The field fungi include fungi of the toxin-producing genus, Fusarium, but not Aspergillus. They typically require moisture contents greater than 22% for growth and toxin production. The field fungi produce several mycotoxins of significant animal health and economic concern *[e.g., T-2 toxin, deoxynivalenol (vomitoxin, DON), zearalenone]*.

2. The answer is 1 *[II A 2]*. Aflatoxins are typically produced when persistent high environmental temperatures are present for 1 week or more, and some stress (e.g., drought or insect damage) opens the pollen tubes or seed coat to allow fungal invasion in the presence of temperatures and moisture ranges optimal for toxin production. Low to moderate temperatures or alternating and fluctuating temperatures are more likely to favor the growth of *Fusarium,* which produces trichothecenes, especially deoxynivalenol (vomitoxin, DON). Deficiency of soil fertility factors (e.g., nitrogen, phosphorus) are not associated with aflatoxin production. Wheat and barley are not common substrates for aflatoxin production compared to corn, milo, cottonseed, and peanuts. Aflatoxin-producing fungi are aerobic and will neither grow nor produce mycotoxins under anaerobic conditions.

3. The answer is 1 *[II C]*. Aflatoxins are metabolized by microsomal mixed function oxidases (MFOs) to an epoxide that can bind covalently to the N7 guanine of deoxyribonucleic acid (DNA) as well as to ribonucleic acid (RNA) and proteins. This binding modifies DNA and may induce carcinogenesis. In addition, aflatoxins disrupt protein synthesis, leading to a loss of essential enzymes and causing cellular damage and necrosis. Deoxynivalenol (vomitoxin, DON) and T-2 are metabolized to hydroxylated metabolites, which are less toxic than the parent epoxide. They are rapidly excreted in bile and, to a lesser extent, in urine. Ergot alkaloids and fumonisins appear to be toxic in their natural and unmetabolized form, and there is no evidence that MFO activity alters or enhances toxicosis.

4. The answer is 5 *[II G 1 a]*. Hydrated sodium calcium aluminosilicate (HSCAS) adsorbs aflatoxin and prevents its absorption from the intestinal tract. Bentonite is of limited value

for the adsorption of aflatoxin as well as zearalenone. However, bentonite is much less effective than HSCAS. Anhydrous ammonia destroys aflatoxin by chemical alteration of the aflatoxin molecule, rather than by adsorption. Fullers earth or other forms of clay have not been effective for adsorbing aflatoxin.

5. The answer is 3 *[II H]*. Marketing of milk should be suspended until the source of aflatoxin has been determined, and regulatory officials should be contacted. After adding aluminosilicates to the feed to reduce contamination, the milk should be tested to determine when marketing can resume. Aflatoxins are carcinogens and are of serious regulatory concern. Removal of aflatoxin from the feed in combination with feeding of an effective adsorbent will significantly reduce further absorption of aflatoxin and hasten return to a residue-free status. Milk from dairy cattle fed feed containing more than 20 ppb aflatoxin will contain residues in excess of the current Food and Drug Administration (FDA) action level, which is 0.5 ppb.

6. The answer is 4 *[II F 2]*. The aflatoxins interfere with hepatic protein and enzyme synthesis and the activity and production of serum proteins. Their predilection for the liver leads to hepatic fatty change, hepatic necrosis, and increases in plasma levels of hepatocellular enzymes as well as bilary retention with increases in serum bile acids and bilirubin. Ochratoxins cause primarily renal damage with resultant azotemia and hyposthenuria. Fumonisins inhibit enzymes of sphingolipid biosynthesis, altering the plasma sphinganine:sphingosine ratio and causing elevated serum cholesterol as well as cholestatic liver damage (characterized in part by hyperbilirubinemia). Leukopenia, thrombocytopenia, and coagulopathy in the absence of significant liver damage are characteristics of the trichothecene mycotoxins (e.g., T-2 toxins).

7. The answer is 4 *[I E 6]*. Mycotoxins are stable to the acid conditions produced by propionic acid mold inhibitors, so preformed mycotoxins are not destroyed. Acids lower the pH, forming an unfavorable environment for mold growth and thus helping to prevent mycotoxin formation. In addition, propionic acid is a fatty acid that can be utilized as a nutrient by ruminants.

8–17. The answers are: 8-1 *[II F 2]*, **9-2** *[IV 1–2]*, **10-3** *[VIII E 1 a]*, **11-4** *[VI F 1 b]*, **12-1** *[II F 3]*, **13-1** *[II F 2 c (1)]*, **14-5** *[III F 1 a (4)]*, **15-3** *[VIII E 1 b (1)]*, **16-5** *[III F 1 a (2)]*, **17-1** *[II F 1 b]*. Aflatoxin inhibits protein synthesis in the liver and leads to diminished weight gain, liver dysfunction characterized by hepatocellular damage (indicated by both nonspecific and specific liver enzymes), and icterus as a result of both hepatocellular damage and bile retention associated with bile duct hyperplasia.

Deoxynivalenol, also known as DON or vomitoxin, is a trichothecene mycotoxin that affects brain neurochemistry (e.g., dopamine and 5-hydroxyindolacetic acid), leading to nausea and appetite suppression. Feed refusal or decreased feed intake occurs through a learned response known as "taste aversion."

Fumonisins are strongly associated with severe equine central nervous system (CNS) disease. These toxins cause massive liquifaction necrosis of the cerebral white matter, leading to cavitation and the condition known as equine leukoencephalomalacia. A differential diagnosis could be severe aflatoxicosis, which could lead to hepatic encephalopathy as a result of hepatic failure. However, the moderate elevations of alanine aminotransaminase (AST) and the increase in γ-glutamyl transpeptidase (GGT) suggest mild hepatocellular damage and cholestatic liver damage, respectively. If aflatoxicosis were causing hepatic encephalopathy, evidence of severe liver damage would be an important indicator.

The signs of end-stage renal disease, confirmed by typical lesions of chronic nephrosis, are typical of the nephrotoxic damage induced by ochratoxins. Gastric ulcers may result from the direct effects of the ochratoxin, or they may be the result of azotemia following severe nephrosis and terminal renal failure.

The pattern of heptacellular damage described is typical of aflatoxin, including the distinct centrilobular pattern and the bile duct hyperplasia. Fumonisins are also hepatotoxic mycotoxins, but liver damage from fumonisins is typically mild to moderate and characterized by a more disorganized hepatic structure and little or no evidence of bile duct hyperplasia.

Only aflatoxin is potentially detected by direct fluorescence, a yellow-green glow known as BGYF (bright yellow-green fluorescence) that really results from a coincidental metabolite of *Aspergillus flavus* known as kojic acid. Kojic acid acts as a marker to suggest the probability of aflatoxin. The presence of aflatoxin can only be confirmed by analysis using classic chemical testing or immunoadsorption techniques. The other mycotoxins listed do not fluoresce directly under ultraviolet light.

Zearalenone possesses properties typical of estrogens such as estradiol. Feminization has been seen in young boars that are not sexually mature. Older, sexually mature boars are not affected by high levels of zearalenone, presumably because of their high endogenous testosterone production.

Fumonisins at high dosages produce severe interlobular edema and hydrothorax that culminates rapidly in respiratory embarassment, cyanosis, and death (due to anoxia) in swine. There is typically a 3- to 5-day latent period, followed by rapid progression of dyspnea, pulmonary edema, and death from anoxia over a clinical course of just a few hours.

In sexually mature sows, the estrogenic effect of zearalenone is luteotropic and causes the corpus luteum to be maintained for as long as 40–60 days after the zearalenone consumption has stopped. This condition is sometimes called pseudopregnancy. Affected sows may appear to be gravid and show udder development, but then they spontaneously return to estrus. If anestrus is caused by zearalenone, the retained corpora lutea can be expressed by administering 10 mg of prostaglandin $F_{2\alpha}$. Generally, sows return to estrus 2–4 days following treatment.

Among the many effects of aflatoxins is their ability to interfere with pancreatic lipase, reducing fat absorption and increasing lipid in the feces (i.e., causing steatorrhea). Spontaneous bruising or bruising in response to mild handling or trauma may result from decreased hepatic synthesis of clotting factors or capillary damage, although the exact mechanism of this effect is unknown.

Chapter 30
Zootoxins

I. GENERAL CONSIDERATIONS

A. Zootoxins are found in many classes of the animal kingdom, and occur throughout the world. Only the zootoxins of major importance to animals in North America are covered in this chapter.

B. Delivery of venom can occur by a variety of physical methods, and is often parenteral rather than oral.

C. Reactions are often acute, severe, and life-threatening.

II. INSECTS

A. *Hymenoptera* (bees, hornets, wasps)

1. **Geographic range and habitat.** Various species of bees, wasps, and hornets are found throughout North America.
   a. They are generally found in greater numbers in mild climates.
   b. They are usually located in secluded places.
   c. They usually build nests of mud, papery material, or wax.

2. **Exposure.** Exposure most commonly occurs when animals unintentionally disturb a nest or a swarm.

3. **Toxic principle.** The toxins of *Hymenoptera* are not well-characterized. Venom may contain **formic acid,** which may induce mild or severe pain.

4. **Toxicity.** In sensitive individuals or in the presence of multiple stings, systemic anaphylaxis and death can occur. All animal species are susceptible.

5. **Diagnosis**
   a. Clinical signs include mild to severe pain and heat and swelling around the sting. Some species may leave a venom sac with the stinger.
   b. Laboratory evaluation is not usually of value, except that stress-related leukocytosis may be present. Chemical analysis for toxins is not usually performed.
   c. Lesions are usually localized and include a small puncture site, possible intercalation of a stinger in the epidermis or dermis, and redness, swelling, heat, and eosinophilic accumulation in a 0.5- to 2-cm region around the sting. Lesions persist for 24–48 hours in most cases.

6. **Treatment**
   a. Emergency supportive therapy (i.e., respiratory support and treatment of anaphylaxis, shock, and secondary bacterial infections) may be necessary. Epinephrine has commonly been used in emergency response to *Hymenoptera* bites.
   b. Specific antidotes are not available.

B. *Epicauta* species (blister beetles) and *Pyrota insulata*

1. **Geographic range and habitat**
   a. More than forty species of blister beetle are found throughout the United States. Clinical toxicoses appear to be more common in the southern and southeastern United States.
   b. Blister beetles usually feed on leaves or flowers and may be found in gardens, crop fields, and hay fields.

2. **Exposure** usually occurs when numerous beetles are trapped and crushed in crimped hay that is then stored as baled hay. The crushed beetles remain in the hay and are eaten by ruminants and horses.

3. **Toxic principle.** Blister beetle toxin, **cantharidin,** is strongly irritating to mucous membranes, the gastrointestinal mucosa, and the urinary tract. In some cases, heavy exposure may lead to hypocalcemia by an unknown mechanism.

4. **Toxicity** of cantharidin is approximately 500 mg/kg.

5. **Diagnosis**
   a. **Clinical signs**
      (1) **Acute, severe colic** may be accompanied by shock. Death may occur within 2–3 days.
      (2) Gastrointestinal ulceration may cause **diarrhea, bloody feces,** or both.
      (3) Urinary irritation results in **frequent urination, straining,** and **rubbing of the perineum.**
      (4) **Physical evidence** of blister beetles may be present **in hay.**
   b. **Laboratory diagnosis**
      (1) **Hematologic** and **clinical chemistry changes** include hemoconcentration, stress leukocytosis, hypocalcemia, elevated blood urea nitrogen (BUN), and hyposthenuria.
      (2) **Gas chromatography** or **mass spectrometry** of urine, intestinal contents, or contaminated hay may reveal cantharidin.
   c. **Lesions** include congestion, ulceration, and hemorrhage of the gastrointestinal tract. There may also be congestion and irritation of the urinary bladder and urethra.

6. **Treatment**
   a. **Administration of fluids** and **bicarbonate** may be necessary to alleviate shock and acidosis.
   b. **Activated charcoal** and a **saline cathartic** may provide some protection; specific antidotes are not available.

7. **Prognosis** for recovery depends on the dosage. High levels of exposure may cause severe signs and death before intervention is possible.

III. ARACHNIDS

A. *Latrodectus mactans* (black widow spider) and *L. hesperus*

1. **Description.** The spiders are 1–2 centimeters in size. They are shiny and black with a red hourglass mark on the abdomen.

2. **Geographic range.** Black widow spiders are indigenous to the eastern and southwestern United States, and are especially prominent in the Southwest. They are generally more prolific in climates that are warm to arid with mild winters.

3. **Exposure.** Black widows may invade suburban lawns and gardens, presenting a risk to pets and humans that accidentally encounter a nesting area. Both females and males are toxic, but only the female is large enough to envenomate an animal.

4. **Toxic principle and mechanism of action**
   a. **Toxins.** α-**Latrotoxin,** a potent, labile neurotoxin, is produced in higher amounts in the fall.
   b. **Mechanism of action.** The toxins of the black widow are proteinaceous and are believed to exert their effects by binding to calcium channels.
      (1) Calcium-channel binding increases the membrane's permeability to calcium and enhances depolarization.

(2) Large amounts of both epinephrine and norepinephrine may be released, and presynaptic neurotransmitter uptake is inhibited.

5. Toxicity. A single bite may be serious to adult humans and could kill a small animal.

6. Diagnosis
  a. Clinical signs occur almost immediately after the bite. There is **intense pain,** due in part to the release of acetylcholine (ACh), which stimulates contraction of major muscle groups. There may be **ascending motor paralysis, muscle spasms** and **muscle rigidity,** and **salivation.** Death may result from respiratory or cardiovascular failure.
  b. Laboratory evaluation is not helpful.
  c. Lesions are not conclusive or distinctive.

7. Treatment
  a. Muscle relaxants (e.g., **methocarbamol**) should be administered.
  b. Atropine will reduce salivation.
  c. Therapy for shock (e.g., **corticosteroids, fluids**) should be initiated.
  d. A **specific antivenin** that reduces pain and brings relief within 15 minutes of intravenous administration is available for humans and has been used in small animals.

8. Prognosis for recovery is reasonably good in dogs, but may be guarded in cats.

B. *Loxosceles reclusa* **(brown recluse spider)**

1. Description. Brown recluse spiders are brown, 1–4 centimeters long, with a fiddle-shaped mark on the dorsal aspect of the thorax.

2. Geographic range and habitat. At least twelve species of *Loxosceles* are found throughout the United States; however, most attention has been given to *L. reclusa*.

3. Exposure. Spiders tend to stay in secluded, dark places, and bite mainly when their area is invaded.

4. Toxic principle and mechanism of action. The toxin consists of at least eight proteins, including hyaluronidase, proteases, other spreading factors, and hemolysins. The mechanism of action is not well defined, but the toxin damages endothelial cell membranes, leading to intravascular coagulation, capillary thrombi, and tissue necrosis.

5. Toxicity is unclear, but less than 5 µl of the venom causes clinical lesions.

6. Diagnosis
  a. Clinical signs are not apparent immediately after the bite, and often the victim does not feel the bite. If not treated, the lesions may persist for weeks.
    (1) An erythematous area develops around the bite.
    (2) Rarely, systemic signs of fever, nausea, and seizures develop.
  b. Laboratory evaluation may reveal hemolysis followed by hemoglobinuria, but is not generally useful.
  c. Lesions are localized to the bite area and include endothelial damage, necrosis that may penetrate to the underlying muscle, vasculitis, hemorrhage, and leukocyte accumulation.

7. Treatment. Specific antidotes are not available.
  a. Dapsone, a leukocyte inhibitor, may reduce inflammation at the envenomation site.
  b. Corticosteroids may reduce systemic effects.
  c. Fluids and **bicarbonate,** which reduce renal precipitation of hemoglobin, should be administered to treat hemolysis and hemoglobinuria.
  d. Surgical excision of the affected area has been recommended for chronic lesions, but results have been variable.

8. Prognosis for recovery is generally good to fair, although results may be delayed for several weeks.

IV. **REPTILES.** Widespread problems are more frequently associated with the poisonous snakes (as opposed to the toxic lizards).

A. Snakes

1. **General considerations**
   a. **Incidence and exposure**
      (1) Snake bites occur most often when animals graze, hunt, or play in infested areas.
         (a) Among small animals, snake bites are reported most frequently in dogs. More than 90% of the bites are located on the head or extremities (i.e., the muzzle and legs).
         (b) Among large animals, horses are most often reported bitten.
      (2) The incidence of poisonous snake bites is higher in the southwestern and southeastern United States; snake populations are much lower in the northern latitudes.
   b. **Not all bites from poisonous snakes actually result in envenomation.** Fewer than 50% of bites cause envenomation and clinical response.
   c. **Factors affecting the response to envenomation** include the toxicity of the venom, the amount of venom injected, the size of the animal, and the availability of prompt appropriate therapy.

2. **Crotalidae.** In North America, the most significant family of poisonous snakes is the Crotalidae family, which includes **rattlesnakes (*Crotalus horridus*), water moccasins (*Agkistrodon piscivorus*),** and **copperheads (*Agkistrodon contortix*).**
   a. **Description.** Specific characteristics are summarized in Table 30-1. General characteristics are as follows:
      (1) The **head** is **broad** and **triangular**. The neck immediately behind the head is noticeably narrower than the head.
      (2) The **pupils** are **vertically elliptical slits,** rather than round (as in nonpoisonous snakes).
      (3) Crotalidae are also known as **"pit vipers"** because there is a **deep pit between the eye and the nostril** where a heat-sensing organ used to detect prey is located.
      (4) **Prominent curving fangs** at the front of the maxilla retract against the maxilla when the snake is swallowing prey.
   b. **Exposure.** Horses are usually exposed inadvertently while grazing, and dogs often elicit snake bites through aggressive or curious challenges.
   c. **Toxic principle and mechanism of action**
      (1) **Toxic principle.** Multiple complex toxins are produced by the pit vipers. Examples of specific toxic fractions are given in Table 30-2.

TABLE 30-1. Crotalidae

Snake	Maximum Length (m)	Distinguishing Characteristics	Geographic Range
Rattlesnake (*Crotalus*)	2	Dried rings of skin at tip of tail produce characteristic rattle	New England to Florida, lower two-thirds of the United States
Water moccasin (*Agkistrodon piscivorus*)	6	Heavy-bodied, dark brown or olive less prominent crossbands, most likely to challenge humans or animals	Swamps, rivers, and lakes across southeastern United States as far west as Texas
Copperhead (*Agkistrodon contortix*)	0.6–1.2	Distinctive coppery color, tail vibrates when snake is alarmed but lacks "rattles"	Massachusetts to Florida, westward to Texas and northward to Missouri; dry, rocky areas and margins between forests and open fields

TABLE 30-2. Examples of Toxic Fractions in Crotalid Venom

Fraction	Effects
Collagenase	Degrades structural components dependent on collagen for tissue structure and orientation
Hyaluronidase	Acts against glucoside bonds of mucopolysaccharides, allowing venom to penetrate tissues
Phospholipases A and B	Hydrolyzes phospholipids, releasing saturated and unsaturated fatty acids
Ribonucleases, DNA-ase, 5'nucleotidase	Act against nucleic acids and phosphate monoesters
Polypeptides	May induce neurotoxicosis, cardiotoxicity, shock, and vascular permeability
Procoagulants	Enhance coagulation factor activity
Anticoagulants	Inhibit coagulation factor activity

DNA = deoxyribonucleic acid.

        (2) Mechanism of action. The mechanism of action is complex and not fully documented.
           (a) In general, the toxins are designed to incapacitate the prey and to aid the process of tissue digestion.
           (b) Tissue destruction commencing with loss of integrity of blood vessels, impaired coagulation, and altered cardiac function can contribute to cardiac insufficiency, edema, shock, and hemorrhage. Central nervous system (CNS), respiratory depression, or both may occur.
                (i) Severe hypotension may develop and is often considered the proximate cause of death.
                (ii) Bites near the nostrils, on the tongue, or in the throat area may be life-threatening if airway occlusion develops as a result of severe edema and swelling.
     d. Toxicity of crotalid venoms can vary substantially (e.g., from less than 2 mg/kg of body weight (rattlesnake venom) to greater than 10 mg/kg of body weight (copperhead venom). Risk for toxicosis depends both on the toxicity of the venom and on the amount of venom injected. The size of the snake affects venom yield— large rattlesnakes can yield more than 500 mg of venom, compared with copperheads, which may yield less than 75 mg of venom.
     e. Diagnosis
        (1) Clinical signs may develop differentially, depending on the dosage of venom, location of the bite, age of the victim, and physical activity post-envenomation. Generally expected clinical signs include:
           (a) Extreme pain, especially in the area of the bite
           (b) Fang marks
           (c) Rapid swelling around the bite
           (d) Ecchymotic to suffusion hemorrhages in the area of the bite
           (e) Salivation, hyperpnea, tachycardia, and dilated pupils, possibly as a reaction to severe pain
           (f) Secondary infections
        (2) Laboratory diagnosis
           (a) Hematology and **clinical chemistry changes** include hemoconcentration, hemolysis, increased or decreased coagulation times, and, possibly, disseminated intravascular coagulation.
           (b) Analysis for crotalid toxins in tissues is not practical because of the complex nature of the toxins and their similarity to many natural enzymes.
        (3) Lesions include fang marks, acute swelling, edema, ecchymotic to suffusion hemorrhages, and hematomas in the affected area.

f. Treatment. If the snake bite occurs some time before it is noticed by the owner, the clinical response will be advanced and may be difficult to treat.

(1) Acute corrective therapy

(a) Polyvalent crotalid antivenins are available for dogs and humans. Antivenin should be administered as soon as possible after envenomation; delaying administration for more than 4 hours diminishes its effectiveness. Local poison control centers may be helpful in locating antivenin.

(b) Diphenhydramine (10–25 mg IV or SC for dogs) reduces anxiety and helps prevent allergic reactions associated with antivenin.

(c) Treatment of shock and maintenance of a patent airway may be necessary. Fluids (e.g., lactated Ringer's solution) should be used as needed. Corticosteroids may be helpful for counteracting shock, but they are generally not recommended against the bite reaction itself because their use has been associated with increased mortality.

(d) Transfusions help to correct anemia and hemorrhage.

(2) Supportive therapy

(a) Fluid maintenance therapy should follow the acute corrective therapy.

(b) Treatment of pain may be helpful.

(c) Antibiotics will control secondary infections.

g. Prognosis for recovery depends on the area of the bite, the size of the animal, the time since envenomation, and the level of supportive care.

3. Elapidae. This family of snakes includes **coral snakes (*Micrurus*)** and **cobras**. Coral snakes are the only members of the toxic elapid snakes that are indigenous to the United States.

a. Description. The poisonous coral snakes have **adjacent red and yellow transverse bands**. A nonpoisonous snake often confused with the coral snake has yellow rings separated by a black band; in order to differentiate the two, one might remember the old adage, **"Red and yellow kill a fellow/ Red and black, venom lack."**

b. Geographic range. Coral snakes are found primarily in the southeastern coastal states and west to Texas.

c. Incidence of toxicosis. Toxicosis in small animals is relatively uncommon. Coral snakes have small mouths, making envenomation physically unlikely.

d. Toxic principle and mechanism of action. Major toxins include cholinesterase, which has parasympathetic effects, and a neurotoxic polypeptide that induces paralysis.

e. Toxicity. Less than 1 mg/kg body weight of venom can produce toxicosis, but the venom yield is small (i.e., less than 6 mg per snake).

f. Diagnosis

(1) Clinical signs

(a) Numbness of the limbs, weakness, disorientation, paralysis, and respiratory failure may occur.

(b) Fang marks are small, and local swelling is minimal or absent.

(c) Parasympathetic signs include salivation, vomiting, and defecation or diarrhea.

(2) Laboratory diagnosis does not reveal distinctive changes.

(3) Lesions (both gross and microscopic) are minimal, and not likely to help with diagnosis.

g. Treatment

(1) Specific antivenin is produced for humans, but availability for animals may be limited.

(2) Atropine may be used to a limited extent to correct cholinesterase activity.

h. Prognosis. Envenomation is rare, and recovery may be expected if treatment is early and aggressive.

B. Lizards

1. Description. The **Gila monster (*Heloderma suspectum*)** and **Mexican beaded lizard (*H. horridum*)** are large, slow-moving, boldly patterned lizards of the desert Southwest. They have grooved upper teeth and venom glands that bathe the area over the teeth.

2. Exposure. These reptiles are not aggressive, but will bite if provoked. They reportedly do not release the victim immediately following the bite.

3. **Toxic principle and mechanism of action.** The venom is apparently similar to crotalid venom (see IV A 2 c). Toxins have a necrotizing effect, similar to that of crotalid venom.

4. **Toxicity** is not well described.

5. **Diagnosis**
   a. **Clinical signs** include pain and swelling of the affected area, shock, vomiting, and CNS depression.
   b. **Laboratory diagnosis** is usually not helpful.
   c. **Lesions** include local swelling, edema, erythema, and hemorrhages.

6. **Treatment** is similar to that for crotalid bites (see IV A 2 f), but clinical reports indicate that meperidine should not be used to control pain. The efficacy of crotalid antivenin for *Heloderma* bites has not been established.

V. AMPHIBIANS

A. *Bufo marinus* (marine toads)

1. **Geographic range and habitat.** In the United States, *Bufo marinus* is found mainly in Florida and Hawaii. They are large, lethargic toads that may inhabit settled areas.

2. **Exposure** occurs mainly when dogs attack or mouth the large, slow-moving toads.

3. **Toxic principle and mechanism of action**
   a. **Toxic principle. Bufotoxins** and **bufotenins** are cardioactive glycosides that have digitalis-like and oxytocic (vasopressor) action. **Epinephrine** and **5-hydroxytryptamine** may also be present.
   b. **Mechanism of action.** The toxins are produced in the parotid glands of the toad and absorbed by the mucous membranes of the dog. Excessive stimulation by the cardio-active glycosides causes ventricular fibrillation and hypertension.

4. **Toxicity.** A dog can die following one exposure to *B. marinus* toxin, and morbidity rates are high.

5. **Diagnosis**
   a. **Clinical signs** include immediate salivation, vomiting or retching, shaking of the head, apparent blindness or disorientation, and seizures. Ventricular fibrillation precedes death from heart failure.
   b. **Laboratory diagnosis**
      (1) **Hematology** and **clinical chemistry** changes include increased packed cell volume (PCV), glucose, and BUN, hyperkalemia, and hypercalcemia. The leukocyte count decreases as a result of reduced polymorphonuclear leukocytes.
      (2) **Analysis for the toxin** is not practical because of the route of exposure and lack of concentration of the toxin in organs.
   c. **Lesions.** Distinctive lesions are not present.

6. **Treatment.** Specific antidotes are not available.
   a. Owners may be instructed to carefully flush the mouth with a **slow-moving stream** from a garden hose.
   b. Detoxification with **activated charcoal** and an **osmotic cathartic** is recommended.
   c. A large dose of up to 2 mg/kg **propranolol** may be used to control cardiac arrhythmia and potential fibrillation.
   d. **Atropine** may help control salivation and potential bronchoconstriction.
   e. Control of seizures may be critical to successful therapy.

7. **Prognosis** for recovery is good to guarded if prompt intervention and detoxification are followed by appropriate supportive therapy.

B. *Bufo alvarius* (**Colorado river toad**) is found primarily in the desert Southwest. Toxicosis caused by *B. alvarius* is similar to that caused by *B. marinus,* except that mortality from *B. alvarius* is much lower than that caused by *B. marinus.*

STUDY QUESTIONS

1. In which one of the following toxicoses would analysis for the toxin in gastrointestinal contents or body fluids be useful?

(1) *Bufo marinus* (marine toad)
(2) *Crotalus horridus* (rattlesnake)
(3) *Epicauta* (blister beetle)
(4) *Heloderma horridum* (Mexican beaded lizard)
(5) *Latrodectus mactans* (black widow spider)

2. Antivenin is available for all of the following zootoxins *except*:

(1) *Micrurus* (coral snake)
(2) *Crotalus* (rattlesnake)
(3) *Latrodectus mactans* (black widow spider)
(4) *Agkistrodon piscivorus* (water moccasin)
(5) *Hymenoptera* species (bees, wasps, hornets)

3. Which one of the following does *not* cause an immediate and severe physiologic response as part of the toxic syndrome?

(1) *Crotalus horridus* (rattlesnake)
(2) *Latrodectus mactans* (black widow spider)
(3) *Bufo marinus* (marine toad)
(4) *Loxosceles reclusa* (brown recluse spider)
(5) *Hymenoptera* species (bees, wasps, hornets)

4. Which one of the following is generally *not* recommended as treatment for envenomation by *Crotalus* species?

(1) Antibiotics
(2) Administration of antivenin
(3) Administration of corticosteroids
(4) Blood transfusion
(5) Administration of meperidine

1. The answer is 3 *[II B 5 b (2)]*. *Epicauta* (blister beetles) produce cantharidin, a potent irritant and vesicant that irritates the intestinal and urinary tracts. The toxin is excreted in the urine and may also be found in the gastrointestinal tract after the beetles are consumed. Gas chromatography or mass spectrometry may be used to analyze animal specimens if contaminated hay is no longer available. *Crotalus horridus* (rattlesnake), *Heloderma horridum* (Mexican beaded lizard), *Latrodectus mactans* (black widow spider), and *Bufo marinus* (marine toad) toxicoses result from complex proteinaceous or glycoside toxicants that do not accumulate readily in tissues and are difficult or impossible to detect in biological samples.

2. The answer is 5 *[II A 6 b; III A 7 d; IV A 2 f (1) (a), 3 g (1)]*. There is no effective antivenin for stings from *Hymenoptera* (bees, hornets, wasps). The Elapidae and the Crotalidae are major families of poisonous snakes, and each has a polyvalent commercially available antivenin. Coral snakes (*Micrurus*) are members of the Elapidae family, and rattlesnakes (*Crotalus*) and water moccasins (*Agkistrodon piscivorus*) are members of the Crotalidae family. Poisoning by *Latrodectus mactans*, the black widow spider, is also treated with antivenin.

3. The answer is 4 *[III B 6 a]*. *Loxosceles reclusa*, the brown recluse spider, produces proteinaceous toxins and injects them by biting the victim. However, the victim is rarely aware of the bite, and neither pain nor the necrotizing effects are apparent for up to several hours. The necrotizing effects are persistent and may not resolve for several weeks or until corrected by surgical intervention. Immediate pain and rapid swelling or some other physiologic response occur as a result of bites or other exposure to rattlesnakes, black widow spiders, marine toads, bees, wasps, and hornets.

4. The answer is 3 *[IV A 2 f]*. Recommended treatment for rattlesnake bites includes immobilization to reduce spread of the venom, blood transfusion and fluids to treat shock, and administration of drugs to control the intense pain (e.g., meperidine) and anxiety (diphenhydramine). Antibiotics are used to control secondary infections. Corticosteroids are not recommended because they have been associated with increased mortality and they may alter parameters of the complete blood count and serum chemistry that are used to assess prognosis.

COMPREHENSIVE EXAM

QUESTIONS

DIRECTIONS: Each of the numbered items or incomplete statements in this section is followed by answers or by completions of the statement. Select the **one** numbered answer or completion that is **best** in each case.

1. The term that most clearly defines a poisonous chemical produced by a bacterium is:

(1) toxicant.
(2) toxicosis.
(3) toxicity.
(4) toxin.
(5) toxic.

2. An animal is being treated for a suspected toxicosis caused by organophosphate insecticides. Augmenting treatment with an aminoglycoside antibiotic would likely:

(1) enhance toxicosis, because the organophosphate reduces the amount of acetylcholine (ACh) at the neuromuscular junction.
(2) reduce toxicosis, because the aminoglycoside increases the amount of ACh at the neuromuscular junction.
(3) have no effect, because neither the organophosphate nor the aminoglycoside affects the release of ACh.
(4) enhance toxicosis, because both the organophosphate and the aminoglycoside increase the amount of ACh at the neuromuscular junction.
(5) reduce toxicosis, because the aminoglycoside prevents both presynaptic release of ACh and postsynaptic receptor receptivity.

3. "Alkali disease," primarily seen in cattle and horses in the Great Plains region of the United States, results from ingestion of plants that contain which of the following?

(1) Molybdenum
(2) Selenium
(3) Copper
(4) Arsenic
(5) Zinc

4. "Aging" is a term applicable to which of the following?

(1) Irreversible binding of metals to sulfhydryls before administration of an antidote
(2) Irreversible oxidation of methylene blue, which colors the urine blue
(3) Loss of activity of pralidoxime because of instability in light
(4) Irreversible binding of organophosphates to receptor sites
(5) Loss of antidote effectiveness because of metabolism of ethylene glycol to toxic intermediates

5. Why is the hypothesis of tubular leakage as a cause of acute renal failure not considered valid?

(1) Tubular cells do not lose their differential absorptive ability until late in renal failure.
(2) Damaged tubules that might leak filtrate are usually found in nephrons that are not forming filtrate.
(3) Tubular damage can occur only after casts form to obstruct urine flow in the nephron.
(4) Most solutes in the filtrate are bound to proteins and cannot leak back across cell membranes.
(5) Tubular damage is induced by ischemia, but not by toxicants.

6. Lead-induced porphyria does not cause photosensitization because:

(1) porphyrin levels are too low to induce photodynamic reactions.
(2) porphyrin forms a complex with zinc and hemoglobin that prevents the porphyrin from reaching the skin.
(3) porphyrins in domestic animals are so rapidly excreted that they do not accumulate in plasma.
(4) high endogenous glutathione concentrations prevent the oxidative damage induced by sunlight.

7. Classic LD_{50} studies depend on which of the following?

(1) A graded response in individual animals
(2) A comparison of effects in poisoned animals versus controls
(3) A quantal response in a group of treated animals
(4) A single dosage given to a defined number of animals
(5) A comparison of the effects of a poison among different species

8. Which factors are most important regarding the response of ruminants to toxicants?

(1) The large relative size of the rumen and the high secretory rate of buffers from the rumen wall.
(2) The large relative size of the rumen and its capacity for microbial activity.
(3) The inability of rumen epithelium to detoxify chemicals and the lack of xenobiotic absorption from the rumen.
(4) The adsorption of xenobiotics to natural fibers in the rumen and their subsequent passage through the intestine.
(5) The interaction of volatile fatty acids with xenobiotics in the rumen, which produces nonabsorbable complexes.

9. Which statement regarding the effect of weather conditions on susceptibility to poisons is true?

(1) Low environmental temperatures decrease biotransformation of foreign compounds.
(2) High environmental temperatures increase susceptibility to chemicals that uncouple oxidative phosphorylation.
(3) High environmental temperatures reduce blood flow to the skin and cause reduced susceptibility to dermal poisons.
(4) Atmospheric pressure has no known effect on susceptibility to toxicants.
(5) Weather conditions have no significant effect on susceptibility to toxicants.

10. Which of the following would not be useful in the prevention or therapy of nonsteroidal anti-inflammatory drug (NSAID) toxicosis?

(1) Cimetidine
(2) Misoprostol
(3) Dopamine
(4) Intravenous sodium bicarbonate
(5) Parenteral potassium chloride

11. Which class of herbicides may promote plant toxicosis by altering the palatability or toxin content of plants?

(1) Activated amine herbicides
(2) Dipyridyl herbicides
(3) Phenoxy acetic acid derivatives
(4) Substituted urea herbicides
(5) Triazine herbicides

12. Which procedure is considered most effective for removing ingested toxic materials from the stomach?

(1) Emesis
(2) Gastric lavage
(3) Osmotic catharsis
(4) Antacid therapy
(5) Endoscopic retrieval

13. A high total dissolved solids (TDS) level in a water sample would likely cause clinical effects similar to those caused by excessive amounts of which one of the following?

(1) Calcium
(2) Magnesium
(3) Iron
(4) Nitrate
(5) Sulfate

14. Which agent is most likely to cause central nervous system (CNS) depression as a side effect in poisoned animals?

(1) Ammonium chloride
(2) Apomorphine
(3) Atropine
(4) Naloxone
(5) Yohimbine

15. Which chlorinated organic compound is considered the most toxic synthetic molecule known?

(1) Hexachlorodibenzodioxin (HCDD)
(2) Polybrominated biphenyl (PBB)
(3) Polychlorinated biphenyl (PCB)
(4) Trichloroethylene
(5) Tetrachlorodibenzodioxin (TCDD)

16. Bentonite is preferred as an oral adsorbent instead of activated charcoal for which one of the following chemicals?

(1) Chlorinated phenoxy herbicides
(2) Carbamate insecticides
(3) Organochlorine insecticides
(4) Paraquat herbicide
(5) Strychnine

17. Data from efficacy and toxicity trials for a drug indicate that the LD_1 is 100 mg/kg and the ED_{99} is 20 mg/kg. Which statement below is true?

(1) The therapeutic index (TI) is 5.
(2) The standard safety margin (SSM) is 5.
(3) The LD_{50} is less than 200 mg/kg.
(4) The drug is likely to be cumulative.
(5) The drug has a high risk ratio.

18. A pathologist reports that a lung specimen contains mostly cuboidal alveolar type II epithelium. What is the probable reason for the presence of these cells?

(1) They are normal inhabitants of the alveolar lining.
(2) They are the precursors of pulmonary adenocarcinoma.
(3) They have proliferated to protect against pulmonary edema.
(4) They are defense against a high concentration of particulates.
(5) They have proliferated to replace damaged type I epithelium.

19. Cancer chemotherapeutic agents may induce the radiomimetic syndrome. The intestinal effects of this syndrome result from:

(1) hyperosmolarity effects that are caused by the inhibition of solute absorption by the chemotherapeutic agent.
(2) increased vascularization of the submucosa as a result of vasodilation that is caused by the chemotherapeutic agent.
(3) rapid death of villous epithelial cells caused by direct necrotizing effects on the epithelial cells.
(4) necrosis and suppression of mitosis in intestinal crypt cells, leading to loss of replacement intestinal epithelium.
(5) interference with prostaglandins, resulting in a loss of vascular dilation and leading to mucosal ischemia.

20. When is a two-compartment model needed to define the elimination of a toxicant?

(1) When the agent is metabolized to an ionized compound
(2) When first-order kinetics is the mode of elimination
(3) When plasma binding of the drug occurs
(4) When the toxicant can accumulate in body tissues
(5) When absorption is delayed and produces a biphasic blood concentration

21. Which one of the following statements regarding mycotoxins is true?

(1) Mycotoxins are primary and essential products of fungal growth.
(2) They are produced only under optimal growth conditions for the fungus.
(3) They are predictably present when certain fungi are present in grains.
(4) They are often produced in response to host plant or fungal stress.
(5) They are only produced in stored grains.

Questions 22–23

A farmer reports that several of his cows have died suddenly. Investigation of the premises reveals an empty pesticide container in a trash pile near the herd's grazing territory. The label identifies the pesticide's active ingredient as O,O-diethyl S-[(ethylthio) methyl] phosphorodithioate.

22. What is the most likely toxicologic mechanism of this pesticide?

(1) Alteration of the sodium channels of the nerve axon
(2) Uncoupling of oxidative phosphorylation by substituting for phosphates in the tricarboxylic acid cycle (TCA)
(3) Inhibition of neurotoxic esterase in the peripheral nerves
(4) Inhibition of acetylcholinesterase (AChE)
(5) Formation of lipid free radicals in the cell membrane

23. Assuming the pesticide is the cause of the cattle deaths, which combination of samples from the dead cows would provide the most useful information in confirming a tentative diagnosis?

(1) Blood and intestinal contents
(2) Intestinal and rumen contents
(3) Rumen contents and brain tissue
(4) Brain and liver tissue
(5) Liver and kidney tissue

24. The highly toxic *Nerium oleander* (oleander) has clinical effects most similar to which one of the following plants?

(1) *Cassia occidentalis* (coffee senna)
(2) *Digitalis purpurea* (digitalis)
(3) *Eupatorium rugosum* (white snakeroot)
(4) *Lilium* (Easter lily)
(5) *Microcystis aeruginosa* (blue-green algae)

25. Fetal death of two animals in a litter of eight during the second trimester of gestation is likely to cause:

(1) abortion of the entire litter.
(2) resorption of the dead fetuses and death of the remaining fetuses.
(3) resorption of the dead fetuses without any effect on the remainder of the litter.
(4) mummification of the dead fetuses without any effect on the remainder of the litter.
(5) mummification of the dead fetuses and death of the remaining fetuses.

26. Which statement about the biotransformation of xenobiotics is true with respect to the effects of toxicants on cells?

(1) Foreign compounds are usually strongly electrophilic before they encounter the microsomal mixed function oxidase (MFO) system.
(2) Electrophilic intermediates bind preferentially to cell macromolecules and secondarily to glutathione (GSH).
(3) Electrophilic intermediates formed by the MFOs bind covalently to cell macromolecules.
(4) Covalent binding is highly correlated with GSH levels.
(5) GSH binding promotes cell damage by attracting toxicants to the cell and increasing their concentration in the cell.

27. Which characteristic is most likely associated with type II hepatotoxicosis?

(1) Distinctive lesions
(2) Similar lesions among different species exposed to the same hepatotoxin
(3) Non–dose-related response
(4) Experimentally reproducible response
(5) A brief latent period preceding onset of lesions and following exposure to the toxicant

28. The best initial approach to providing respiratory support for an intoxicated animal with severe bradypnea is to:

(1) administer an analeptic such as yohimbine to stimulate respiration.
(2) anesthetize with pentobarbital and administer artificial respiration.
(3) examine the respiratory system, anesthetize lightly, insert an endotracheal tube, and provide mechanical ventilation if needed.
(4) avoid stress by handling the animal as little as possible, give pentobarbital, and place the animal in an oxygen cage.
(5) administer intravenous fluids and bicarbonate to maintain pulmonary vascular tone and combat the acidosis of respiratory failure.

29. Which of the following mechanisms allows renal tubular cells to incorporate high-molecular-weight materials into the cell?

(1) Osmoregulation
(2) Clearance
(3) Endocytosis
(4) Entropy
(5) Tubular transport

30. A herd of cattle in New Mexico has consumed a plant that exudes a whitish, milky sap when the stem is broken. The leaves are narrow. The cattle are salivating and incoordinated and many have been exhibiting seizures. Signs appeared abruptly and have been present for 24 hours. Upon auscultation of the chest, the heart sounds are arrhythmic and slow. The most probable plant cause of the poisoning:

(1) *Asclepias labriformis*
(2) *Astragalus lentigenosus*
(3) *Centaurea solstitialis*
(4) *Datura stramonium*
(5) *Ricinus communis*

31. One microgram per gram (1 μg/g) is equivalent to:

(1)   0.1 part per billion (ppb).
(2)   1 ppb.
(3)   100 ppb.
(4)   1000 ppb.
(5) 100,000 ppb.

32. Which one of the following statements is true?

(1) Adverse effects from use of antidotes are more likely if the toxicant affected by the antidote is present in high concentrations.
(2) Antidotes should be administered before general decontamination therapy so the decontamination process does not inactivate the antidote.
(3) Antidotes are given primarily as prophylactic agents to prevent adverse effects from suspected toxicants.
(4) Relatively few antidotes are cleared for veterinary use.
(5) Adverse effects of antidotes usually result from hypersensitization and are not dose-related.

33. Which one of the following statements regarding the organic ion transport system is true?

(1) The organic ion transport system provides a means for transport of nutrients into the tubule cells to maintain energy metabolism.
(2) The organic ion transport system detoxifies materials by moving them quickly out of the glomerulus during glomerular filtration.
(3) The organic molecules that enter the system are made more polar and less lipophilic by the organic ion transport system.
(4) The organic ion transport system may concentrate agents in tubular cells, increasing toxicant access to the tubules.
(5) The organic ion transport system has little significance because most toxicant excretion in the kidney occurs by glomerular filtration.

34. A litter of pigs born normal and active at term act hungry and try to nurse, but rapidly lose weight and die within a few days. The sow is normal, except there is little or no mammary development. The most likely cause is:

(1) direct toxicosis of the piglets resulting from the secretion of aflatoxin in the milk.
(2) inhibition of lactation by zearalenone.
(3) inhibition of prolactin release resulting from ergot contamination of the feed.
(4) reduced protein synthesis resulting from trichothecene inhibition of transcription and translation.
(5) reduced milk production resulting from deoxynivalenol (vomitoxin, DON)-induced feed refusal.

35. Which drug is a specific reversal agent for an overdosage or excessive clinical response to xylazine?

(1) Apomorphine
(2) Cimetidine
(3) Doxapram
(4) Naloxone
(5) Yohimbine

36. A horse exhibits weakness, dark red-brown urine, pale mucous membranes, and dyspnea. The symptoms began acutely 2 days ago. Which of the following would be a probable cause?

(1) Ingestion of fertilizer stored in a nearby building
(2) Ingestion of leaves from maple tree with branches hanging over the paddock fence
(3) Ingestion of peeling white paint from the fence
(4) Nitrates in the shallow well that supplies drinking water
(5) Bracken fern growing in the woods at the back of the pasture

37. Identify the correct combination of agent, species, and adverse effect.

(1) 4-Methylpyrazole (4-MP), cats, methemoglobinemia
(2) Ammonium molybdate, sheep, acute hemolytic crisis
(3) Acetylcysteine, cats, Heinz body anemia
(4) D-Penicillamine, dogs, hypocalcemia
(5) Methylene blue, cats, methemoglobinemia and Heinz body anemia

38. The cellular organelle most prominently damaged by excessive exposure of animals to monensin or other ionophores is the:

(1) endoplasmic reticulum.
(2) Golgi complex.
(3) mitochondria.
(4) nucleus.

39. Which one of the following situations most accurately describes circumstances of exposure to *Epicauta*?

(1) The family dog accidentally encounters it in its nesting place in a suburban back yard.
(2) A dog accompanying a teenage boy on a hike in the rocky foothills of the mountains challenges it.
(3) A horse eats it in a flake of baled hay.
(4) A horse encounters it as a contaminant in grain screenings.
(5) A young dog in Florida discovers it in his back yard and tries to catch it and eat it.

40. Assume a 100-kg pig in a confinement building is exposed to hydrogen sulfide at a concentration of 0.1 mg/L of air for the entire day. The pig's respiratory rate is 30 respirations/min and the tidal volume is 1.0 L. What is the approximate daily dosage of hydrogen sulfide?

(1) 20 mg/kg
(2) 40 mg/kg
(3) 60 mg/kg
(4) 80 mg/kg
(5) 100 mg/kg

41. What structural (morphological) feature is common to the toxic laurels of rhododendrons?

(1) Both have a vining or climbing growth habit.
(2) Both have green berries that are toxic, but become harmless when they ripen.
(3) Both have characteristic spines on the midrib of the leaves.
(4) Both have broad, flat, oval leaves that stay green all winter.
(5) Both have distinctive hollow stems with linear, purple spots.

42. Which of the following toxicoses results in elevated levels of incompletely formed heme (i.e., porphyria)?

(1) Cadmium toxicosis
(2) Iron toxicosis
(3) Arsenic toxicosis
(4) Mercury toxicosis
(5) Lead toxicosis

43. Male secondary sexual characteristics and libido would most likely be affected by a toxicant that damaged which type of cell?

(1) Sertoli cells
(2) Germinal epithelium
(3) Leydig cells
(4) Myoepithelial cells
(5) Spermatozoa

44. A herd of dairy cows has experienced intermittent lameness, weight loss, and reduced milk production. Some of the cows appear to lap water, rather than drinking with their muzzles immersed in the water. Some of the older cows have noticeable thickening of the proximal metacarpals and metatarsals. What would be the next step in arriving at a diagnosis?

(1) A rectal examination to evaluate kidney size
(2) Auscultation of the abdomen for evidence of rumen stasis
(3) Examination of the hooves for evidence of laminitis
(4) Examination of the teeth for evidence of enamel mottling and pitting
(5) A complete neurologic exam

45. Animal size has been related to which one of the following factors?

(1) Body surface area and metabolic activity
(2) Passage of chemicals across the blood–brain barrier
(3) Body fat and storage of xenobiotics
(4) Efficiency of renal excretion
(5) Rate of intestinal passage of ingesta

46. A pulmonary response characterized by the long-term focal accumulation of pulmonary macrophages containing visible particles, the release of hydrolases and cytokines, and a progression to pulmonary fibrosis is known as:

(1) asphyxiation.
(2) allergy.
(3) carcinogenesis.
(4) emphysema.
(5) pneumoconiosis.

47. Which of the following would be most likely to accumulate in the fat of animals during long-term, low-level exposure?

(1) Organophosphate insecticides
(2) Organochlorine insecticides
(3) Pyrethrins and pyrethroids
(4) Chlorophenoxy herbicides
(5) Bipyridyl herbicides

48. Necropsy of a group of turkeys reveals that most of the birds have markedly enlarged hearts with a distinctly rounded ventricular outline. The farmer indicates that the birds were experiencing diarrhea, so he had started mixing some "old antibacterial powder" into the feed "3 or 4 weeks ago." Based on the lesion, the most likely cause is:

(1) amprolium.
(2) ethylenediamine dihydroiodide (EDDI).
(3) furazolidone.
(4) monensin.
(5) nitrofurazone.

49. What conditions characterize the diuretic phase of acute toxicant-induced renal failure?

(1) Hyperkalemia, hyponatremia, hyperphosphatemia, low urine specific gravity, elevated blood urea nitrogen (BUN) level
(2) Hypokalemia, hyponatremia, hypophosphatemia, elevated urine specific gravity, normal BUN level
(3) Hyperkalemia, hypernatremia, hypophosphatemia, increased urine specific gravity, elevated BUN level
(4) Hypokalemia, hyponatremia, hyperphosphatemia, decreased urine specific gravity, normal BUN level
(5) Hypokalemia, hyponatremia, hyperphosphatemia, normal urine specific gravity, normal BUN level

50. Which sequence best describes the progression from free radical formation to cell death?

(1) Xenobiotic metabolism, cell swelling, lipid peroxidation, free radical formation, phospholipase activation, calcium sequestration, loss of membrane function, necrosis
(2) Lipid peroxidation, free radical formation, xenobiotic metabolism, free radical formation, phospholipase activation, loss of calcium sequestration, loss of membrane function, cell swelling, necrosis
(3) Free radical formation, xenobiotic metabolism, lipid peroxidation, phospholipase activation, loss of calcium sequestration, loss of membrane function, cell swelling, necrosis
(4) Xenobiotic metabolism, lipid peroxidation, free radical formation, phospholipase activation, loss of calcium sequestration, loss of membrane function, cell swelling, necrosis
(5) Xenobiotic metabolism, free radical formation, lipid peroxidation, covalent binding, reduced membrane function, loss of calcium sequestration, phospholipase activation, cell swelling, necrosis

51. The best therapeutic choice for a lead-poisoned animal with high blood levels and serious clinical signs is:

(1) calcium disodium ethylenediaminetetra-acetic acid (EDTA).
(2) D-penicillamine.
(3) dimercaprol.
(4) EDTA and D-penicillamine.
(5) EDTA and dimercaprol.

52. Which of the following pairs of pesticidal compounds have similar mechanisms of action?

(1) Organophosphate insecticides and rotenone
(2) Rotenone and pyrethrins
(3) Pyrethrins and DDT
(4) DDT and paraquat
(5) Paraquat and 2,4-D

53. Which one of the following is the preferred approach for sampling grain?

(1) Sampling of the most severely molded specimen in the storage unit
(2) Sampling from the surface of the storage bin, where oxygen and moisture are most abundant
(3) Probe sampling from the center of a grain storage unit
(4) Collecting multiple samples from a moving stream of grain
(5) Collecting samples over a period of 7–10 days

54. If 2 pounds of a drug containing 4 ounces of active ingredient per pound are added to 1 ton of livestock ration, how many parts per million (ppm) of the drug are present in the ration?

(1)   25 ppm
(2) 100 ppm
(3) 250 ppm
(4) 1000 ppm
(5) 2500 ppm

55. Within the body, the linking of an activated foreign chemical to an endogenous agent to form a less lipophilic, more water-soluble, and readily excreted product is called:

(1) antagonism.
(2) bioactivation.
(3) conjugation.
(4) potentiation.
(5) synergism.

56. Feed-grade urea contains 45% nitrogen. If a feed tag states that the feed contains 21% equivalent crude protein from urea, what is the actual urea concentration in the feed?

(1) 2.5%
(2) 5.0%
(3) 7.5%
(4) 10.0%
(5) 20.0%

57. What type of toxicant is most likely the source of toxicosis in an animal that is weak and has a high fever?

(1) An inhibitor of γ-aminobutyric acid (GABA)
(2) An uncoupler of oxidative phosphorylation
(3) A toxicant that interferes with ribosomal-dependent protein synthesis
(4) A toxicant that causes oxygen deficiency
(5) A toxicant that reduces lipoprotein synthesis needed to transport high-energy lipids from the liver

58. Which hepatic structure is most closely associated with cholestatic liver damage?

(1) Kupffer cells
(2) Disse's space
(3) Bile canaliculi
(4) Hepatic sinusoids
(5) Common bile duct

Questions 59–60

On a Friday afternoon, a client brings a cat to the veterinarian because the cat has seemed "depressed" and has refused to eat since Thursday morning. In addition, the owner noted that the urine in the cat box was "coffee-colored." Physical examination reveals cyanotic mucous membranes, dyspnea, and mild icterus. The palpebrae, conjunctiva, and face are slightly swollen. The urinary bladder is empty and the cat is dehydrated. The laboratory report on a blood sample contains the following information: hemoglobin, 6.8 g/dl; packed cell volume (PCV) 18%; total bilirubin, 2.1 mg/dl; and blood urea nitrogen (BUN), 35 mg/dl. The plasma and serum are a red-brown color.

59. All of the following laboratory findings would be compatible with this history *except:*

(1) Heinz bodies in the blood smear
(2) Markedly elevated serum alanine aminotransferase (ALT) levels
(3) Markedly elevated serum creatinine phosphokinase levels
(4) Methemoglobinemia
(5) Increased erythrocyte fragility

60. Which of the following would be most useful for countering toxicosis in this cat?

(1) Activated charcoal
(2) Sodium sulfate
(3) Methylene blue
(4) Acetylcysteine
(5) Oxygen therapy

DIRECTIONS: Each of the numbered items or incomplete statements in this section is negatively phrased, as indicated by an italicized word such as *not, least,* or *except.* Select the **one** numbered answer or completion that is **best** in each case.

61. All of the following enhance absorption of a chemical *except:*

(1) High lipid solubility
(2) Nonpolar
(3) Un-ionized state
(4) Low molecular weight
(5) Protein-bound

62. All of the following are reasonable differential diagnoses to consider against the possibility of acute caffeine toxicosis in a dog *except:*

(1) Amphetamine toxicosis
(2) Cholecalciferol toxicosis
(3) Lead toxicosis
(4) Metaldehyde toxicosis
(5) Strychnine toxicosis

63. The metal toxicosis *least* likely to cause signs of gastroenteritis or colic is:

(1) arsenic.
(2) cadmium.
(3) lead.
(4) molybdenum.
(5) zinc.

64. A cat walked through some spilled granular materials in a home owner's garage, then groomed its paws. Within a few minutes, the cat began to salivate moderately, made licking and champing motions, and vomited twice. Upon examination, the attending veterinarian finds erythema and mild ulceration of the interdigital skin and pale white patches on the tongue and gingiva. All of the following could have caused the problem *except:*

(1) Drain cleaner
(2) Fireplace colors
(3) Garden fertilizer
(4) Garden herbicide
(5) Thawing salt

65. Which of the following factors is *least* likely to contribute to plant toxicosis?

(1) Nutrient deficiency
(2) Overgrazing
(3) Undergrazing
(4) Recent shipping or confinement of animals
(5) Boredom

66. All of the following characteristics are typical of a toxic snake of the family Crotalidae *except:*

(1) a broad, triangular head.
(2) alternating red and yellow bands.
(3) vertical, elliptical pupils.
(4) long, curved, retractable fangs.
(5) a deep pit between the nostril and the eye.

67. All of the following are true about urea toxicosis in ruminants *except:*

(1) Acidic ruminal conditions predispose animals to ammonia toxicosis by promoting absorption of urea across the ruminal wall.
(2) Excessive ammonia released from ruminal microbial activity on urea is absorbed across the ruminal wall where it interferes with intermediary metabolism and causes metabolic acidosis.
(3) Urea toxicosis is more likely if animals are fasted and unaccustomed to urea in the diet.
(4) Ammonia toxicosis runs its full clinical course within 24 hours of exposure.
(5) Autolysis and proteolysis of poorly preserved rumen contents or blood samples from urea-poisoned animals may alter ammonia concentrations and give false diagnostic values.

68. The sudden death of swine with lesions typical of clay pigeon poisoning would have to be carefully differentiated from all of the following *except:*

(1) *Amaranthus retroflexus* toxicosis
(2) Hepatosis dietetica
(3) *Xanthium strumarin* (cocklebur) toxicosis
(4) Gossypol toxicosis
(5) Acute aflatoxicosis

69. A client calls the veterinarian because his dog is "acting strange." The dog is disoriented and barking for apparently no reason. Which one of the following would be *least* likely to be included on a differential diagnosis list?

(1) Marijuana
(2) Jimson weed seeds
(3) Mescal bean seeds
(4) Morning glory seeds
(5) Rhubarb leaves

DIRECTIONS: Each group of items in this section consists of numbered options followed by a set of numbered items. For each item, select the **one** numbered option that is most closely associated with it. Each numbered option may be selected once, more than once, or not at all.

Questions 70–73

Match each clinical presentation with the causative agent.

(1) Dimethyl(2,2,2 trichloro-1-hydroxyethyl) phosphonate
(2) Cyclodiene-type chlorinated hydrocarbon insecticide
(3) Pyrethrin
(4) Strychnine
(5) Metaldehyde

70. Clinical signs include salivation, vomiting, polyuria, dyspnea, diarrhea, miosis, and bradycardia. Affected animals are ataxic, weak, and have muscle tremors and, occasionally, seizures.

71. Toxicosis is characterized by the sudden onset of muscle tremors and stiffness, followed by tonic to tetanic seizures and marked hyperesthesia.

72. Typical signs include salivation, mydriasis, tremors, and hyperthermia, but no vomiting or diarrhea.

73. The typical seizure pattern is intermittent cranial to caudal epileptiform seizures with little or no hyperesthesia. Hyperthermia may be present during or after seizures.

Questions 74–77

Match each clinical presentation with the most likely toxicosis.

(1) Copper
(2) Lead
(3) Molybdenum
(4) Sodium arsenite
(5) Zinc

74. A dog with gastroenteritis, moderate anemia, and basophilic stippling, but no neurologic signs

75. A cat with acute intractable vomiting, projectile fluid diarrhea, and dehydration

76. A cat with colic, vomiting, central nervous system (CNS) depression, and mild anemia

77. A dog with a history of weight loss, vomiting, depression, and an increasing yellowish tinge to the sclera

Questions 78–82

Match each clinical syndrome with the most likely plant-related cause.

(1) *Delphinium barbeyi* (larkspur)
(2) *Sorghum* (Sudan grass)
(3) *Tetradymia glabrata* (horsebrush)
(4) *Pteridium aquilinum* (bracken fern)
(5) *Festuca arundinacea* (Kentucky 31 tall fescue)

78. Anemia, thrombocytopenia, leukopenia hematuria, ventral edema, and urinary bladder neoplasms (cattle)

79. Swollen coronary bands, lameness, dry gangrene, and loss of hooves (cattle)

80. Dark brown blood accompanied by weakness, dyspnea, depression, and death (cattle)

81. Muscle tremors, excitement, disorientation, bloat, cardiac arrhythmia, prostration and death within 24 hours (cattle)

82. Photophobia, conjunctivitis, sunburn, weeping and exudation of serum from light-skinned areas, swollen eyelids and ears, and exfoliation of the epidermis from the muzzle and udders (sheep)

Questions 83–87

For each toxicant, choose the best sample for postmortem confirmation of toxicosis.

(1) Stomach contents
(2) Renal or hepatic tissue
(3) Brain tissue
(4) Stomach contents and renal or hepatic tissue
(5) Stomach contents and brain tissue

83. Carbamate insecticides

84. Cholecalciferol

85. Strychnine

86. Brodifacoum

87. Zinc phosphide

Questions 88–89

Match each description with the antidote it best describes.

(1) Ammonium molybdate
(2) Calcium disodium ethylenediaminetetraacetic acid (EDTA)
(3) Desferoxamine
(4) D-Penicillamine
(5) Dimercaprol

88. Used for long-term removal of both lead and copper

89. Used for both lead and arsenic

Questions 90–94

Reproductive and teratogenic effects of poisonous plants can cause considerable economic loss in grazing animals. Match each clinical reproductive problem with the plant that causes it.

(1) *Astragalus* (locoweed)
(2) *Nicotiana tabacum* (tobacco)
(3) *Lupinus* (lupine, bluebonnet)
(4) *Pinus ponderosa* (Western yellow pine, ponderosa pine)
(5) *Veratrum californicum* (veratrum, false hellebore)

90. Prolonged gestation in ewes followed by delivery of larger-than-normal lambs; many lambs are stillborn with craniofacial malformations including a shortened maxilla and an enlarged, single ocular orbit containing one or two eyes

91. Late-term abortions in cattle accompanied by edema of the udder, retained placentas, and metritis

92. Contracted tendons and excessive carpal flexure accompanied by a moderate arthrogryposis in lambs

93. "Crooked calf disease" (i.e., twisted necks, twisted and bowed limbs, and cleft palate)

94. Twisting and arthrogryposis of the limbs in piglets

ANSWERS AND EXPLANATIONS

1. The answer is 4 *[Chapter 1 I B 2]*. Toxin is the term used to identify poisons of natural or biologic origin. Snake venoms, toxic mold metabolites, and poisonous principles in plants are examples of toxins. The term toxicant is synonymous with poison.

2. The answer is 5 *[Chapter 14 I C 2 a]*. Administering aminoglycoside antibiotics to an animal with a suspected organophosphate insecticide toxicosis would help to alleviate the effects of the insecticide. Organophosphate insecticides are cholinesterase inhibitors; therefore, they permit accumulation of excess of acetylcholine (ACh) at the neuromuscular junction. The aminoglycoside antibiotics cause neuromuscular blockade by inhibiting the presynaptic release of ACh and reducing postsynaptic receptivity to ACh. Therefore, they reduce the availability and influence of ACh at the neuromuscular junction.

3. The answer is 2 *[Chapter 17 VIII A 3 b, B 1; Table 17-5]*. The high and dry alkaline soils of much of the Great Plains are noted for their high selenium content. Obligate indicator plants which grow well in the Great Plains region, absorb selenium from the soil and convert it to a more soluble form that is readily available to animals.

4. The answer is 4 *[Chapter 6 III M 2]*. By definition, "aging" is the formation of a stable or nearly irreversible bond between the organophosphate and cholinesterase. This effect occurs within 8–24 hours postexposure, and once it occurs, the pralidoxime is largely ineffective because it cannot attack the organophosphate–cholinesterase bond and bind to the organophosphate. In most situations requiring antidotal therapy, prompt treatment with the antidote is necessary to ensure its effectiveness.

5. The answer is 2 *[Chapter 9 II B 1]*. Renal micropuncture studies done with direct measurement of tubular filtrate flow and pressure showed that tubules with damaged epithelium usually do not contribute to the formation of filtrate. Thus, if no filtrate is present in the tubule, fluid and electrolytes cannot leak through the cells of the nephron.

6. The answer is 2 *[Chapter 16 III B 2 b (1) (c)]*. Porphyrins that are produced after δ-aminolevulinic acid dehydrase (δ-ALAD) is inhibited would be photodynamic if they reached the fluids of the subcutaneous tissue and dermis. Protoporphyrins, the porphyrins resulting from lead toxicosis, are chelated by zinc, which prevents them from exiting the erythrocytes. Thus, photosensitization is not a clinical feature of the porphyria produced by lead poisoning.

7. The answer is 3 *[Chapter 1 I F 1 b (4)]*. Classic LD_{50} studies use the quantal, or all-or-none response (e.g., the number dead per group, or, for efficacy studies, the number affected per group). Multiple dosages are used to construct a dose–response curve, and the studies are not done across species but with a well-defined homogeneous group of animals.

8. The answer is 2 *[Chapter 10 V A–B]*. The relatively large size of the rumen and its capacity for microbial activity are two factors that cause ruminant toxicology to differ from that of other domestic animals. The large rumen acts as a physical buffer; however, it also acts as a reservoir and prolongs the presence of toxicant when the rumen is heavily contaminated. In addition, a major factor in ruminant response to toxicants is the ability of microbes in the rumen to either detoxify toxicants or to produce metabolites that are more toxic than the parent compound. Other factors (e.g., xenobiotic metabolism and secretion of buffers by the epithelium) are not significant because the rumen is a modification of the esophagus.

9. The answer is 2 *[Chapter 3 IV C, D]*. High environmental temperatures increase susceptibility to substances that alter metabolism, such as oxidative uncouplers. Oxidative uncouplers increase the internal body temperature of animals because metabolic energy is lost as heat and not stored as high energy phosphate bonds. High environmental temperatures increase blood flow to the skin, causing increased absorption of chemicals, such as pesticides. Low environmental temperatures have been shown to increase the biotransformation of xenobiotics, possibly because of increased food intake and general increases in metabolic demands. Atmospheric pressure affects response to toxicants primarily through changes in environmental oxygen tension.

10. The answer is 5 *[Chapter 24 III F]*. Because renal damage and oliguria can be a significant factor in nonsteroidal anti-inflammatory drug (NSAID) toxicosis, potassium-containing fluids that could aggravate hyperkalemia during an oliguric crisis should be avoided. Excessive NSAID use is associated with gastric irritation and mucosal damage. These complications are routinely treated with histamine-receptor antagonists, such as cimetidine and ranitidine. In addition, exogenous prostaglandins (e.g., misoprostol) have been useful in preventing NSAID-induced gastric ulcers. The complications of hypotension and reduced urine output may be prevented or lessened by the intravenous administration of fluids (with or without dopamine). The addition of sodium bicarbonate to the intravenous fluid therapy combats acidosis and enhances urinary elimination of the NSAIDs.

11. The answer is 3 *[Chapter 28 I E 2 c]*. The phenoxy acetic acid herbicides (e.g., 2,4-D) are plant hormones that cause changes in plant metabolism. Both enhancement of palatability and increases in toxin content (e.g., nitrates) have been demonstrated for some toxic plants treated with these herbicides. The other classes of herbicides also alter plant metabolism, but do not seem to affect toxin content or the response of animals to poisonous plants.

12. The answer is 1 *[Chapter 5 II B 1, 2]*. Emesis in animals that can readily vomit provides an effective means for removing both liquid and solid materials, often as much as 80 percent, from the stomach. Early emesis (within 2–4 hours of ingestion) prevents access to the intestine, where a major portion of absorption occurs. Gastric lavage is, at best, an alternative to emesis and is almost never as effective at removing solids from the stomach. Endoscopic retrieval is effective mainly for dense solids such as metals, which may remain in the stomach and be slowly absorbed as the gastric acids dissolve the metal. Osmotic cathartics are effective at increasing passage of ingesta through the intestine, but they do not cause gastric emptying. Antacids do not empty the stomach. In addition, antacids may even enhance absorption of acidic poisons by changing the pH of the stomach contents.

13. The answer is 5 *[Chapter 27 II C 4 c; Table 27-2]*. Sulfates in excessive amounts cause an osmotic catharsis resulting in mild to moderate diarrhea that is usually transient and appears similar to the osmotic effect of excessive total dissolved solids (TDS). Calcium and magnesium cause no clinical effects in the concentrations found in water. Iron at the usual concentrations in water causes esthetic and, possibly, nutritional effects, but does not affect the gastrointestinal tract. Nitrate causes methemoglobinemia, not diarrhea.

14. The answer is 2 *[Chapter 5 II B 1 c (1) (a)]*. Apomorphine is a narcotic derivative; therefore, a prominent side effect is central nervous system (CNS) depression. Ammonium chloride and atropine generally stimulate the nervous system. Naloxone and yohimbine are reversal agents against CNS depressants, such as narcotics and xylazine, respectively. Overdosage or repeated use of apomorphine is likely to induce prolonged vomiting as well as excessive CNS depression.

15. The answer is 5 *[Chapter 18 III A 2 a (1), E 1 c]*. Tetrachlorodibenzodioxin (TCDD) is considered the most toxic synthetic molecule in existence, with chronic cumulative toxicity caused by dosages of only a few micrograms per kilogram body weight. Because of their extreme toxicity, cumulative nature, and persistence in the environment, dioxins, especially TCDD, are still of some concern, although most contemporary products are manufactured in a way to prevent contamination by TCDD. Hexachlorobenzodioxin (HCDD) has 6 chlorines; compounds with more than 4 chlorines are generally less toxic.

16. The answer is 4 *[Chapter 20 III H 1 a (2)]*. Paraquat is strongly bound to colloidal clays, both in soil, in vitro, and in vivo. Because this binding for parquat to bentonite or clays is stronger than to charcoal, and because prevention of paraquat signs is extremely important, the preferred oral detoxicant for paraquat is bentonite or clay compounds. Chlorinated phenoxy herbicides, carbamate insecticides, organochlorine insecticides, and strychnine are adsorbed by activated charcoal.

17. The answer is 2 *[Chapter 1 I D 2]*. Standard safety margin (SSM) is the ratio of LD_1 to the ED_{99} and is a more conservative estimate of safety than the therapeutic index (TI), which is the LD_{50} divided by the ED_{50}.

Acute toxicity values are not used to define chronic toxicity, and whether the drug is too dangerous is a decision that cannot be made from the information available. Risk analysis is a comprehensive process that considers conditions of use, environmental contamination, and long-term harmful effects to evaluate a chemical's potential for harm to humans, animals, or the environment.

18. The answer is 5 *[Chapter 11 I A 1 c (2); II B 1 b (2) (a)].* When alveolar epithelium is injured and lost, the type II cells proliferate rapidly to replace the lost type I cells. In their immature state, type II cells are cuboidal. Within a few days, they mature to the flattened epithelium characteristic of the alveolar epithelial cell, but until that time, they transfer oxygen less effectively than type I cells. If large numbers of type II cells are present, the diffusion of essential respiratory gases may be impaired. Type II cells are normal inhabitants of the alveolar epithelium, but they generally only comprise 10% of the total surface area.

19. The answer is 4 *[Chapter 10 IV B 1 b (2)].* Radiomimetic syndrome, which is a complex of effects that result from excessive radiation exposure, can also be caused by some cancer chemotherapeutic agents. These agents are powerful antimitotic chemicals that may also cause necrosis, especially of metabolically active and rapidly dividing cells. Intestinal crypt cells are in actively mitotic and serve as the source of mature cells that populate the villous intestinal epithelium. Loss of crypt cells causes eventual loss of the epithelial lining of the intestines, with resultant diarrhea and intestinal hemorrhage.

20. The answer is 4 *[Chapter 1 III D 3 b (3)].* One-compartment models mainly describe elimination from the blood. When storage or accumulation in other tissues (e.g., fat) occurs, each compartment will have a depletion curve that must be accounted for in the kinetic evaluation.

21. The answer is 4 *[Chapter 29 I A].* Mycotoxins may be produced when conditions for growth create fungal stress, rather than under optimal conditions. Many fungi capable of and known for producing mycotoxins do not produce them consistently, because environmental conditions as well as the fungal species and variety affect the potential for mycotoxin production. Mycotoxins can be produced both in stored grains and in growing grains. Mycotoxins are secondary products of fungal growth, as opposed to primary products, which would be necessary for fungal growth or reproduction.

22–23. The answers are 22-4 *[Chapter 19 I E; Figure 19-1],* **23-3** *[Chapter 19 I G 2 a (2), b (2)].* The chemical formula found on the bag clearly identifies the material as an organothiophosphate, a very common form of organophosphate insecticide. This is readily evident from the designator word "phosphorodithioate." Furthermore, the chemical name indicates a diethyl ester (O,O diethyl), which is typical of the basic structure of organophosphates. The organophosphates are well-known cholinesterase inhibitors. The other mechanisms listed are associated with DDT (altered sodium channels), pentachlorophenol and metaldehyde (uncoupling oxidative phosphorylation), paraquat (formation of lipid free radicals), and tri-ortho-cresyl phosphates (inhibition of neurotoxic esterase).

The available evidence suggests that the pesticide bag is a potential source of toxicosis and that oral exposure is most likely. Confirming oral exposure depends, in part, on finding the toxicant in the rumen, abomasum, or intestinal tract. The organophosphate compounds are relatively stable under mildly acidic conditions (e.g., in the rumen), but they are unstable under alkaline conditions (e.g., in the intestinal tract). Thus, the rumen would provide a better sample than the intestines. In addition, absorption from the intestine reduces the amount of organophosphate remaining there. The second major confirmatory test is evidence of cholinesterase depression. Blood will be clotted in the dead animal and difficult to collect as a representative sample. In addition, blood cholinesterase values may be decreased in organophosphate toxicosis, but generally, these values correlate less strongly with the severity of the toxicosis than samples from the brain or caudate nucleus. Liver and other tissues often contain very little or no detectable organophosphate residues and thus, are unreliable indicators of toxicosis. Therefore, the best combination is collection of a stable specimen that represents intake of pesticide (rumen contents) as well as a biologically relevant indicator of effect (brain tissue).

24. The answer is 2 *[Chapter 28 VI B 1 c, d].* *Nerium oleander* (oleander) and *Digitalis purpurea* (digitalis) both contain cardioactive glycosides that interfere with the sodium-potassium-ATPase pump and affect calcium exchange in the heart. At excessive dosages these glycosides cause conduction block and asystole. *Cassia species* (coffee senna) can cause cardiac myonecrosis. *Eupatorium rugosum* (white snakeroot) also may affect the heart, especially in horses, but the mechanism is unclear and appears to involve cardiac muscle damage. *Lilium* (Easter lily) is known to cause nephrotoxicity in cats, but it has no known cardiotoxic effects. *Convallaria majalis* (lily-of-the-valley) does contain cardioactive glycosides, however. *Microcystis aeruginosa* is one of the blue-green algae and is most likely associated with hepatic damage.

25. The answer is 4 *[Chapter 12 III C 2 c (2)].* Mummification of a fetus occurs after calcification of the skeleton takes place. At this stage, the dead fetus becomes dehydrated, but the calcified skeletal remains and the dermis may remain until delivery. Because only a small portion of the litter dies, the fetal influence in maintenance of pregnancy is not eliminated and the pregnancy is maintained.

26. The answer is 3 *[Chapter 2 I D 2].* Electrophilic intermediates produced by metabolic transformation bind to cell macromolecules and denature or damage them, reducing their structural or enzymatic integrity. Glutathione (GSH), by binding preferentially with electrophiles, acts as a major protective molecule against toxicants. Covalent binding is positively correlated with cell damage but not with GSH status.

27. The answer is 3 *[Chapter 8 III A 2].* Type II (idiosyncratic, unpredictable, drug-related) hepatotoxicosis is probably caused by individual differences in the ability to metabolize and detoxify xenobiotics. These differences may be hereditary and are not detected by routine experimental toxicity testing. Thus, excessive susceptibility may occur at very low dosages and a dose–response relationship is not demonstrable. Prior sensitization (e.g., by an allergic-type reaction) may also be a factor.

28. The answer is 3 *[Chapter 5 III B 1].* The best approach is to assure a patent airway, using a cuffed endotracheal tube if necessary and relying on mechanical ventilation. Drugs should be avoided as much as possible in poisoned animals, even in respiratory support, and anesthesia should be avoided without the

security of artificial ventilation. Central respiratory stimulants are used only if spontaneous respiration does not return. Respiratory stimulants may cause seizures, or animals may respond and then relapse into a depressed or comatose state.

29. The answer is 3 *[Chapter 9 I B 1 b].* Endocytosis (i.e., the uptake, via invagination of the cell membrane, of particulate materials or high-molecular-weight complexes) allows materials that would not normally be reabsorbed to enter renal tubule cells. The endocytosed complexes are exposed to the enzymes inside the cell; in some cases these complexes are metabolized, leaving the toxic molecule in a free state. The toxic molecule can then interact with susceptible cellular receptors or structures.

30. The answer is 1 *[Chapter 28 II A].* The milky juice (latex) of *Ascelpias* (milkweed) contains a resinoid toxin that causes neurotoxis and a cardiotoxic glycoside that has digitalis-like activity. Milkweed grows throughout the United States, but the more toxic narrowleafed (whorled) varieties are more likely in the western states. *Astragalus lentigenosus, Centaurea solstitialis, Datura stramonium,* and *Ricinus communis* can be eliminated by the fact that they do not secrete a milky juice; however, one must remember that other toxic plants may have been eaten as well and the milkweed is only a confounding factor. A more accurate means of eliminating choices would be on the basis of clinical effects. *Astragalus* (locoweed) would not likely cause salivation or bradyarrhythmia. Signs usually develop gradually rather than explosively. *C. solstitialis* (yellow star thistle) is only known to affect horses with a depressive neurologic syndrome caused by necrosis of the substantia nigra and globus pallidus. Therefore, the clinical syndrome is not characteristic or documented for cattle. *Datura* (Jimson weed) is an anticholinergic and would not cause salivation, even though disorientation and seizures may be seen. The atropine-like action would be expected to produce tachycardia, not bradycardia. Cattle could be poisoned by *R. communis* (castor bean) following accidental access to the seeds or to contaminated castor bean meal; however, this would be unlikely under range conditions because castor bean is a cultivated plant which would not survive under natural conditions of the desert southwest. It contains a toxalbumin or phytotoxin that is associated with serious gastroenteritis and diarrhea followed by renal damage. Therefore, from the available evidence concerning location, affected species, and clinical response, *Asclepias* is the logical choice.

31. The answer is 4 *[Chapter 1 II B 1 b].*
One microgram per gram (1 μg/g) is 1 part per million (ppm), which is equivalent to 1000 parts per billion (ppb).

32. The answer is 4 *[Chapter 6 I B 2 c, 3 a].*
Effective antidotal therapy in veterinary medicine is limited to approximately 12 to 14 drugs. Of these, only atropine, vitamin K_1, and ascorbic acid are cleared for veterinary use. Others are effective, but not available except from human sources or by preparing the antidote from basic chemicals [e.g., 4-methylpyrazole (4-MP), ammonium tetrathiomolybdate]. Adverse effects of antidotes are more likely when levels of the toxicant are low or nonexistent; therefore, antidotes should not be used as prophylactic agents or when the toxicant has not been clearly identified. General decontamination therapy should be carried out prior to antidote administration.

33. The answer is 4 *[Chapter 9 I B 2 b].*
The organic ion transport system is responsible for tubular secretion or excretion of endogenous or exogenous normal metabolites or toxicants. During the secretion process, toxic chemicals may concentrate in the renal tubules at levels that cause binding of macromolecules, interference with protein synthesis, impaired energy metabolism, or peroxidative damage of organelle or cell membranes. Thus, the intended benefit of excretion can become a lethal effect when highly toxic chemicals are concentrated in the tubules.

34. The answer is 3 *[Chapter 29 V D 1 c].*
The ergot alkaloids are potent blockers of prolactin release in many species of animals during late pregnancy. Failure of prolactin release prevents the initiation of lactation, so the dam is healthy and normal, but does not develop an udder and secrete milk. As a result, the young are born normal but quickly die from starvation. Estrogens (e.g., zearalenone) have been implicated in the reduction of lactation, but they are far less potent than ergot alkaloids in this respect, and they do not inhibit prolactin release. If the effects were the result of aflatoxin or trichothecene toxicosis, the sow would likely be clinically affected before or during the time the pigs were affected.

35. The answer is 5 *[Chapter 5 II B 1 c (2)].*
Yohimbine is a recently developed commercially available reversal agent for xylazine. It acts mainly by blocking central α_2-adrenoreceptors, thereby countering the α_2-agonist effect of xylazine. Although approved only for dogs, yohimbine has been used in other animals, including cats, birds, rabbits, chinchillas, and laboratory rats. Intravenous dosage for both dogs and cats has been 0.1 mg/kg.

36. The answer is 2 *[Chapter 16 IV B 3].*
The clinical signs point clearly to a potential hemolytic anemia, because the mucous membranes are pale and the urine is dark and reddish-brown. These signs could also suggest azoturia or ionophore toxicosis, but there is no history of abnormal exercise and feeding (which would be consistent with azoturia) or access to ionophore-contaminated feeds. Red maple ingestion by horses has been documented to produce acute Heinz body hemolytic anemia by an unknown mechanism. Fertilizers are usually composed of nitrates or urea. Nitrates could cause methemoglobinemia, but not hemolytic anemia. White paint on the fences suggests lead toxicosis, but there are no associated neurologic or gastrointestinal signs, which are more prominent than the hematologic signs in lead toxicosis. Furthermore, the hematologic signs for lead include only very mild non-hemolytic anemia (i.e., anemia resulting from failure of heme synthesis). Nitrates in the well water would also cause methemoglobinemia, but high concentrations are required for that effect in a monogastric animal such as a horse. Bracken fern might be suspected in cattle that develop anemia; however, anemia caused by bracken fern is aplastic and accompanied by granulocytopenia (the radiomimetic syndrome). In addition, the horse usually develops neurologic signs in response to bracken.

37. The answer is 5 *[Chapter 6 Table 6-1].*
The well-known effect of methylene blue, an azo dye, in cats is either oxidation of their hemoglobin, producing methemoglobin, or oxidative damage to hemoglobin with production of Heinz bodies (i.e., denatured hemoglobin), leading to decreased pliability of the red blood cell and either hemolysis or premature removal of the cell from the vascular system. 4-Methylpyrazole (4-MP) is not an effective antidote for cats experiencing ethylene glycol toxicosis; however, it does not lead to methemoglobinemia. Ammonium molybdate

lessens the risk of acute hemolytic crisis in sheep. Acetylcysteine is not contraindicated in cats. D-Penicillamine does not chelate calcium; therefore, hypocalcemia is not an adverse effect of penicillamine therapy. Although adverse effects associated with penicillamine have been reported in humans, similar problems have not been reported in dogs.

38. The answer is 3 *[Chapter 26 IV A 2 a]*. Mitochondria are damaged in ionophore toxicosis. Ionophores facilitate the transport of sodium and potassium across cell membranes at the sodium channels, which alters calcium transport by changing the sodium component of the sodium–calcium exchange mechanism. As a result, calcium accumulates in the organelles. In the mitochondria, the excess calcium inhibits adenosine triphosphate (ATP) hydrolysis and reduces cellular energy metabolism leading to cell death, especially of cardiac and skeletal muscle cells. The sensitivity of mitochondria is primarily a result of their dominant role in energy metabolism.

39. The answer is 3 *[Chapter 30 II B 2]*. Blister beetles (*Epicauta*) commonly inhabit legume forages or other plants and may be present in large numbers when the hay is cut and crushed. The flakes of hay may contain many crushed beetles that cause toxicosis when fed to ruminants and horses. Black widow spiders (*Latrodectus mactans*) may invade suburban lawns and gardens in the eastern and southwestern United States. They are not aggressive but may present a risk to animals or humans that accidentally encounter their nesting places. *Agkistrodon contortix* (copperheads) inhabit dry, rocky areas and would be likely to respond to a challenge from a curious dog or boy by biting. *Bufo marinus,* marine toads, may inhabit settled areas and are found most frequently in Florida and Hawaii. A marine toad is a slow-moving target that a curious dog may view as a plaything; unfortunately, bufotoxin is extremely toxic and just one exposure can kill a dog.

40. The answer is 2 *[Chapter 11 II C 4]*. The approximate daily dosage of hydrogen sulfide received by the pig is 40 mg/kg. The 24-hour respiratory volume is the product of the tidal volume, the respiratory rate, and the amount of time:

1.0 L × 30 respirations/min × 60 min/hr × 24 hr/day

or 43,200 L/day. If there is 0.1 mg of hydrogen sulfide per liter of air, then the total daily dose

is 43,200 L/day x 0.1 mg/L, or 4,320 mg/day. The dosage is 4,320 mg/day divided by the weight of the pig (100 kg), or 43.2 mg/kg/day.

41. The answer is 4 *[Chapter 28 VI A 1]*. The Ericaceae (laurel or heath) family contains plants such as mountain laurel, rhododendron, and azalea. These plants are found mainly in temperate climates where winters are mild. The broad, green leaves are shiny or waxy in appearance, somewhat thickened, and present all year, including during the winter. Few of the common toxic plants exhibit this feature.

42. The answer is 5 *[Chapter 17 V E 2 c]*. Lead inhibits the activity of several key enzymes in heme synthesis, especially δ-aminolevulinic acid dehydrase (δ-ALAD), coproporphyringogenase, and heme synthetase, leading to the accumulation of several precursor molecules in the heme pathway (e.g., aminolevulinic acid and free erythrocyte porphyrins). Elevations of these molecules is detectable by clinical laboratory testing and signifies porphyria, which could be from other causes, but is also typical of lead toxicosis. Although iron may affect the vascular system and erythrocytes, heme synthesis is not interrupted. Cadmium, arsenic, and mercury are strong epithelial poisons, but they do not affect enzymes of heme synthesis.

43. The answer is 3 *[Chapter 12 II A 3 a]*. Testosterone, which is responsible for both secondary sexual characteristics and libido, is produced by Leydig cells. In addition, testosterone supports the function of the Sertoli cells, which are closely involved in nutrition and developmental support of spermatocytes. Thus, testosterone is important in the development and delivery of spermatozoa.

44. The answer is 4 *[Chapter 18 IV F 1 b]*. The general signs of lameness, exostoses (i.e., excess periosteal bone formation), and lapping of water are highly suggestive of fluorosis. A dental examination revealing pitted, mottled, or discolored tooth enamel and excessive tooth wear would further strengthen the diagnosis of fluorosis. Tooth sensitivity, resulting from the excessive wear that eventually exposes the pulp cavity, is part of the reason affected animals lap cold water. Dental lesions are only evident in the younger animals (i.e., those that had active tooth formation during the period of fluoride exposure). Animals that had fully erupted teeth when the fluoride exposure began will have no dental effects, but they still will exhibit lameness and lesions of the long bones.

45. The answer is 1 *[Chapter 3 III F 2].* The metabolic body weight (mbw) of an animal is influenced by the surface area and the relationship of surface area to body weight (bw) is shown by the formula $mbw = bw^{2/3}$. Smaller animals have a high metabolic activity relative to body weight when compared to larger animals. Thus, both bioactivation and detoxification may proceed more rapidly in small animals, which means that large animals may be affected by lower body weight dosages compared to those for small animals.

46. The answer is 5 *[Chapter 11 III D 1].* Pneumoconiosis is the generalized pathologic response of the lung to particulates. The accumulation, activation, and death of macrophages containing particulate material releases enzymes and cytokines that stimulate fibroblasts. Fibroblasts produce fibrous connective tissue that surrounds major areas of particulate reaction. The characteristic response to specific agents such as asbestos or silica may be somewhat different; each response is named for the principal agent encountered (e.g., asbestosis, silicosis). Asphyxiation occurs when toxic gases or vapors either crowd out oxygen (simple asphyxiation) or interfere with oxygen transport or utilization (chemical asphyxiation). Carcinogenesis is believed to be the response to chronic covalent binding and deoxyribonucleic acid (DNA) damage in the lung. Emphysema occurs when the activation of macrophages causes them to burst, releasing hydrolases and proteases, which destroy the elastin in the alveolar walls. Allergic responses do not progress to pulmonary fibrosis.

47. The answer is 2 *[Chapter 19 II B 1 b].* Organochlorine insecticides are highly lipophilic and accumulate in adipose tissue over time, even at small dosages. Organophosphate insecticides, pyrethrins and pyrethroids, chlorophenoxy herbicides, and bipyridyl herbicides have short half-lives and low lipid solubility; thus they are excreted daily, or within a few days to weeks after acute exposure.

48. The answer is 3 *[Chapter 26 II B 2 c (2) (a) (iv)].* There is a strong association between the use of furazolidone and the appearance of "round heart disease" in turkeys. Furazolidone inhibits the tricarboxylic acid (TCA) cycle in intermediary metabolism; however, it is not known exactly how this causes "round heart disease." Amprolium and nitrofurazone cause clinical effects and lesions in the central nervous system (CNS), not the heart. Ethylenediamine dihydroiodide (EDDI) affects the skin, eyes, and respiratory tract. Acute monensin toxicosis causes a cardiac lesion in horses and ruminants. Monensin may also be considered a potential cardiotoxicant in turkeys, but it has not been linked to cardiac hypertrophy as has furazolidone.

49. The answer is 4 *[Chapter 9 IV B 1–3].* The diuretic (subacute) phase of acute toxicant-induced renal failure is characterized by hypokalemia, hypernatremia, hyperphosphatemia, decreased urine specific gravity, and a normal blood urea nitrogen (BUN) level. The immature cells of the recovering tubule lack the ability to control potassium and sodium balance through the normal sodium pump and exchange mechanisms, producing dilute urine. Because urea is freely filtered, the BUN level may be kept within a normal range because of the high rate of filtration and formation of dilute urine.

50. The answer is 5 *[Chapter 2 I E 3].* The order of damage or pathogenesis of cellular injury begins with the metabolic transformation of chemicals to free radicals. Free radicals have an unpaired electron that can interact with the hydrogen supplied by polyunsaturated lipids, which leads to lipid peroxidation, which, in turn, damages cell or organelle membranes. As a result, calcium is released to the cytosol from sequestered sites (e.g., mitochondria). Calcium can activate phospholipases, which further damage organelle and cellular membranes, releasing acid hydrolases that aid in the loss of membrane function, cell swelling, and eventual cell death.

51. The answer is 5 *[Table 6-1].* The best therapeutic choice for a lead-poisoned animal with high levels of lead in the blood and serious clinical signs is calcium disodium ethylenediaminetetraacetic acid (EDTA) and dimercaprol. Calcium disodium EDTA promotes removal of lead from the tissues; however, high blood lead levels may contribute to continuing toxicosis. Dimercaprol appears to bind to circulating lead made available from the tissues by calcium disodium EDTA, preventing the circulating lead from interacting with susceptible receptors until it can be excreted in the urine. D-Penicillamine may be used as an alternative to calcium disodium EDTA therapy; however, it is not the antidote of choice in this situation.

52. The answer is 3 *[Chapter 19 II E 1; III D 1].* Both pyrethrins and DDT affect the sodium channels of nerve membranes, altering sodium currents and changing the threshold for an action potential. Both compounds result in excitatory effects, leading to tremors and seizures. The organophosphate insecticides are cholinesterase inhibitors and rotenone is an uncoupler of oxidative phosphorylation. Paraquat causes formation of activated oxygen, leading to lipid peroxidation and cell membrane damage. The herbicide 2,4-D uncouples oxidative phosphorylation, and it also causes myotonia by affecting muscle membranes by an unknown mechanism.

53. The answer is 4 *[Chapter 29 I C 3 b].* United States Department of Agriculture (USDA)-recommended grain sampling techniques include sampling a large portion of grain by reducing the particle size through shelling or grinding, then taking multiple samples from a moving stream of grain that represents a large portion of the supply to be tested. Probe sampling at multiple sites is the best alternative. Unacceptable sampling methods are those that involve selection of biased (e.g., "worst case") samples by taking single samples from only one site in a large storage unit, because mycotoxin contamination is typically quite heterogeneous within a storage facility.

54. The answer is 3 *[Chapter 1 II B 2 a].* Two pounds of drug containing four ounces of active ingredient per pound is eight ounces or one-half pound, per ton. In that 1 lb is 454 g, 0.5 lbs = 227 g. There are 907 kg in one ton. It follows then that there are 227 g, or 0.227 kg, of active ingredient in 907 kg of livestock ration. Therefore, 0.227 kg/907 kg = 0.025%, and when the decimal is moved four places to the right, the calculation becomes 250 parts per million (ppm).

55. The answer is 3 *[Chapter 3 III A 1 b].* Conjugation is the final step in xenobiotic metabolism. Endogenous molecules, such as glucuronide, sulfate, or glutathione, combine with activated molecules from phase I metabolism, forming products that are generally less lipophilic, more water soluble, and more

readily excreted than the parent product. Many animals with notable susceptibility to specific chemicals have deficiencies of the enzymes or metabolites needed to complete conjugation and detoxication.

56. The answer is 3 *[Chapter 26 V A 3 a–b].* In order to solve this problem, it is necessary to determine the protein equivalent supplied from the urea first. Protein is approximately 16% nitrogen. Therefore, the protein equivalent equals the amount of nitrogen in the urea multiplied by 6.25 (100/16): 45 x 6.25 = 281%. That is, the nitrogen from 1 gram of urea is capable of supplying the nitrogen for rumen bacteria to synthesize 2.81 grams of protein. If 21% equivalent protein is divided by 2.81%, the quotient is 7.5%, meaning that the feed actually contains 7.5% urea.

57. The answer is 2 *[Chapter 2 II D 1].* Lack of energy, fatigue, and high fever are expected from agents that uncouple or inhibit oxidative phosphorylation, reducing the formation of high-energy phosphate bonds stored as adenosine triphosphate (ATP). Instead, the energy of intermediary metabolism is lost as heat, resulting in the typical clinical sign of fever.

58. The answer is 3 *[Chapter 8 II B 2].* Cholestatic agents alter the ability of the bile canaliculi to transport bile salts. This activity may be related to osmotic changes caused by the secreted bile salts or to energy-dependent osmotic control accomplished through the sodium-potassium-adenosine triphosphatase (ATPase) pump. Cholestasis occurs in the bile canaliculi, and not in the common bile duct. Kupffer cells, Disse's space, hepatic sinusoids, and the common bile duct are part of the hepatic parenchyma and are not directly involved in bile salt formation.

59–60. The answers are 59-3 *[Chapter 24 I F 2 a–b],* **60-4** *[Chapter 24 I G].* The cat's history is strongly suggestive of exposure to an oxidant chemical, such as acetaminophen. Because at least 36 hours have passed since the initial toxicosis, there is likely involvement of both the blood and the liver. The acetaminophen toxic metabolite oxidizes hemoglobin to form methemoglobinemia and Heinz bodies, and initiates cellular necrosis in the liver. Therefore, it is likely that bloodwork would reveal Heinz bodies, methemoglobinemia, and markedly increased serum hepatic enzyme [e.g., alanine aminotransferase (ALT)] levels. The oxidant activity that causes Heinz body formation also increases erythrocyte fragility, leading to hemolysis. Although the blood urea nitrogen (BUN) level is slightly elevated, this is probably a result of dehydration and reduced glomerular filtration, and does not necessarily signal renal damage. Creatine phosphokinase is primarily an enzyme associated with striated muscle. Although the facial swelling could suggest damage to muscle tissue there, acetaminophen toxicosis is not characterized by significant muscle necrosis.

Acetylcysteine, which replenishes or substitutes for glutathione, should be administered to this cat, even though 36 hours have passed since exposure. The next best therapy would be to try to provide a substrate for conjugation or to alleviate the effects of the toxicosis. Sodium sulfate has been effective for treating acetaminophen toxicosis if given early because it provides a source of sulfur for conjugation with acetaminophen. Neither methylene blue nor sodium sulfate are highly effective after 24 hours have passed since exposure, because most of the acetaminophen has been metabolized and has already produced significant clinical effects. In addition, the use of methylene blue in cats has been associated with the development of Heinz body anemia. Activated charcoal given 24 hours or more after the onset of clinical signs is relatively ineffective because the drug has already been absorbed. This cat should be started on intravenous fluids to combat the dehydration, and tested for possible renal necrosis.

61. The answer is 5 *[Chapter 3 II B 1, 2, 4].* Small molecules that are lipid-soluble, nonpolar, and un-ionized usually pass readily through pores or channels of the bimolecular lipid protein mosaic of the cell membrane. Large charged molecules, such as proteins, are generally not absorbed, and if toxicants are bound to the protein, only the unbound toxicant is available for absorption.

62. The answer is 2 *[Chapter 24 IV E, G 1].* Methylxanthine alkaloids stimulate the central nervous system (CNS) and increase irritability of the sensory cortex. Major effects of methylxanthine toxicosis are hyperactivity, hyperreflexia, stiffness, muscle tremors, and twitching, and, sometimes, tetanic seizures. Tachycardia, tachyarrhythmias, and polypnea are also life-threatening aspects of methylxanthine toxicosis. All of the agents listed except cholecalciferol (i.e., lead, metaldehyde, strychnine, amphetamine) cause some degree of CNS stimulation or neuromuscular activity, or both. The weakest of these four differential diagnoses is lead poisoning, although lead still has a significant CNS component that can include seizures and hysteria in dogs. Cholecalciferol increases active vitamin D levels in the body and its toxic effects are mediated through renal damage and hypercalcemia. Hypercalcemia produces cardiac signs nearly opposite those produced by the methylxanthines.

63. The answer is 2 *[Chapter 17 X A 4].* Because of its predilection for renal tissues and the relative infrequency of exposure, cadmium presents the least threat to the gastrointestinal tract. Lead causes colic, vomiting, or both. Arsenic causes severe gastroenteritis with vomiting and fluid diarrhea. Molybdenum in ruminants causes a prominent intractable diarrhea. Zinc is associated with vomiting and variable degrees of gastroenteritis.

64. The answer is 4 *[Table 25-1].* Herbicides are of relatively low toxicity, and their toxicity is most often caused by systemic effects after consumption and absorption. In this case, the obvious route of exposure is from the contaminated paws of the cat. The product is a direct irritant because both the feet and the mouth are affected with direct irritation, necrosis, and ulceration. The other potentially available products are all irritant to some degree. Drain cleaners are highly caustic, containing mainly sodium hydroxide. Fireplace colors are combinations of metalloids and heavy metal salts that can be direct irritants and also systemic toxicants. Garden fertilizers contain high concentrations of urea, or salts of potassium and phosphate, and these are direct irritants, as are the calcium chloride or potassium chloride found in thawing salts.

65. The answer is 3 *[Chapter 28 I B].* Factors that increase the risk of plant toxicosis are numerous. Animals that are bored by confinement, or have unusual appetites as a result of starvation or malnutrition are highly likely to consume toxic plants, as are animals that are hungry or thirsty following extended transportation or trailing. Overgrazing decreases the percentage of desirable grasses and legumes in a pasture by favoring the overgrowth of weeds, which may be toxic. Undergrazing, on the other hand, favors beneficial plants, which crowd out weedy competition and reduce access to toxic plants.

66. The answer is 2 *[Chapter 30 IV A 2 a, 3 a].* All of the characteristics described are typical identifiers for poisonous members of the Crotalidae family, except for the bright red and yellow alternating bands. The coral snakes of the southern and southeastern United States, members of the Elapidae family, are characterized by brightly colored rings of red and yellow. The crotalids have irregular or diamond-shaped patterns of more muted colors ranging from tan to olive. Their pupils are vertical, elliptical slits, and their prominent, curving fangs retract so the snake can swallow its prey. Crotalids are also known as "pit vipers" because of the pit between the nostril and the eye that houses a heat-sensing organ used to detect prey. Their heads are broad and triangular.

67. The answer is 1 *[Chapter 26 VI V B 1–2, 4].* Acidic rumen conditions supply protons and maintain the ammonia released from urea in an ionized state (NH^{4+}), which increases its solubility in water and retards its absorption and transport across epithelium. This is a form of ion trapping, and is, in part, why acidification of the rumen with acetic acid or vinegar helps to alleviate ammonia toxicosis from urea. All other statements are true statements and reinforce the important points that ammonia toxicosis results in metabolic acidosis, is most likely to occur in fasting animals that are unaccustomed to urea, and is a rapidly progressing acute to peracute disease. Proper preservation of samples is necessary to prevent changes in ammonia concentrations.

68. The answer is 1 *[Chapter 25 III E 1 f; Chapter 26 VIII D; Chapter 28 IV A 4; V D 1; Chapter 29 II D].* Clay pigeon poisoning in swine is characterized by acute illness or sudden death with lesions of massive centrilobular hepatic necrosis. *Amaranthus retroflexus* toxicosis causes acute tubular nephrosis with no liver lesions, so it would be easily differentiated from clay pigeon poisoning. Hepatosis dietetica (vitamin E/selenium deficiency), cocklebur toxicosis, and acute aflatoxicosis all produce marked hepatic damage that could appear similar to clay pigeon poisoning. Gossypol causes both cardiac and liver lesions.

69. The answer is 5 *[Chapter 28 II B 4, C 1, D 2, F 6; V A 1 d].* Marijuana, Jimson weed, mescal bean, and morning glory all contain a hallucinogenic principle that could cause hallucinogenic signs in dogs. Only rhubarb is not a hallucinogen. Oxalates in rhubarb form a complex with plasma calcium, causing functional hypocalcemia and tubular nephrosis.

70–73. The answers are 70-1 *[Chapter 19 I G; Figure 19-1],* **71-4** *[Chapter 22 V G 1],* **72-5** *[Chapter 19 VIII F],* **73-2** *[Chapter 19 II G 1].* Judging from the chemical name [dimethyl(2,2,2 trichloro-1-hydroxyethyl) phosphate], the agent is an organophosphate ester. It is a cholinesterase inhibitor that produces strong signs of parasympathetic stimulation (e.g., bradycardia). Other agents (e.g., pyrethrins, metaldehyde) may cause some similar external signs, but they would not cause bradycardia.

Strychnine causes loss of the inhibitory effect of the internuncial neurons in the spinal reflex arc. Loss of these inhibitory effects allows excessive reaction to stimuli. The extensor muscles predominate, leading to rigidity and tetanic seizures that are worsened by stimuli because there is no control over the spinal reflexes.

A history of salivation, mydriasis, tremors, and hyperthermia could suggest organophosphate toxicosis because of the salivation and tremors, but, in fact, metaldehyde poisoning would be the correct diagnosis. Mydriasis would not result from the cholinergic stimulation characteristic of the organophosphate insecticides. Furthermore, the absence of vomiting or diarrhea suggests that cholinergic or muscarinic stimulation is not present. In cases where the distinction is not clear, blood cholinesterase levels can be evaluated to differentiate organophosphate toxicosis from metaldehyde poisoning.

The classic reaction to the cyclodiene insecticides (e.g., chlordane, toxaphene, heptachlor) is intermittent cranial to caudal epileptiform seizures with little or no hyperesthesia. There is rarely, if ever, any vomiting as would be seen with metaldehyde or the organophosphates toxicosis, and the seizures are not tetanic or hyperesthetic as with strychnine toxicosis.

74–77. The answers are 74-5 *[Chapter 17 IX G 1–2],* **75-4** *[Chapter 17 II F 1 a],* **76-2** *[Chapter 17 V F],* **77-A** *[Chapter 17 III C].* Both zinc toxicosis and lead toxicosis cause some gastroenteric signs and mild regenerative anemia; however, the lack of neurologic signs makes zinc the best choice in this case.

Trivalent arsenic is found in herbicides and ant baits, which are used to kill ants in homes and businesses. Cats are especially sensitive to both trivalent arsenicals (e.g., arsenites) and to pentavalent arsenicals. Signs of acute toxicosis include colic and severe vomiting and diarrhea; death occurs within 8–12 hours in most cases. Because of the severity of the toxicosis, many ant baits are now using carbamates or other, less potent insecticides.

Lead toxicosis in cats causes colic, vomiting, central nervous system (CNS) depression, and mild anemia.

Chronic copper accumulation in dogs is characterized by colic, vomiting, depression, and clinical icterus (as evidenced by the yellow discoloration of the eyes). Bedlington terriers are the best known species of dog susceptible to a familial accumulation of liver copper, but this condition has also been recognized in West Highland white terriers and in Doberman pinschers.

78–82. The answers are 78-4 *[Chapter 28 VIII A 4 a]*, **79-5** *[Chapter 28 VI E 2 d]*, **80-2** *[Chapter 28 VIII; Table 28-6]*, **81-1** *[Chapter 28 II F 2]*, **82-3** *[Chapter IV C 1 f]*. *Pteridium aquilinum* (bracken fern), a classic radiomimetic toxin, causes pancytopenia and often induces intestinal epithelial damage as well, leading to anemia, hemorrhage, and diarrhea. In addition, hematuria associated with urinary bladder neoplasms has been observed in cattle eating bracken fern.

Festuca arundinacea (Kentucky 31 tall fescue) causes "fescue foot," a major clinical toxicosis of cattle in the southeastern and south central United States. The vascular constriction caused by ergopeptide alkaloids reduces peripheral circulation, causing dry gangrene of the distal limbs, especially at the coronary band. Early signs of lameness progress to loss of the hooves. Gangrene may necessitate amputation of the digits. An endophyte fungus, *Acremonium coenophialum*, that inhabits the fescue is believed to be responsible for this response.

Sorghum (Sudan grass) can cause methemoglobinemia, which is characterized by dark brown blood. Nitrites that are reduced from nitrates in plants oxidize ferrous iron in hemoglobin to ferric iron, rendering the hemoglobin unable to carry oxygen. Anoxia and cyanosis result.

Delphinium barbeyi (larkspur) is a major cause of cattle loss. The toxic principle, a diterpene alkaloid, is a neuromuscular blocking agent that acutely affects postsynaptic cholinergic and nicotinic receptors. Effects include muscle tremors, excitement, disorientation, bloat, arrhythmia, prostration, and death.

Tetradymia glabrata (horsebrush) is an example of a secondary (hepatogenous) photosensitizing plant. It causes liver damage that interferes with the biliary excretion of phylloerythrin, a photodynamic metabolite of chlorophyll. Photoactivation of the phylloerythrin results in epithelial damage and subcutaneous edema.

83–87. The answers are 83-5 *[Chapter 19 I G 2 a (2), b (2)]*, **84-2** *[Chapter 22 III G 3]*, **85-4** *[Chapter 22 V G 1 b (3), 2 b]*, **86-2** *[Chapter 22 II G 2 d]*, **87-1** *[Chapter 19 VIII F 2 c]*. Carbamate insecticides inhibit cholinesterase; therefore, evaluation of cholinesterase activity in the whole brain or caudate nucleus is commonly used for postmortem diagnosis. Because the inhibition is labile and spontaneous hydrolysis may occur before or during testing for the enzyme, chemical analysis of the stomach contents is often performed in addition to cholinesterase evaluation.

Cholecalciferol toxicosis is best confirmed by sampling of renal or hepatic tissue. Poisoning by cholecalciferol is usually delayed at least 24 hours, so stomach contents are not representative. Vitamin D metabolism takes place initially in the liver and then in the kidney, and the lesions of tubular necrosis and tissue calcification are prominent in the kidney.

Strychnine is a basic compound that ionizes and partitions well in an acidic environment such as the stomach. In addition, strychnine toxicosis often occurs rapidly and causes no vomiting, so the stomach contents are often readily available for inspection and analysis. In the rare case where stomach contents are not available, hepatic tissue may contain detectable residues.

Brodifacoum is an anticoagulant rodenticide. The greatest concentration is likely in the liver, where metabolism takes place, because ingestion likely occurred more than 24 hours prior to the onset of signs. Metabolites are more water-soluble and may also be found in the renal tissue.

Metaldehyde is difficult to diagnose by laboratory means, but sampling should include the stomach contents because the toxicosis is relatively acute and some of the metaldehyde may still be present. Tissue analysis is not reliable.

88–89. The answers are 88-4 *[Chapter 6 III K]*, **89-5** *[Chapter 6 III G]*. Of the commonly available heavy metal antidotes listed, only D-penicillamine has been found consistently effective for chelation of both lead and copper. D-Penicillamine is a natural chelator that provides binding sites at both an amino group and a sulfhydryl group, forming a soluble chelate that strongly enhances urinary elimination of lead or copper. Calcium disodium ethylene diamine tetraacetic acid (EDTA) and desferoxamine are only active parenterally against lead and iron, respectively. Ammonium molybdate effectively aids the excretion of copper by forming a copper–molybdate complex that is more readily excreted in urine, but ammonium molybdate has no useful value as a chelator for lead.

Dimercaprol is a disulfhydryl three carbon compound (2,3-dimercapto-1-propanolol) that can form a disulfide linkage with either lead or arsenic. Dimercaprol, also known as British antilewisite (BAL), was originally developed in Great Britain to counteract the vesicant war gas Lewisite. When used in combination with calcium disodium EDTA, dimercaprol enhances the mobilization of lead from tissues, especially the brain, and speeds the excretion of lead in the urine and bile. Ammonium molybdate, desferoxamine, and D-penicillamine have little or no activity against arsenic.

90–94. The answers are 90-5 *[Table 28-7]*, **91-4** *[Chapter 28 IX A 3]*, **92-1** *[Chapter 28 IX A 1; Table 28-7]*, **93-3** *[Table 28-7]*, **94-2** *[Table 28-7]*. *Veratrum calcifornicum* (veratum, false hellebore) produces a congenital cyclopian malformation in lambs born to ewes exposed on the fourteenth day of gestation. Prolonged gestation and brachygnathia are also part of the syndrome.

Pinus ponderosa (ponderosa pine, loblolly pine) needles cause an abortion syndrome ("pine needle abortion syndrome") in cattle exposed during the third trimester. The toxin is unknown, but it is water-soluble and often causes udder edema, retained placenta, and metritis as well.

Astragalus (locoweed) causes abortion in a high percentage of cattle, but in lambs, it is associated with congenital flexure of the joints and contracted tendons. Swainsonine, the same toxin responsible for the neurologic manifestations of locoweed, is suspected as the teratogen.

Lupinus species are acutely toxic to sheep, and chronically toxic to cattle. Calves are born with "crooked calf disease," which is characterized by torticollis, scoliosis, twisted limbs, and cleft palate. Calves may be born alive and survive.

Nicotiana tabacum (tobacco) contains an alkaloid, anabasine, which is the suspected teratogen in tobacco plants. Effects, which include twisting and arthrogryposis, are likely in the offspring of sows that ingested stalks of the plant during the first trimester of gestation.

Index

Note: Page numbers in *italic* indicate illustrations; those followed by *t* indicate tables; Q denotes questions; E denotes explanations.

A

Abdominal distension, 113
Abdominal pain, 93, 113
   in intestinal toxicosis, 115
   in NSAID toxicosis, 307
Abortion, 136
   in carboxyhemoglobinemia, 172
   causes of, 137, 401
Abrus precatorius (rosary pea, precatory
      bean), 377
Acacia berlandieri (guajillo), 80*t*, 373
Acepromazine in treating
      4-methylimidazole toxicosis, 344
Acer rubrum (red maple), 397
Acetamides, 258*t*
Acetaminophen, 60*t*, 304
   chemistry of, 303
   diagnosis of, 303–304
   exposure to, 303
   mechanism of toxicologic damage, 303
   sources of, 303
   toxicity of, 303, 314Q, 316E
   toxicosis of, 315Q, 316E
      acetylcysteine for, 58–59
   treatment of exposure to, 304
Acetates, 29
Acetylation of aromatic amino
      compounds, 30
Acetylcholine (ACh), 71, 76, 233
   toxic action of inhibitors, 233
Acetylcholinesterase (AChE), 70, 226,
      450Q, 461E
Acetylcoenzyme A, 159
Acetylcysteine, 58, 60*t*, 264, 304, 455Q,
      466–467E
   absorption, metabolism, excretion and,
      58–59
   overdose effects, 59
   storage of, 58
Achromotrichia in molybdenum
      toxicosis, 200
Acid(s), 143
   definition of, 10
   protonated, 10, 15E
   weak, 14Q, 15E
Acid–base disturbances, 52
Acid–base dysfunction, 105
Acidemia, lactic, 342
Acidic agents, 53, 54
Acidic ruminal conditions, 456Q, 468E
Acidity (pH), 352
Acidosis, 105, 162, 283
   correction of, 113
   metabolic, 342
   in NSAID toxicosis, 307
Acid urine, 54
Acinar model of liver, 87
Aconitine, 393
Aconitum napellum (monkshood), 393
Acremonium lolii, 429

Acrosomes, 133, 139Q, 140E
Actin, 159
Action potentials, 67, 85Q, 86E
   generation of, 69–70
Activated partial thromboplastin time
      (APTT), 278
Activated prothrombin time, 278
Active ingredients, 28
Active oxygen (superoxide), 18
Acyl coenzyme A, 159
Adenosine diphosphate (ADP), 167
Adenosine triphosphate (ATP), 159
Adenylate cyclase activation, 114
α-Adrenergic receptors, toxicant
      stimulation of, 163
β-Adrenergic agonists, toxicant
      stimulation of, 163
Adsorption therapy with activated
      charcoal, 50–51
Adverse reactions versus toxicosis, 297
Aerobic metabolism, 159
   toxicants affecting, 162
Aerosols, 127
Aesculin, 365
Aesculus glabra (Ohio buckeye, horse
      chestnut), 365–366
Aflatoxicosis, 419
Aflatoxin, 21, 139Q, 140E, 409, 410*t*,
      433Q, 434Q, 435E, 436E
   chemical characteristics of, 417
   diagnosis of, 419
   mechanism of toxicologic damage,
      417, 417–418
   public health considerations for, 420
   sources of, 416–417
   toxicity of, 418, 418*t*
   toxicokinetics of, 417
   treatment and prevention of toxicosis,
      420
Agalactia, 402
Agave, 386
Agave lechiguilla (Agave), 386
Agent Orange, 28
Aging, 447Q, 459E
   biotransformation and, 29, 31, 34Q,
      35E
   role of organophosphorus compounds
      in, 233
Agkistrodon contortix (copperheads),
      440
Agkistrodon piscivorus (water
      moccasins), 440, 444Q, 445E
Agranulocytes, 167
Agriculture, herbicides in, 257
Agrostemma githago (corn cockle), 377
Alachlor, 260*t*
Alcohols, 74*t*
   absolute, 347Q, 349E
Alfalfa, 402
Aliphatic hydrocarbons, 213
Aliphatic phosphorus esters, 226

Alkali disease, 447Q, 459E
Alkalies, 143
Alkaline phosphatase (AP), 90, 262
   in urine, 104
Alkaline urine, 53, 54
Alkaloids, 362*t*
Alkalosis, 53, 84
Alkyl mercurials, 199
Allergic contact dermatitis, 146, 147*t*
Allergic effects, 27, 34Q, 35E
Allium (onions, garlic), 397–398
Alopecia, 148
Alpha-chloralose, 74*t*, 290*t*
Alpha-chlorohydrin
      (3-chloro-1,2-propanediol),
      290*t*
Alpha naphthyl-thio urea, 290*t*
Altered membrane integrity, 17
Altered pharmacologic effects of drugs,
      94
Altered protein synthesis, 92
Aluminum, phosphides of, 282–284
Alveolar-capillary membrane, 121
Alveolar epithelium, 130Q, 131E
Alveolar macrophage, 130Q, 131E
Amanita muscaria, 78*t*
Amanita pantherina, 78*t*
Amanita phalloides (deadly amanita,
      death angel), 377, 383
Amanita toxins (amatoxins), 383
Amantine, 21
Amaranthus retroflexus (redroot
      pigweed), 389–390, 404Q, 406E
   toxicosis from, 456Q, 468E
Amaurosis, 144
Ambient air, toxicants from, 123
Amimal size, 453Q, 464–465E
Amino acids, 29
   transport of, into central nervous
      system, 67
γ-Aminobutyric acid (GABA), 71, 76,
      252Q, 254–255E
Aminoglycoside, 447Q, 459E
   antibiotics, 82*t*, 84, 153, 235
Aminolevulinic acid (ALA), 172
α-Amino β-methyl aminopropionic acid,
      384
β-Amino propionitrile (BAP), 374
4-Aminopyridine, 72*t*
Amitraz
   chemical structure of, 245
   diagnosis of
      clinical signs of, 246
      laboratory, 246
      lesions, 246
   exposure to, 245
   mechanism of toxicity of, 245
   prevention of, 246
   prognosis of, 246
   public health concerns from, 246
   sources of, 245